The Research Process in Nursing

The Research Process in Nursing

SEVENTH EDITION

Edited by

Kate Gerrish
CBE, PhD, MSc, B.Nurs, RN, RM, NDN Cert, FRCN
Professor of Nursing Research, University of Sheffield and Sheffield Teaching Hospitals NHS Foundation Trust

Judith Lathlean
DPhil (Oxon), MA, BSc (Econ) (Hons)
Professor of Health Research, Faculty of Health Sciences, University of Southampton

WILEY Blackwell

Registered Office
John Wiley & Sons, Ltd, The Atrium, Southern Gate, Chichester, West Sussex, PO19 8SQ, UK

Editorial Offices
9600 Garsington Road, Oxford, OX4 2DQ, UK
The Atrium, Southern Gate, Chichester, West Sussex, PO19 8SQ, UK
Main Street, Malden, MA 02148-5020, USA

For details of our global editorial offices, for customer services and for information about how to apply for permission to reuse the copyright material in this book please see our website at www.wiley.com/wiley-blackwell

Library of Congress Cataloging-in-Publication Data

The research process in nursing. – Seventh edition/edited by Kate Gerrish, Judith Lathlean.
p. ; cm.
Includes bibliographical references and index.
ISBN 978-1-118-52258-5 (pbk.)
I. Gerrish, Kate, 1955– , editor. II. Lathlean, Judith, editor.
[DNLM: 1. Nursing Research–methods. 2. Data Collection–methods. 3. Research Design. WY 20.5]
RT81.5
610.73072–dc23

2014030766

A catalogue record for this book is available from the British Library.

Wiley also publishes its books in a variety of electronic formats. Some content that appears in print may not be available in electronic books.

Set in 10/12pt Times by SPi Publisher Services, Pondicherry, India
Printed and bound in Malaysia by Vivar Printing Sdn Bhd

2 2016

Contents

Contributors

Leanne M. Aitken
PhD, B HSc (Nurs) (Hons), Int Care Cert, Grad Cert Mgt, Grad Dip Sc Med (ClinEpi), FACN, FAAN
Professor of Critical Care Nursing, Griffith University & Princess Alexandra Hospital, Brisbane, Australia and Professor of Nursing, City University London, London, UK

Claire Beecroft
MA, BA (Hons), DPS, FHEA, MCLIP
Information Specialist and University Teacher, School of Health and Related Research (ScHARR), University of Sheffield, Sheffield, UK

Andrew Booth
PhD, MSc, Dip Lib, BA, MCLIP
Reader in Evidence Based Information Practice, School of Health and Related Research (ScHARR), University of Sheffield, Sheffield, UK

Jo Booth
PhD, BSc (Hons), BA, RGN, RNT
Reader, School of Health and Life Sciences, Glasgow Caledonian University, Glasgow, UK

Tracey Bucknall
PhD, RN, BN, ICU Cert, PGD Adv Nurs
Professor and Associate Head of School (Research), School of Nursing & Midwifery, Deakin University; Foundational Chair in Nursing, Alfred Health, Melbourne, Australia

Charlotte Clarke
DSocSc, PhD, MSc, PGCE, BA, RN
Professor of Health in Social Science and Head of the School of Health in Social Science, University of Edinburgh, Edinburgh, UK

Julie Cooper
PhD, PG Cert Academic Practice, BSc (Hons), DipHE, RGN
Senior Lecturer Primary and Community Care, Faculty of Education & Health, University of Greenwich, London, UK

Kara DeCorby
MSc
Formerly Managing Director and Knowledge Broker – Health Evidence, School of Nursing, Faculty of Health Sciences, McMaster University, Hamilton, ON, Canada

Jo Dumville
PhD, MSc
Senior Lecturer in Applied Health Research, School of Nursing, Midwifery & Social Work, University of Manchester, Manchester, UK

George T.H. Ellison
DSc, PhD, MSc (Med), BSc (Hons)
Associate Professor, Division of Epidemiology & Biostatistics, Faculty of Medicine & Health, University of Leeds, Leeds, UK

Catherine Evans
PhD, MSc, BSc, RN, RHV, DN
NIHR Clinical Lecturer in Palliative Care/CNS, King's College London, London, UK

Jenny Freeman
PhD, MSc, BSc (Econ), CSTAT, FHEA, CertLT
Associate Professor of Biostatistics, University of Leeds, Leeds, UK

Dawn Freshwater
PhD, BA (Hons), RN RNT, FRCN
Professor of Mental Health, University of Leeds, UK; Senior Deputy Vice Chancellor, University of Western Australia, Crawley, Australia

Kathleen T. Galvin
PhD, BSc (Hons), RN
Professor of Nursing Practice and Associate Dean, Research and Enterprise, Faculty of Health and Social Care, University of Hull, Hull, UK

Leslie Gelling
PhD, MA, BSc (Hons), RN MICR FRSA
Reader in Research Ethics, Faculty of Health, Social Care and Education, Anglia Ruskin University, Cambridge, UK

Kate Gerrish
CBE, PhD, MSc, B.Nurs, RN, RM, NDN Cert, FRCN
Professor of Nursing Research, School of Nursing and Midwifery, University of Sheffield and Sheffield Teaching Hospitals NHS Foundation Trust, Sheffield, UK

Claire Goodman
PhD, RN, FQNI
Professor of Health Care Research, Centre for Research in Primary and Community Care, University of Hertfordshire, Hertfordshire, UK

Peter Griffiths
PhD, BA (Hons), RN
Chair of Health Services Research, Centre for Innovation and Leadership in Health Sciences, University of Southampton, Southampton, UK

Carol A. Haigh
PhD, MSc, BSc (Hons), RGN
Professor in Nursing, Faculty of Health, Psychology and Social Care, Manchester Metropolitan University, Manchester, UK

Felicity Hasson
PhD, MSc, PgDip, BA (Hons)
Senior Lecturer, Institute of Nursing Research, School of Nursing, University of Ulster, Ulster, UK

Immy Holloway
PhD, MA, BEd, CertEd
Professor Emeritus, School of Health and Social Care, Bournemouth University, Dorset, UK

Katherine Hunt
PhD, MSc, BSc, RN
Senior Research Fellow, Faculty of Health Sciences, University of Southampton, Southampton, UK

Alison M. Hutchinson
PhD, MBioeth, BAppSc (Adv Nsg), RN, Cert Nsg, Cert Midwifery
Professor in Nursing, School of Nursing and Midwifery, Faculty of Health, Deakin University, Melbourne, Australia, and Chair in Nursing, Centre for Nursing Research – Deakin University and Monash Health Partnership, Monash Health, Melbourne, Australia

Martin Johnson
PhD, MSc, RN, RNT
Professor in Nursing, School of Nursing, University of Salford, Salford, UK

Martyn Jones
PhD, CPsychol, BSc (Hons), RNMH, Dip Ed
Professor of Heathcare Research, School of Nursing and Midwifery, University of Dundee, Dundee, UK

Sinead Keeney
PhD, MRes, BA (Hons), PGCHEP, FHEA
Senior Research Fellow, Institute of Nursing and Health Research, School of Nursing, University of Ulster, Ulster, UK

Bridie Kent
PhD, BSc (Hons), PG Cert HE, RNT, RN
Professor in Leadership in Nursing, Plymouth University, Plymouth, UK

Sarah E. Keyes
PhD, BA (Hons)
Research Fellow, Interdisciplinary Social Science in Health, School of Health in Social Science, University of Edinburgh, Edinburgh, UK

Anne Lacey
DPhil. MSc, BSc Hons, RGN, RNT, DipN(Lond)
Formerly Diocesan Health Coordinator, Diocese of Madi and West Nile, Arua, Uganda

Judith Lathlean
DPhil (Oxon), MA, BSc (Econ) (Hons)
Professor of Health Research, Faculty of Health Sciences, University of Southampton, Southampton, UK

Tony Long
PhD, MA, BSc (Hons), RNT, SRN, RSCN
Professor of Child and Family Health, School of Nursing, University of Salford, Salford, UK

Susie Macfarlane
BSc (Hons), GCertHigherEd
eLearning Educational Developer, School of Exercise and Nutrition Sciences, Deakin University, Melbourne, Australia

Brendan McCormack
DPhil (Oxon), BSc (Hons), FEANS, PGCEA, RMN, RGN
Professor and Head of the Division of Nursing, School of Health Sciences, Queen Margaret University, Edinburgh, UK

Hugh McKenna
CBE, PhD, BSc (Hons), RMN, RGN, RNT, DipN(Lond), AdvDipEd, FFN, RCSI, FEANS, FRCN, FAAN
Pro-Vice Chancellor, Research & Innovation, University of Ulster, Ulster, UK

Julienne Meyer
PhD, MSc, BSc, Cert Ed (FE), RN, RNT
Professor of Nursing, Care for Older People; Executive Director: *My* Home Life programme, City University London, London, UK

Andrea E. Nelson
PhD, BSc (Hons), RGN
Head of School and Professor of Wound Healing, School of Healthcare, University of Leeds, Leeds, UK

Anne Marie Rafferty
CBE, DPhil (Oxon), MPhil, BSc, RN, FRCN, FAAN, FQNI, FKC, LLD (Hon)
Professor of Nursing Policy & Director of Academic Outreach, Florence Nightingale School of Nursing and Midwifery, King's College London, London, UK

Janice Rattray
PhD, MN, Cert Ed, RGN, SCM
Reader in Acute and Critical Care Nursing, School of Nursing and Midwifery, University of Dundee, Dundee, UK

Jan Reed
PhD, BA, Cert Ed
Emeritus Professor, Northumbria University, Newcastle upon Tyne, UK

Angie Rees
MA, BA (Hons), DPS, FHEA, MCLIP
University Teacher and Information Specialist, School of Health and Related Research (ScHARR), University of Sheffield, Sheffield, UK

Jo Rycroft-Malone
PhD, MSc, BSc (Hons), RN
Professor of Implementation Research and Head of School, Bangor University, Gwynedd, UK

Sarah Salway
PhD, MSc, BSc (Hons) (Oxon)
Senior Research Fellow, NIHR School for Public Health Research, School of Health & Related Research (ScHARR), University of Sheffield, Sheffield, UK

Janey Speers
EdD, MA, BSc (Hons), RMN, RGN
Senior Lecturer, Mental Health Nursing, Institute of Health and Social Care Studies, St Martin, Guernsey, Channel Islands

Julie Taylor
PhD, MSc, BSc (Hons), RN, FRCN
Professor of Child Protection, Child Protection Research Centre, University of Edinburgh, Edinburgh, UK

Angela Tod
PhD, MSc, MMedSci, BA (Hons), RN
Professor of Clinical Nursing Practice Research, University of Manchester, Manchester, UK

David Torgerson
PhD, MSc
Professor and Director, York Health Trials Unit, Centre for Health Economics, University of York, York, UK

Annie Topping
PhD, PGCE, BSc (Hons), RGN
Assistant Executive Director of Nursing – Nurse Education, Hamad Medical Corporation, Qatar and Visiting Professor of Nursing, University of Huddersfield, Huddersfield, UK

Joanne Turnbull
PhD, MSc, PCAP, BSc
Senior Research Fellow, Faculty of Health Sciences, University of Southampton, Southampton, UK

Stephen J. Walters
PhD, MSc, PGCE, BSc (Hons), CStat
Reader in Medical Statistics, School of Health and Related Research (ScHARR), University of Sheffield, Sheffield, UK

Introduction to the 7th Edition

Since the 6th edition of *The Research Process in Nursing* was published in 2010, there have been some significant developments in nursing research in the United Kingdom. A framework for Clinical Academic Careers in nursing has been implemented across the United Kingdom creating for the first time the opportunity for nurses to progress through masters preparation, doctoral and postdoctoral research fellowships whilst combining research activity with clinical practice. At the same time, the pace of change in nursing research has been rapid, with a broader range of research approaches and methods being used to answer research questions arising from nursing practice. Finally, the drive to ensure that research evidence is used to inform practice has continued to gain momentum in both policy and in the everyday work of practising nurses. Patients expect to receive high-quality health care informed by the very best evidence. Nursing research is central to this endeavour.

As editors, we have felt it necessary to ensure that this well-established research text reflects these developments in nursing research. In compiling the 7th edition of *The Research Process in Nursing*, we have made some changes to the content of the book, although the overall structure remains unchanged. There are two completely new chapters, one on the use of digital technologies in research and the second examining future trends in nursing research, and five chapters on established topics have been prepared by new authors. The remaining chapters have been revised and updated to ensure that the reader is provided with the very latest information on research processes and methods. In order to engage readers, we have included for the first time a number of reflection activities in each chapter which encourage the reader to think more broadly about what they have read and apply their learning to practice. In addition, we have extended the resources available on the web site associated with the book (www.wiley.com/go/gerrish/research), enabling readers to complement their studies by accessing the many web resources that are available in the field of health care research and highlighting work being undertaken by some of the chapter authors.

We, the editors, have been privileged to continue to work with chapter authors who are leaders of nursing research and other disciplines across the United Kingdom and also in Australia and Canada. We are indebted to our team of authors for their wide-ranging and authoritative contributions to the research methodology literature. We have continued to target the book at novice researchers, be they pre-registration students or those embarking on a postgraduate research degree, but the book should also be of value to many who are further on in their research careers. We have encouraged authors to write in an accessible style, but not to shrink away from complex debates and technical issues.

The book is structured into six sections.

Section 1, *Setting the Scene*, deals with the background issues of nursing research in the current policy context in the United Kingdom, the nature of the research process and ethics. Two chapters encouraging inclusive approaches to the research process are also included in this section. The chapter on user involvement has been rewritten by new authors and the chapter on research in a multi-ethnic society has been substantially updated. A new and innovative chapter on technologies in research has been included in this edition to reflect the increasing use of a range of digital technologies at different stages of the research process. Readers new to the context in which nursing research is taking place will find themselves orientated to the subject by this section and, we hope, enthused to engage with an activity that has the potential to change and improve the provision of health care.

Section 2, *Preparing the Ground*, includes chapters that take the reader through the essential steps that are necessary before a research project can begin. The chapters outlining how research evidence can be accessed and appraised in order to inform research have been updated, especially in terms of the use of technologies to assist in these processes. Subsequent chapters guide the reader through the process of developing a research proposal and subsequently planning and managing the research project. Regulatory frameworks governing research in the United Kingdom have continued to evolve, and the chapter on this issue has been revised to reflect these changes.

Section 3, *Choosing the Right Approach*, is the longest section and in many ways the heart of the book. It starts by providing an introduction to the philosophical debates underlying the different research approaches available to nurses and is followed by a chapter on sampling that has been prepared by new authors. The remainder of this section presents 14 research approaches used in nursing research and explores each of them in detail. Whereas these qualitative and quantitative approaches were included in the previous edition, they have each been revised to reflect recent developments, with the chapters on practitioner research and mixed methods prepared by new authors, thus providing a fresh perspective. In addition to commonly used approaches such as surveys, systematic reviews and grounded theory, the inclusion of other approaches such as practitioner research and realist synthesis represents new ways of thinking about doing research. They are commended to the reader as possible ways into difficult-to-research areas, particularly those related closely to nursing practice.

Section 4, *Collecting Data*, and Section 5, *Making Sense of Data*, are both practical sections dealing with the skills required in data collection and analysis. Here the emphasis is upon research tools, such as interviewing and statistical analysis, common to many different research approaches.

Section 6, *Putting Research into Practice*, concludes the book by taking the reader through the process of disseminating research findings and getting them implemented into policy and practice. As well as addressing active researchers, these chapters will be of use to nurses who, though not wanting to engage themselves in research, want to incorporate it into their professional lives through evidence-based practice. The final chapter is new to this edition and introduces the reader to current trends in nursing research which will be important for nurse researchers to consider in the future.

Although the book is designed in a logical fashion, as outlined above, each chapter is also intended to be complete in itself. Many readers will dip in and out of different sections as necessary. For this reason, we have included cross-references wherever possible to other chapters that might be helpful and have provided key point summaries at the beginning of each chapter. We have also compiled a glossary of research terms to help the reader with new language with which they may be unfamiliar.

Throughout the book, we have adopted certain generic terms to assist readability and reduce repetition. Foremost among these is the term 'nursing'. By this we mean to include all the professions of nursing, midwifery, health visiting and related specialisms. We hope that members of these professions will forgive our shorthand, but we have tried to ensure that examples given are taken from a wide range of health care settings. We have also used the terms 'evidence' and 'evidence-based practice' to denote the plethora of resources and implementation activities that have become so important in health care today.

This book is intended to be used primarily by nurses, midwives and health visitors, but it has much wider application to any health and social care practitioner who wishes to learn about research. Members of the allied health professions, particularly, face many of the same debates and dilemmas as nurses in developing research capacity. The contributors of the book are not all nurses but include statisticians, social scientists and information specialists.

We trust that this 7th edition of a well-established book will continue to make a valuable contribution to research capacity building in nursing and health care.

Kate Gerrish and Judith Lathlean
Editors to the 7th edition
2015

About the Companion Website

This book is accompanied by a companion website:

www.wiley.com/go/gerrish/research

The website includes:
- Interactive multiple-choice questions
- Key points of each chapter
- End-of-chapter web resources

SECTION 1

Setting the Scene

Nursing research does not exist in a vacuum but is an applied discipline set in the context of a dynamic academic community and relating to a complex health care system. This section explores this context and introduces the reader to the nature of nursing research.

Chapter 1 presents the fundamental concepts of the discipline, reviews the current context of nursing research and emphasises the essential connection between nursing research and the practice of the profession. Even those who do not see themselves as active researchers should be users of the knowledge generated by research, and so need to understand much of what follows in the sections of this book. Chapter 2 takes the reader through the essential steps in the research process, each of which will be dealt with in much more depth in later sections, but with the aim of giving an overview of the entire undertaking, that is research. Recent examples from the literature are used to illustrate the varied nature of nursing research.

Research in nursing, as in health care generally, is complicated by the fact that it is involved with vulnerable human beings, and ethical principles need to be observed from the outset of any research project. Chapter 3 therefore tackles this moral obligation on the researcher, drawing out the practical implications, and setting the context for the more specific ethical regulations dealt with in Section 2.

The next two chapters, Chapters 4 and 5, deal with the need for nursing research to be inclusive in scope. User involvement in research has been advocated from within and outside the profession for more than a decade now, and Chapter 4, which has been written by new authors, argues for the full inclusion in the research process of those to whom the outcomes might apply. Chapter 5 examines research in a multi-ethnic society. Although there are many minority groups that deserve special consideration when designing nursing research, ethnicity perhaps merits particular consideration as a major factor impacting upon health care in UK society.

Chapter 6 is new to the seventh edition of the book and reflects the growth in digital technologies in recent years. This chapter introduces the reader to a range of digital technologies and considers how they can be used to support different stages of the research process.

The Research Process in Nursing, Seventh Edition. Edited by Kate Gerrish and Judith Lathlean.

Companion Website: www.wiley.com/go/gerrish/research

CHAPTER 1

Research and Development in Nursing

Kate Gerrish

Key points

- Research is concerned with generating new knowledge through a process of systematic scientific enquiry, the research process.
- Research in nursing can provide new insights into nursing practice, develop and improve methods of caring and test the effectiveness of care.
- Whereas comparatively few nurses may undertake research, all nurses should develop research awareness and use research findings in their practice.
- Evidence-based practice involves integrating the best available research evidence with professional expertise whilst also taking account of patient preferences, the patient's state, setting and circumstances and health-care resources.

INTRODUCTION

Significant changes in health care have taken place in the three decades since the first edition of this book was published, and these changes are set to continue. Technological developments have led to improved health outcomes and at the same time have raised public expectations of health-care services. Increased life expectancy and lower birth rates mean that the population in the United Kingdom is ageing. An older population is more likely to experience complex health needs, especially in regard to chronic disease, and this places additional demands on an already pressurised health service. At the same time, the escalating cost of health care is leading to a shift from expensive resource-intensive hospital care to more services being provided in the primary and community care sectors. In response to these changes, government health policy is increasingly focused on improving the clinical and cost-effectiveness of health care while at the same time reducing the burden of ill health through active public health and health promotion strategies. These changes in the United Kingdom are reflected in other high-income countries internationally.

In order to respond to these challenges, the UK government has identified a number of priorities that need to be progressed in order to provide high-quality care for patients and promote the health of

The Research Process in Nursing, Seventh Edition. Edited by Kate Gerrish and Judith Lathlean.

Companion Website: www.wiley.com/go/gerrish/research

the population at large. These include improving health outcomes by preventing illness as well as enhancing the quality of care provided to people with particular needs, for example, patients with common long-term conditions such as diabetes or those in need of palliative and end-of-life care (Department of Health 2012a, 2013a). In order to achieve the aspirations for enhancing quality and improving health and health outcomes, there is a need to change the way health-care professionals work and the way health services fit together and ensure that patients have access to the best available treatments. However, achieving quality in health care is a moving target. What was considered high-quality care in 1948 when the NHS was first founded is no longer considered to be the case nearly seven decades later. Knowledge about effective health-care interventions has increased by leaps and bounds, and this is certainly the case with nursing interventions.

It is essential that nurses respond proactively to the developments in nursing and health-care delivery outlined earlier in order to provide high-quality care in response to the needs of the individuals and communities with whom they work. To do this, they need up-to-date knowledge to inform their practice. Such knowledge is generated through research. This chapter introduces the concept of nursing research and considers how research contributes to the development of nursing knowledge. In recognising that nursing is a practice-based profession, the relevance of research to nursing policy and practice is examined within the context of evidence-based practice, and the responsibilities of nurses are explored in respect of research awareness, research utilisation and research activity.

NURSING RESEARCH AND DEVELOPMENT

The definition of research provided by Hockey (1984) in the first edition of this book is still pertinent today:

> *Research is* an attempt to increase the sum of what is known, usually referred to as a 'body of knowledge' by the discovery of new facts or relationships through a process of systematic scientific enquiry, the research process. (Hockey 1984: 4)

Other definitions of research emphasise the importance of the knowledge generated through research being applicable beyond the research setting in which it was undertaken, that is, that it is generalisable to other similar populations or settings. The Department of Health, for example, defines research as

> the attempt to derive generalisable new knowledge by addressing clearly defined questions with systematic and rigorous methods. (Department of Health 2005: 3, section 1.10)

Research is designed to investigate explicit questions. In the case of nursing research, these questions relate to professional activities and concerns that are primarily the responsibility of nurses. The International Council of Nurses' (ICN) definition of nursing research captures these broad areas of interest that are relevant to nurse researchers:

> Nursing research is a systematic enquiry that seeks to add new nursing knowledge to benefit patients, families and communities. It encompasses all aspects of health that are of interest to nursing, including promotion of health, prevention of illness, care of people of all ages during illness and recovery or towards a peaceful and dignified death. (ICN 2009)

The ICN has identified nursing research priorities in two broad areas, namely, health and illness and the delivery of care services. These priority areas are outlined in Box 1.1. In further developing the nursing research agenda, various organisations have identified priorities for specific areas of nursing practice. For example, a recent consultative exercise in the United Kingdom involving patients, carers, health-care professionals and researchers identified 12 research priorities into the prevention and management of pressure ulcers (James Lind Alliance Pressure Ulcer Partnership 2013). Box 1.2 shows that these priorities are broad ranging and cover not only aspects of nursing care but also education, service delivery, surgical interventions and patient/carer involvement.

Research in the field of nursing education is also important, for unless nurses are prepared appropriately for their role, they will not be able to respond to the needs of patients, families and communities.

Box 1.1 Priorities for nursing research identified by the International Council of Nurses

Health and illness

Nursing research priorities in health and illness focuses on:

- health promotion
- prevention of illness
- control of symptoms
- living with chronic conditions and enhancing quality of life
- caring for clients experiencing changes in their health and illness
- assessing and monitoring client problems
- providing and testing nursing care interventions
- measuring the outcomes of care

Delivery of care services

Nursing research priorities in delivery of care services focus on:

- quality and cost-effectiveness of care
- impact of nursing interventions on client outcomes
- evidence-based nursing practice
- community and primary health care
- nursing workforce to include quality of nurses' work life, retention and satisfaction with work
- impact of health-care reform on health policy, programme planning and evaluation
- impact upon equity and access to nursing care and its effects on nursing
- financing of health care

ICN (2009)

Box 1.2 Top 12 pressure ulcer research priorities

1. How effective is repositioning in the prevention of pressure ulcers?
2. How effective at preventing pressure ulcers is involving patients, family and lay carers in patient care?
3. Does the education of health and social care staff on prevention lead to a reduction in the incidence of pressure ulcers, and, if so, which education programmes are most effective?
4. What is the relative effectiveness of the different types of pressure-relieving beds, mattresses, overlays, heel protectors and cushions?
5. What impact do different service models have on the incidence of pressure ulcers including staffing levels, continuity of care and the current organisation of nursing care in hospitals?
6. What are the best service models to ensure that patients with pressure ulcers receive the best treatment outcomes?
7. For wheelchair users sitting on a pressure ulcer, how effective is bed rest in promoting pressure ulcer healing?
8. How effective are wound dressings in the promotion of pressure ulcer healing?
9. Does regular turning of patients in bed promote healing of pressure ulcers?
10. Does improving diet and hydration promote pressure ulcer healing?
11. How effective are surgical operations to close pressure ulcers?
12. How effective are topical skin care products and skin care regimes at preventing pressure ulcers?

James Lind Alliance Pressure Ulcer Partnership (2013)

Box 1.3 Priorities for research in nursing education

Education–practice linkages

- Education models focused on delivery of team-based patient-centred care to diverse patient populations in a variety of clinical settings
- Education–practice partnerships designed to relate innovative teaching models to quality patient care outcomes
- New curriculum models related to inter-professional education and practice

Knowledge acquisition

- The effectiveness of various creative teaching–learning approaches to foster development of clinical reasoning in patient care contexts
- Teaching–learning approaches that relate knowledge acquisition and evidence-based practice to the patient's actual care experience

Technology in nursing education

- The effectiveness of emerging technologies in the teaching of nursing decision-making skills
- The relationship between simulated learning experience, programme outcomes and graduate nurse competencies

Adapted from National League for Nursing (2012)

Some examples of priorities for research in nursing education are identified in Box 1.3.

Most nursing research investigates contemporary issues; however, some studies may take a historical perspective in order to examine the development of nursing by studying documentary sources and other artefacts. Rafferty (2010) points out that studying what happened in the past can contribute to our understanding of the contemporary problems we face and give insight into human behaviours and the forces influencing social change.

The questions that nursing research may address vary in terms of their focus. Over 30 years ago, Crow (1982) identified four approaches that research could take; these remain pertinent today:

1. Research that will provide new insights into nursing practice
2. Research that will deepen an understanding of the concepts central to nursing care
3. Research that is concerned with the development of new and improved methods of caring
4. Research that is designed to test the effectiveness of care

Reflection activity

Think about your own area of nursing practice. What priority areas for nursing research can you identify? You may be aware of aspects of your own practice that are underpinned by research, but there may be other areas of practice that require further research. The list of research priorities identified by the ICN (Box 1.1) may help you to think more broadly about areas for research. From the list you have compiled, identify the area that you think is the most important to research.

Nursing research does not necessarily need to be undertaken by nurses. Indeed, sociologists and psychologists undertook some important early studies into nursing practice and nurse education from the 1950s to 1970s. However, research expertise amongst nurses has developed considerably in the past 40 years, to the extent that research examining nursing practice is most likely to be undertaken by nurses themselves or nurses collaborating with other disciplines.

Likewise, nurses who engage in research may not confine their area of enquiry to nursing research. The growing emphasis on multidisciplinary, multiagency working means that nurse researchers may choose to examine questions that extend beyond the scope of nursing into other areas of health and social care. Nurse researchers may find themselves working in multidisciplinary teams including statisticians, health economists, psychologists, sociologists and other health professionals, working on research areas such as rehabilitation that encompass a wide range of disciplines. Nurse researchers work appropriately in a number of university departments such as social science and health services research as well as in departments of nursing and midwifery.

Whereas the generation of new knowledge is valuable in its own right, the application and utilisation of knowledge gained through research are essential to a practice-based profession such as nursing. This latter activity is known as 'development' and may take the form of practice or service development. Thus, research and development ('R&D') go hand in hand.

R&D can be divided into three types of activity:

1. *Basic research* is original, experimental or theoretical work, primarily for the purpose of obtaining new knowledge rather than focusing on the specific use of the findings. For example, biomedical laboratory-based research falls within this category.
2. *Applied research* is also original investigation with a view to obtaining new knowledge, but it is undertaken primarily for practical purposes. Much nursing research falls within this category and is undertaken with the intention of generating knowledge that can be used to inform nursing practice and can involve both clinical and non-clinical methods.
3. *Development* activity involves the systematic use of knowledge obtained through research and/or practical experience for the purpose of producing new or improved products, processes, systems or services.

Development activity that focuses on the use of knowledge generated through research can take different forms. The most common activities include clinical audit, practice development and service evaluation (see Box 1.4). Like research, these activities often employ systematic methods to address questions arising from practice. Research, however, is undertaken with the explicit purpose of generating new knowledge that has applicability beyond the immediate setting. By contrast, clinical audit, practice development and service evaluation are primarily concerned with generating information that can inform local decision-making (Health Research Authority 2013). Yet, the boundaries between some forms of research, for example, action research (see Chapter 23) and practice development and evaluation research (see Chapter 22) and service evaluation, are often blurred (Gerrish & Mawson 2005). It is, however, important to be able to differentiate between these activities as they require very different approval processes before the work can begin (see Chapter 11).

DEVELOPING NURSING KNOWLEDGE

Nursing research is concerned with developing new knowledge about the discipline and practice of nursing. Nursing knowledge, like any other form of knowledge, is never absolute. As the external world changes, nursing develops and adapts in response. In parallel, nursing knowledge develops and changes. This year's 'best available evidence' has the potential of being superseded by new insights and discoveries. Therefore, nursing knowledge is temporal and will always be partial and hence imperfect. This does not mean, however, that nurses should not continually strive to develop new knowledge to inform nursing and health-care policy and practice.

Box 1.4 Definitions of research, clinical audit and practice development

Research seeks to create generalisable new knowledge to answer clearly defined questions by undertaking a systematic and rigorous process of enquiry (Department of Health 2005).

Clinical audit is the process that helps ensure patients and service users receive the right treatment from the right person in the right way. It does this by measuring the care and services provided against evidence-based standards and then narrowing the gap between existing practice and what is known to be best practice (Health Quality Improvement Partnership 2009).

Practice development encompasses a broad range of innovations that are initiated to improve practice and the services in which that practice takes place. It involves a continuous process of improvement towards increased effectiveness in patient-centred care. This is brought about by helping health-care teams to develop their knowledge and skills and to transform the culture and context of care (Garbett & McCormack 2002).

Service evaluation seeks to assess how well a service is achieving its intended aims. It is undertaken to benefit those who use a particular service and is designed and conducted solely to define or judge current service (Health Research Authority 2013).

Whereas the focus of this book is on the generation of knowledge through research, it is important to recognise that nursing knowledge may take different forms. In addition to empirical knowledge derived through research, nurses use other forms of knowledge, such as practical knowledge derived from experience and aesthetic or intuitive knowledge derived from nursing practice (Thompson 2000). Nurses use these different forms of knowledge to varying degrees to inform their practice (Gerrish *et al.* 2008). It is beyond the scope of this book to examine in detail the various forms of nursing knowledge; however, Chapter 38 introduces the reader to some of these within the context of promoting evidence-based practice.

The definitions of research given earlier in this chapter emphasise the role of systematic scientific enquiry – the research process – in generating new knowledge. The research process comprises a series of logical steps that have to be undertaken to develop knowledge. Different disciplines may interpret the research process in different ways, depending on the specific paradigms (ways of interpreting the world) and theories that underpin the discipline. A biological scientist's approach to generating new knowledge will be different from that of a sociologist. However, the basic principles of the systematic research process will be followed by all disciplines. Nursing, as a discipline in its own right, is relatively young in comparison to more established professional groups such as medicine and is in the process of generating theories that are unique to describing, explaining or predicting the outcomes of nursing actions. Nursing theories are generated through the process of undertaking research and may also be tested and refined through further research. However, nursing also draws upon a unique mix of several disciplines, such as physiology, psychology and sociology, and any of these disciplines may be appropriate for research in nursing. For example, the management of pain can be studied from a psychological or physiological perspective; whichever approach is chosen will be influenced by the theories relevant to the particular discipline.

The research process in nursing is no different from other disciplines, and the same rules of scientific method apply. Chapter 2 sets out a systematic approach to research – the scientific method in action – and subsequent chapters consider the various components of the research process in detail.

At this stage, it is worth noting that in some texts, the 'scientific method' is taken to reflect a particular view of the world that values the notion that we can be totally objective in our research endeavours. In this book, the term 'scientific method' is not restricted in this way and is used to mean a rigorous approach to a systematic form of enquiry. Chapter 12 introduces the reader to the different ways in which the scientific method can be interpreted depending on the assumptions that the researcher holds about the nature of the social world and reality. These can be broadly classified as quantitative and qualitative approaches to research. Quantitative research is designed to test a hypothesis and generally involves evaluating or comparing interventions, particularly new ones, whereas qualitative research usually involves seeking to understand how interventions and relationships are experienced by patients and nurses (Health Research Authority 2013).

RESEARCH AWARENESS, UTILISATION AND ACTIVITY

Research-based practice is arguably the hallmark of professional nursing and is essential for high-quality clinical and cost-effective nursing care (ICN 2009). It is now over 45 years since the Report of the Committee on Nursing (1972) stressed the need for nursing to become research based to the extent that research should become part of the mental equipment of every practising nurse. Although considerable progress has been made in the intervening period, this objective still remains a challenge. In order for nursing to establish its research base, nurses need to develop an awareness of research in relation to their practice, they need to be able to use research findings, and some nurses need to undertake research activity.

Research awareness implies recognition of the importance of research to the profession and to patient care. It requires nurses to develop a critical and questioning approach to their work and in so doing identify problems or questions that can be answered through research. Nurses who are research aware will be able find out about the latest research in their area and have the ability to evaluate its relevance to practice. They will also be open to changing their practice when new knowledge becomes available. Research awareness implies a willingness to share the task of keeping abreast of new developments by sharing information with colleagues. It also entails supporting and co-operating with researchers in an informed way. Nurses need to understand the implications for patients arising from research being undertaken in the clinical area in which they work. For example, nurses may need to provide care according to an agreed research protocol, and deviating from the protocol may jeopardise the research. However, they must ensure that the well-being of patients remains paramount and report promptly any concerns they may have regarding the research to more senior clinicians and managers as well as the researchers. Nurses should develop research awareness as part of preregistration nurse education programmes and continue to develop their knowledge and skills following registration.

Research utilisation is concerned with incorporating research findings into practice so that care is based on research evidence. Not all research, even that which is published in reputable journals, is necessarily of high quality. Before findings can be applied, a research study needs to be evaluated critically in order judge the quality of the research undertaken. All nurses should be able to appraise a research report although specialist advice may need to be sought in regard to judging the appropriateness of complex research designs or unusual statistical tests. Chapter 8 provides guidance on how to appraise research reports.

Research studies do not always provide conclusive findings that can be used to guide practice. Indeed, different studies examining the same phenomenon may produce contradictory results. Wherever possible, a systematic review of a number of studies examining a particular phenomenon should be undertaken in order to provide more robust guidance for practice than the findings of a single study would allow. Chapter 25 outlines the procedures for undertaking a systematic review. It is a time-consuming process and requires a good understanding of research designs and methods together with knowledge of techniques for analysis, including statistical tests. Whereas some nurses may develop the skills to undertake a systematic review as part of a postgraduate course, many systematic reviews are undertaken by people who are experts in the technique. For example, The Joanna Briggs Institute, which is based in Australia, is a collaborative involving over 70 teams in different parts of the world who are involved in undertaking detailed reviews of the best available evidence to inform nursing care (www.joannabriggs.org).

The findings from a systematic review then need to be incorporated into clinical guidelines or care protocols that can be applied to practice. Whereas some guidelines may be developed at a national level, nurses may need to adapt national guidelines for application at a local level or develop their own guidelines where no national ones are available (see Chapters 38 and 39 for more information).

All nurses should be research aware and use research finding in their practice; however, not all nurses need to undertake research. To carry out rigorous research, nurses need to be equipped with appropriate knowledge and skills. Undergraduate nursing programmes tend to focus on developing research awareness and research utilisation. It is generally not until nurses embark on a master's programme, or a specialist research course, that they will learn how to undertake a small-scale research study, under the supervision of a more experienced researcher. This represents the first step in acquiring the skills to become a competent researcher. Comparatively, few nurses progress to develop a career in nursing research in which they undertake large-scale studies that are funded by external agencies. It generally requires study at doctoral level followed by an 'apprenticeship' working within a research team with supervision and support from experienced researchers before being able to lead a large-scale study.

Within the United Kingdom, initiatives are underway to support nurses, midwives and a range of allied health professionals to develop their competence as researchers whilst still maintaining and developing their clinical role. The clinical academic training pathway creates opportunities for practitioners to progress from master's programmes in clinical research through doctoral and postdoctoral clinical research opportunities with the aim of ultimately holding a senior clinical academic appointment between a university and a health-care organisation (Department of Health 2012b).

Although relatively few nurses progress to lead large research studies, many more nurses participate in research led by nurse researchers, doctors and other health professionals. Nurses working in clinical practice may be asked to undertake data collection for researchers, and their clinical nursing experience can be valuable to the research enterprise. Even if they are not leading a study, nurses who assist other researchers should have a sound understanding of the research process in order to collect valid and reliable data and to adhere to the research governance and ethical requirements outlined in Chapter 11.

Reflection activity

A number of research studies have identified the barriers that nurses experience in using research findings in practice. From your own experience of nursing, what do you think are the main barriers to nurses using research in their everyday practice? How can these barriers be overcome? After undertaking this exercise, you might like to refer to Chapter 38, which provides more details of the barriers to research use.

RESEARCH AND NURSING PRACTICE

Current policy initiatives seek to promote a culture of evidence-based practice in which nurses use the best available evidence to inform their decision-making. There are several components to evidence-based practice, namely, the knowledge derived from research, the clinical expertise of practitioners, the insights that patients contribute about their condition and their preferences for different treatment options, the patient's clinical state, setting and circumstances and health-care information and resources (DiCenso *et al.* 2005). In recognising that knowledge derived from research is never absolute, nurses should draw upon their own expertise and that of other more experienced colleagues when deciding on an appropriate intervention. However, clinical expertise should not be seen as a substitute for research evidence but rather as contributing to the decision about the most appropriate intervention for a particular patient. Nurses have a responsibility to share their knowledge of the best available evidence with patients in order to help them make informed choices about the care they receive. This is particularly important where there are alternative courses of action that can be selected. However, the patient's clinical state (e.g. severity of illness or disability), the setting in which they are receiving care (e.g. hospital or community settings) and their social and economic circumstances may affect the delivery of evidence-based care. Finally, decision-making can also be influenced by other sources of information available, for example, national policy documents or local clinical audit information, and by the resources available to provide care. These issues are examined in more detail in Chapters 38 and 39.

Nursing's progress towards becoming evidence based needs to be viewed within the context of wider influences on health care. The UK (England, Northern Ireland, Scotland and Wales) governments are actively promoting standards for health care through major policy reforms. For example, the NHS Outcomes Framework 2014/15 for England (Department of Health 2013b) identifies key priorities in terms of preventing premature deaths, enhancing the quality of life for people with long-term conditions, supporting recovery from episodes of ill health or injury, ensuring positive experiences of care for patients and protecting people from harm by providing a safe environment for care. All of these priorities have implications for nursing care. Quality improvement, a process whereby health-care organisations and the people who work in them are responsible for continually improving the quality of services and safeguarding high standards of care, is central to these initiatives (Batalden & Davidoff 2007). Clearly, improvements in the quality of care and health-care services need to be based on the best available evidence. Research is therefore essential to making progress towards achieving quality improvement.

Reflection activity

Consider your own area of practice. What mechanisms are in place to ensure that patients receive care that is based on the best available evidence?

Are there any specific initiatives underway to improvement quality of patient care, the patient experience or patient outcomes?

As outlined earlier in this chapter, the knowledge generated through nursing research should be used to develop evidence-based practice, improve the quality of care and maximise health outcomes (ICN 2009).

In order to enhance the quality of nursing care, it is important to ensure that care is clinically effective. Often referred to as 'doing the right thing right', clinical effectiveness involves providing the most appropriate intervention in the correct manner at the most expedient time in order to achieve the best outcomes for the patient. Nurses need to draw upon knowledge generated through research in order to decide which intervention is most appropriate and how and when to deliver it. Research may also highlight reasons for non-compliance. A particular dressing may have been shown through research to be effective in promoting wound healing, but if it is unacceptable to the patient, problems with compliance may arise.

As mentioned earlier in this chapter, the findings from a single study may not provide sufficient evidence to direct practice, and wherever possible, nurses should rely on knowledge generated through systematic reviews of research evidence drawn from several research studies. There are a number of national initiatives to assist nurses and other health professionals to provide clinically effective care. These include the development of clinical guidelines based on the research evidence by, for example, the National Institute for Health and Care Excellence (NICE) and the Scottish Intercollegiate Guidelines Network (SIGN). In addition, the NHS Evidence portal provides health-care professionals with access to a comprehensive evidence base to inform clinical practice. It is intended to provide a 'one-stop shop' for a range of information types, including primary research literature, practical implementation tools, guidelines and policy documents. The websites listed at the end of this chapter provide some useful links to these resources.

Increasing demands on the finite resources within the NHS have resulted in the need to ensure that health-care interventions are not only clinically effective but also cost-effective. There is little point pursuing a costly intervention if a cheaper one is seen to be equally as effective. The field of health economics is concerned with examining the financial and wider resource implications of providing a specific intervention or service. Economic evaluations can be undertaken to evaluate different treatments or alternative ways of providing services from an economic perspective and providing information that can be used to inform judgements about the clinical and cost-effectiveness of a particular intervention or service (Jackson 2012). NICE and SIGN guidelines take account of both clinical and cost-effectiveness when making recommendations for best practice.

CONCLUSION

Research is necessary to develop the knowledge base to inform nursing policy and practice. In an era of evidence-based practice, nurses are constantly challenged to identify new and better ways of delivering care that is grounded in knowledge derived from research (ICN 2009). Nurses have a professional obligation to their patients and to wider society to provide care that is based on the best available evidence. Whereas relatively few nurses will develop a career in nursing research, all nurses should become research aware. This means developing a critical and questioning approach in order to identify areas where practice could be improved on the basis of research findings or areas where research evidence is lacking and new knowledge needs to be generated through research. Nurses also need to utilise research findings in their day-to-day practice. However, in order to provide evidence-based care, nurses should be able to evaluate the quality of published research reports. This requires a sound understanding of the research process, together with knowledge of different research designs and the methods that can be used to collect and analyse data. The following chapters of this book examine the research process, designs and methods in detail in order to equip nurses with the knowledge base to critically appraise research reports and to engage in the process of undertaking research under the supervision of a more experienced researcher.

References

Batalden P, Davidoff F (2007) What is 'quality improvement' and how can it transform healthcare? *Quality and Safety in Health Care* **16**(1): 2–3.

Committee on Nursing (1972) *Report of the Committee on Nursing*. London, Her Majesty's Stationary Office. (not Stationary)

Crow R (1982) How nursing and the community can benefit from nursing research. *International Journal of Nursing Studies* **19**(1): 37–45.

Department of Health (2005) *Research Governance Framework for Health and Social Care*, 2nd edition. London, Department of Health.

Department of Health (2012a) *The Public Health Outcomes Framework for England, 2013–2016*. London, Department of Health. https://www.gov.uk/government/uploads/system/uploads/attachment_data/file/216159/dh_132362.pdf (accessed 6 January 2014).

Department of Health (2012b) *Developing the Role of the Clinical Academic Researcher in the Nursing, Midwifery and Allied Health Professions*. London, Department of Health.

Department of Health (2013a) *The Mandate: a mandate from the government to the NHS Commissioning Board April 2013 to March 2015*. London, Department of Health.

Department of Health (2013b) *The NHS Outcomes Framework 2014/15*. London, Department of Health.

DiCenso A, Ciliska D, Guyatt G (2005) *Evidence-Based Nursing: a guide to clinical practice*. Philadelphia, Elsevier Publishing & AMA Press.

Garbett R, McCormack B (2002) A concept analysis of practice development. *Nursing Times Research* **7**(2): 87–100.

Gerrish K, Mawson S (2005) Research, audit, practice development and service evaluation: implications for research and clinical governance. *Practice Development in Health Care* **4**(1): 33–39.

Gerrish K, Ashworth P, Lacey A, Bailey J (2008) Developing evidence-based practice: experiences of senior and junior clinical nurses. *Journal of Advanced Nursing* **62**: 62–73.

Health Quality Improvement Partnership (2009) *What Is Clinical Audit?* London, HQIP. http://www.hqip.org.uk/assets/Images/Uploads/HQIP-What-is-Clinical-Audit-Nov-09.pdf (accessed April 2014).

Health Research Authority (2013) *Defining Research: NRES guidance to help you decide if your project requires review by a Research Ethics Committee.* London, Health Research Authority.

Hockey L (1984) The nature and purpose of research. In: Cormack DFS (ed) *The Research Process in Nursing*, 1st edition. London, Blackwell Science, pp 1–10.

International Council of Nurses (2009) *Nursing Research: a tool kit*. Geneva, International Council of Nurses. http://www.icn.ch/matters_research.htm (accessed February 2014).

Jackson D (2012) *Healthcare Economics Made Easy*. Banbury, Scion.

James Lind Alliance Pressure Ulcer Partnership (2013) *Top 12 Pressure Ulcer Research Priorities*. York, University of York. http://www.york.ac.uk/media/healthsciences/documents/wounds-research/12priorities.pdf (accessed April 2014).

National League for Nursing (2012) *Research Priorities for Nursing Education*. New York, National League for Nursing. http://www.nln.org/researchgrants/researchpriorities.pdf (accessed April 2014).

Rafferty AM (2010) Historical research. In: Gerrish K, Lacey A (eds) *The Research Process in Nursing*, 6th edition. Oxford, Wiley Blackwell, pp 321–330.

Thompson DR (2000) An exploration of knowledge development in nursing – a personal perspective. *NT Research* **5**(5): 391–394.

Websites

http://www.evidence.nhs.uk – The NHS Evidence website provides access to a comprehensive evidence base to inform clinical practice. It provides a 'one-stop shop' for a range of information types, including primary research literature, practical implementation tools, guidelines and policy documents.

http://www.joannabriggs.org – An international research and development collaborative, led by the University of Adelaide, Australia, that undertakes systematic reviews of best evidence for nursing interventions and draws up recommendations for practice, based on the best available evidence.

http://www.nice.org.uk – The National Institute for Health and Care Excellence (NICE) publishes recommendations on treatments and care using the best available evidence of clinical and cost-effectiveness.

http://www.rcn.org.uk/development/research_and_innovation – The RCN Research and Innovation Co-ordinating Centre website provides links to a range of resources to support nursing research and evidence-based practice.

http://www.sign.ac.uk – The Scottish Intercollegiate Guidelines Network (SIGN) publishes national clinical guidelines containing recommendations for effective practice based on current evidence.

http://www.york.ac.uk/inst/crd – The Centre for Reviews and Dissemination (CRD) undertakes and publishes reviews of research about the effects of interventions used in health and social care.

CHAPTER 2

The Research Process

Anne Lacey

Key points

- The research process is a series of steps that needs to be undertaken to carry out any piece of research.
- The precise stages of the research process, and the order in which they are undertaken, will vary depending on the nature of the research but will always follow a systematic pattern from initial ideas through to dissemination and implementation.
- Rigour in research is essential if the work is to be trustworthy and free from bias.

INTRODUCTION

The process of undertaking research is essentially the same, whether the subject matter of the research is pure science, medicine, history or nursing. The following rather expansive definition from Graziano and Raulin (2004) sums up the breadth of scope of the research process:

> Research is a systematic search for information, a process of inquiry. It can be carried out in libraries, laboratories, schoolrooms, hospitals, factories, in the pages of the Bible, on street corners, or in the wild watching a herd of elephants. (Graziano & Raulin 2004: 31)

In all cases, the researcher must ascertain the extent of existing knowledge, define his or her own area of enquiry, collect data and analyse it and draw conclusions. For the pure scientist, however, the research might take place in the context of a laboratory, where experimentation is relatively straightforward as the researcher is in control of the environment and can eliminate potential confounding factors that might invalidate the research. Unless using animals or human tissue, there are few ethical considerations to take into account.

For the student of nursing research, or any research in a social context, the process is complicated by practical and ethical constraints of working in the 'real world' (Robson 2011). There is no single universally accepted way of carrying out research in the social world, but a plethora of different designs and methodologies ranging from phenomenology to randomised controlled trials, from epidemiology to action research. The range of approaches derives

The Research Process in Nursing, Seventh Edition. Edited by Kate Gerrish and Judith Lathlean.
 Published 2015 by John Wiley & Sons, Ltd.
Companion Website: www.wiley.com/go/gerrish/research

Box 2.1 The research process

Stages in the research process	Chapters in this book
Developing the research question	2
Searching and evaluating the literature	7, 8
Choice of methodology, research design	12, 14–27
Preparing a research proposal	9
Gaining access to the data	11
Sampling	13
Pilot study	2
Data collection	28–33
Data analysis	34–36
Dissemination of the results	37
Implementation of research findings	38, 39

from different paradigms, or ways of seeing the world. However, all are valid ways of conducting research, provided the methodology used is appropriate for the research question and is applied in a rigorous, systematic fashion.

In this chapter, the research process that is common to all nursing research will be explored, and subsequent chapters in Section 2 will look at each of the stages of research in more detail. In Section 3 of this book, different methodologies or research designs are discussed in turn and in detail.

Although the research process will be presented as a linear, sequential process, the stages are often revisited several times during the process. In qualitative research, in particular, it is likely that the 'stages' of the research process are modified to take account of the emergent nature of the enterprise. Qualitative researchers sometimes find it difficult or even inappropriate to formulate a precise research question until they have begun to collect, and possibly even analyse, data.

However, it is helpful in the first instance to think through the entire research process in a systematic way. Many authors (Parahoo 2006; Moule & Goodman 2009; Moule & Hek 2011) have described the research process, and each comes up with a different number of stages, but essentially they contain the same elements. Box 2.1 illustrates this process as it will be described in this chapter, and indicates the principal chapters in the book that deal with each stage. In this chapter, a brief overview of the various stages will be given to enable readers to see the whole before looking in more detail at each stage in subsequent chapters.

DEVELOPING THE RESEARCH QUESTION

Most research questions begin with a 'hunch' or initial idea that is not precisely defined. The idea might arise from clinical practice, from professional discussion among colleagues, from an issue in the media or from reading an article or book. Alternatively, the question may be derived from a 'call for proposals' from a funding body that asks researchers to develop a proposal on a specific topic. Box 2.2 provides an example of such a call, in this case from the National Institute for Health Research

Box 2.2 NIHR call health services and delivery research programme

Information obtained from **HS&DR Communications** <hsdrinfo@soton.ac.uk> on 24 October 2013

Health Services and Delivery Research Programme

NHS
National Institute for Health Research

Funding opportunities with the Health Services and Delivery Research (HS&DR) Programme

Commissioned call for proposals

Applicants are invited to submit proposals on the following commissioning brief by **1pm on 16 January 2014:**

- 13/156 - Effectiveness and cost-effectiveness of integrated homeless health and care services

Applicants are also invited to submit proposals on the following commissioning brief by **1pm on 15 May 2014:**

- 13/157 - Research on improving performance and productivity at the clinical microsystem (team) level

The commissioning briefs, application forms and guidance notes for these topics are all available on the HS&DR commissioned call webpage.

HTA researcher-led call on homeless population

The Health Technology Assessment (HTA) Programme is also interested in receiving applications to their researcher-led workstream, to advance existing knowledge on the clinical and cost-effectiveness of particular therapeutic interventions in the homeless population. For more information please visit the HTA researcher-led webpage, where the information will be available shortly.

New website for NIHR Evaluation, Trials and Studies Programmes and activities

As a part of wider developments of NIHR websites, the HS&DR website has now become part of a new NETS website with improved functionality. Visit the site at http://www.nets.nihr.ac.uk and let us know what you think of it!

Contact us
Tel: 023 8059 4304
Email: hsdrinfo@southampton.ac.uk
Web: www.nets.nihr.ac.uk/hsdr

Follow us  | Sign up  | NIHRtv 

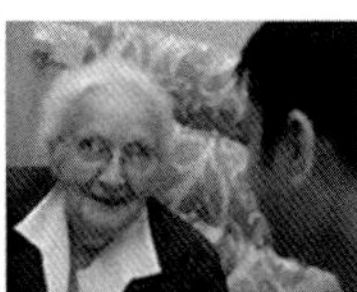 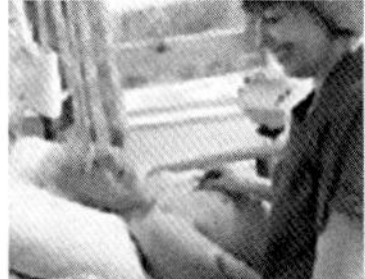 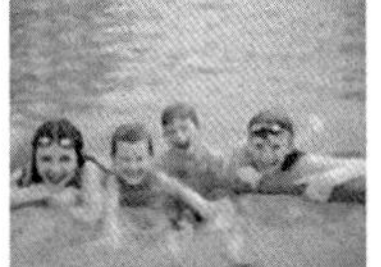 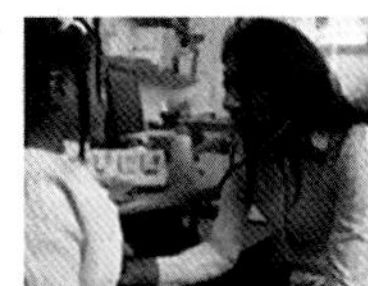

To find out more visit
www.nets.nihr.ac.uk/hsdr

Health Services and Delivery Research (HS&DR) Programme. The call is specific about the research areas to be investigated and a deadline by which proposals have to be submitted. Full details about the commissioning brief are available from the HS&DR website, together with a standard application form.

However, most nurse researchers begin with an initial idea that is not yet well defined. Let us consider how research questions might be developed, using some real examples from the nursing literature to illustrate our discussion (see Research Examples 2.1–2.3).

RESEARCH EXAMPLE

2.1 A Quantitative Experimental Study

Stafne SN, Salvesen KA, Romundstad PR, Torjusen IH, Morkkved S (2012) Does regular exercise including pelvic floor muscle training prevent urinary and anal incontinence during pregnancy. *British Journal of Obstetrics and Gynaecology* **19**(10): 1270–1280.

This study used a quantitative experimental approach to assess whether pregnant women who followed an exercise course that included pelvic muscle floor training were less likely to experience urinary and anal incontinence towards the end of pregnancy than women who received standard care.

Researchers in Norway recruited 855 pregnant women and randomly allocated them to either a training group (who received a 12-week exercise programme delivered by a physiotherapist) or the control group (who received normal antenatal care). Patients in the training group received a weekly group session led by a physiotherapist and were encouraged to exercise at least twice each week. Self-reported urinary incontinence and anal incontinence were measured for the two groups. Results showed that fewer women in the training group experienced urinary incontinence (11% compared to 19% $P=0.004$) and anal incontinence (3% compared to 5% $P=0.18$). The researchers concluded that pregnant women should exercise, and in particular do pelvic floor exercises, to prevent and treat urinary incontinence.

RESEARCH EXAMPLE

2.2 A Quantitative Questionnaire Survey

Chevalier I, Benoit G, Gauthier M, Phan V, Bonnin A, Lebel M (2008) Antibiotic prophylaxis for childhood urinary tract infection: a national survey. *Journal of Paediatrics and Child Health* **44**: 572–578.

A national survey of Canadian paediatricians was conducted to assess their practice in prescribing prophylactic antibiotics for children with urinary tract infections, with and without vesicoureteral reflux. A self-completion questionnaire was mailed to a sample of 1136 paediatricians and 42 paediatric nephrologists. A response rate of 58.1% was obtained. Although a majority of respondents prescribed prophylaxis for children with reflux, only 15% felt that this practice was evidence based. A quarter of respondents also prescribed prophylaxis for children under 1 year with a first febrile urinary tract infection, without evidence of reflux. Again, only 19% felt that this practice was evidence based. The overall conclusion was that practice in this area varies widely in Canada, because of a lack of solid evidence about prophylaxis.

RESEARCH EXAMPLE

2.3 A Qualitative Study

Hasson F, Kernohan W, Waldron M, Whittaker E, McLaughlin D (2008) The palliative care link nurse role in nursing homes: barriers and facilitators. *Journal of Advanced Nursing* **64**: 233–242.

This descriptive qualitative study explored the views and experiences of link nurses for palliative care working in nursing homes in Northern Ireland. A purposive sample of 14 link nurses from 10 nursing homes was selected and interviewed using focus groups. Data from the focus groups were recorded, transcribed and analysed. Link nurses identified a number of barriers to their role as educators and facilitators of palliative care, including lack of management support, a transient workforce and lack of adequate preparation for the role. Facilitators included external support, peer support and access to a resource file. The researchers concluded that the link nurse role had considerable potential to improve care in this area, but managers needed to be aware of the sustained support needed for the role, and more work needs to be done to find ways of developing the role further.

Question 1

Perhaps, a research team has a 'hunch' that the use of a general exercise programme involving pelvic floor exercises might reduce the likelihood of women experiencing urinary and anal incontinence during late pregnancy. This hunch is probably based on knowledge of the anatomy of the pelvic muscles and the process of micturition and defaecation. It might also be supported by the professional experience of midwives. There are several ways in which the question could be developed. The following are examples of research questions derived from this area of interest:

- *Q1(a) Are pelvic floor exercises taught to women during antenatal classes?*
- *Q1(b) Do pregnant women understand what pelvic floor exercises are, and are they willing to learn the skills of doing them?*
- *Q1(c) Does the use of pelvic floor exercises as part of a general exercise programme reduce the experience of (i) urinary incontinence and (ii) anal incontinence?*

Obviously, each of these research questions will give us very different kinds of information and will require different research methods to be employed. They would also need to be refined further – the precise pelvic floor exercises to be taught need to be clarified, for example, and the stage of pregnancy at which they are taught needs to be defined. Q1(b) suggests the need to measure understanding and willingness to learn – neither of these concepts are straightforward, and tools to measure them would need to be developed. Perhaps, a qualitative study needs to be undertaken to explore the concepts first. Research Example 2.1 (Stafne *et al.* 2012) describes an experimental study that is related to Q1(c); in this case, the outcome measure was defined as self-reported urinary and faecal incontinence during late pregnancy.

Question 2

Alternatively, a research team might be interested in the evidence base used by doctors in their prescribing practice. Overuse of antibiotics in children, for instance, is known to cause problems with the development of drug resistance, and it is important that clinical practice is based on sound clinical evidence. Again, a number of research questions could be asked:

- *Q2(a) How reliable is the research evidence about prophylactic antibiotic prescription in children with urinary disease?*
- *Q2(b) How effective are prophylactic antibiotics in preventing urinary tract infections in children at risk?*

Q2(c) What is the prescribing practice of paediatric doctors regarding antibiotic prophylaxis?

Again, these three questions lead to very different types of study, and each question needs further clarification and refinement. What is meant by 'urinary disease'? How do we decide that research evidence is reliable? What ages of children are concerned? Which children are 'at risk'? Research Example 2.2 (Chevalier *et al.* 2008) is an example of a survey to answer Q2(c), but it was undertaken with a specific group of paediatric doctors in Canada. Is it appropriate to apply the answers gained from this study to doctors in Europe or China?

Question 3

In our last example, research questions might be generated concerning the best way to deliver palliative care in nursing homes. This setting is known to be a common one in which palliative care is delivered, but formal training and facilities are not always available. Three questions could be constructed to investigate this:

Q3(a) Is patient satisfaction with palliative care delivered in nursing homes lower or higher than that delivered in a hospital setting?
Q3(b) What is the level of knowledge about palliative care among nurses working in nursing homes?
Q3(c) What is the experience of link nurses for palliative care working in nursing homes?

Before setting out with any of these questions, the researcher would need to be clear how 'nursing home' was to be defined, and for Q3(b), a validated tool to measure knowledge would need to be available. Q3(a) suggests a comparative survey of samples of nursing homes and hospitals, but would the underlying question be answered by asking patients' views alone? Palliative care is needed up to and after the point of death, and so it might be necessary to extend the survey to satisfaction of next of kin who can give a full picture of care given. Q3(c) suggests a research design that needs a more in-depth approach, and the answer will be contained in words rather than numbers – Research Example 2.3 (Hasson *et al.* 2008) describes a study to answer this question using a qualitative approach.

Reflection activity

Identify a potential research topic from your own area of practice. Write down three research questions that could address this topic. What ideas do you have for how each of these questions might be answered by undertaking a research study?

USING A HYPOTHESIS

A hypothesis is a statement that can be tested and is used mostly in experimental research. Qualitative designs and surveys do not usually have a hypothesis, although sometimes surveys do test for differences between groups and so might use one. Statistics are required to test the hypothesis, which has to be very precisely written. The hypothesis expresses the predicted outcome of the experiment, either in positive or negative terms. As an example, Q2(b) could be answered by testing a hypothesis, which would be something like the following:

> *Children under 5 years of age with reflux given prophylactic antibiotics will experience fewer episodes of urinary tract infection in 1 year than children with reflux not given prophylactic antibiotics.*

The hypothesis might even express the magnitude of the expected difference – in this case, it might be predicted that children given antibiotics will experience, on average, at least 50% less infections than those not given antibiotics. But for the purpose of statistical testing, the hypothesis is more often expressed in negative terms, or as a null hypothesis, as in the following example:

> *Children under 5 years of age with reflux given prophylactic antibiotics will experience the same*

number of urinary tract infections in 1 year as those not given prophylactic antibiotics.

In this case, the experiment would aim to find the null hypothesis false, assuming that prophylactic antibiotics are effective in such cases. Chapter 36 gives more information about how such hypotheses are tested for statistical significance.

SEARCHING AND EVALUATING THE LITERATURE

The next stage is to find out what evidence already exists in the chosen research area. It is a waste of time and money to conduct research where the answer to the question is already known. What is already known about a subject can be found from a variety of sources. Books may be a starting point, but quickly get out of date if the subject matter is topical. Academic journals are a better place to start, and access to online databases such as Cumulative Index of Nursing and Allied Health Literature (CINAHL; see Chapter 7 for more details) makes this task speedy and relatively simple. If anything, the problem is that there will be too much information, and Chapter 7 discusses how to refine the search. Beyond written sources, evidence may be found on the Internet and various online resources. As well as locating the evidence, it must be appraised and evaluated. Not all that is written is of good quality, and evidence from one country or in one population may not necessarily generalise to other cultures or situations. Chapters 7 and 8 discuss this stage in considerable detail.

Sometimes, the research process may consist entirely of a review of the literature. A well-designed systematic review is an accepted research approach in its own right, systematically searching out and evaluating all the research that has been published on a particular topic. In an increasingly complex and fragmented world of information, it is important to develop an evidence base that is well validated and on which practice can be based. Q2(a) earlier would suggest the need for a systematic literature review, and Chapter 25 deals with this specialised form of research. Box 2.3 gives an example of a systematic review.

Box 2.3 Example of systematic review

Coleman S, Gorecki C, Nelson A, Closs SJ, Defloor T, Halfens R, Farrin A, Brown J, Schoonhoven L, Nixon J (2013) Patient risk factors for pressure ulcer development: systematic review. *International Journal of Nursing Studies* **50**(7): 974–1003.

This research study used established methods of systematic review to identify risk factors that could predict pressure ulcer development in adult patients. Fourteen electronic databases were searched for relevant articles published from the period when the database was created to 2010. In addition, hand searching of specialist journals and conference proceedings was undertaken. A total of 5462 abstracts were retrieved and 365 were identified as potentially eligible. Of these, 54 met the criteria for review, but only 17 were judged as high or moderate quality. The remaining 37 studies had inadequate numbers of pressure ulcers and other methodological limitations.

The most frequent risk factors identified that could predict pressure ulcer development included mobility/activity, perfusion and skin/pressure ulcer status. In addition, skin moisture, haematological measures, age, nutrition and general health status were also important. Further research was required to confirm whether body temperature and immunity were relevant. The review concluded that no single factor could be identified to explain pressure ulcer risk; rather, the interplay between a number of factors increased the risk of pressure ulcer development.

Most of the questions in the earlier examples would require a literature review before being able to refine the question further. It might be, for example, that a study has already been conducted to test the effectiveness of pelvic floor exercises undertaken during antenatal classes and found them to be effective in reducing urinary incontinence. But can this be applied to women who undertake the exercises at home? And can a study conducted in, say, the United States be applied in the United Kingdom? A literature search on palliative care in nursing homes might show that nurses in this setting have very low levels of knowledge or interest in palliative care. But the studies are few, out of date and somewhat contradictory. Is it justifiable to conduct a further piece of research in the area?

CHOICE OF METHODOLOGY AND RESEARCH DESIGN

The majority of this book (Section 3) is devoted to a description of different research designs. In many ways, the choice of research design is the most important stage of the research process, for it affects all the others. Some questions are more appropriate for an experimental approach; others are entirely suited to an in-depth ethnographic study. Researchers often make explicit a *conceptual framework* within which they are working, which will determine the overall research approach. A conceptual framework makes clear the researcher's 'world view' – their assumptions and preconceptions about the subject under consideration. In Question 1 earlier, for example, the researchers may have a conceptual framework that emphasises women's right to autonomy in decisions and policies relating to their pregnancy. Consequently, any research study would be concerned to gather the experiences and feelings of women about their pregnancy, rather than purely objective clinical data. The kind of data collected, the types of analysis that are possible and the way in which the results can be applied to practice will all depend upon the research design.

Some research designs are *quantitative*. This means they ultimately collect numerical data and are amenable to statistical analysis. Such research designs may or may not have a hypothesis, but experimental studies always require such a statement to be tested statistically. Research Example 2.1 (Stafne *et al.* 2012) and Research Example 2.2 (Chevalier *et al.* 2008) both describe quantitative studies. Quantitative designs may be experimental such as Stafne *et al.* (2012) but may also be observational, such as Chevalier *et al.*'s (2008) survey using a questionnaire. In the latter, structured answers such as ticked boxes enable the data to be coded and translated into numerical form. Surveys may also use medical records or laboratory tests as their data source, to estimate the numbers of patients in a community who have measles, for example. Epidemiological studies of the incidence and distribution of diseases also use quantitative methods.

Other research designs are *qualitative*. These designs use narrative, words, documents or graphical material as their data source and analyse material to identify themes, relationships and concepts and, in some cases, to develop theory. Such research approaches explore an experience, culture or situation in depth, taking account of context and complexity. Qualitative designs may be used where comparatively little is known about a subject, so no hypothesis can be formulated. The purpose is exploratory rather than explanatory, although qualitative studies may certainly contribute much to our understanding of phenomena and many also develop theory. An example of a qualitative study is given in Research Example 2.3 (Hasson *et al.* 2008).

Both approaches are valid ways of advancing nursing knowledge. A quantitative study may be very good at finding out the extent of compliance with diabetic therapy, for instance, by measuring levels of the blood glucose in a sample of diabetic patients. A qualitative study, on the other hand, may tell us why it is that certain diabetic patients do not take their insulin as prescribed by observing and talking to them and gaining understanding of the context in which the insulin is (or is not) taken.

More than this, qualitative and quantitative methodologies are based on different philosophical assumptions and derive from different historical traditions. Chapter 12 discusses these issues in much more detail, and the reader is encouraged to get to grips with this academic debate. Nursing needs to embrace all research methodologies in order to engage with the breadth of questions that need to be asked. Ours is a discipline drawing on many different traditions of academic enquiry.

The research design (or *methodology*) is distinct from the *methods* used for data collection. A single data collection method, for example, interview or observation, may be used for many different research designs.

So we can return to our hypothetical questions generated in Examples 1–3 and consider the research methodology that might be appropriate to answer each one. In the example relating to pelvic floor exercises for pregnant women, Q1(a) and Q1(b) are both essentially asking for information that can be gathered in a quantitative survey, but Q1(a) might also be answered by observation of antenatal classes or examination of the women's records. Q1(c) will require an experimental design in order to compare outcomes in two groups (Research Example 2.1). With regard to a potential study examining the prescribing of prophylactic antibiotics, Q2(a) suggests a literature review as described earlier, but Q2(b) would require a rigorous experimental design to answer the question about effectiveness. Q2(c) requires a survey, as described in Research Example 2.2. Finally, in relation to examining the best way to deliver palliative care in nursing homes, Q3(a) and Q3(b) both suggest a quantitative survey design, but Q3(a) will require a comparative survey, measuring satisfaction in the two types of care settings. It might also be answered using qualitative methods, asking in-depth questions of palliative care patients and their relatives in two types of settings. Indeed, this question might require mixed methods, as discussed in Chapter 27 of this book. Q3(c) certainly needs a qualitative approach (Research Example 2.3).

Reflection activity

Select one of the research questions you identified in the earlier reflection activity and sketch out the various stages of the research process you would need to undertake to answer the question. Provide as much detail as you can for each stage.

What knowledge and skills would you need to develop to undertake your proposed study?

PREPARING A RESEARCH PROPOSAL

Whether a large-scale, multi-centre study costing many thousands of pounds is planned, or a small, unfunded study for an educational degree, a formal research proposal is likely to be needed.

Such a proposal is a written statement of *what* the researcher intends to do, *why*, *how*, *when* and, often, *how much it will cost*. It is used to gain approval for the research, to secure funding if that is required and then to guide the research process during its execution. It will often be modified in the light of pilot studies or practical difficulties, but it is important that the detailed intentions are clear at the outset. It has been said that if you don't know where you are going, you are unlikely to get there!

Chapter 9 sets out the content of a research proposal in detail, but the precise form of the proposal will vary according to the nature of the research and the purpose of the written proposal. A proposal written in response to a funding call from the National Institute of Health Research or the Medical Research Council is likely to be a substantial document of many pages, written by a team of experienced researchers. One written for the purpose of outlining a small study for a master's degree may be only a few pages, written by the postgraduate student themselves with some guidance from their supervisor.

Whatever the context, however, the proposal will certainly include a section on each stage of the research process outlined in Box 2.1. It will also include a section detailing the ethical issues raised by the research and how the researcher will ensure that confidentiality, informed consent and other ethical principles are respected. Chapter 3 discusses these issues in more detail. It is usual to include a table or Gantt chart showing the timescale of the project. Table 2.1 shows such a chart for a complex evaluation study involving a survey, documentary analysis, case studies and focus groups. It is also helpful to identify milestones, stating the date by which each stage of the research will be completed, though this is obviously subject to change as the inevitable obstacles and delays come into play. It is customary to include a breakdown of resources required and a justification of why they are needed.

Table 2.1 Example of a Gantt chart for a mixed method piece of research

Timetable	**Year one July 2015–June 2016**						**Year two July 2016–June 2017**					
Months of evaluation	2	4	6	8	10	12	14	16	18	20	22	24
Key tasks												
1. **Baseline survey**												
Development of survey instrument												
Baseline survey data collection												
Baseline survey data analysis												
2. **Analysis of routine activity data and resource use data**												
Activity and resource use data collection (after 1 year and after 2 years)												
Data analysis												
3. **Case studies**												
Pilot case study												
Case study data collection												
Case study analysis												
4. **Focus groups**												
Focus groups with project co-ordinators at prearranged workshops × 2												
Transcription and analysis of focus groups												
Dissemination												
Interim report to Regional Advisory Group												
Feedback to project sites, dissemination and writing of final report for Regional Advisory Group												

Clearly, the research proposal cannot be written until the researcher has thought through all the stages of the research process in some detail. However, the proposal is of necessity one of the early stages in the process, as it is impossible to proceed without one.

GAINING ACCESS TO THE DATA

Because of the sensitivity of much of the research that takes place in health care and the vulnerability of many of its subjects, a complex system of governance has been developed in the United Kingdom to ensure all research is approved for its ethical soundness, scientific quality and legal propriety. NHS organisations are also concerned to ensure that all research that takes place within the organisation is properly funded and insured against liability. A system of ethical regulation via the National Research Ethics Service (www.nres.nhs.uk) is in place, and all applicants carrying out research in health care must follow this system. In addition, since 2001, a system of research governance has been developed to guard against research that has not been properly scrutinised and approved, after various high-profile scandals concerning NHS research (Department of Health 2005). Chapter 11 deals with this topic in depth. Suffice it to say at this stage that the system is necessary but rather bureaucratic and time-consuming. It is important to factor in the time required to gain such approvals when planning a research study.

In addition to formal permission, however, access to the data may require negotiation of a more informal nature with local personnel who act as 'gatekeepers'. If access to patients or their records is needed, for example, it may be necessary to gain the co-operation of the appropriate consultant, practice manager or audit department in addition to ethical and research governance committees. Access to a nursing home or school will require the permission of the appropriate senior manager. Chapter 11 also deals in more depth with this informal process of negotiating access.

SAMPLING

Once the research begins, the first stage is likely to be selecting the sample. Unless it is a complete census, researchers collect data from a selected group, rather than an entire population. In our earlier examples, samples might be taken from antenatal clinic attenders, nursing homes in a particular region of the country, consultants in paediatric medicine or relatives of patients requiring palliative care. How are the samples to be selected, and how many is enough? These questions are dealt with in detail in Chapter 13, but the answers are rarely simple, particularly about sample size.

A quantitative study involving a comparison between two groups is likely to require a *power calculation*, a statistical technique to estimate minimum sample size. This is comforting to the researcher as it gives a scientific answer to the question but is also based on various assumptions and decisions that any statistician making the calculation will ask the researcher to make. In qualitative research, samples tend to be smaller, but again, there is no hard and fast rule as to how big they must be. Data saturation, or achieving the stage where no new information is being revealed by additional data collection, may be the stated goal, but it is impossible to predict beforehand when that stage may be reached.

As to the method of selection of the sample, there is a range of well-developed methods to choose from (see Chapter 13). The type of sampling will depend on the research design. Random sampling, and its variants, is the method of choice in traditional survey research, whereas theoretical sampling may be more appropriate for grounded theory. Whatever approach is adopted, it is essential for the validity of the research that the sample is chosen in a rigorous way, and sampling techniques adopted are adhered to closely.

The size and selection of the sample will have an effect on the timescale and cost of the research. Usually, the cost increases with sample size, although this is less significant for, say, a postal survey than for a randomised controlled trial. Similarly, in-depth interviewing and subsequent transcription of tape recordings are resource intensive, and each increase in sample size will require significant extra resources. A realistic assessment of how quickly a particular sample size can be obtained is necessary before embarking on a piece of research – all too often patients with the relevant condition seem to disappear as soon as a research study starts recruiting!

PILOT STUDY

It is always advisable to conduct a pilot study before embarking on the research. This may take the form of a 'dummy run' to see if the whole recruitment process works or may simply involve testing out a data collection instrument. Questionnaires are usually piloted on a small sample of people with similar characteristics to those in the full study, to pick up questions that are misinterpreted, or items that are frequently missed out. Modifications can then be made to the questionnaire before large numbers are printed and money wasted. If interviews are to be used, a wise researcher will conduct one or two pilot interviews to test out the interview schedule, to ensure technical equipment (such as an audio digital recorder) works satisfactorily and to assess how long the interview is likely to take. Data collected in a pilot study is not usually included with the main results, but may be reported separately and even published if the pilot study is a substantial one.

DATA COLLECTION

A wide range of data collection techniques and methods is available, and Chapters 28–33 describe the commonest of these. Nursing research relies heavily on interviews, focus groups and questionnaires as methods of choice, but observation, clinical measurement and the use of documents as data are also appropriate methods to be considered. In our earlier boxed examples, data collection methods would include clinical self-reporting and documents (occurrence of urinary and faecal incontinence), questionnaires (prescribing practice of doctors) and focus groups (experience of palliative care link nurses). The stage of data collection is, in many ways, the most straightforward and rewarding stage of research. It frequently involves interaction with patients, the public or other research participants after a long stage of filling in forms and writing research proposals. At last, the researcher gets to ask the questions he or she started out with.

Data collection tools will usually have been selected at the research proposal stage. Ethical and research governance committees like to see the intended instruments or at least to have a draft of an interview schedule or questionnaire. The instruments will need to be refined and developed ready for use, however, and practicalities of how the data will be collected, by whom and when are often done as data collection begins.

It is at this stage that the researcher needs to keep tight control over the data collection process. Failure to keep index numbers on documents, or to record the time of a clinical observation, can render data collected useless. It is also important to consider who should be involved in data collection. Using our earlier example in Question 1, it might be unwise to use the same physiotherapist who was teaching the pelvic floor exercises to collect the data, as he/she might feel some conscious or unconscious interest in showing that his/her teaching was effective.

All data collected needs secure storage, whether this is in hard copy (paper records or audiovisual material) or in electronic form. Paper copies need to be locked in a cabinet or drawer to preserve confidentiality, and electronic records and digital recordings need to be stored on a secure computer and backed up on a separate disc or server. Many researchers will preserve both paper and electronic records, as either can be destroyed or corrupted by unexpected events such as fire, theft or computer breakdown.

Reflection activity

Identify three different types of data collection that you are familiar with from reading research articles. What are the advantages and disadvantages of each method? How suitable might they each be for studying the research topic you have identified?

DATA ANALYSIS

This is perhaps the most crucial phase of any research project. Once data are collected, they need to be assembled and organised in such a way that conclusions can be drawn from them. A huge spreadsheet of numbers or multiple pages of narrative cannot be disseminated to others or used in practice until some analysis has taken place. It is also the phase that is most demanding from an intellectual point of view. Whether using qualitative or quantitative methods, data analysis is hard work. Contrary to many people's expectations, computer software analysis packages such as NVivo (for qualitative analysis) and SPSS (for quantitative analysis) do not do the analysis; they simply provide practical tools to manage the data more easily. The researcher still has to manage and guide the process and do some serious thinking about the meaning of the data.

If the data collected are qualitative, data analysis techniques such as those described in Chapter 34 can be used. The exact methods used will vary according to the qualitative methodology adopted. In practice, there are few universally accepted methods of analysing qualitative data, but the researcher must make the process 'transparent' by describing in detail how the results were derived.

Quantitative data are usually analysed statistically, and Chapters 35 and 36 provide guidance on the standard techniques available. With anything other than a small project, a quantitative piece of research should include a statistician in the research team, or at least be able to access professional statistical advice.

Some research projects use 'mixed methods' that include both qualitative and quantitative approaches. Here, the analysis may attempt to combine the two sets of results, perhaps using the qualitative data to provide interpretation of the quantitative results. See Chapter 27 for more on this issue.

DISSEMINATION OF THE RESULTS

Of course, there is little point in conducting any research if the results are never made known to anybody except the researcher. Dissemination can take many forms. At the local level, research can be presented to colleagues at team or unit meetings or as a more formal seminar to local professionals who may be interested. The study in Research Example 2.1 about pelvic floor exercises might be of interest to pregnant mothers, consultant obstetricians, general practitioners and physiotherapists, as well as to midwives themselves. Many nurses have access to a specialist group of health professionals in their discipline at local or national level, and this is also a suitable forum in which to disseminate the results of small- or large-scale research.

The increasing use of the Internet has provided opportunities for researchers to post details of their research on a website, perhaps hosted by a healthcare organisation or university. This ensures that research results are widely and freely available, but, like most online resources, provides no guarantee of quality. Increasingly, however, information is being disseminated via the web, and social media such as Twitter and online discussion groups are also enabling informal exchange of ideas.

Publication in written form, in academic and professional journals, remains the most widely accepted method of dissemination of research, but presentation of results at conferences, by oral presentation or by poster, is also common. All of these media enable fellow researchers and practitioners to discuss the results and provide some feedback about the usefulness of the research and possible avenues for further studies. Chapter 37 in this book discusses methods of dissemination more thoroughly.

IMPLEMENTATION OF THE RESULTS

This topic is dealt with in depth in Chapters 38 and 39 of this book. Needless to say, the purpose of nursing research is to improve practice in some way, whether by direct application of the results of a trial, by better informing practitioners of the culture in which they are working or by evaluating the effects of an innovation. While it is not the direct responsibility of the research community to ensure implementation of the findings of research, it is incumbent upon researchers to ensure that their findings are

Reflection activity

To what extent do you think researchers are effective in promoting the uptake of their research findings into practice? What might they do differently?

being shared with those who implement nursing policy and engage in clinical practice. This implies that research findings should be published in places where practitioners, managers and policymakers will read them and taken to professional as well as academic conferences. The findings from the study in Research Example 2.3, for example, will not be implemented unless they reach the managers and owners of nursing homes, who may not attend the research conferences or read the academic journals where the results are first presented.

ENSURING RIGOUR

Rigour refers to the strength of the research design in terms of ensuring that all procedures have been followed scrupulously, that all possible confounding factors have been eliminated and that the user can be confident that the conclusions are dependable. Of course, this is always a relative concept; social research can very rarely be said to have eliminated all possible sources of error, but the quality of the research will be judged by the extent to which this has been done.

There are two key concepts that concern the quality of research: validity and reliability. *Validity* concerns the extent to which the research measures what it purports to measure without bias or distortion. A study to assess the health effects of air pollution in a community would not be valid if it simply collected people's views about the air quality, without measuring actual levels of disease, or even mortality rates. In the study in Research Example 2.1, validity would be reduced if the pelvic floor exercises were taught poorly, or if some women were given additional written materials while others were not. Validity would also be affected by the representativeness of the sample chosen – if this included only well-educated middle-class women from the United Kingdom, for example, it would not be valid to apply the results to a mixed community living in Brazil.

Reliability refers to the consistency of measurement within a study. A set of weighing scales that gave a person's weight as 52 kg at 10:00 am and 55 kg at 10:05 am could not be said to be reliable. Repeated measurement is the usual test of reliability and can be done by second administration of a questionnaire under similar conditions or by two researchers making the same set of observations and comparing results. Data collection tools such as quality of life scales are extensively tested for reliability before being used as a standard measure in research studies. Unreliable measurement tools will always mean that the validity of a research study is compromised, as confidence in the quality of data collection is reduced. A study might use perfectly reliable instruments, however, and still not be valid. Meticulous collection of body mass index of patients in primary care, for example, will not generate a valid measure of the prevalence of diabetes in the practice, though the two may be related. In the study in Research Example 2.2, a poorly designed questionnaire that gave ambiguous answers or low completion rates would have made the results unreliable.

Some qualitative researchers reject the terms validity and reliability because of the association of the terms with the quantitative research tradition and the assumption implicit in their definition that research can be entirely objective and free from bias (Holloway & Wheeler 2010). Such researchers may prefer to use concepts such as credibility, trustworthiness and transparency to describe the quality of the research, but the underlying concept of rigour and the use of a systematic approach remain the same. Chapters 12 and 14–16 of this book will discuss these issues further.

Reflection activity

Select a published research paper that is of interest to you. How have the authors ensured rigour in the research process?

CONCLUSION

The research process outlined in this chapter will be adapted according to the research design, the scale of the undertaking, the resources available and the context in which the research is conducted. However, all research needs to be systematic and rigorous in its approach. This chapter has discussed the relative complexity of conducting research in a social, rather than a laboratory, context. One of the particular complexities is the need to conduct research that involves people according to ethical principles, and this requirement frequently impinges on the design and conduct of the research process. This question is addressed in the next chapter.

References

Chevalier I, Benoit G, Gauthier M, Phan V, Bonnin A, Lebel M (2008) Antibiotic prophylaxis for childhood urinary tract infection: a national survey. *Journal of Paediatrics and Child Health* **44**: 572–578.

Coleman S, Gorecki C, Nelson A, Closs SJ, Defloor T, Halfens R, Farrin A, Brown J, Schoonhoven L, Nixon J (2013) Patient risk factors for pressure ulcer development: systematic review. *International Journal of Nursing Studies* **50**(7): 974–1003.

Department of Health (2005) *Research Governance Framework for Health and Social Care*. London, Department of Health.

Graziano AM, Raulin ML (2004) *Research Methods: a process of inquiry*, 5th edition. Boston, Pearson.

Hasson F, Kernohan W, Waldron M, Whittaker E, McLaughlin D (2008) The palliative care link nurse role in nursing homes: barriers and facilitators. *Journal of Advanced Nursing* **64**(3): 233–242.

Holloway I, Wheeler S (2010) *Qualitative Research in Nursing*, 3rd edition. Oxford, Wiley-Blackwell.

Moule P, Goodman M (2009) *Nursing Research: an introduction*. London, Sage.

Moule P, Hek G (2011) *Making Sense of Research: an introduction for health and social care practitioners*, 4th edition. London, SAGE.

Parahoo K (2006) *Nursing Research: principles, process and methods*, 2nd edition. Basingstoke, Macmillan.

Robson C (2011) *Real World Research: a resource for social scientists and practitioner-researchers*, 3rd edition. Oxford, Wiley.

Stafne SN, Salvesen KA, Romundstad PR, Torjusen IH, Morkkved S (2012) Does regular exercise including pelvic floor muscle training prevent urinary and anal incontinence during pregnancy. *British Journal of Obstetrics and Gynaecology* **19**(10): 1270–1280.

Websites

http://www.hra.nhs.uk – The NHS Health Research Authority where you can find information about ethical approval and research governance.

www.rdinfo.org.uk – The RDinfo 'Support and Help' section gives information about the research process, writing research proposals and getting approval.

http://www.nres.nhs.uk/ – The National Research Ethics Service gives full information about the system of ethical regulation for the NHS and social care research.

CHAPTER

3 Research Ethics

Martin Johnson and Tony Long

Key points

- The main ethical issues that require attention when planning and conducting research include the importance of respecting participants, responding to the needs of vulnerable individuals and groups, gaining consent and maintaining confidentiality.
- Strategies for conducting ethical research include balancing the potential disadvantages of participation in the research with the likely benefit to participants, minimising the risk of harm to participants, formal ethical scrutiny of research proposals and acceptance of individual responsibility.
- When evaluating a research report, consideration needs to be given to the ethical conduct of the study.

THE IMPORTANCE OF ETHICS IN RESEARCH

Early nurse researchers paid scant attention to ethics as such. Nurses were assumed to be professionals with integrity and a vocation in which putting patients' interests before their own could be assumed. Even from these times, however, researchers were confronting moral dilemmas and sometimes used methods that, when made public, were seen to have infringed human rights and possibly caused harms.

As a result of increasing public concern that not all health professionals have behaved with complete integrity, procedures to assure ethical probity of research programmes have become increasingly rigorous – some might even say tiresome (Howarth & Kneafsey 2003, 2005; Pollock 2012). Chapter 11 examines these procedures in some detail. Arguments regarding the adequacy and appropriateness of some approaches are provided by Long and Fallon (2007), while examples of studies where the ethical issues are controversial are considered elsewhere (Johnson 2004).

In this chapter, we introduce basic issues that researchers need to think about in the design of their studies. We will suggest that while it is essential to keep the core principle of respect for individuals firmly in mind, it will also be necessary in most cases to focus carefully on balancing potential disadvantages

The Research Process in Nursing, Seventh Edition. Edited by Kate Gerrish and Judith Lathlean.

Companion Website: www.wiley.com/go/gerrish/research

of participating in the research study with the likely benefits for participants. The chapter has two main parts: issues that require the researcher's attention and strategies that may be employed to deal adequately and ethically with these issues. This chapter can present only a brief introduction to the key ideas, and a wide range of resources are available, some of which we refer to here. Elsewhere, we have dealt with most of the issues and some of their solutions at much greater length and with more concrete examples (Long & Johnson 2007).

ISSUES FOR RESEARCHERS TO ADDRESS

Respect for participants

This key principle is based on the belief that every individual matters and has the right to be treated with respect. Most adults are autonomous: that is, they have the mental ability to deliberate about issues that affect them and to make decisions (however wise, foolish or capricious) for themselves. Respecting the individual implies respecting their decisions. Many factors may conspire to limit the autonomy of an individual.

Adequate information on which to base choices

Many decisions in life would be flawed if vital elements of relevant information were not available – or even deliberately withheld. A constant concern for researchers in health care is how much information to give people (particularly about unlikely risks) without worrying them unduly. However, the key aspects of participation should be made clear to potential recruits for them to make an informed choice, together with at least the most important risks in terms of likelihood of occurrence or extent of potential impact.

Understanding and evaluating the issues involved

While most adults (and, indeed, many children) are able to understand a sufficient depth of information or detail to allow for rational decision-making, this is not the case for all. It is possible for this ability to be temporarily or permanently lost through illness, trauma or degenerative processes of ageing or disease. Under normal circumstances, potential participants need to know what harms, if any at all, might result. However, in circumstances where this is simply not possible and when the research results might be important, different approaches may need to be adopted (see Research Example 3.1).

Perceived or actual coercion

Health professionals generally accept a role in persuading their patients to do what they consider to be good for them. Nurses regularly encourage and cajole people to mobilise after surgery, to take medication and to abstain from harmful behaviours. Coercion, however, involves using 'undue' pressure or leverage to engage compliance. In practice, the distinction is often blurred, particularly in circumstances of increased vulnerability of the patient, when the consequences of a poor choice are potentially disastrous or at times when staff are under strain. These pressures are easily transferred to the research arena, too.

Freedom from undue social restriction

While the individual's ability to make decisions may be compromised genuinely by severe intellectual disability resulting, for example, from dementia or head injury, it may also be limited by the social diminution of status that is inherent in the stereotyping and stigmatisation of some forms of illness or disability (Johnson 1997; Ben-Zeev *et al.* 2010). Health researchers therefore need to be aware that personal autonomy can become limited for both pathological and social reasons rendering the individual more vulnerable and less autonomous.

Vulnerable individuals and groups

Every recipient of health care is in some way vulnerable, but those with more limited ability to act autonomously can also be more vulnerable to the impact of research activity. For example, those whose first language is not English, notably some members of minority ethnic communities, can find it difficult to

RESEARCH EXAMPLE

3.1 Practical Ethics

Lawton J (2000) The Dying Process: patients' experiences of palliative care. London, Routledge.

Julia Lawton used open participant observation in order to avoid long and possibly exhausting interviews with the dying people in a hospice. In this edited extract from her book, she illustrates how, while attempting to get consent, wherever possible, she had to be practical:

> *Formal interviews not only seemed to be too obtrusive to many patients and their families; in a substantial number of cases they were simply not viable. Some patients, for example, were heavily sedated during their stay in the hospice, whilst others experienced changes in their mental state, such as becoming very paranoid or confused. It was, of course, impossible to interview a patient in a coma.*
>
> *I worked as an 'in-house' volunteer within the hospice because this particular role enabled me to have substantial and regular contact with patients and their visitors in the wards, side rooms and other communal areas within the building...*
>
> *I often found that performing a practical task, such as making a bed, gave me an ideal excuse to enter a ward and make observations in situations when it might have been too awkward and obtrusive to have a researcher present; for instance, when one of the patients had just died. ...*
>
> *Whenever possible, patients were informed by staff about my research and given the option of 'opting out' of any observations I made. In cases where a patient was admitted in a coma, or was suffering from confusion, the consent of his or her relatives was obtained instead.*
>
> (Lawton 2000: 30–31)

make their preferences known or to understand the issues (Royal College of Nursing 2007). Similar difficulties may attach to other individuals, such as some deaf people who use only sign language, whether using English or some other language in the written form (Breivik 2005).

Most young children are self-evidently vulnerable. In the light of several scandals in the United Kingdom in which the poor standard of care of children has led to their deaths, great prominence has been given to safeguarding children, and responsibility has been passed to the independent body Office for Standards in Education, Children's Services and Skills (Ofsted), which reports directly to Parliament. It inspects and regulates services that care for children and young people and those providing education and skills for learners of all ages (Ofsted 2008). Continued failures, however, mean that concern for the safety and well-being of children and young people must remain high on the agenda of all professionals, including researchers. The ability to act and decide autonomously develops with maturity, but even very young children of primary school age can be capable of holding reasoned, well-informed views on issues that affect them. When children are unable to determine what is in their best interests, parents are normally the best alternative decision-makers.

In situations where the planned research participants are children under local authority care, special care needs to be taken to be sure that decisions are made by the appropriate legal guardian. Despite the difficulties inherent in researching with children and young people, such research is essential if advances in treatment and better understanding of their needs are to be achieved (Long 2004) and if their unique perspectives are to be recognised (Livesley & Long 2013). Without such efforts to find ways to make inclusion in a study compatible with the best interests of children and young people, we risk double jeopardy by adding denial of the chance of improvement to the misfortune of suffering from a health or social problem.

It is equally tempting to assume that older people are automatically vulnerable to inappropriate clinical or research interventions. On the other hand, the majority of health care recipients *are* older people, and this trend will continue. Although it may sometimes be more convenient, excluding people from research on the grounds of age alone is not equitable and constitutes ageism (Watts 2012).

The same applies to other groups that might require extra efforts and resources to reach, but that should not be excluded inappropriately from studies. Minority ethnic populations are sometimes difficult to involve in research, especially where there are language and cultural differences, but with determination and sensitivity, the problems can often be overcome (Finigan & Long 2012) (see Chapter 5 for more information on undertaking research in a multi-ethnic society). For this reason, sensitive efforts should be made to include people with such backgrounds where possible, since everyone should have the opportunity to take part in and potentially to benefit from research. This applies both to individuals and to whole groups defined by ethnicity, age or gender.

In some cases, nurses care for, and may need to be involved in research with, individuals who are considered to be no longer cognitively competent to give consent. For example, some patients may have severe stroke, progressive dementia or brain damage to a degree that leaves them in a persistent vegetative state (Brady *et al.* 2012). Leslie Gelling (2004) discusses approaches that he and colleagues took to doing research with patients in the vegetative state and their families. Gelling carefully discusses the different degrees of loss of competence and autonomy through brain damage. He shows that research with this group and their families can help to clarify diagnosis and prognosis and help in arriving at more appropriate plans of care and treatment. He argues that despite the complexity involved, it would be quite wrong to avoid doing research with this group of individuals who have been largely ignored by the research community. In England and Wales, the provisions of the Mental Capacity Act 2005 have clarified the position that already pertained in Scotland, that an appropriate advocate, such as a relative, can make decisions on behalf of those who lack capacity such as for treatment or to participate in research (HM Government 2005).

Nurse researchers commonly wish to study their own clients, students or staff. In this context, it is important to ask why these particular participants are more appropriate, given the possibility for an existing power relationship (e.g. teacher/student) that might affect the individual's decision to participate or the outcomes of the study. Even those who are not affected by illness may become vulnerable in circumstances of power differential.

To summarise, research samples should be inclusive of and represent the diversity of society across all relevant groupings. In particular, vulnerable people should not be excluded from participation in research except for well-justified reasons, which do not include mere convenience to the researcher. A mature approach to such cases is needed in which extra efforts are made to ensure protection of vulnerable individuals without denying them the chance to participate and to benefit potentially from the research.

Reflection activity

In one study of a group of young people who were vulnerable as a result of their lack of family stability and their indulgence in risky sexual behaviours, some participants who were 14–15 years old were keen to take part but insisted on their parents or GP not knowing this information. What would you have done as a researcher?

You would probably think about the risk and potential benefits of taking part. You might try to weigh up how well the young people understood what was involved in taking part and what the risks and benefits might be. Is age everything? How do you gauge maturity? Do young people have the right to make capricious decisions just as adults do?

You might think about the consequences of denying such individuals the opportunity to take part. How would you ever know what their perspectives and needs were? Would these needs ever be met if research failed to provide the evidence?

Gaining consent

People who are able to consider what participation will involve should be able to decide whether or not to take part in a study. Researchers should provide full information that is easy to understand, and software is now available to evaluate the readability of such information, while standard tests of readability based on sentence length and other criteria are also available. A number of helpful electronic resources in this area are provided at the end of this chapter. The consent of the participant should be freely given, and opportunities should be provided for consent to be withdrawn at a later stage. In some studies, it may be necessary to ensure continuing consent on several occasions over a long period. However, it should be noted that an excess of concern in this respect could make respondents feel that research is more harmful than it really is. It is important to establish a sense of balance here. Engaging participation in a trial of a new anti-cancer drug carries far greater dangers than a focus group to evaluate a new service. The potential harms and possible benefits are of a different order of magnitude.

Consent freely given to a research design that might have dangers does not absolve the researcher of accountability for these dangers. It has long been established that responsibility for the welfare of research participants rests with the researcher who must prioritise the best interests of participants. Perhaps less serious, but no less challenging, is what to do when the researcher discovers a clear and present need, for example, for pain relief. In such cases, where demands of the research design and more immediate needs of participants conflict, the researcher needs to be clear in advance what they will do. It is debatable whether or not registered nurses retain an overriding professional duty to pursue the best interest of patients and clients when acting solely as a researcher. Such issues cannot be left until the point at which a decision is needed, but must be resolved clearly by the individual before embarking on the study.

In practice, obtaining consent should involve giving clear unambiguous information to potential respondents so that they (or their advocate) can make an autonomous decision. An example of participant information sheet and consent form is given in Chapter 11. Further guidance is available for nurses from the Royal College of Nursing (2007).

Reflection activity

Imagine that you want to undertake research with young adults who have lost the ability to move their limbs purposefully through degenerative disease. They cannot hold a pen to sign a consent form. Their intellectual ability is unimpaired, but communication may be problematic. What would you do to gain consent and evidence that this was done?

The first step would be to establish the state of ability for each individual and work from that. You would need to ensure that information about the study was provided in a format that was helpful to the potential recruits. If printed sheets are not helpful, then perhaps electronic media might serve better.

A consent form is not consent, and neither is a signed form. Consent is the explicit act of agreeing to participate. You might, for example, record verbal consent in response to verbal explanation and invitation to participate. You might involve a carer or friend whom the participant trusts to communicate with them and witness their verbal or signed consent. Research sometimes requires some innovation and the determination to find a way for people to be included rather than excluded.

Maintaining confidentiality

The collection of data, usually about people, is the principal strategy of nursing research. Often, these data include personal, biographical and demographic information that, while essential to the analysis, should normally be used for this purpose only. In some cases, such as focus groups, research participants and others may need to be asked to keep matters discussed confidential to the group. This is illustrative of the need to be responsive to the nature of the data and address issues of confidentiality accordingly. The possibilities for collecting and holding data of a novel or non-standard nature have expanded to a large degree to include still photography; video images and voices; computerised patient records; paintings, sculpture, drama and other forms of expression; and human tissues. Each of these forms of data poses different problems for the researcher, and sometimes creative means are required for both analysis and safe storage (Haigh & Jones 2005). However, there is nothing inherently unethical about their use, and we feel that the potential of some of these tools is insufficiently exploited in nursing research where the semi-structured interview seems to predominate (Long & Johnson 2002).

Collected data must be stored securely, and in many cases, arrangements are made to dispose safely of data once used for their main purpose on the grounds, some feel, that data used for one purpose should not, without permission, be used for any other. The Data Protection Act 1989 has a bearing upon this. Certainly, there is a convention that data should not normally be put to a use that has not previously been made clear to research participants. However, it seems to us that the value of data, suitably anonymised and carefully stored, should never be underestimated. There is no way to know what great benefit it may offer in the future. What is important is that generally people know that data may be kept and that it might be used to support research in due course. It is wise to make clear that such data may be used on more than one occasion for research and publication purposes. Before data is destroyed, we must ask what undertakings were made regarding storage or destruction of data and what harm such data could do now.

It has become traditional in much nursing and health research to assure research participants and organisations of the confidentiality of the data collected. However, researchers need to be aware that in a research context (as in a clinical one), they may become privileged with information of great importance, for example, in a criminal matter. We take the view that in an overriding interest such as personal safety or the protection of vulnerable people, confidentiality cannot be considered an absolute duty. This should also, however, be made clear to participants. Declarations by participants that suggest the potential for harm to themselves or third parties should prompt the serious consideration of the researcher divulging the essential information to an appropriate authority or professional.

Reflection activity

What do you think participants would make of your intention to destroy their data on completion of the project? They might be reassured to know that the matter will be closed off and their participation clearly ended. They might, alternatively, be shocked to think that the time and effort that they have contributed will be used once and then discarded.

Try asking participants or colleagues first what they think happens to data on completion of a study and then what they would hope would be done with the data. Explain about the potential for meta-analysis to produce convincing evidence from many smaller studies that cannot offer such confident evidence in isolation. Does this change their view?

The place of anonymity

A common way of assuring confidentiality of responses is to anonymise both individuals and organisations. In large surveys, this may be relatively straightforward. In smaller qualitative studies, anonymising data can be much more difficult. Certainly, erring on the side of safety, it has become common to remove identifying characteristics and to assign pseudonyms to respondents and organisations in much health and social care research. However, we need to remember that in some research traditions, like nursing history, the preservation of anonymity is inappropriate and may even be contrary to respondents' interests. An historian of British nursing research would inevitably collect data from, and name, key individuals and reserve the right to evaluate their contribution critically.

The Unlinked Anonymous Prevalence Monitoring Programme (UAPMP) began in the United Kingdom in 1990 and has tested millions of samples of human tissue (mostly blood) from pregnant women, substance-misusing adults and attendees at genito-urinary clinics since then (Health Protection Agency 2013). Much of the activity is related to genito-urinary medicine clinic attendees, injecting drug users and pregnant women – all potentially vulnerable groups. Consent is not sought, but the samples are acquired through a process that irreversibly removes any link to the identity of the donor. The purpose of the programme is to measure the distribution of undiagnosed infection, particularly human immunodeficiency virus (HIV), in parts of the adult population. This programme – essentially a public health data collection activity – meets with the ethical requirements laid down by the National Research Ethics Service, the Department of Health, the Medical Research Council and English law, and it is a prime example of large-scale data collection in which consent is not sought but otherwise the research subjects are protected by the maintenance of their anonymity. Although this position seems defensible, one might reasonably ask why, when a potentially harmful blood result is found, the patient and people they have intimate relations with may in some cases never hear of it.

STRATEGIES FOR ETHICAL RESEARCH

Balancing risks and benefits

We would argue that, in general, decisions about health-care interventions, and about research, are ones in which we weigh the possible risks and benefits in the interests of individuals and wider society. A problem with this notion of balancing risks and benefits, however, is that this implies a degree of certainty about what these may be. It suggests a calculation that cannot actually be performed. Instead, a human judgement needs to be made that accepts the disadvantages of an approach and takes account of the benefits research may bring either now or in the future.

In some forms of experimental research, the evidence for and against the planned intervention may already be substantial and can be summarised both for approval bodies and for research participants. Certainly, obvious risks (such as allergic reaction) and discomfort or pain should be made very clear to all concerned in the context of a rationale that includes the likely benefits of the research. In exploratory research, which is often qualitative, these outcomes may be less clear. Nevertheless, compared to the quite profound iatrogenic risks of much health care, serious physical or emotional harms are rare in nursing research.

Potential benefits from participation in research

Before any research project is undertaken, the possible benefits should be clear to all concerned. First among these might be a direct improvement in the health or care of individuals participating in the study. Second are longer-term benefits for others. Third, as a report by Len Doyal (2004) has argued, is the development of research skills, which is itself a legitimate aim of research. Each of these possible benefits must be carefully balanced with any likely disadvantages.

Predicting the benefits of a particular study can be difficult even with the most rigorous of experiments. In qualitative research with less foreseeable outcomes, this estimation can be even harder to make. For this reason, approval committees and other gatekeepers sometimes find it difficult to approve such studies. However, the more that such studies are undertaken, the greater the likelihood that some may be very beneficial, and few would doubt the influence and importance of works of this kind by Glaser and Strauss (1965), which drew attention to the way the dying were treated; by Stockwell (1984) who explored the inappropriate labelling of patients; and more recently by Lawton (2000) who shows clearly how grim, even in a hospice, the process of dying can actually be.

Minimising harm

Most patient care and treatment contains an element of risk of harm or, at the very least, discomfort. Nurses give injections, dress painful wounds and detain patients with a clear sense of proportion between the discomfort or denial of liberty and the likely future benefit. Research is little different but the level of risk depends on the nature of the research.

The trial of new products may cause harm, such as allergic reaction or worsening of the condition, to particular individuals. Other risks are less obvious, such as the possibility of upsetting people in research about sensitive subjects or inadvertently stimulating or revealing cause for conflict between participants. It is therefore important to be clear about harms and discomforts and to discuss these openly with research participants. In many cases, nursing research will involve minor inconvenience at most. This should be kept to a minimum, but complete avoidance may be impossible.

Watson (1996) argues that 'the concept of a test or trial immediately raises ethical issues' (Watson 1996: 7). Above and beyond the risk of actual harm, he argues that it is almost impossible to conduct a clinical trial without a measure of deceit. For example, even though respondents know they are in a trial, they may be blinded to which, if any, intervention they are receiving. Once again, the risk of harm must be minimised, and in such cases, truly informed involvement means that the subject accepts this element of potential deception.

It may be that this situation of conflict – between ensuring high-quality research that can result in positive outcomes and protecting participants – is compounded by being a health professional. It could be argued that non-professionals would feel less responsibility to rescue research subjects from minor discomforts and dangers. With the aim of minimising harm, health professional researchers now more clearly see that they should intervene to prevent or reduce harms in certain circumstances. Occasionally, the issue is potentially too serious for a nurse to ignore. Researchers learn, however, that many dilemmas are much less clear-cut and some tolerance of standards and procedures different to one's own is part and parcel of doing research in practice settings. Such issues are best discussed with experienced research colleagues or supervisors.

Personal integrity and professional responsibility

Although there are many safeguards such as research ethics committees, NHS research governance procedures and university approval arrangements, the protection of participants' interests in matters of research still often relies on the professionalism and personal integrity of the members of the research team.

Promises to keep data safely should be kept, and research processes should be carried out rigorously. Research approval processes increasingly have a brief reporting procedure, but sadly this can hardly be relied upon to assure quality and proper adherence to high standards of research conduct. Perhaps more reliable, although far from foolproof, is effective training of researchers and accountability to departmental or unit-based supervisors. Being overseen by a steering committee that contains suitably briefed representatives of the population being studied and a genuine peer review process are also usually of great help, if time-consuming. Additional guidance on personal responsibility for nurses in research is provided by the Royal College of Nursing (2007).

The ethical evaluation of research studies

The methodological literature in nursing research is expanding, but it is clear that despite the current fashion in the United Kingdom for procedural control of research in an attempt to prevent problems, little exists by way of ethical evaluation of the nursing research literature. An edited collection of essays (de Raeve 1996) examined some dilemmas and legal problems that researchers have faced themselves, but there is a general reluctance to debate the issues and problems faced by others. Matthews and Venables (2004) offered areas or criteria that might be used for such a purpose as the degree to which participation was

Box 3.1 Questions to ask about research conduct

For each question, the reviewer ought to consider: Did this exert any impact on the worth of the findings?

- What were the aims of the study? How important were they and why?
- Who undertook the study and how did their background prepare them?
- Who supervised or monitored the study?
- What sort of ethics approval was given, if any?
- What information were participants given and how readable and accurate was this?
- What checks were made to ensure that consent was given and remained in force?
- What opportunities were given for participants to withdraw?
- How were issues of power between researcher and respondents dealt with?
- Were any social groups excluded, and if so, how powerful was the justification?
- Were participants deprived of a known helpful intervention? If so, on what grounds?
- What risks/harms were associated with the study? Were these acceptable in the context of the potential benefits?
- What benefits were likely from the study and for whom?
- Did the effort made to disseminate the study outcomes to all concerned match the promises made?

voluntary, whether informed consent was achieved and the risk–benefit ratio. Unfortunately, they shrink from identifying genuine studies to illustrate their use of this approach. Instead, they offer four brief hypothetical examples. Their general intention is sound, however.

It is important that as part of the reader's and especially the advanced student's evaluation of any research report, they give thought to its ethical conduct. Achieving this may sometimes require the reader to dig a little deeper than the published article, since not all authors are equally robust in reporting the mistakes made and problems encountered while undertaking research. In Box 3.1, we offer a list of questions that might be asked about studies being reviewed or developed. It would be useful if more attention was given to these issues in the review of literature than has been customary in the past. It is possible to bring moral theory such as consequentialism, duty and 'ethics of care' to bear on these discussions (Long & Johnson 2007), but much can be achieved generally by critical debate of the issues raised by these questions.

CONCLUSION

Despite the developing bureaucracy that is meant, at least in part, to assure ethical conduct of research, much will continue to rely on the integrity and training of the researchers themselves and their supervisors. They should try not to be intimidated from undertaking an important study by myths that the proposed study may be unethical. Such myths include the involvement of children or the very ill as participants and the use of technology to record data. The ethics approval mechanisms should really review what, if any, real harm might result and, in balance with this, what benefits might accrue. Provided that these are addressed clearly in the proposal and the approach defended with rigour and obvious integrity, it should be possible to negotiate the bureaucracy.

Of course, for those who are less experienced, it is wise to work with a supervisor to design a study that is realistic and avoids putting the approval mechanisms, and the researcher, under too much strain. Reading widely and considering some of the more difficult issues that we can refer to only briefly here can also help. Certainly, novice researchers should try to develop the skill of identifying the ethical issues in every study they read or hear about, but they should also maintain a realistic sense of proportion.

References

Ben-Zeev D, Young M, Corrigan P (2010) DSM-V and the stigma of mental illness. *Journal of Mental Health* **19**(4): 318–327.

Brady M, Frederick A, Williams B (2012) People with aphasia: capacity to consent, research participation and intervention inequalities. *International Journal of Stroke* **8**(3): 193–196.

Breivik JK (2005) Vulnerable but strong: deaf people challenge established understandings of deafness. *Scandinavian Journal of Public Health* **33**(Suppl 66): 18–23.

de Raeve L (ed) (1996) *Nursing Research: an ethical and legal appraisal*. London, Baillière Tindall.

Doyal L (2004) *The Ethical Governance and Regulation of Student Projects: a draft proposal*. Working group on ethical review of student research in the NHS, Chair: Professor Len Doyal. London, Central Office for Research Ethics Committees.

Finigan V, Long T (2012) The experiences of women from three diverse population groups of immediate skin-to-skin contact with their newborn baby: selected outcomes relating to establishing breastfeeding. *Evidence Based Midwifery* **10**(4): 125–130.

Gelling L (2004) Researching patients in the vegetative state: difficulties of studying this patient group. *NT Research* **9**(1): 7–17.

Glaser BG, Strauss AL (1965) *Awareness of Dying*. Chicago, Aldine.

Haigh C, Jones N (2005) An overview of the ethics of cyber-space research and the implications for nurse educators. *Nurse Education Today* **25**: 3–8.

Health Protection Agency (2013) *The Unlinked Anonymous Prevalence Monitoring Programme*. London, Health Protection Agency.

HM Government (2005) *The Mental Capacity Act*. London, The Stationery Office.

Howarth ML, Kneafsey R (2003) Research governance: what future for nursing research? *Nurse Education Today* **23**: 81–82.

Howarth ML, Kneafsey R (2005) The impact of research governance in healthcare and higher education organisations. *Journal of Advanced Nursing* **49**: 1–9.

Johnson M (1997) *Nursing Power and Social Judgement*. Aldershot, Ashgate.

Johnson M (2004) Real world ethics and nursing research. *NT Research* **9**: 251–261.

Lawton J (2000) *The Dying Process: patients' experiences of palliative care*. London, Routledge.

Livesley J, Long T (2013) Children's experiences as hospital in-patients: voice, competence and work. Messages for nursing from a critical ethnographic study. *International Journal of Nursing Studies* **50**(10): 1242–1303.

Long T (2004) *Excessive Crying in Infancy*. London, Whurr.

Long T, Fallon D (2007) Ethics approval, guarantees of quality, and the meddlesome editor. *Journal of Clinical Nursing* **16**(8): 1398–1404.

Long T, Johnson M (2002) Research in Nurse Education Today: do we meet our aims and scope? *Nurse Education Today* **22**(1): 85–93.

Long T, Johnson M (2007) *Research Ethics in the Real World: issues and solutions for health and social care*. Edinburgh, Churchill Livingstone-Elsevier.

Matthews L, Venables A (2004) Critiquing ethical issues in published research. In: Crookes P, Davies S (eds) *Research into Practice*, 2nd edition. Edinburgh, Baillière Tindall, pp 129–142.

Ofsted (2008) *The Annual Report of Her Majesty's Chief Inspector of Education, Children's Services and Skills* 2007/08. London, Ofsted.

Pollock K (2012) Procedure versus process: ethical paradigms and the conduct of qualitative research. *BMC Medical Ethics* **13**: 25.

Royal College of Nursing (2007) *Research Ethics: RCN guidance for nurses*. London, RCN. Available at http://www.rcn.org.uk/__data/assets/pdf_file/0007/388591/003138.pdf (accessed 1 September 2014).

Stockwell F (1972, 1984) *The Unpopular Patient*. London, Croom Helm.

Watson R (1996) Product testing on trial. In: de Raeve L (ed) *Nursing Research: an ethical and legal appraisal*. London, Baillière Tindall, pp 3–17.

Watts G (2012) Why the exclusion of older people from clinical research must stop. *British Medical Journal* **344**: e3445.

Websites

www.hra.nhs.uk – The Health Research Authority has a role to protect and promote the interests of patients and the public in health research and to streamline ethical review and approval of health research.

www.nres.nhs.uk – The UK National Research Ethics Service offers comprehensive guidance to researchers.

www.gov.uk/government/publications/health-research-ethics-committees-governance-arrangements – This document outlines the policy of the UK health departments, describing the role of research ethics committees that review research proposals that relate to areas of the departments' responsibility. The policy covers the principles, requirements and standards for research ethics committees, including their remit, composition, functions, management and accountability. It also describes the Research Ethics Service in which the research ethics committees operate the review function they provide.

www.invo.org.uk – INVOLVE is a national advisory group that supports greater public involvement in NHS, public health and social care research. INVOLVE is funded by and part of the National Institute of Health Research (NIHR). It shares knowledge and learning on public involvement in research.

Sources of standard tests for readability: *www.literacytrust.org.uk/campaign/SMOG.html* and *www.usingenglish.com/glossary/readability-test.html.*

CHAPTER 4

User Involvement in Research

Janey Speers and Judith Lathlean

Key points

- User involvement in research is more than a political and policy imperative; there are clear reasons why it genuinely adds value.
- Knowledge derived from users forms an essential part of the knowledge needed by contemporary researchers and practitioners. Without it, practice is not properly evidence based.
- A continuum exists in research between consultations with users through partnerships in a collaborative model through to complete user control. This results in different models of user involvement in research.
- There are an increasing number of examples to illustrate the different ways in which users can take part in and have a major impact upon research.

INTRODUCTION

There is general agreement that the engagement of people referred to as service users, patients and the public is an important facet of research. Indeed, in the United Kingdom, the Department of Health (DH) and the funding body, the National Institute for Health Research (NIHR), require information from researchers submitting bids for funding regarding 'how patients and the public have been involved in the development of the application as well as the plans for involvement in the proposed research' (see http://www.crncc.nihr.ac.uk). Other nations too require similar commitment to patient and public engagement, for example, the Australian Research Council (www.arc.gov.au). For the purposes of this chapter, the term 'user' will be mainly employed and will include those who have been or are currently in receipt of health/social services, as well as potential users, normally referred to as the public or 'consumers of services'. Nevertheless, several authors that are cited emphasise the *service* user aspect, and so this will be the term of choice in places.

The value of user involvement in research will be considered and the relevance to practice of user involvement, alongside examples from the literature.

The Research Process in Nursing, Seventh Edition. Edited by Kate Gerrish and Judith Lathlean.

Companion Website: www.wiley.com/go/gerrish/research

Reflection activity

Whilst there is a political, social and policy imperative to involve users in all aspects of research, why might this genuinely add value to the research? In terms of the impact they may have and the knowledge they bring, you may find it helpful to look at Chapter 37.

It will provide practical guidance on different approaches that can be adopted and advice on the challenges of engaging users in a meaningful way.

WHY SHOULD USERS BE INVOLVED IN RESEARCH?

The nature of knowledge for research

Most researchers would agree that there are different sorts of legitimate knowledge. For example, Bradbury and Reason (2003) suggested four interdependent ways of knowing:

- **Experiential** knowledge: gained from life experience
- **Presentational** knowledge: concerned with narrative – how our story is told
- **Propositional** knowledge: informed by concepts and theories
- **Practical** knowledge: draws on all of the above to inform what action to take

None of the above is the preserve of the professional. This is one example of many typologies available that illustrate the important point that the definition of knowledge has widened over the last decades (see also Chapter 37). Nevertheless, in terms of what knowledge counts, 'patient knowledge' has often been relegated to that of least value in the evidence-based hierarchy (Simons *et al.* 2007).

Knowledge and power are linked concepts. Two seminal theorists have strongly influenced thinking about the connections. As Foucault (2001) suggested, once a powerful position has been achieved, this dominant position can be exploited through the repetition of certain language and actions. This often results in embedded change and a broad acceptance of the supremacy of the 'knowledge' subscribed to by this dominant group. Freire (1972) also led the way by showing that it is possible to gain knowledge from the oppressed, as well as the powerful. What is clear is that the powerful can privilege and propagate their own version of the truth (Hui & Stickley 2007).

More recently, Beresford (2010) made a case for recognising diversity within the umbrella term of 'service user'. For example, particularly unequal and disempowered users (such as mental health service users) seldom have their direct voice heard. Rather, their views are reported on by others, and Beresford suggested that 'significant fault lines can be expected between these views and those of professionals' (p. 496).

User knowledge versus professional knowledge

It can be argued that one culturally constructed truth (the positivist evidence base) has achieved a dominance that has been perpetuated through the system. This dominant discourse has added to the power of those who create this knowledge whilst diminishing the influence and status of other legitimate truths (such as the voice of relatively powerless service users). This matters for the reasons shown in Box 4.1.

Henderson and Henderson (2010) argued effectively that the consideration of everyday knowledge from the patients' perspective provides added value, complementing the propositional knowledge afforded by dispassionate, objective (and arguably reductionist) research methods and outcome measures traditionally used in health care. The fact that inferior status is still given to non-propositional, experiential subjective information ensures that the balance of power remains seriously skewed. Warne and McAndrew (2007) suggested taking steps to ensure that the patient experience is recognised as a primary source of knowledge.

Box 4.1 Why overlooking the value of service user knowledge matters

Service user expertise – its added value	The impact of overemphasis on professional expertise
• The knowledge held by service users is often complementary to that held by professionals. Jordan and Court (2010) suggest that consultation with service users is crucial as they have knowledge, understanding and experience of the diagnosis and management of the illness process, which is different to that of professionals. • There are often 'significant fault lines' between the views of professionals and those of service users (Beresford 2010). • Failure to actively seek out this knowledge would be 'missing a trick'. • In setting up the first service user and carer-led research group in Wales, Wilson and Fothergill (2010) described a therapeutic shift in self-perception for service users towards that of useful, 'expert citizen'.	• Evidence suggests that this has been harmful. For example, Happell *et al.* (2003) identified that service users often found the attitudes of mental health professionals to be even more debilitating than their mental illness. • A culture of superiority acts as an obstacle to partnership. McAllister *et al.* (2004) provide a compelling link between the dominance of a culture that places emphasis on problem-identifying, solution-prescribing professional experts and its corollary – powerless, depersonalised, passive or therapy-resistant patients.

Sociopolitical drivers for user involvement in research

There is a convincing argument for seeking out the expertise of users. Indeed, this principle has achieved mainstream acceptance, with a plethora of policies and reports stressing an expectation of user/carer involvement in all types of research (e.g. INVOLVE 2012). Consumerism, and its underlying doctrine that recipients of services have a better grasp of their needs than professionals, has been around for a long time. For example, it was mentioned in the Citizen's Charter (Cabinet Office 1991). This has resulted in political and professional imperatives requiring that service users are involved (e.g. National Institute for Health Research 2013; Social Care Institute for Excellence 2007). The drive for this change is supported by two of the main political positions in the United Kingdom, the Left and the Right, for different reasons. The Right favours consumerism, self-reliance and individual choice, whereas the Left emphasises voice, democracy, equity and advocacy (Ward *et al.* 2010). Beresford and Branfield (2006) added that a contemporary emphasis on human rights, outcome measurement and choice have reinforced this thrust. The recommendations of the Francis Report (2013), which looked into serious failures in services provided in Mid Staffordshire (United Kingdom),

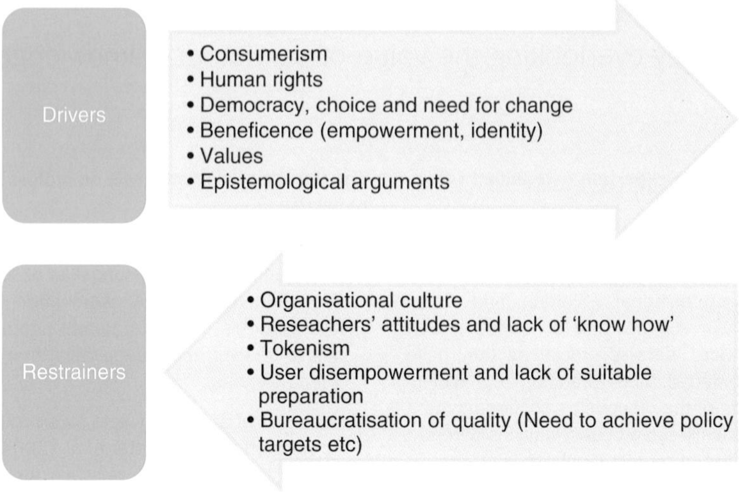

Figure 4.1 Key drivers and restrainers of user involvement in research

highlighted the need for an improved patient focus and better harnessing of stakeholder opinions and feedback.

However, although user involvement is now part of the mainstream rhetoric, there is evidence that the views of users are given unequal credence (Beresford 2007) and that they can be involved in research in a merely tokenistic manner (Simons *et al.* 2007; Elstad & Eide 2009). There are a number of reasons why this may be so. Figure 4.1 illustrates some of the drivers and restrainers to involvement.

Reflection activity

Who do you consider to be the users of services with connections to your workplace or research area? Would they bring perspectives of having engaged in services or from a forum that encourages users (and carers) to come together? What might be the benefits of involving these different types of people?

WHO SHOULD BE INVOLVED?

'Involvement' entails the active engagement of users in the design, delivery, dissemination and evaluation of research (Staley & TwoCan Associates 2012). Depending on the research field, specific users will have a particular experiential knowledge. This specificity may be linked to life stage, life events or perhaps to a health or social care need with which they were or are living. Returning to the earlier argument for positive discrimination in terms of what knowledge counts, some researchers make a particular effort to engage with users whose voices are seldom heard. Such people may be part of marginalised, stigmatised or especially powerless groups. Beresford and Carr (2012) and Nolan *et al.* (2007) provide some useful examples.

Another consideration is whether these are people who have experience of being patients or consumers or whether they have decided to join a group or forum to give 'voice' to consumers.

Representativeness

Davies (2005) cited the common perception that the views of user 'activists' are often unrepresentative, arguing that experienced representatives become socialised into the structures and processes of involvement, thereby becoming less 'ordinary'. Beresford and Carr (2012) put forwards the pejorative term of 'the usual suspects'. There is a lack of consensus about the accuracy of this perception. For example, Ward *et al.*'s (2010) qualitative study analysed this and other issues in the context of participation in research. They question whether consumers who opt to be involved in research are really representative or objective, given their 'lifeworlds' ('bigger things to worry about'). They also explore the term 'professional layperson' as the notion that people with economic, cultural and social capital are more likely to get involved with research. In contrast, Rose *et al.* (2010) conducted a user-led study in which semi-structured interviews were conducted with both activists and non-activists in two London boroughs. They found little difference between the views articulated by activist and non-activist groups, thus offering reassurance about the representativeness of those putting themselves forwards for involvement.

HOW ARE USERS INVOLVED?

It has already been established that there is an expectation that all research, regardless of methodology, will have service user involvement. Staley and TwoCan Associates (2012) selected 45 studies at random from England's NIHR's mental health research portfolio. Lead researchers were interviewed, and the findings are outlined in Research Example 4.1.

Service users have also been involved in exercises to identify priorities for research in cancer. For example, Corner *et al.* (2007) undertook a study, using a nominal group technique, to identify priorities for research for those attending UK cancer treatment centres. Additionally, an Ipsos MORI

RESEARCH EXAMPLE

4.1 Service User Involvement in Mental Health Research

Staley K, TwoCan Associates (2012) *An evaluation of service user involvement in studies adopted by the Mental Health Research Network*. London, The Mental Health Research Network.

This evaluative study of completed projects found the following engagement of users:

Planning, design and delivery

- 40% of projects involved service users in a steering committee deciding on design and recruitment, for example. There was considerable variation in how well this worked. Although some users had a major impact, others found it difficult to contribute in committee meetings.
- About 20% of projects consulted service users at the design stage, perhaps shaping the research question and/or design. More commonly noted was their useful practical contribution, for example, setting limits of questionnaire length.
- 20% of projects had users as co-researchers or members of advisory panels, contributing to all decisions. Advantages included keeping the research grounded and focused on issues important to users, boosting recruitment and retention rates and the quality of interview data.

Dissemination

- Lead researchers were considering how best to achieve this, for example, through communication of findings to a lay audience.

Reflection activity

The research journey usually involves planning, data collection, data analysis, writing up and dissemination of findings. When undertaking research, when would it be appropriate to involve users? What does this depend upon?

survey of 1295 adults, published by the NHS Health Research Authority (HRA) (www.hra.nhs.uk) in November 2013, showed that public confidence in health research studies can be increased by knowing that patients have been consulted in the design of the study.

Approaches to involvement

It is important to acknowledge the diversity of options for user engagement in research. This is best expressed in terms of a continuum, and there are variations. Guidance from INVOLVE, a DH-funded national advisory group that promotes active public involvement in NHS, public health and social care research, suggests that 'approaches' to involvement is the preferred term to 'levels'. Different types of research design support the opportunity for varying kinds of user involvement. Box 4.2 illustrates this by suggesting that, in this respect, research operates within three paradigms: traditional, participatory and emancipatory. The traditional paradigm encompasses both quantitative and many qualitative designs where the research is not considered to involve participation. However, there is a fine dividing line, or overlap, between traditional approaches and research that has some element of participation and is characteristically described as 'action research' (see Chapter 23). Similarly, emancipatory research, which seeks to empower participants including service users, patients and carers, also comes under the umbrella of forms of action-orientated research, commonly referred to as participatory action research (PAR) or co-operative inquiry (see Research Examples 4.2, 4.3 and 4.4).

CONSIDERATIONS OF USER INVOLVEMENT

Challenges

Key challenges identified by Staley and TwoCan Associates (2012) included a lack of resources, 'know-how' and skills (such as how to recruit the right service users, chair meetings involving researchers and service users, managing dissent, etc.). As service user involvement in research has become more mainstream, so a growing bank of concrete, practical, accessible and encouraging advice has become available in the literature (such as that provided by Nolan *et al.* 2007; Beresford & Carr 2012; Morrow *et al.* 2012). When undertaking their preparatory reading, researchers are urged to pay as much attention to this issue as to other methodological considerations.

Also highlighted by Staley and TwoCan Associates (2012) was the challenge presented by avoiding tokenism, maintenance of involvement through periods of ill health and the antagonistic attitudes of some colleagues. On this latter note, Ward *et al.* (2010) described a 'do-know gap' when examining the reasons for the discrepancy between researchers' perceptions and their actual practice in terms of involving service users and carers. They found that the underlying issues revealed by those interviewed were complex. Nevertheless, there was a sense that there remained a lack of recognition that service users' knowledge (emanating from experience) was as valid as researchers' knowledge (emanating from expertise).

Finding the 'right' degree of participation is challenging. Throughout the research process, judgements need to be made relating to how many issues can or should be dealt with in an executive fashion (e.g. by the lead researcher) and how many in a democratic fashion (using the combined expertise of the group). For example, Cotterell (2008) undertook a participatory research project that involved working together with service users, conducting 32 group meetings over 3 years. On the other hand, Speers (2012) negotiated eight meetings over 2 years. The degree of involvement in both studies differed in part because it was negotiated in the light of personal

Box 4.2 Parameters of traditional, participatory and emancipatory research

Parameter	Traditional	Participatory	Emancipatory
Ownership of research	Held by academic researchers	Joint/shared	Held by service users
Values	Value neutral	Shared/negotiated	Political, partisan, reflecting user interests
Accountability	To academic peers, host organisation, funding agency	To research group, host organisation, funding agency	To co-researchers (service users), host organisation, funding agency
Focus of enterprise	Science and accumulation of generalisable knowledge; an emphasis on limited forms of research dissemination	Articulation of user voice; an emphasis on research dissemination and utilisation	Orientation towards changing or improving people's lives and opportunities; an emphasis on research utilisation to bring about change in people's everyday lives
Locus of control for change	External	Internal and external	Internal, generated by service user research group
Concepts, methodology	Imposed	Product of process, evolutionary	Product of process, evolutionary
Research dissemination	Written for academic audiences, therefore likely to be published in academic journals	Could be written for a multiplicity of audiences, therefore found in academic and popular outlets and grey literature	Likely to be written mostly for user audiences, often located in grey literature and on user organisation websites
Costliness	Can be costly	Can be costly	Expensive
Sources of funding	Widespread	Growing	Very limited; still constrained by lack of official backing for putting evidence into practice

RESEARCH EXAMPLE

4.2 Involving Mental Health Service Users in Co-operative Inquiry Research

Tee S, Lathlean J, Herbert L, Coldham T, East B, Johnston T (2007) User participation in mental health nurse decision-making: a co-operative enquiry. *Journal of Advanced Nursing* **16**(2): 135–145.

This study attempted to encourage participants to work together to identify strategies for increasing user participation in clinical decisions and to evaluate the value of co-operative inquiry as a vehicle for supporting learning in practice. It was based on the premise that user involvement is essential for good practice. The research design – a co-operative inquiry – engaged all participants ($n = 17$), who were mental health nursing students and service users, as co-researchers, with repeated cycles of action and reflection, over a 2-year period. It used multiple data collection methods (e.g. observation, interviews and reflective discussions). Factors inhibiting participation included stigmatising and paternalistic approaches, where clinical judgements were made solely on the basis of diagnosis. Enhancing factors were a respectful culture that recognised users' 'expertise' and communicated belief in individual potential. Inquiry benefits included insight into service users' perspectives, enhanced confidence in decision-making, appreciation of power issues in helping relationships and deconstruction of decision-making within a safe learning environment.

RESEARCH EXAMPLE

4.3 Participatory Action Research with Mental Health Service Users and Nursing Students

Speers J (2012) Student nurses' feedback from mental health service users: A participatory action research study. Unpublished EdD Thesis, Open University.

In this doctoral research, service users contributed in two ways:

- Firstly, they gave students feedback and then talked about their experience afterwards.
- Secondly, along with other stakeholders such as mentors and lecturers, they formed part of a group that met regularly to help the lead researcher to 'look, think and act' (see Koch and Kralik 2006).

Key aspects of the research journey, from the user perspective, were:

- receipt of letter inviting involvement and explaining its gist and purpose. It made it clear that the letter could be ignored, without any repercussions.
- a preliminary 2 hour (or 2hr) meeting to:
  - give interested stakeholders the chance to find out whether they thought longer-term involvement was for them or not
  - negotiate ground rules and start 'talking about talking about' (i.e. how we were going to work together, the group's preferred degree of participation and how we were going to review our performance as a group).
- formation of a stakeholder participation group – two meetings to collaboratively plan a draft mechanism for students to ask service users in practice for feedback.
- thereafter, and over 2 years, the group met every 3 months or so to:
  - collectively make sense of data (reduced in amount by the lead researcher). The data emanated from interview transcripts and related to students', service users' and mentors' experience of the feedback system.
  - collectively decide, in the light of the data, what changes to make to the feedback system in order to improve it.
  - discuss everyone's perceptions of the quality of involvement and working relationships, using a modified version of Morrow *et al.*'s (2010) tool.

RESEARCH EXAMPLE

4.4 Reflections on Experiences in a Participatory Action Research Project

Reproduced from Speers J (2012) *Student nurses' feedback from mental health service users: A participatory action research study*. EdD Thesis, Open University, with permission from Janey Speers.

Our experience of user involvement in research

Participatory action research has been experienced as complex and messy, but ultimately the input of service users added immensely to the quality of the research. This 'added value' related to both practical and philosophical aspects of the project. For example, service users and mentors gave useful advice about the use of plain English, catering for people when unwell and on the content of feedback tools devised. Our combined expertise enabled us to make sound decisions about the next cycle of research. All participants enjoyed this transforming, constructive and collaborative partnership approach, concluding that both the journey and the destination were worthwhile.

As lead researcher, working in this new way meant the conscious eschewing of typical nursing roles. This demanded advanced reflexivity, assisted by the likes of a reflective diary and supervision. For example, a deliberate emphasis was placed on facilitation rather than prescription, on the avoidance of 'rescuing' behaviour and on humility – the open exposure of dilemmas, uncertainties and mistakes. I learned that owning my own expertise was not the same as privileging it, and I found that being transparent about the sources of my knowledge was helpful in engendering more equal relationships.

Achieving representation of all stakeholders became less important to us. In contrast, discovering whether it was possible to move beyond custom and practice to find new ways of working became more important. When service users and nurses engage in participatory action research, we found it was possible to develop new, more reciprocal ways of working together. The conventional relationship dynamics were slowly reinvented and developed into new ways of interacting. There were occasional times when more stereotypical roles were transiently returned to. This was usually during a period of personal or collective emotional difficulty, rather than when there was a research-related challenge facing the group as a whole. However, for the most part, members of the group acknowledged feeling 'freed up to be themselves'.

A strength of participatory action research lies with the opportunity it provides to develop safe, effective working relationships between participants over time. In turn, this enables deeper exploration and for complex issues to be gradually and thoroughly uncovered and explored. Equally, it allows the researcher(s) to refine their approach over time, learning from mistakes as few initial plans are perfect.

Service user participants noticed that their confidence, sense of influence and credibility grew over time. Whether lecturer, mentor or service user, we all gained a sense of well-being from working in this new way. For the most part, the atmosphere was one of good-natured collaboration and purposeful enjoyment. This was particularly evident when, as frequently occurred, there was evidence of change.

As a group, our knowledge of participatory action research grew as a result of our experience. In conclusion, we learned that as the size of the group is likely to diminish, particularly initially, it is wise to recruit a bigger than desirable group. We concluded that the research becomes more ethical when the balance between the executive function of the lead researcher and the democratic input of the group is negotiated rather than prescribed. This situation-specific approach enables contributions that target meaningful involvement and provide a good match with their individual resources. The collaborative analysis of data that had already been reduced by the lead researcher can work well if this is the group's preference. Finally, because of the relationships that develop over time, it is important to pay attention in the group to ending and 'saying goodbye'.

preferences and individual circumstances. In the same way, another part of the research journey, data analysis, lends itself to a flexible approach. Some researchers (Cashman *et al.* 2008; Cotterell 2008) support the value of wholly collaborative data analysis. However, Cashman *et al.* also concede that, given the magnitude and complexity of most qualitative data, a compromise option could involve the lead/academic researcher(s) in 'reducing' the data to a more manageable form. Thereafter, they would engage with the user participants, working together to arrive at insights and discoveries from the reduced data. This conclusion is appropriately nonprescriptive, recognising the importance of negotiating where best research participants' input should be directed. The key point here is that the whole research team will need to collectively reflect on the research *process*, as well as the research *product*, ideally on a regular basis as, in real life, circumstances change.

Ethics

Research involving users will need to be authorised by the relevant ethics committee(s) (see Chapter 3 for a discussion of ethics). Consent, and its attendant ethical principle (respect for autonomy), is complicated in this context, particularly when considering exclusion criteria. There is a risk that the values underpinning user involvement in research could be compromised through a return to a more expert professional – vulnerable patient-type dynamic in making judgements about exclusion. This may be experienced as patronising and disempowering. A common expectation is that service users will opt in to a project, having been furnished with balanced, accessible information through an 'easy-to-reject' invitation. Such information will include a sense of the necessary time commitment and duration of the project. Potential challenges as well as possible benefits will be included, along with the assurance that, whatever their decision, their services will not be affected.

If service user organisations are approached, then they can organise their own system for identifying potential participants and/or co-researchers. Whilst there is a duty to protect vulnerable adults and ethics committees will expect professional researchers to demonstrate a responsible approach to this, invoking the concept of 'service user-hood' is insufficient to justify paternalistic measures, which could lead to exclusion and undermine service user autonomy unnecessarily (Roberts 2004). For example, although mental illness can affect capacity, there is also evidence to support a poor link between psychopathology and the ability to engage in the consent process (Tee & Lathlean 2004). As user participants are usually involved over time, even if they were assessed as having the capacity to consent at the outset, it is possible that their capacity would fluctuate thereafter. A formal ad hoc reassessment of capacity mid-project could lead to a sense of rejection and a loss of trust (Tee & Lathlean 2004). If an individual service user lacks the cognitive ability to give valid consent or had been coerced in any way, then the research objectives would have to be suspended in a gentle and non-abrupt manner. In reality, it is often the case that service user participants regulate their own involvement, temporarily suspending engagement in research if they do not feel up to it (Speers 2012).

In terms of protection against inadvertent maleficence in the form of distress caused by disclosure or trauma, for example, the opportunity for 'behind the scenes' support is important. This follows for all researchers, professional or lay. Thus, an ongoing awareness of vulnerability and sensitivity to people's levels of distress (on the part of the whole research team) may be adopted as a more measured protective approach to this potential problem.

Payment and training

There is broad agreement that the adequate remuneration of service users volunteering to contribute to research is essential (Lammers & Happell 2004). The UK DH document 'Reward and Recognition' (Department of Health 2006) provides guidance on the reimbursement of expenses and payment for service user/carer involvement in research. Although, for participants, the value of involvement cannot be reflected entirely through monetary reward (McKeown *et al.* 2012), contingency in the research budget will usually need to be made.

Training to prepare and support users to engage in research is recommended, both for the users themselves and for researchers. Briefing notes, compiled by a combined team of service users and researchers and issued by INVOLVE (2012), are an invaluable source of practical information that will be of interest to more experienced researchers as well as to novices.

Reflection activity

Whilst not all research will utilise an action research approach, whereby users and other stakeholders are an integral part of the research design, all studies require users to engage in meaningful ways. What ways might be appropriate when planning and undertaking other types of research such as experimentation, surveys, mixed methods and other qualitative designs?

EXAMPLES OF RESEARCH INVOLVING USERS

There are now many examples of research to be found that actively involve users. Morrow *et al.* (2012) provide a useful chapter on international perspectives including Europe, the United States, Canada, Australia, New Zealand and developing countries. In these countries and in the United Kingdom, health and social care research involving users is conducted in a range of different fields, such as learning disability, older adult care, survivors of childhood abuse, midwifery, health visiting, mental health, long-term conditions, primary care and children in need.

Case studies and research examples

Staley and TwoCan Associates (2013) provide seven user-friendly case studies illustrating ways in which users may be involved in an eclectic range of projects (including a randomised control trial and a systematic review). You might find reference to these helpful.

For many busy health and social care professionals, conducting research might seem like an unachievable luxury, or something best left to professional researchers. However, certain approaches lend themselves to research in the workplace and are highly accessible to hard-pressed practitioners. One such approach is action research, with its emphasis on service improvement and change. One form of action research is referred to as 'co-operative' enquiry, a label that emphasises the co-operation and collaboration between participants in the research, some of whom are service users. Tee *et al.* (2007) provide an example of this approach, whereby mental health students and service users came together in research designed both to enable students to learn more about users' views and for service users to appreciate the challenges of being a student (see Research Example 4.2).

Research Example 4.5 is an example of a PAR study – a variant on co-operative inquiry (Speers 2012). It was conducted in an educational and a mental health practice setting and sought to explore the experiences of those involved when student nurses asked mental health service users for feedback. The feedback was about the service users' perception of the students' interpersonal skills, and it was sought in a practice setting whilst students were on placement.

It is unusual to read reflective accounts of research engagement, but Research Example 4.4 details the experience of the group in Speers' (2012) study, from the perspective of the lead researcher.

CONCLUSION

There is an expectation, identified by policy requirements and good research practice, that service users, patients and members of the public will be engaged in a range of different aspects of health-care research. There is evidence that this is not only beneficial to the outcomes of the research but that users can bring vital perspectives to the commissioning, design, running and evaluation of research. User and public involvement can be achieved in a variety of ways, and there is now considerable guidance on how this can be done effectively and what needs to be taken into account.

References

Beresford P (2007) User involvement, research and health inequalities: Developing new directions. *Health and Social Care in the Community* **15**(4): 306–312.

Beresford P (2010) Public partnerships, governance and user involvement: A service user perspective. *International Journal of Consumer Studies* **34**: 495–502.

Beresford P, Branfield F (2006) Developing inclusive partnerships: User-defined outcomes, networking and knowledge – A case study. *Health & Social Care in the Community* **14**(5): 436–444.

Beresford P, Carr S (2012) *Social Care, Service Users and User Involvement.* London, Jessica Kingsley Publishers.

Bradbury H, Reason P (2003) Action research: An opportunity for revitalizing research purpose and practices. *Qualitative Social Work* **2**(2): 155–175.

Cashman S, Adeky S, Allen A, Corburn J, Israel B, Montano J, Rafelito A, Rhodes S, Swanston S, Wallerstein N, Eng E (2008) The power and the promise: Working with communities to analyse data, interpret findings and get to outcomes. *American Journal of Public Health* **98**(8): 1407–1415.

Cabinet Office (1991) *The Citizen's Charter: raising the standard (Cm.1599).* London, HMSO.

Corner J, Wright D, Hopkinson J, Gunaratnam Y, McDonald JW, Foster C (2007) The research priorities of patients attending UK cancer treatment centres: Findings from a modified nominal group study. *British Journal of Cancer* **96**(6): 875–881.

Cotterell P (2008) Exploring the value of service user involvement in data analysis: Our interpretation is about what lies below the surface. *Educational Action Research* **16**(1): 5–17.

Davies BR (2005) Coercion or collaboration? Nurses doing research with people who have severe mental health problems. *Journal of Psychiatric and Mental Health Nursing* **12**(1): 106–111.

Department of Health (2006) *Reward and Recognition.* London, Department of Health, Her Majesty's Stationery Office.

Elstad T, Eide A (2009) User perspectives in community mental health services: Exploring the experiences of users and professionals. *Scandinavian Journal of Caring Sciences* **23**: 674–681.

Foucault M (2001) *Madness and Civilisation.* London, Routledge.

Freire P (1972) *Pedagogy of the Oppressed.* Harmondsworth, Penguin Education.

Francis R (2013) *Report of the Mid Staffordshire NHS Foundation Trust Public Inquiry*, London, The Stationery Office.

Happell B, Pinikahana J, Roper C (2003) Changing attitudes: The role of a consumer academic in the education of postgraduate psychiatric nursing students. *Archives of Psychiatric Nursing* **17**(2): 67–76.

Henderson A, Henderson P (2010) The recognition and valuing of patient knowledge: A way forward. *International Journal of Consumer Studies* **34**: 613–616.

Hui A, Stickley T (2007) Mental health policy and mental health service user perspectives on involvement: A discourse analysis. *Journal of Advanced Nursing* **59**(4): 416–426.

INVOLVE (2012) *Briefing Notes for Researchers: public involvement in NHS, public health and social care research.* Eastleigh, INVOLVE.

Jordan Z, Court A (2010) Reconstructing consumer participation in evidence-based health care: A polemic. *International Journal of Consumer Studies* **34**: 558–561.

Koch T, Kralik D (2006) *Participatory Action Research in Health Care.* Oxford, Blackwell.

Lammers J, Happell B (2004) Research involving mental health consumers and carers: A reference group approach. *International Journal of Mental Health Nursing* **13**(4): 262–266.

McAllister M, Matarasso B, Dixon B, Shepperd C (2004) Conversation starters: Re-examining and reconstructing first encounters within the therapeutic relationship. *Journal of Psychiatric and Mental Health Nursing* **11**(5): 575–582.

McKeown M, Malihi-shoja L, Hogarth R, Jones F, Holt K, Sullivan P, Lunt J, Vella J, Hough G, Rawcliffe L, Mather M, CIT (2012) The value of involvement from the perspective of service users and carers engaged in practitioner education: Not just a cash nexus. *Nurse Education Today* **23**: 178–174.

Morrow E, Ross F, Grocott P, Bennet J (2010) A model and measure for quality service user involvement in health research. *International Journal of Consumer Studies* **34**: 532–539.

Morrow E, Boaz A, Bearley S, Ross F (2012) *Handbook of Service User Involvement in Nursing and Healthcare Research.* Oxford, Wiley-Blackwell.

National Institute for Health Research (2013) *Central Commissioning Facility National Institute for Health*

Research and Policy Research Programme Patient and Public Involvement Plan (April 2013 to March 2015). London, NIHR. Available from: http://www.nihr.ac.uk/CCF/PPI/CCF_PPI_Plan_2013-15.pdf (accessed 26 March 2014).

Nolan M, Hanson E, Grant G, Keady J (2007) *User Participation in Health and Social Care Research. Voices, Values and Evaluation.* Maidenhead, Open University Press.

Roberts M (2004) Psychiatric ethics: A critical introduction for mental health nurses. *Journal of Psychiatric and Mental Health Nursing* **11**(5): 583–588.

Rose D, Fleischmann P, Schofield P (2010) Perceptions of user involvement: A user-led study. *International Journal of Social Psychiatry* **56**(4): 389–401.

Simons L, Tee S, Lathlean J, Burgess A, Herbert l, Gibson C (2007) A socially inclusive approach to user participation in higher education. *Journal of Advanced Nursing* **58**(3): 246–255.

Social Care Institute for Excellence (2007) *SCIE Position Paper 9: Developing Measures for Effective Service User and Carer Participation.* London, SCIE.

Speers J (2012) Student nurses' feedback from mental health service users: A participatory action research study. EdD Thesis, Open University.

Staley K, TwoCan Associates (2012) *An Evaluation of Service User Involvement in Studies Adopted by the Mental Health Research Network.* London, The Mental Health Research Network.

Staley K, TwoCan Associates (2013) *A Series of Case Studies Illustrating the Impact of Service User and Carer Involvement on Research.* London, The Mental Health Research Network.

Tee SR, Lathlean J (2004) The ethics of conducting a co-operative inquiry with vulnerable people. *Journal of Advanced Nursing* **47**(5): 536–543.

Tee S, Lathlean J, Herbert L, Coldham T, East B, Johnston T (2007) User participation in mental health nurse decision-making: A co-operative enquiry. *Journal of Advanced Nursing*, **16**(2): 135–145.

Ward P, Thompson J, Barber R, Armitage C, Boote J, Cooper C, Jones G (2010) Critical perspectives on 'consumer involvemen't' in health research: Epistemological dissonance and the know-do gap. *Journal of Sociology* **46**(1): 63–82.

Warne T, McAndrew S (2007) Passive patient or engaged expert? Using a Ptolemaic approach to enhance mental health nurse education and practice. *International Journal of Mental Health Nursing* **16**(4): 224–229.

Wilson C, Fothergill A (2010) A potential model for the first all Wales mental health service user and carer-led research group. *Journal of Psychiatric and Mental Health Nursing* **17**: 31–38.

Further reading

Barber R, Boote J, Cooper C (2007) Involving consumers successfully in NHS research: A national study. *Health Expectations* **10**: 380–391.

Caldon L, Marshall-Cork H, Speed G, Reed M, Collins K (2010) Consumers as researchers – innovative experiences in UK National Health Service Research. *International Journal of Consumer Studies* **34**: 547–550.

Carr S (2004) *Has Service User Participation Made a Difference to Social Care Services?* Position paper 3, London, Social Care Institute for Excellence.

Morrow E, Boaz A, Bearley S, Ross F (2012) *Handbook of Service User Involvement in Nursing and Healthcare Research.* Oxford, Wiley-Blackwell.

Smith E, Manthorpe J, Brearley S, Ross F, Donovan S, Sitzia J, Beresford P (2006) *User Involvement in the Design and Undertaking of Nursing, Midwifery and Health Visiting Research*, London, Report to the National Co-ordinating Centre for NHS Service Delivery and Organisation R&D. Available from http://www.nets.nihr.ac.uk/__data/assets/pdf_file/0004/64471/FR-08-1305-069.pdf (accessed on 21 March 2014).

Wright D, Foster C, Amir Z, Elliott J, Wilson R (2010) Critical appraisal guidelines for assessing quality and user impact in research. *Health Expectations* **13**(4): 359–368.

Websites

http://www.invo.org.uk/ – INVOLVE is a national advisory group, funded by the Department of Health, which aims to promote and support active public involvement in NHS, public health and social care research.

http://www.peopleinresearch.org/ – People in Research provides information to members of the public who want to find out more about public involvement in research and has a database of opportunities for the public to get involved in the research in the United Kingdom.

http://www.invo.org.uk/invonet/ – invoNET is a network of people working to build evidence, knowledge and learning about public involvement in NHS public health and social care research.

http://www.mhrn.info/ – The Mental Health Research Network is an organisation that supports research studies carried out in England with the help of people who used NHS services and people who work in them.

https://www.evidence.nhs.uk/search?q=Patient+and+Public+Engagement+in+research – Links to a broad range of publications of relevance to patient and public involvement in research.

http://healthtalkonline.org/peoples-experiences/medical-research/clinical-trials/topics – Healthtalkonline provides information designed for the public on involvement in clinical trials, including accounts of people's experiences of participating in research.

CHAPTER 5

Research for a Multiethnic Society

Sarah Salway and George T.H. Ellison

Key points

- Conducting ethnicity and health research presents important challenges and demands particular competencies.
- Researchers must recognise the multifaceted nature of ethnicity and the varied ways in which health-related experiences and outcomes may be associated with ethnicity.
- Ethnic identities are complex, fluid and increasingly 'mixed' so that using fixed ethnic categories in research requires careful consideration.
- Describing and explaining differences between ethnic 'groups' demand careful attention to sampling, data generation and analysis so that misleading interpretations are avoided.
- Research needs to move beyond simply describing ethnic inequalities to understanding their underlying causes and evaluating interventions aimed at redressing such disparities.
- Researchers should be alert to the potential for research to do more harm than good and should ensure that their research focus and approach is informed by the experiences and priorities of minority groups.

INTRODUCTION

Ethnic diversity, linked to both historical and more recent patterns of migration, is a common feature of most high-income countries. This presents both opportunities and challenges for health policy and health-care practice. For instance, the United Kingdom is now widely regarded as a multiethnic society, with the 2011 Census of England and Wales reporting a rise in ethnic diversity over the previous 10 years: 19.5% of the population now self-identify as belonging to an 'ethnic group' other than White British and 14% as belonging to a non-White ethnic group. Similarly, in 2006, Statistics Canada reported the 'visible minority' population as comprising 16.3% of the total Canadian population and expected this to rise to 30.6% by 2031 (Statistics Canada 2010).

The Research Process in Nursing, Seventh Edition. Edited by Kate Gerrish and Judith Lathlean.

Companion Website: www.wiley.com/go/gerrish/research

Box 5.1 Cultural competence in research

Papadopoulos and Lees (2002) suggest the following model of cultural competence in research.

Cultural awareness: examining and challenging your own personal value base and behaviours and reflecting on how these may affect the research process.

Cultural knowledge: understanding the similarities, differences and inequalities between and across ethnic 'groups' and the multiplicity of factors that might account for these patterns. Such knowledge should help to avoid stereotyping, prejudice and discrimination in research.

Cultural sensitivity: challenging power relationships and oppressive practices to offer true partnership to the participants of research studies founded upon trust, respect and empathy.

Cultural competence: synthesis and application of awareness, knowledge and sensitivity, enabling racism, discrimination and ethnocentricity to be recognized and challenged.

Both culture-generic and culture-specific competences are considered necessary, the former being the acquisition of knowledge and skills that are applicable across ethnic groups and the latter being the knowledge and skills that relate to a particular ethnic 'group' and enable an understanding of particular values and behaviours.

Words such as 'ethnic group', 'visible minority' and 'ethnicity' are commonly heard in public policy, the media and even everyday conversation. Likewise, health and social research pays increasing attention to ethnic inequalities in both experiences and outcomes. However, the meaning of such terms remains ambiguous and research that engages with these issues is inherently politicised and often controversial in nature. Conducting research that appropriately and sensitively pays attention to ethnicity presents an important challenge to researchers and demands particular competencies (see Box 5.1).

Notwithstanding the underlying complexity, there is substantial evidence that minority ethnic groups are often disadvantaged on a range of health indicators in many different geographical contexts, including the United Kingdom (Gill *et al.* 2007), Germany (Zeeb & Razum 2006), Canada (Wu *et al.* 2005) and the United States (Williams 2001). Despite variation in the extent to which health policy and practice has responded to these patterns of disadvantage, the importance of understanding and tackling ethnic health inequalities is increasingly recognised across Europe, North America (Salway *et al.* 2011) and further afield, for example, Australia (Davis *et al.* 2012) and South Africa (Kon & Lackan 2008). Furthermore, nursing has been identified as a key profession to contribute to this endeavour (Drevdahl 2013).

Clearly, there is a need for researchers to generate an evidence base that reflects the needs of increasingly ethnically diverse populations. This requirement is federally mandated in the United States (Iqbal *et al.* 2013) and has been formally acknowledged by the United Kingdom's Department of Health in its Research Governance Framework for Health and Social Care (Department of Health 2005: para 2.2.7).

However, much health research does not include participants from minority ethnic groups and/or fails to give considered attention to ethnicity as a factor in any analyses (Hussain-Gambles 2003). Furthermore, despite recent improvements in some areas, routine data collection systems – such as the Hospital Episodes Statistics in the United Kingdom – still often fail to collect any information on ethnicity or achieve low coverage and poor quality information, thereby limiting the potential for analysis (Salway *et al.* 2011).

A number of factors appear to contribute to the inadequate attention to ethnicity in health and nursing research including:

- a lack of awareness of the potential significance of ethnicity
- a tendency to consider ethnicity as a specialist area of investigation
- conscious exclusion of minority ethnic individuals on the grounds of added cost and complexity (particularly a reluctance to include participants who do not speak the majority language)
- a lack of researcher confidence and skills to engage with individuals from ethnic groups that are perceived to be 'hard to reach'

At the same time, growing awareness of past abuses and negative experiences of research may also make some individuals from minority ethnic groups fearful of participating in health research, though the picture is complex (Fischer & Kalbaugh 2011).

Research interest in ethnicity and health is, however, growing in many countries (Drevdahl *et al.* 2006). Yet, as the volume of research addressing ethnicity and health expands, so too do concerns regarding the *quality* of this research, its potential to inform changes in policy and practice that benefit minority ethnic populations and its potential role in stereotyping and stigmatising ethnic minority populations. Indeed, a number of persistent pitfalls have been identified including the use of outdated, inappropriate models of ethnicity that present ethnic 'groups' as stable, discrete entities; a failure to research issues that are of concern to minority ethnic people; a lack of cultural competence in research practice; and a failure to incorporate a broader social, historical and political analysis of ethnicity (Mir *et al.* 2013).

Against this rather unpromising background, it is important to stress that poorly designed and poorly conducted research will, at best, fail to contribute to a better understanding of the links between ethnicity and health and how ethnic inequalities in health might be addressed. At worst, such research may perpetuate the stereotyping and disadvantage experienced by minority ethnic groups. Indeed, conducting research into ethnicity and health appropriately and sensitively raises a range of theoretical, methodological and practical issues. Researchers therefore require support and guidance if their work is to make a positive contribution.

This chapter introduces the reader to some of the most important issues for consideration. We encourage researchers to recognise that there are often no simple, 'cook book' solutions to the complex issues that arise in researching ethnicity and health and to aim instead for heightened critical reflexivity in their work.

THE CONCEPT OF ETHNICITY

So far, our discussion has employed the term 'ethnicity' without further elaboration. However, frequent, everyday reference to 'ethnicity' and 'ethnic groups' belies the complex and contentious nature of these terms.

In health research (as well as wider societal and policy discourse), the term 'ethnicity' is employed in diverse and contradictory ways. This is particularly the case when looking across countries and over time, since understandings relating to ethnicity and the language employed to describe ethnic identities are socially and historically situated (Salway *et al.* 2011). At its most generic, 'ethnicity' represents a form of social or group identity, which draws on notions of shared origins or ancestry. However, different conceptualisations of 'ethnicity' tend to emphasise different aspects of such group identity and to view processes of identification very differently. Some conceptualisations emphasise the cultural commonality within ethnic groups, identifying shared beliefs and behaviours, sameness and belonging – essentially an *internal* identification. In contrast, other ideas about ethnicity place emphasis on geographical origins and shared biological features among the members of ethnic groups. Still, others focus on sociopolitical dimensions, viewing ethnicity as the *process* through which boundaries between hierarchically organised 'groups' are constructed and symbolised – the emphasis here being on the imposition of categories and labels by external forces. Indeed, some conceptualisations appear to invoke a combination of all three of these dimensions. This is

Box 5.2 Ethnicity or race?

The terms 'ethnicity' and 'race' are used variably across different international contexts. For instance, while 'ethnicity' is currently more often employed in UK health research than the term 'race', both terms are in common usage in the United States. Despite these variations, it is useful to recognise that the two concepts are closely related. It is commonly suggested that while 'race' refers to biological features (such as skin colour) to distinguish different groups of people, 'ethnicity' focuses primarily on differences in cultural practices and beliefs. In practice, however, this neat distinction is not consistently applied in either research practice or social discourse. As Gunaratnam (2003) and others have noted, 'race' may often emphasise differences in physical characteristics (such as skin colour), but 'race' has always been a far broader concept that *also* sought to reflect differences in a range of social and cultural characteristics. Likewise, though ethnicity tends to emphasise cultural and religious attributes, these characteristics are frequently represented as relatively fixed and inherent, being passed down from one generation to the next through endogamous marriage as well as processes of socialisation. Given the complex interrelationships between the two terms, it is not surprising that there is little standardisation of research practice, and there are disparate opinions as to which of these two terms should be employed by health researchers. While some advocate avoiding the use of the term race because of its association with discredited 19th century work labelled 'scientific racism', other researchers retain its use as a biological, social and/or biosocial construct. Some researchers go one step further and place the term race in scare quotes – 'race' – both to signal its contested meaning and to acknowledge that as long as racism exists within society, then 'race' (however problematic) will be needed in research. Few comparable concerns have been raised over the use of the term 'ethnicity' in health research. However, some researchers have argued that 'race' is preferable to 'ethnicity' since the latter tends to obscure the importance of external forces, power and exploitation in the lives of people from minority ethnic groups and instead (mis)leads researchers to ascribe disadvantage to the internal attributes of the groups themselves. Other researchers have suggested a compromise of sorts, in which the two terms are conflated in a joint formulation – 'race/ethnicity' – to encapsulate and signal the diverse biosocial character of both terms while retaining a focus on the role each have played in stereotyping, discrimination and disadvantage.

why some have called ethnicity a 'biosocial' or 'biocultural' concept. Similar variability exists in the ways in which the term 'race' is employed (see Box 5.2).

There is also variation across research contexts in the extent to which the boundaries and characteristics of ethnic 'groups' are seen as fixed. Recent years have witnessed increasing criticism of health-focused research that portrays ethnic identities as immutable and ethnic groups as distinct, homogenous and unchanging. On the one hand, researchers who have taken the discredited view that ethnic groups display wholesale genetic differences (attributed to their different geographical and sociocultural ancestries) have tended to interpret ethnic disparities in health as resulting primarily from biological differences. This approach thereby ignores or downplays the importance of culture, socioeconomic status and discrimination. On the other hand, there are researchers who portray the culture of ethnic groups (together with related beliefs and behaviours) as homogeneous, distinct, immutable and, in some respects, 'innate'. Such 'cultural determinism' ignores the diverse, fluid and context-dependent nature of cultural characteristics, overlooks the potential role of socioeconomic status and discrimination and thereby contributes to the stereotyping and stigmatisation of minority ethnic populations as culturally deviant or inferior (Gerrish 2000).

Researchers must therefore recognise the multi-faceted, dynamic and context-dependent nature of ethnicity and the varied ways in which health-related experiences and outcomes may be associated with ethnicity. It is useful to think of two broad modes of impact: first, the ways in which an individual's experience of their own ethnic identity informs their health-related attitudes, beliefs and behaviours (and thus their risks and responses to ill health) and, second, the role of ethnic identification in processes of inclusion and exclusion that can importantly determine exposure and access to a wide range of risks and resources relevant to health (including appropriate health services). Researchers must take care to 'unpack' the concept of ethnicity so that it is clear which of its various biosocial dimensions are being explored in their work.

Adopting this inherently reflexive approach will frequently require researchers to explore not only the implications of ethnic identities for health experiences and outcomes but also the mechanisms through which ethnic identification occurs (at both the interpersonal level and between groups within society at large) (Gunaratnam 2003).

IDENTIFYING A RESEARCH FOCUS

Before embarking on the details of study design, researchers should give careful consideration as to whether or not attention to ethnicity is warranted within a particular study. Clearly, there are some research issues in which ethnic identity is unlikely to play a role, such as studies exploring the functioning of a new medical device or the effects of new technologies on health-care policies. There may also be reasons for excluding attention to ethnicity in some studies on the grounds of cost and/or complexity. Nonetheless, since ethnicity is such an important axis of identity and inequality in contemporary societies, there are unlikely to be convincing arguments for overlooking ethnicity in most areas of nursing research.

Where the topic of inquiry makes a case for paying attention to ethnicity, the researcher then needs to carefully consider how to focus the research. As Johnson notes:

> from the perspective of minority populations there may be both 'too much' research – insofar as their particular ('peculiar') specific characteristics may attract research attention that is unwelcome or serves to stigmatise their community – or 'too little', insofar as they may be excluded from research that has measureable benefits or informs policy and practice shaping the provision of services they want or need. Johnson (2006: 49)

Framing research questions in such a way that the knowledge generated contributes positively to understanding and tackling ethnic inequalities in health requires careful thought.

Engagement with people from minority ethnic backgrounds can help ensure that research is adequately informed by the experiences and perspectives of these groups. However, this requires careful planning to achieve adequate representation of diverse views and experiences, as well as cultural sensitivity and meaningful involvement (Johnson 2006).

Reflection activity

Identify a potential research topic from your own area of practice that relates to an aspect of ethnic inequality. Write down two research questions that could address this topic. Now, reflect on the following questions in relation to these potential research questions:

- Does the framing of the research avoid presenting ethnic 'groups' as static or homogenous?
- Does the study go beyond description to explore the causes of inequalities?
- Does the research focus too narrowly on any particular dimension(s) of ethnicity and/or overlook other aspects of difference and disadvantage?
- Is the focus important and meaningful to those who are the subject of the research? How could you ensure this?

Recent reviews have highlighted the low volume and narrow focus of interventional research that considers ethnicity. Liu *et al.* (2012) reviewed UK guidelines and international evidence relating to health promotion and found little specific guidance on which health promotion interventions are effective for minority ethnic populations. Meanwhile, Clarke *et al.*'s (2013) review of 30 years of interventional research in the United States concluded that researchers have predominantly focused on the patient as the target for change rather than investigating how to improve the health system serving minority ethnic people. These findings indicate the need for a clearer focus on developing and evaluating interventions that can address persistent inequalities.

ETHNIC CATEGORIES AND LABELS

In studies that gather new data, the researcher must decide how to operationalise, or measure, ethnicity within their research. Studies that explore ethnic identification as a process will need to examine the multiple and diverse constructions of ethnicity and will most often employ qualitative, inductive approaches (though some quantitative studies provide important insights, e.g. Nandi & Platt 2012). Here, the researcher will generally avoid the use of predetermined, fixed ethnic categories and will instead operationalise ethnicity as a fluid property of individuals and groups. Nevertheless, there is clearly a need to start somewhere and, in most studies, to identify potential respondents. Researchers will therefore often be guided by 'real-life' categories (Mason 2002), using, for instance, self-reported ethnicity, physical appearance or perhaps membership of an ethnically affiliated organisation to identify respondents who seem likely to have a range of relevant social positions and experiences.

Studies that seek to understand ethnicity as a potentially important determinant of health experiences and outcomes tend to be framed differently. Here, the focus is usually on the characteristics, outcomes or experiences of a set of individuals categorised as belonging to an ethnic 'group'. Frequently, comparisons are made between two or more such 'groups', and these can be useful in identifying areas of inequality or minority ethnic disadvantage. These studies usually need to operationalise ethnicity as a discrete categorical variable, and this can be challenging for those researchers who regard ethnicity as a fluid and context-specific concept. Furthermore, attempts at categorisation, and the labels employed for specific categories, vary over time and place. This variation calls into question the meaningfulness of such categories and makes the comparison and synthesis of findings from different studies difficult (Morning 2008; Salway *et al.* 2011). However, while accepting that ethnic classifications will *always* be crude, researchers can nonetheless seek to identify the best available categorisation for the study in hand (Ellison 2005).

It is important to consider the extent to which the categories chosen can serve as adequate proxies for the components of interest in the research at hand (whether cultural, sociopolitical and/or genealogical factors). As such, it should be recognised that particular categorisations will have utility in some research studies but will be less helpful in others. For instance, Bhopal *et al.* (1991) argue that the collective ethnic category 'Asian' or 'South Asian' is inappropriate for understanding coronary heart disease risk and treatment in the United Kingdom, advocating instead the use of more refined categories: Indian, Pakistani and Bangladeshi. In contrast, Ali *et al.* (2006) employed the grouping 'South Asian' and found that these finer distinctions were not relevant within their study of patient–general practitioner interactions.

Notwithstanding the observation that some categorisations will be more or less useful depending on the research topic, any attempt at categorising ethnicity will not get over the fundamental tension that exists in 'fixing' socially mediated categories that are inherently complex and variable.

In many instances, researchers interested in exploring ethnic variation in health and health care will be forced to rely on secondary data collected using standardised and statutory classifications, categories and labels (such as those developed for use in the 2011 UK Census, see Box 5.3). When undertaking new data collection, other options are often available, but there will be pros and cons associated with adopting bespoke, as opposed to standard, classifications.

Box 5.3 Measurement of ethnic group in the UK census

The most recent census in England, carried out in 2011, asked people:

What is your ethnic group?

Choose **one** section from A to E, and then tick **one** box to best describe your ethnic group or background.

A White

☐ English/Welsh/Scottish/Northern Irish/British
☐ Irish
☐ Gypsy or Irish Traveller
☐ Any other White background (please write in)

B Mixed/multiple ethnic groups

☐ White and Black Caribbean
☐ White and Black African
☐ White and Asian
☐ Any other mixed/multiple ethnic background (please write in)

C Asian or Asian British

☐ Indian
☐ Pakistani
☐ Bangladeshi
☐ Chinese
☐ Any other Asian background (please write in)

D Black or Black British

☐ Caribbean
☐ African
☐ Any other Black background (please write in)

E Other ethnic group

☐ Arab
☐ Any other ethnic group (please write in)

Questions were also asked on religion and country of birth.

Data source: Office for National Statistics (2012). http://www.ons.gov.uk/

The disadvantages of standardised schemes include the fact that they may not be precise measures of the key dimension(s) of ethnicity that the study aims to examine. They may also be insufficiently refined to differentiate between important ethnic subgroupings (such as those with different religious, socioeconomic or ancestral characteristics). For instance, the category 'Black African' that is frequently employed in UK national surveys has doubtful utility in many contexts because of the substantial heterogeneity with respect to national origins, religion and language concealed therein (Aspinall & Chinouya 2008). However, statutory categories have often gone through substantial testing and development to ensure that they are

Reflection activity

Revisit the research topic and questions you identified in the earlier reflection activity. Consider the following questions:

- What will be your source of data on ethnicity?
- What ethnic categories will you be working with? What are the pros and cons of this approach?

both acceptable and meaningful to respondents – something that may affect how research findings are received and acted upon. Moreover, statutory classifications and categories are often used by a large number of studies and agencies and therefore facilitate aggregation and comparison. Nonetheless, when studies (only) use these types of classifications, they are often constrained in the analyses and explanations they can offer.

A final issue for consideration is how ethnic categories should be assigned. An individual's self-reported ethnicity will best reflect their own perceptions of who they are, and some would argue that this is the only ethical way to measure ethnicity. Nonetheless, assignment of ethnicity by a third party may also be appropriate, particularly when the focus of a study is on how one person's view of other people's ethnicity (e.g. a health-care practitioner's view of a patient's ethnicity) affects the way they treat those people.

Regardless of the approach to categorisation and labelling adopted, it is important to be explicit about the methods employed, and the rationale behind these, so that any inherent problems and potential limitations are clearly articulated.

SAMPLING

Researchers interested in exploring the ways in which health experiences and outcomes are influenced by ethnicity will commonly engage with individual people, be they patients, providers or members of the public, to elicit data that are relevant to their focus of inquiry. Though the logic behind sampling in qualitative and quantitative research is very different, the approaches share important elements. First, the sample's purpose is to provide access to data that will allow answers to specific research questions. Second, a sample must have an explicit and meaningful link with a 'wider universe' – a larger population to whom the results of the research can then be applied. Third, the act of sampling indicates that selection is possible and therefore demands a clear rationale as to why that particular sample (and not another) was chosen. Sampling must therefore clearly link to both the study's research questions and any planned analyses.

As suggested earlier, studies that seek to understand *processes* of ethnic identification will usually adopt sampling strategies that access a diversity of individuals capable of capturing the full range of ethnic identity as understood and experienced by the populations of interest. Such sampling schemes tend not to be predetermined, but, rather, are flexible and involve the selection of participants in a purposive manner. In these studies, data analysis and theory building often take place alongside data collection, so that new participants are chosen intentionally to fill gaps in understanding or to test emerging hypotheses.

Studies that are framed more in terms of describing the experiences and circumstances of ethnic 'groups' and those that aim to explain any differences (or similarities) found can essentially adopt one of three different sampling strategies: exclusive, comparative and representative.

Exclusive sampling strategies aim to recruit participants from just one ethnic 'group' and can be justified on two grounds: first, for studies that aim to generate evidence on an issue that only, or disproportionately, affects the population concerned and, second, for studies that aim to generate evidence for an ethnic 'group' that has not previously been adequately studied with regard to the topic concerned. In quantitative work such exclusive samples should be representative of the wider population that could be categorised as belonging to the ethnic 'group' concerned. In qualitative work, the exclusive sample drawn will relate to the wider ethnic 'group' in a more theoretical or interpretive way. Such samples will often deliberately aim to capture a diverse set of respondents to explore the full diversity of experience.

Comparative sampling strategies aim to recruit participants from two or more ethnic 'groups' so that any similarities and/or differences in the outcome of interest (e.g. health or health care) can be identified among different ethnic groups. An important consideration in such quantitative designs is the need to ensure that the ethnic categories used are equally diverse and capture an equivalent focus on ethnic identity (and on the cultural, sociopolitical and/or genealogical dimensions of ethnicity) and that the samples of each ethnic group are of a comparable size. These are complicated technical issues that need not undermine simple *descriptive* comparisons, but are worthy of consideration when designing studies that aim to explore causal relations between health/health care and ethnicity (including those exploring differential effectiveness of interventions). Similar concerns arise in qualitative work when comparisons are drawn between predefined ethnic 'groups' that do not necessarily include individuals with uniform or meaningful experiences and thereby lead to misleading or partial interpretations. However, qualitative researchers have substantial flexibility to investigate ethnic group identification and, if appropriate, to modify the sampling strategy used as analysis proceeds. For instance, a study initially designed as a comparison between two ethnic 'groups' might, as analyses proceed, be reconfigured as a three-way comparison if the findings reveal important unforeseen diversity within one of the 'groups' as originally delineated.

Comparative sampling strategies, whether qualitative or quantitative in nature, also need to generate an equivalent volume of data relating to each of the ethnic 'groups' of interest. This is necessary to ensure that any comparisons are not compromised by spurious or inaccurate data that are more likely to arise from smaller samples. To this end, quantitative surveys often include the so-called 'boosted' samples to generate adequate data from minority ethnic 'groups'.

Researchers using comparative sampling also need to consider how many different ethnic 'groups' to include. Qualitative studies should generally avoid trying to include too wide a range of ethnic 'groups' because they are likely to provide greater clarity and depth of understanding when fewer categories are considered (Atkin & Chattoo 2006). Practical considerations may also limit the number of 'groups' that a quantitative study can sample, particularly since costs can be considerable when seeking to access 'boosted' samples from small and geographically dispersed populations. Nonetheless, the choice of groups included, and the analytical consequences of excluding the groups that are not, should be carefully considered and justified in terms of what the study aims to achieve.

Finally, representative sampling strategies aim to ensure that the ethnic diversity found within the study's sample is the same as that found in the wider 'target' population (to which the study's results are intended to apply). This notion is fundamental to quantitative research and researchers should strive to ensure that their samples are representative of their target populations, even when the decision has been made to use exclusive or comparative samples of just one or two ethnic groups (as described earlier). However, the fluid and context-specific nature of ethnicity means that careful consideration should always be given to specifying the target population to which findings can be most safely extrapolated, not least when applying the results of one study to an ostensibly similar population in a very different context (e.g. from UK-based 'Black African' samples to US-based 'African American' populations). Meanwhile, a final word of caution is warranted: representative samples from ethnically diverse populations will ordinarily include participants from a range of different ethnic groups, and it is important to recognise that samples of this sort are often inappropriate to use for comparative analyses. This is because, except in the case of extremely large study samples, representative sampling strategies inevitably generate samples of each of the different ethnic groups that are of very different size and therefore very different statistical power.

For qualitative research, the principle that a sample should be empirically representative of the wider (target) population is rarely adopted on both theoretical and practical grounds. Nevertheless, qualitative researchers should consider whether their samples adequately offer the potential to generate data that is generalisable. Indeed, even when there is no intention to perform systematic comparative analyses across ethnic 'groups', it will often be desirable for qualitative research to generate findings that have a wider resonance with the diverse experiences of multiethnic communities.

DATA COLLECTION

Researchers have a wide range of methods to choose from when deciding how to generate the data needed to address their research questions. Here, we highlight some general issues worth consideration when researching the field of ethnicity and health.

First, ethnicity is a multifaceted concept that can be a marker or proxy for a wide range of factors. Studies that seek to do more than simply describe differences between ethnic 'groups' will therefore need to adopt data generation methods that yield information on a variety of potentially important dimensions of ethnicity. In particular, there are concerns that health-related research has often failed to address the sociopolitical dimensions of ethnicity (including the effects of racism) and that innovative tools are needed to effectively capture these dimensions (Porter & Barbee 2004). Studies that exclude attention to one or more particular dimensions of ethnicity run the risk of producing partial and superficial findings.

Second, ethnicity research will frequently imply the need for researchers to work across languages and cultural contexts. In quantitative work, this means that careful attention is needed to ensure the equivalence of standardised measurement tools/questionnaires, and caution should be exercised when employing measures and tools for which cross-cultural/cross-language validity and reliability have not been established. Standard guidelines exist for translating between languages (Behling & Law 2000), but in general, the focus should be on ensuring conceptual equivalence (Atkin & Chattoo 2006). To this end, we recommend the inclusion of multilingual researchers within the research team rather than reliance upon interpreters who are unfamiliar with the context and purpose of the research.

More generally, researchers must be alert to the possibility that their data generation methods may operate differently among different sets of participants. For instance, methods that depend heavily on respondents' narratives may lead to erroneous interpretations if there is significant diversity in forms of expression among 'groups' of study participants. Further, the identity of the researcher/data gatherer and their interactions with research participants deserve attention. Notions of 'insider' and 'outsider' status are complex, and there are no simple rules regarding ethnic matching (Gunaratnam 2003). Indeed, the personal characteristics and skills of the data gatherer are likely to be just as important as any marker of social identity in gaining the trust of participants and generating credible findings.

DATA ANALYSIS AND INTERPRETATION

As we have seen, much health-related research that pays attention to ethnic diversity takes a comparative approach, often comparing outcomes and experiences of minority ethnic groups to the majority (such as the White British group in the United Kingdom or the White group in the United States). While this approach may be a useful way of flagging up inequalities, caution is needed in both the analytical procedures employed and the interpretations drawn.

First and foremost, researchers should recognise, and counter, any tendency for *associations* to be interpreted as *explanations.* It is important that analyses seek to identify underlying causal factors, rather than simply inferring their existence. Where data on potential causal attributes are not available, analysis and interpretation must be cautious and speculative. It is also important that researchers are aware of factors that may importantly shape minority or majority experiences but may be beyond the scope of their analysis (such as geographical concentration of particular ethnic groups, historical factors or wider social structures). As described earlier, researchers should also recognise that analyses taking an ethnicity-focused approach may fail to capture the diversity of experiences *within* groups. In both qualitative and quantitative research, it is useful to explore the ways in which other factors (such as age, gender, class/economic status and so on) interrelate with ethnicity to create divergent experiences and circumstances within delineated groups.

Finally, it is important that analyses explore absolute levels of particular outcomes and experiences, in addition to relative differences between 'groups', and that comparisons are drawn with a range of 'groups' rather than solely with the majority category alone. This approach helps to avoid the tendency to overlook important issues facing minority ethnic people just because they are similar to those experienced by the majority.

Reflection activity

Revisit the research topic and questions you identified earlier. Consider the following questions:

- In what ways might the findings of your research be sensitive or controversial? Could your work do more harm than good for the minority ethnic groups who are involved?
- What steps could you take to actively involve patients and/or members of the public from minority ethnic groups in the design, conduct and dissemination of your research project?

ETHICAL ISSUES

Many general issues of research ethics apply quite straightforwardly to research that gives attention to ethnicity. However, a further point worth emphasising is the potential for group harm that can ensue from research that includes minority ethnic individuals. Attention to this issue is warranted at all stages in the research process, but particular care is needed in the presentation and dissemination of findings. Researchers must be alert to, and should manage from the outset, the ways in which the findings of their work might be interpreted, distorted and (mis)used by the media and others, particularly in establishing or contributing to the stereotyping and stigmatisation of ethnic groups and the threat of breaching the confidentiality of data collected from very small ethnic groups.

In general, researchers should consider carefully the best way to represent and disseminate the findings of their research. As with all good research, it is important to ensure effective communication to all stakeholders, but particularly to ensure that the minority ethnic individuals and communities who are the subject of the research have ready access to the findings in a format that is appropriate and relevant. Standard reports and academic publications may usefully be supplemented with innovative dissemination media such as participatory workshops, radiobroadcasts and use of the arts.

CONCLUSION

Many of the issues raised earlier relate fundamentally to sound research practice. Clear conceptualisation, careful measurement, strategic sampling, rigorous analyses and accurate representation are all generic elements of good research. However, the dangers of poor research are much greater when the focus of the research is ethnicity. Indeed, there is substantial concern that such research, if poorly executed, may do more harm than good. While there are no simple answers to some of the issues raised in this chapter, critical reflexivity and a cautious approach to interpretation can go a long way to improving the quality of research and the usefulness of findings.

We urge nursing researchers not to shy away from these complex and contentious issues, but rather to accept their responsibility to generate an evidence base that informs positive change in nursing policy and practice for all members of contemporary multiethnic societies.

References

Ali N, Atkin K, Neal RD (2006) The role of culture in the general practice consultation process. *Ethnicity and Health* **11**(4): 389–408.

Aspinall P, Chinouya M (2008) Is the standardised term 'Black African' useful in demographic and health research in the United Kingdom? *Ethnicity & Health* **13**(3): 183–202.

Atkin K, Chattoo S (2006) Approaches to conducting qualitative research in ethnically diverse populations. In: Nazroo J (ed) *Health and Social Research in Multiethnic Populations*. London, Routledge, pp 95–115.

Behling O, Law KS (2000) *Translating Questionnaires and Other Research Instruments: problems and solutions*. (Quantitative Applications in the Social Sciences) London, Sage.

Bhopal RS, Unwin N, White M, Yallop J, Walker L, Alberti KG, Harland J, Patel S, Ahmad N, Turner C, Watson B, Kaur D, Kulkarni A, Laker M, Tavridou A (1991) Heterogeneity of coronary heart disease risk factors in Indian, Pakistani, Bangladeshi, and European origin populations: cross sectional study. *BMJ (Clinical research ed.)* **319**: 215–220.

Clarke AR, Goddu AP, Nocon RS, Stock NW, Chyr LC, Akuoko JA, Chin MH (2013) Thirty years of disparities intervention research: what are we doing to close racial and ethnic gaps in health care? *Medical Care* **51**(11): 1020–1026.

Davis TM, Hunt K, McAullay D, Chubb SA, Sillars BA, Bruce DG, Davis WA (2012) Continuing disparities in cardiovascular risk factors and complications between Aboriginal and Anglo-Celt Australians with type 2 diabetes: The Fremantle Diabetes Study. *Diabetes Care* **35**(10): 2005–2011.

Department of Health (2005) *Research Governance Framework for Health and Social Care*, 2nd edition. London, Department of Health.

Drevdahl DJ (2013) Injustice, suffering, differences: how can community health nursing address the suffering of others? *Journal of Community Health Nursing* **30**(1): 49–58.

Drevdahl DJ, Philips DA, Taylor JY (2006) Uncontested categories: the use of race and ethnicity variables in nursing research. *Nursing Inquiry* **13**(1): 52–63.

Ellison GTH (2005) 'Population profiling' and public health risk: when and how should we use race/ethnicity? *Critical Public Health* **15**: 65–74.

Fischer JA, Kalbaugh CA (2011) Challenging assumptions about minority participation in US clinical research. *American Journal of Public Health* **101**(12): 2217–2222.

Gerrish K (2000) Researching ethnic diversity in the British NHS: methodological and practical concerns. *Journal of Advanced Nursing* **31**(4): 918–925.

Gill PS, Kai J, Bhopal RS, Wild S (2007) Black and minority ethnic groups. In: Stevens A, Raftery J, Mant J, Simpson S (eds) *Health Care Needs Assessment: the epidemiologically based needs assessment reviews*. Abingdon, Radcliffe Medical Press, pp 227–239.

Gunaratnam Y (2003) *Researching Race and Ethnicity: methods, knowledge and power*. London, Sage.

Hussain-Gambles M (2003) Ethnic minority under-representation in clinical trials: whose responsibility is it any way? *Journal of Health Organisation and Management* **17**(2): 138–143.

Iqbal G, Dunn J, Thorogood M (2013) Systematic review of interventions to increase recruitment and retention of black, minority and ethnic patients into randomised controlled trials. *Trials* **14**(Suppl 1): P83.

Johnson M (2006) Engaging communities and users: health and social care research with ethnic minority communities. In: Nazroo J (ed) *Health and Social Research in Multiethnic Populations*. London, Routledge, pp 48–64.

Kon ZR, Lackan N (2008) Ethnic disparities in access to care in post-apartheid South Africa. *American Journal of Public Health* **98**(12): 2272–2277.

Liu J, Davidson E, Bhopal RS, White M, Johnson MRD, Netto G, Deverill M, Sheikh A (2012) *Adapting Health Promotion Interventions to Meet the Needs of Ethnic Minority Groups: mixed-methods evidence synthesis*. (Health Technology Assessment, No 16.44) Southampton, NIHR Evaluation, Trials and Studies Coordinating Centre.

Mason J (2002) *Qualitative Researching*. London, Sage.

Mir G, Salway S, Kai J, Karlsen S, Bhopal R, Ellison GTH, Sheikh A (2013) Principles for research on ethnicity and health: the Leeds Consensus Statement. *European Journal of Public Health* **23**(3): 504–510.

Morning A (2008) Ethnic classification in global perspective: a cross-national survey of the 2000 census round. *Population Research and Policy Review* **27**: 239–272.

Nandi A, Platt L (2012) Developing ethnic identity questions for understanding society. *Longitudinal and Life Course Studies: International Journal* **3**(1): 80–100.

Office for National Statistics (2012) *Ethnicity and National Identity in England and Wales 2011*. Office for National Statistics. http://www.ons.gov.uk/ons/dcp171776_290558.pdf (accessed 25 March 2014).

Papadopoulos I, Lees S (2002) Developing culturally competent researchers. *Journal of Advanced Nursing* **37**(3): 258–264.

Porter CP, Barbee E (2004) Race and racism in nursing research: past, present and future *Annual Review of Nursing Research* **22**: 9–37.

Salway S, Higginbottom G, Reime B, Bharj K, Chowbey P, Foster C, Friedrich J, Gerrish K, Mumtaz Z, O'Brien B (2011) Contributions and challenges of cross-national comparative research in migration, ethnicity and health: insights from a preliminary study of maternal health in Germany, Canada and the UK. *BMC Public Health* **11**:514. DOI: 10.1186/1471-2458-11-514.

Statistics Canada (2010) *Projections of the Diversity of the Canadian Population.* http://www5.statcan.gc.ca/bsolc/olc-cel/olc-cel?catno=91-551-X&lang=eng (accessed 25 March 2014).

Williams DR (2001) Racial variations in adult health status: patterns, paradoxes and prospects. In: Smelser NJ, Wilson WJ, Mitchell F (eds) *American Becoming: racial trends and their consequences.* Washington, DC, National Academy Press, pp 371–410.

Wu Z, Penning MJ, Schimmele CM (2005) Immigrant status and unmet health care needs. *Canadian Journal of Public Health* **96**: 369–373.

Zeeb H, Razum O (2006) Epidemiological research on migrant health in Germany. An overview. *Bundesgesundheitsblatt Gesundheitsforschung Gesundheitsschutz* **49**: 845–852.

Further reading

Bhopal RS (2014) *Migration, ethnicity, race, and health in multicultural societies.* Oxford, Oxford University Press.

Websites

https://www.jiscmail.ac.uk/cgi-bin/webadmin?A0=MINORITY-ETHNIC-HEALTH – International discussion list on minority ethnic health.

http://mighealth.net/index.php/Main_Page – Information network on good practice in minority and migrant health care.

CHAPTER 6

Digital Technologies in Research

Susie Macfarlane and Tracey Bucknall

Key points

- Digital literacy is a vital skill for 21st-century nurse researchers. Social media and Web 2.0 tools can assist researchers to identify, create, filter and disseminate knowledge more rapidly than traditional research tools.
- Social media and Web 2.0 tools foster engagement, communication and collaboration among researchers, patients, communities, funding bodies and policy-makers in the planning, implementation and dissemination phases of research.
- An integrated social media strategy not only facilitates networking and the transfer of knowledge between researchers but also the translation of research to health networks, organisations, practitioners, patients and the broader community.

INTRODUCTION

Digital technologies and the instant access to information, tools, people and resources provided by Web 2.0 platforms and social media have had a dramatic impact on the way we live, work and interact – and even on how we think. The speed, scale and complexity of this new and evolving means of communication, instant access to an enormous and growing volume of information and free access to publishing platforms have put powerful tools for learning and knowledge production into the hands of the majority of people. These tools have also significantly changed how health researchers access and share information, communicate and collaborate, recruit and engage participants, gather and analyse data and disseminate and translate research findings. As Fausto *et al.* (2012) point out:

> The emergence and expansion of information and communication technologies and internet-based tools is opening space for new possibilities to improve both scientific methodology and communication. Fausto *et al.* (2012: 1)

The Research Process in Nursing, Seventh Edition. Edited by Kate Gerrish and Judith Lathlean.

Companion Website: www.wiley.com/go/gerrish/research

Box 6.1 Glossary of common terms

Term	Definition
Altmetrics	Measures of impact that are an alternative to journal impact factor, such as article citations, views and downloads or mentions in social and traditional media.
App	A self-contained program that performs a specialized function that is downloaded by a user to a mobile phone or tablet.
Blog	A self-published online collection of short, regularly updated posts written by one or more authors that contain text, links, images and video.
Crowdfunding	'Funding a project, by raising many small amounts of money from a large number of people, usually via the internet' (Oxford Dictionary).
Curation	Collecting, filtering, organising and maintaining information. Additionally, using Web 2.0 and social media platforms to share the curated collection for the benefit of others.
Digital	Using computer technology to use or store data or information.
Digital literacy	The ability to use digital technologies and networks to navigate, evaluate, communicate and create information.
Microblog	A very short message that may contain text, images or video links. Microblogs are posted on platforms such as Twitter or Tumblr or as status updates on platforms such as Facebook or LinkedIn.
Social media	Websites and applications that enable users to create and share content or participate in social networking.
Social networking	The use of dedicated websites and applications to create a public profile and communicate with other users. Social networks may consist of existing friendship groups or communities who share similar interests or beliefs.
Twitter	A free online social networking microblogging service that allows users to publically broadcast messages up of to 140 characters called Tweets.
Web 2.0	The changing use of the Internet from static web pages to social media and user-generated content.

This chapter explores the key digital technologies that provide new ways to conduct and disseminate healthcare research and provides guidelines to select and use the most appropriate tools for each research activity. In order to assist the reader who may be unfamiliar with some of the new technologies, a glossary of the key terms is provided in Box 6.1.

DIGITAL TECHNOLOGIES: SOCIAL MEDIA AND WEB 2.0 PLATFORMS

Web 2.0 platforms

Over the last decade, there has been a significant change in the way we use and interact with websites and Web platforms, characterised as the shift from Web 1.0 to Web 2.0. Websites built on Web 1.0 technologies provide static content, with the flow of information in a one-way direction. Visitors to the site can therefore only *read* information – they are unable to communicate with others or create content. Web 2.0 technologies, however, allow users to contribute information and interact with other users. These Web 2.0 technologies form the basis of this chapter. Examples of popular Web 2.0 platforms include social networking sites such as Facebook and Twitter, video-sharing sites such as YouTube and Vimeo, wikis such as Wikipedia, blogs such as Blogger and Web-based services such as Google docs. Web 2.0 platforms harness high-speed Internet connectivity and interactive technologies to enable visitors to interact, participate, collaborate and produce and share user-generated content. The flow of information shifts from *one to many*, an expert disseminating knowledge (Web 1.0), to *many to many*, a community of peers who collaborate to share experiences, filter and evaluate information and construct new knowledge (Web 2.0).

Social media

Social media are methods of communication used by members of online networks and communities to create and share information. Communication in social media is not a one-way process of broadcasting or dissemination; communication occurs in the form of conversations – listening to, acknowledging and building on the contributions of others – with the aim of connecting, sharing, establishing relationships and trust and ultimately community building.

Social media place the power to communicate and publish in real time on a large scale in the hands of individuals, groups and communities. Social media such as blogging and Tweeting are now established ways for researchers to engage in conversations and share their research. The open access, scale and velocity of social media communication provides researchers with a potent medium for consulting, engaging and collaborating with patients, communities and other stakeholders in ways that differ fundamentally from traditional approaches to research.

As with any well-designed research project, the use of social media requires careful planning. It is important to:

- identify the project activities such as communication and engagement, participant recruitment, surveillance or other data collection methods, as well as dissemination of project outcomes
- identify the various stakeholder groups and how and where they communicate
- identify the appropriate traditional and social media channels and platforms to achieve these goals

There are significant advantages to using social media for research. Firstly, communication is significantly faster than traditional communication and engagement approaches. For example, using Twitter, hundreds of research participants can be recruited and have completed a survey within hours. Secondly, there is the opportunity to access people with an enormous diversity of experience, cultures and perspectives. Thirdly, research projects using social media can be informed by and are responsive to patients' and community needs and preferences. Fourthly, social media and Web 2.0 platforms allow research findings to be rapidly disseminated across a wide range of audiences. Finally, the power of social media analytics in measuring the reach, re-sharing and impact of social media activities means that the effectiveness of each communication approach can be evaluated and adapted in real time, enhancing project rigour and effectiveness.

Web 2.0 and social media tools

There is an enormous array of social media tools researchers can use to engage and consult stakeholders, secure funding, collect data and disseminate findings. Table 6.1 lists various social media tools and Web 2.0 platforms and identifies the research activity for which each tool is best suited.

Table 6.1 Web 2.0 and social media tools and their research functions

Web 2.0 and social media tools		**Professional profile and networking**	**Collaboration and project management**	**Information retrieval, filtering and management**	**Data collection and storage**	**Dissemination and translation**
Activity	**Example tools**					
Online presence and professional networking	LinkedIn, Academia.edu, ResearchGate	✓		✓		✓
Crowdfunding	Petridish.org, Pozible, Experiment.com	✓	✓			
Project and document management	Basecamp, Evernote, Good reader, Papers		✓	✓		
Cloud services (software)	Google docs	✓	✓		✓	
Cloud storage	Dropbox, Google Drive, MS Office 365		✓		✓	
Information retrieval	RSS feeds, Google alerts			✓		
Reference managers	Mendeley, Zotero, Endnote web, CiteULike		✓	✓	✓	
Video conferencing	Skype, Google hangouts, MS Lync	✓	✓			
Clinical databases and registries				✓	✓	
Survey tools	Surveymonkey, Qualtrics, Poll Daddy, Google forms		✓		✓	
Mobile devices	Text messaging, apps				✓	✓
Social networking	Facebook, Google circles, Yammer	✓	✓			✓
Blogging	Wordpress, Blogger	✓	✓			✓
Microblogging	Twitter, Hootsuite TweetDeck, Tumblr	✓	✓	✓		✓
Curation	Scoop.it, Pinterest			✓		✓
Video hosting	YouTube, Vimeo	✓			✓	✓
Altmetrics	Impactstory.org, altmetrics.com	✓				✓

Reflection activity

Consider the quality of your online presence. Could people with similar research interests to your own find useful information about your education, interests, experience and skills? What professional networking platform would best suit your current career stage and future goals? How much and what type of information is it appropriate to share?

DIGITAL TECHNOLOGIES ACROSS PHASES OF THE RESEARCH PROCESS

The following section outlines characteristics and examples of digital technologies that can enhance each phase of the research process:

- Locating and filtering information
- Securing funding
- Project planning and management
- Data collection
- Data storage
- Dissemination and impact

LOCATING AND FILTERING INFORMATION

Historically, medical and scientific information was found primarily in books and academic journals, with access limited to specialists and academics. The Internet has dramatically shifted this problem of information scarcity to one of overabundance. Web 2.0 technologies have empowered anyone with an Internet connection to publish anything at any time. Each day, there are 1 million hours of video uploaded to YouTube, 2 million blog posts written, 4 billion items shared on Facebook, and 2.5 billion gigabytes of data created – 90% of this between 2011 and 2013. As a result, relevant and high-quality information may be concealed by masses of irrelevant, superseded or invalid information; even powerful search engines may be unable to effectively locate and filter quality resources.

The challenge has shifted from one of finding sufficient information to that of filtering and curating high-quality information to produce meaningful insights. Scoop.it and Pinterest are two examples of widely used social curation platforms. These Web 2.0 technologies allow users to locate and upload resources on their areas of interest and share them publicly across social media and blogging platforms. Users can locate other users with expertise, follow their curated topics as they are updated and learn at the pace of the expert.

Social bookmarking, curation and filtering tools allow researchers to undertake the following:

- Store, organise, share and discover research papers and data using reference management tools such as Mendeley, Endnote Web, Zotero and CiteULike.
- Collect, curate, comment on and share collections of resources (articles, news items, blog posts, images and journal articles) on a particular topic of interest using Scoop.it or Pinterest.
- Access a stream of relevant and current information by following people or topics on Twitter.
- Engage with and learn from key leaders in their field by reading their blogs, subscribing to their YouTube channel or following them on Twitter.

These platforms provide the means to connect with experts in many fields. Rather than having to develop expertise across many areas, individuals can now draw on and benefit from others' expertise and curation.

Reflection activity

Reflect on how you store and manage the information you find and the resources you develop. Can others access and learn from your efforts? What are the benefits and challenges in providing to others access to your collections of information and resources? Which of the social curation platforms outlined in this chapter may allow this?

Box 6.2 Successful crowdfunding strategies

The Crowdfunding.org website offers a rich collection of crowdfunding resources and recommends the following strategies for successful crowdfunding:

- Select a topic that will interest the public or a particular community.
- Set an *achievable* target: 87% of projects that hit the goal exceed it.
- Match the research design to the attainable funding level.
- Establish the projects' credibility and that of the research team.
- Aim for 30% of the project target to be achieved before the campaign launch by the project team's friends and family circle, as visitors respond to the sense of progress and momentum.
- Create a meaningful story that communicates the significance of the project and invites public participation.
- Acknowledge and reward contributions.
- Communicate constantly: use an integrated social and traditional media communication strategy to communicate regularly on project progress and outcomes.

(Crowdfunding.org 2012)

SECURING FUNDING

Crowdfunding is an alternative source of funding appropriate when the topic under investigation is of interest to members of the public, and granting bodies and other traditional sources of research funding do not cover the project focus. Crowdfunding is the collective effort of individuals who network and pool financial resources to support others' projects (Parvanta *et al.* 2013). In 2012, over 1 million projects were funded for over $2.7 billion on over 500 crowdfunding platforms including Kickstarter and Indiegogo (Crowdfunding.org 2012). Crowdfunding uses social media and Web 2.0 tools to harness our desire for meaningful social experiences and to be actively involved in something larger than ourselves.

Crowdfunding enables researchers to invite members of the community impacted by or committed to the issue under investigation to fund their research. Science research-based crowdfunding sites include Petridish.org, Experiment.com and Pozible. Researchers pitch their project, often via video, set a fundraising target and timeline and then campaign to attract supporters who donate at a range of specified levels.

Successful crowdfunding requires careful planning, months of preparation and ongoing effort (Box 6.2); however, the benefit is that this longer-term engagement strategy can reap rewards that go beyond solely securing research funds. The engagement with a committed and informed group of supporters can help raise awareness; crowd source the research topic, methods and participants; gain public support; and promote, disseminate and implement the research outcomes.

PROJECT PLANNING AND MANAGEMENT

Planning and coordinating a research project require tools that support communication and collaboration, document sharing and project management. Traditional forms of communication including telephone and email remain effective for some project tasks, but collaborative online tools may be useful when synchronous communication between geographically dispersed team members or input from multiple parties on documents is required. In addition, many people now work on multiple devices in multiple locations, requiring access to communications and documents from a computer, smartphone and tablet.

Video conferencing

Researchers and research students can conduct meetings using video-conferencing tools including Skype and Google hangouts. Some universities and organisations may also provide enterprise tools such as Microsoft Lync that have advanced features including group calls, document sharing and meeting recording. These tools are easy to use and work across multiple operating systems and devices.

Collaboration

Social platforms such as Google circles for social networks and Yammer for organisations provide spaces for sharing and commenting on documents and ideas. Groups can be set up to be public or private – allowing more in-depth discussion. Researchers who are used to more traditional approaches to communication may initially find the social feel of collaboration platforms disconcerting. Thus, choosing the right tool and securing a commitment from team members to use it are important prerequisites for successful implementation.

Document management

Project teams can store, manage and share documents using free file storage sites including Dropbox and Google Drive. Google docs and Microsoft Office365 allow multiple parties to edit documents at the same time. These platforms store files online, so access is available on any computer or device with an Internet connection. It is important to consider the security features and conditions of use before choosing a tool for storage of sensitive data or material.

Task and information management

Task and information management tools vary from sophisticated tools with many functions to those that solely track tasks. For example, Evernote is a sophisticated app that allows storage and annotation of scientific papers, information, links, photos, audio clips and text notes in one place. Once stored, documents are searchable and accessible on multiple devices even in the absence of an Internet connection.

Digital document management

It is no longer necessary to copy or print documents on paper. The following apps allow researchers to scan, create, store and share documents using a smartphone or tablet:

- Scan journal articles with Scanner Pro.
- Take notes that sync with audio recordings using Notability.
- View, store and annotate pdf documents with GoodReader, PDF Expert or ezPDF Reader.
- Download, organise and tag scientific papers with Papers.
- Organise ideas into mind maps with MindNode.

DATA COLLECTION

Mobile devices, such as smartphones and tablets, can be harnessed to collect data using a range of methods that may be referred to as mobile data collection, mResearch or mobile research.

Survey research

Mobile survey research allows data to be collected from participants' own devices or by dedicated devices provided by the research team. One advantage of this approach is that it allows real-time sampling of the patient's experience in the situation under investigation rather than requiring recall via survey, questionnaire or focus group at a later time. For example, a link to a survey of the patient's experience may be sent during their stay in hospital rather than requiring patient recall after the event. Researchers may use free or low-cost Web-based platforms such as Surveymonkey or Qualtrics or develop or purchase customised apps that trigger data collection by location, time or situation.

Mobile-enabled ethnography

Patients can use the audio, text or video features of a mobile device to document their symptoms, treatment or side effects, as well as their mood, behaviour and well-being, by recording their activities or thoughts using speech, photos or video.

Passive data collection

Smartphones allow researchers to unobtrusively capture reliable behavioural data such as the patient's activity levels, location and movements. Passive data collection can be integrated with active data collection in which the user's location or the time of day can trigger responses such as surveys, alerts or location-specific questions that are sent directly to the individual via their own phone.

There are significant challenges in collecting reliable and complete mobile data, some of which include self-selecting participants resulting in biased samples, high costs of devices or app development and inconsistent Internet access. Unreliable devices, surveys longer than 3–7 min or confusing survey interfaces may reduce participation and completion rates. Communicating clearly to participants, the rationale for the project and how their data will be used can increase survey completion. Participants may also be concerned that adequate measures are being taken to ensure confidentiality and secure their data. Pilot testing the reliability of the hardware and the usability of the software with an equivalent cohort is vital. The pilot should also establish the survey frequency and timing that are most convenient for participants. For short surveys of two or three questions, text messaging is an effective method. Box 6.3 outlines some important considerations in mobile research.

In 2013, there were over 100,000 medical or healthcare apps in Apple's iOS and Google's Android platforms (Kamerow 2013). Use of healthcare apps is on the increase – over 25% of young people have downloaded an app of this type. Healthcare apps offer significant potential to translate research into practice in a cost-effective manner; however, there are concerns regarding the lack of evidence for some recommendations or activities and issues regarding potential privacy and security of personal information. Apple has recently instigated a policy requiring

Box 6.3 Considerations in mobile research

- Harness the features of mobile devices by asking participants to describe or visually capture their current thoughts, feelings, experiences and actions rather than rely on recall.
- Most people are unfamiliar with participating in research studies so it is important to anticipate the challenges and areas of confusion participants may encounter and provide detailed instructions and support to prevent this.
- Work within the limitations of the small screens of many mobile devices: be concise so the information is easy to read and understand.
- Reduce the inconvenience and time burden imposed on participants by asking closed-ended questions, allowing speech rather than typing and requesting short responses or videos.
- Thoroughly address any ethical considerations in your research design and recruitment process (ESOMAR World Research 2012). In addition to managing traditional research ethics issues, conducting mobile phone research requires consideration of additional issues including the intrusiveness of the contact or participant safety while engaged in driving and other activities.
- Maintain high reporting standards when publishing your findings (Eysenbach 2011b).

app developers to cite research validating the information the app provides to users and vouching for the effectiveness of any behaviours recommended.

Quick response codes

Mobile devices provide a bridge between the virtual and physical worlds, and technologies such as Quick Response (QR) codes exploit this capacity. A QR code is a two-dimensional matrix barcode that can be read by camera-equipped smartphones. The QR code contains a message that is scanned and read by the smartphone, requesting it to access a website, display information or make a phone call. Free code reader apps such as *QR reader* or *Optiscan* are used to read codes. QR codes of various sizes and complexity can be generated for free online at websites including *Kaywa* or *i-nigma*.

Potential applications of QR codes in health research include patient recruitment, anonymous patient access to research information and online surveys, patient education via text or video, dissemination of health information on posters in hospitals and clinics and engaging colleagues at conference presentations. There are, however, issues to consider in using QR codes in health research, including confidentiality and data security. The current lack of encryption suggests that QR codes should be precluded from aspects of the research process that include access to patients' health records (Bikshandi 2011).

Health informatics, databases and registries

The discipline of health informatics (also called health information systems or clinical informatics) is the application of big data resources, equipment and information management methodologies to health. Health informatics involves the analysis of data and rapid communication of the resulting information to healthcare professionals enabling them to deliver optimal care or to identify trends in disease and treatment. It is one of the fastest growing areas in healthcare. Clinicians collaborate with other healthcare professionals and IT specialists to develop health informatics tools that promote safe and efficient patient care. Competency in informatics is now required as healthcare environments evolve from being paper-based and discipline centred to computerised and patient centred (Goncalves *et al.* 2012).

Clinical databases and registries have become potent instruments for observing and understanding patterns of care received by patients, the effectiveness of care, patient responses to treatment and the monitoring of patient safety during treatment. In addition, information found within registries is used by government organisations such as the US Food and Drug Administration to monitor risks associated with treatments and by reimbursement bodies such as private health insurers to determine the effectiveness of treatments. Clinical informatics has resulted in large integrated datasets stored in clinical data warehouses. The integration of electronic health record data with other datasets provides researchers with significant opportunities for investigation. Largely the information is used to improve patient management by basing decisions on evidence.

DATA STORAGE

Storing digital data securely and safely is an important consideration in planning and conducting research. The data management plan should include an estimation of the volume of data the project will generate; the equipment and budget required; strategies to securely and confidentially store, back up and destroy data; and the personnel responsible.

Data that is subject to privacy or confidentiality laws should be encrypted or stored on a computer that is not connected to a network or to the Internet. TrueCrypt is a free tool that encrypts data in real time and is compatible with all operating systems. Physical security is also important. Store data on an external hard drive that is secured in a locked safe when not in use. Hard drives fail, memory sticks and laptops can be lost or stolen, disks may be damaged by heat and water, and data can be corrupted, so it is vital to back up and regularly refresh a second copy of project data. Create backup copies using high-quality DVDs, CDs or memory sticks stored securely in a different location to the primary copy. Remote

Reflection activity

Consider a research project you are undertaking or may undertake in the future. What role can social media play in each stage of the research project? What privacy, security and ethical considerations are therein using social media and how can these be addressed effectively?

backup services such as Dropbox and Google Drive allow files to be synchronised and stored online. Many online storage tools such as Dropbox now offer an additional layer of security via two-factor authentication (whereby a user, in addition to completing the usual sign on process, is required to authenticate using a second method such as via their mobile phone).

A further consideration is the geographical location of the server that stores the data and the associated legal implications. For example, files that a UK-based researcher stores in an online file storage service may actually be hosted on a server located in the United States. It is therefore important for researchers to check local requirements for data protection and storage and provide details on the research ethics application form of precisely how the data will be stored.

DISSEMINATION AND IMPACT

New models of publishing and dissemination

Research has traditionally been published in academic journals accessible only to individuals and institutions that have paid to access them and understood only by those with expertise in the field. Dr Ben Goldacre – doctor, academic and blogger at Badscience.net – has pointed out the communication gap that exists between researchers and the public, with neither academic journals nor the mainstream media meeting this need (Goldacre 2008). While the public are increasingly accessing medical information via the Internet, the quality of the information varies enormously. The challenge for health researchers is to extend the communication of scientific knowledge beyond academic journals and conferences into the public domain and ultimately to enhance the scientific and health literacy of the general public, for as Small (2011) points out:

> The days of scientists communicating only with each other, in the languages of our individual disciplines, and relying on science journalists to translate for the public, are rapidly coming to an end. Small (2011: 141)

Social media and Web 2.0, in conjunction with the open-access movement (the campaign to make research publications freely available via the Internet), have disrupted traditional dissemination practices. Researchers can harness a range of social media and Web 2.0 tools to disseminate and translate research findings into practice and enhance the health and science literacy of patients and communities by challenging incorrect information and providing high-quality health information.

Dissemination activities may include:

- publishing your profile and research publications on LinkedIn, ResearchGate, Academia.edu or Google scholar
- writing or co-writing an article on Web-based news outlets such as The Conversation (theconversation.com/au) summarising research findings or challenging a policy that is not evidence based
- sharing research findings on a video-sharing platform such as YouTube or Vimeo
- posting a narrated slide presentation on Slideshare
- creating a Facebook page, LinkedIn group or a network or discussion on Google+
- posting a podcast or video summary of a journal publication on the journal's website to accompany the full manuscript
- writing a blog post (blogging is covered in detail in the following section)

Twitter in research

Twitter is an increasingly popular tool that can serve as a useful case study in effectively harnessing social media in research. Twitter is a microblogging service that enables individuals to rapidly post messages of up to 140 characters that are shared with their followers and anyone following the topic posted. On 30 June 2013, Twitter had 218.3 million monthly active users – an increase of 44% in 1 year – and the Twitter timeline is viewed 1.65 billion times per day. Twitter is a powerful platform for connecting with individuals and organisations who curate and share relevant and timely information, resources and ideas. Tweets are messages that may include links to journal articles, Web pages, blogs, images and video. For researchers, there is increasing evidence that journal publications that have been actively tweeted are cited significantly more frequently than those that are not (Eysenbach 2011a). An advantage of Twitter over other communication platforms such as blogs (see the following section 'Blogging') is that the Tweets of any individual on Twitter are received automatically by the Twitter users who follow them. In contrast, blogs require users to remember to visit the blog. One useful way to address this is to use both platforms, sending Tweets that contain a link to the most recently published blog post.

Tweets can be categorised as substantive Tweets written in complete sentences, informal conversational style Tweets or – most commonly used in academia – a middle-ground style. The London School of Economics has published an excellent guide for academics and researchers on using Twitter that outlines the advantages and disadvantages of each category of Tweet (Mollett *et al.* 2011).

Researchers and project teams can harness Twitter across all stage of the research process to:

- participate in and build communities of patients, healthcare consumers and healthcare professionals and researchers
- raise community awareness of the research topic by asking powerful questions or tweeting links to relevant articles and resources
- communicate new project developments to interested stakeholders
- publicise and disseminate project outcomes by tweeting links to new publications, website updates, blog posts or videos
- engage policy-makers and funding bodies to raise awareness of gaps in policy or service delivery or recognise progress in the field
- evaluate the reach and impact of project communications strategies using social media analytics tools

It is important, however, to acknowledge that Tweets (unlike SMS text messages) are public, identified and perpetually searchable and accessible. This means that anyone can access all posted Tweets now or in the future, and therefore, care should be taken to ensure the content of each Tweet is clear, accurate, respectful and useful to others and has an appropriate level of disclosure.

Twitter users tag their Tweets using hashtags (#) to categorise the topic of the Tweet and make it searchable (in the same way journal article keywords support database searching). While some hashtags such as #nurse are perpetual, hashtags may also be created for an event or conference or emerge as a trending topic as it rises in popularity. Researchers can create a hashtag for their project or research area or contribute to a topic using existing hashtags. The website hashtags.org lists existing hashtags and their frequency of use. Nursing hashtags with wide reach include #WeNurses and #rnchat. An example of nursing research conference hashtags is #research2014 for the *RCN International Nursing Research Conference 2014*. Tweets with useful information, resources and support for higher degree by research students and early career researchers are tagged with #hdrchat and #ecrchat. Twitter discussions on mobile health apps and devices use the hashtag #mhealth and for healthcare technology using #hcIT. Box 6.4 provides some guidance on how to use Twitter in research.

Blogging

A blog ('Web log') is a website consisting of a series of entries ('posts') on a particular topic or theme, with features that allow readers to comment and engage with the author and other readers. Blog posts

Box 6.4 Using Twitter in research

- Before tweeting, listen to and learn about the individuals, organisations and community you are engaging with.
- Become familiar with the Twitter rules and your organisation's social media guidelines. Quickly acknowledge and correct mistakes or errors of judgement.
- Tweet regularly to build followers, and establish your credibility and reputation or that of the research project, by being a trusted source of relevant, current and high-quality information. Ensure links are to open-web, full versions of publications or articles (Mollett *et al.* 2011).
- Build trust, strong relationships and a sense of community by engaging authentically in honest and respectful dialogue.
- Twitter is a space for conversation, connecting with the audience and sharing: it is not a broadcast channel or marketing tool. Ask questions and crowdsourcing ideas and contributions, always acknowledging others' feedback and contributions.
- The Twitter website is easy to use, but for more advanced features, choose a programme to manage your Twitter account that offers the features your project requires. Programmes such as Seesmic and Hootsuite integrate multiple social media accounts on one dashboard, and like TweetDeck (another useful Twitter dashboard tool), their features include favourites, lists, scheduled tweets and shared management of the account.
- Evaluate project reach and impact by measuring the engagement with researchers and other stakeholders, the most shared resources, retweets and mentions, the citation rates of promoted articles and other relevant social media metrics.

may consist of text, images, video and links to related resources and other blogs. With 39% of Internet users reading at least one blog and over 112 million blogs on the Internet (Batts *et al.* 2008), blogs offer a powerful mechanism for rapid dissemination of information and communication with others interested in a topic. Researchers may use blogs during all stages of the research process including determining the research question, recruitment, data collection, translation, advocacy and dissemination.

Kouper (2010) proposed that there are four role types a science blogger plays: inform the public about scientific knowledge, explain complex ideas, critically evaluate claims in the scientific and mainstream media and outline their positions on controversial issues of interest. For example, the science and medicine journal *PLoS* published by the Public Library of Science publishes 16 blogs, including the Speaking of Medicine community blog for medical publishing at blogs.plos.org/speakingofmedicine.

Blogging provides scientists, clinicians and researchers with the opportunity to disseminate, evaluate and translate information and ideas more rapidly and more directly to the public than traditional academic publishing allows. However, the current lack of genre conventions in scientific blogging frequently results in writing that is characterised by fragmented parts of a more complex whole, superficial analyses or re-reporting of others' stories. Content consists primarily of informing and explaining; in-depth critique or rigorously argued positions on controversial topics appear less frequently. In contrast, effective research blogs are welcoming to non-scientists and focus on communicating with and engaging the reader. Kouper (2010) recommends scientific bloggers engage in 'explanatory, interpretive and critical modes of communication' rather than only reporting and expressing opinions. PLoS has published a list of 10 qualities that are essential for science bloggers that includes demonstrating humour, heart and a passion for science, giving credit to peers, having a voice and taking a stand and making original research comprehensible to as many readers as possible (Costello 2012).

Measuring research impact

Traditional measures of scholarly impact have significant limitations that are well documented: citation measures are slow and narrowly defined, and influential work may have low citation rates; peer review lacks transparency and accountability; and the Journal Impact Factor is skewed by small numbers of highly cited works and is a poor measure of the impact of an individual paper (Fausto *et al.* 2012). In contrast:

> Tools such as blogs, social bookmarks and online reference managers, Twitter and others offer alternative, transparent and more comprehensive information about the active interest, usage and reach of scientific publications. Fausto *et al.* (2012: 2)

There is an increasing call to track *Altmetrics* such as mentions, views, saves and shares that may provide more accurate measures of the extent to which a paper is being read and shared. Two examples are ImpactStory.org that collates data on audience and type of engagement on platforms including Twitter, Facebook, Mendeley and Scopus and altmetric.com that in addition evaluates a paper's impact on science blogs and mainstream news outlets. Research in this field is just emerging; early findings indicate that higher altmetric scores based on Twitter, Facebook posts, blogs and mainstream media are associated with higher citations (Thelwall *et al.* 2013).

Reflection activity

Consider a research project you are undertaking or may undertake in the future. Who are the key stakeholders with whom you would like to share your findings and what forms of social media communication will engage them most effectively?

DEVELOPING AN INTEGRATED SOCIAL MEDIA STRATEGY

One of the key challenges of using social media for research is the difficulty of reaching people who are not currently engaged in the selected social media platforms. While in some cases it may be straightforward to identify an appropriate platform (e.g. Facebook for young, Internet-connected diabetes patients), in other cases, there may be considerable diversity of connectedness and digital literacy in the target population. It is therefore important to recognise that in general one platform will not successfully engage all stakeholders or achieve all of the goals of the project. A more effective approach is to establish the project's digital presence using several platforms and coordinate communication and engagement activities through an integrated social media strategy.

Developing an integrated communication and engagement strategy involves identifying the social media platforms that are best suited to engage relevant patient communities, practitioners, policymakers and other stakeholders. This process comprises reviewing and selecting the social media platforms based on the project budget, expertise, goals and activities. The selected platforms may include:

- a website to convey information about the project, recruit participants, share news and events and disseminate project findings
- a blog to communicate the progress of the project over time; crowdsource and test ideas for conference presentations and academic publications; build the project community by inviting guest bloggers and linking to related blogs; and seek feedback from research colleagues and other stakeholders
- a Twitter account to connect and update interested stakeholders and link to dissemination publications on other platforms such as blogs, journal articles or news media
- a Facebook page may also be an appropriate platform to reach some groups

Box 6.5 provides some guidance on the elements to include when developing an integrated social media plan.

Box 6.5 Developing an integrated social media plan

A thorough social media plan should include the following elements:

- GOALS: project goals for communication, dissemination and engagement
- TOOLS: the hardware, software, platforms and apps required
- PROCESS: the communication strategies (e.g. resource sharing and polling to raise awareness or establish project rationale, engaging leaders and policy makers in the field through invitations to guest blog)
- GUIDELINES: a set of social media guidelines for preventing and responding to inappropriate sharing of confidential information, security breaches and negative comments posted on public sites
- PERSONNEL: project team member(s) with social media expertise in community building, communications and dissemination
- EVALUATION: identified measures of success of the project communications, engagement and dissemination and the evaluation process

Reflection activity

Devise a research communication and engagement plan for a project you are undertaking or may undertake in the future. What are the criteria for selecting communication platforms that are of most importance to this project?

Selecting appropriate tools and platforms

Choosing the right tools and platforms is an important process that may take some time. This is, however, a worthwhile investment – if a selected platform does not ultimately meet project requirements, considerable time, project progress and stakeholder confidence can be lost. To choose the right tool, list the features the project requires, then consult colleagues and reputable online review sites to identify options and determine the platforms that meet these needs.

When constructing the checklist, the following issues should be considered:

- Privacy – Is the intended audience private or public?
- Security – Where is the data stored, what are the policies and conditions of use, and what security features protect the data?
- Expertise – How difficult is the tool or platform to set up and to use? Can you or other project team members use it or learn to use this tool, and what is the time investment required to do this?
- Functionality – Document all the essential tasks that users and administrators of the platform must be able to perform with the tool, and evaluate each potential tool against this list.
- Budget – Identify the project budget and evaluate the costs of tools available against this figure. A common model is 'freemium' – tools that are free with basic features and limited numbers of users that can be upgraded upon payment of a fee. Note that project plans frequently omit consideration of the labour and financial costs of communications platforms, so it may be necessary for project teams to adapt their initial budget.

CONCLUSION

This chapter has outlined a vast array of digital technologies that provide researchers with powerful tools to enhance the effectiveness and impact of their research activities. With the ubiquity and rapidly evolving nature of these technologies, it is vital for research students and early career researchers to develop and maintain their own digital literacy. Each digital technology and social media platform – and the community that uses it – has specific social, cultural and technical characteristics that need to be understood, practised and mastered. In addition, there are complex challenges in addressing the privacy, security and ethical issues involved in using Web 2.0 platforms and social media to ensure the integrity and successful completion of the research project. With the rapid pace of change that characterises technology in the 21st century, the ability to locate, critically appraise and select appropriate technologies, understand their specific cultural practices and harness the opportunities they provide is a fundamental skill for all researchers.

References

Batts SA, Anthis NJ, Smith TC (2008) Advancing science through conversations: bridging the gap between blogs and the academy. *PLoS Biology* **6**(9): 1837–1841.

Bikshandi B (2011) QR codes in healthcare. *Pulse IT.* http://www.pulseitmagazine.com.au/index.php?option=com_content&view=article&id=751:qr-codes-in-healthcare (accessed on 1 September 2014).

Costello V (2012, December 31) Ten essential qualities of science bloggers. *PLoS Blogs*. http://blogs.plos.org/blog/2012/12/31/ten-essential-qualities-of-science-bloggers (accessed on 1 September 2014).

Crowdfunding.org (2012) *Crowdfunding Industry Report: market trends, composition and crowdfunding platforms.* Crowdsourcing LLC. www.crowdfunding.nl/wp-content/uploads/2012/05/92834651-Massolution-abridged-Crowd-Funding-Industry-Report1.pdf (accessed on 1 September 2014).

ESOMAR World Research (2012) *ESOMAR Guideline for Conducting Mobile Market Research.* Amsterdam, ESOMAR World Research.

Eysenbach G (2011a) Can Tweets predict citations? Metrics of social impact based on Twitter and correlation with traditional metrics of scientific impact. *Journal of Medical Internet Research* **13**(4): e123. DOI: 10.2196/jmir.

Eysenbach G (2011b) CONSORT-eHealth: improving and standardizing evaluation reports of web-based and mobile health interventions. *Journal of Medical Internet Research* **13**(4): e126.

Fausto S, Machado FA, Bento LFJ, Iamarino A, Nahas TR, Munger DS (2012) Research Blogging: indexing and registering the change in science 2.0. *PLoS ONE* **7**(12): e50109.

Goldacre B (2008) *Bad Science*. London, Harper Collins.

Goncalves L, Wolff LDG, Staggers N, Peres AM (2012) Nursing informatics competencies: an analysis of the latest research. *Nursing Informatics* **2012**: 127.

Kamerow D (2013) Regulating medical apps: which ones and how much? *BMJ (Clinical research ed.)* **347**: f6009.

Kouper I (2010) Science blogs and public engagement with science: practices, challenges, and opportunities. *Journal of Science Communication* **9**(1): 1–10.

Mollett A, Moran D, Dunleavy P (2011) *Using Twitter in University Research, Teaching and Impact Activities: a guide for academics and researchers.* London, London School of Economics Public Policy Group. http://issuu.com/amymollett/docs/twitter_guide_academics.

Parvanta C, Roth Y, Keller H (2013) Crowdsourcing 101: a few basics to make you the leader of the pack. *Health Promotion Practice* **14**(2): 263–267.

Small G (2011) Time to Tweet. *Nature* **479**: 141.

Thelwall M, Haustein S, Lariviere V, Sugimoto C (2013). Do altmetrics work? Twitter and ten other social web services. *PLoS ONE* **8**(5): 1.

Further reading

Cann A, Dimitriou K, Hooley T (2011) *Social Media: a guide for researchers.* Research Information Network. http://www.rin.ac.uk/our-work/communicating-and-disseminating-research/social-media-guide-researchers (accessed on 1 September 2014).

Fielding N, Lee RM, Blank G (eds) (2008) *The Sage Handbook of Online Research Methods*. London, SAGE.

Minocha S, Petre M (2012) *Handbook of social media for researchers and supervisors; digital technologies for research dialogues*. Vitae innovate, Open University. https://www.vitae.ac.uk/vitae-publications/reports/

innovate-open-university-social-media-handbook-vitae-2012.pdf/view (accessed on 1 September 2014).

Nunsinger J, Klastrup L, Allen M (2010) *The International Handbook of Internet Research*. London, Springer.

Websites

Audio and video tools

Flickr flickr.com
Vimeo vimeo.com
YouTube youtube.com

Blogging and microblogging tools

Blogger blogger.com
Tumblr tumblr.com
Twitter twitter.com
Wordpress wordpress.com
Yammer yammer.com

Crowd funding platforms

Experiment.com experiment.com
Pozible pozible.com
Petridish.org petridish.org

Dissemination and impact

Academia.edu academia.edu
Altmetric.com altmetric.com
Google scholar google.com/scholar
Impactstory.org impactstory.org
LinkedIn linkedin.com
ResearchGate researchgate.net

Project management and file storage tools

Basecamp basecamp.com
Evernote evernote.com
Good reader goodreader.com
Google Drive drive.google.com
Microsoft Office 365 www.365login.com

Meeting and collaboration tools

Google hangouts google.com/+/learnmore/hangouts
Microsoft Lync office.microsoft.com/en-us/lync
Skype skype.com

Research and writing collaboration tools

Dropbox dropbox.com
Google docs docs.google.com
Papers papersapp.com
Wikispaces wikispaces.com

Social bookmarking, information management and curation tools

CiteULike citeulike.org
Endnote Web myendnoteweb.com
Google alerts google.com.au/alerts
Mendeley mendeley.com
Pinterest pinterest.com
Scoop.it scoop.it
Zotero zotero.org

Social networking services

Facebook facebook.com
Google circles google.com/+/learnmore
Yammer yammer.com

Survey/data collection tools

Google forms docs.google.com
Poll Daddy polldaddy.com
Qualtrics qualtrics.com
Surveymonkey surveymonkey.com

SECTION 2

Preparing the Ground

At the beginning of any research enterprise, a considerable amount of work needs to be undertaken before the active stages of data collection and analysis can begin. This section deals with five major issues that require attention in the early stages of a research project, leading on to research design which will be the subject of Section 3.

Chapters 7 and 8 are linked together and draw on the discipline of information science. Chapter 7 takes the reader through the essential preparatory stage of reviewing existing evidence in the field of interest for research. Chapter 8 builds on this base using the now well-established science of critical appraisal and equipping the reader with tools with which to test the validity and applicability of published research to their own situation. It is impossible to overstate the importance of these preparatory stages in research; unless new knowledge is developed from a sound base of previous well-validated evidence, the credibility of nursing research will be called into question. More than this, those who implement research findings must also develop the skills of finding and appraising the evidence that is available.

Chapters 9, 10 and 11 are concerned with practical issues of preparing to undertake a specific project. Chapter 9 guides the reader through the formal process of writing a research proposal. The proposal might be for an academic dissertation or for a national funding body, but the process is the same in principle. Getting the proposal right is likely to make the difference between obtaining approval and funding or not, but writing the proposal also helps to clarify the researcher's thinking. Chapter 10 deals with planning and managing a research project. The chapter focuses particularly on the needs of students pursuing higher degrees and their relationship with supervisors and other sources of support. Many of the users of this book will be engaged in research in the course of academic study and will find this chapter a valuable source of advice. Chapter 11 completes the section by discussing in detail the complex process of obtaining formal permissions for research and the regulatory frameworks that exist in the United Kingdom for research in health and social care. No research project that takes place in a health care context in the United Kingdom can proceed without going through the ethical and governance approval procedures, and successful negotiation of the regulations depends on careful and informed preparation and planning.

The Research Process in Nursing, Seventh Edition. Edited by Kate Gerrish and Judith Lathlean.

Companion Website: www.wiley.com/go/gerrish/research

CHAPTER 7

Finding the Evidence

Claire Beecroft, Andrew Booth and Angie Rees

Key points

- Effective literature searching is an essential skill for research, audit and evidence-based practice.
- The research literature consists of journals, reports, theses, conference proceedings, government publications and Web-based resources.
- Much literature searching uses electronic databases and the Internet.
- High-quality sources of evidence include systematic reviews, evidence syntheses and critically appraised topics.
- Reference management skills are vital for effective research and evidence review.

INTRODUCTION

As the nursing and health-care literature grows, so does the need for individuals to acquire the skills to search it effectively. While databases such as the Cumulative Index to Nursing and Allied Health (CINAHL) are key for those seeking to access the nursing and health-care literature, specialist resources such as the Cochrane Library (www.thecochranelibrary.com) and 'academic' search engines such as Google Scholar (http://scholar.google.co.uk) complement traditional information sources. There is also increasing use of social media such as Twitter for the sharing of knowledge (Skibba 2008). The vast array of information available and the ever-growing access to research evidence via open-access journals makes developing searching skills more vital than ever.

Before carrying out research, you should undertake a systematic search of the literature to identify previous studies that are similar or identical to the proposed study. Searching the literature is also essential when developing policy or guidelines, evaluating practice or attempting to implement change. When auditing a service, up-to-date, high-quality evidence is required on which to base the proposed standards. So, consider the ability to search the literature as a skill to support you throughout your career.

The Research Process in Nursing, Seventh Edition. Edited by Kate Gerrish and Judith Lathlean.

Companion Website: www.wiley.com/go/gerrish/research

ELECTRONIC INFORMATION RESOURCES AND THE INTERNET

Nurses need to be able to access electronic and Internet-based information resources if they are to obtain timely, high-quality information to support evidence-based practice. UK National Health Service (NHS) staff have access via the Internet to a host of specialist resources via the NHS Evidence service (www.evidence.nhs.uk). Similar resources in other countries underpin the use of high-quality research.

In this chapter, the 'Internet' is primarily a means of delivering access to information. It is increasingly the 'go-to' source for information of all kinds, and many databases that nurses have access to, such as MEDLINE and CINAHL, are accessed via the Internet. However, caution should be exercised when searching for research evidence via search engines such as Google, as search results can number in the hundreds of thousands, with many results of no direct relevance. However, with the emergence of academic search engines such as Google Scholar and the wider availability of citation data, it is possible to conduct a complete and thorough search for research evidence via the Internet and obtain full-text articles electronically. The key to a successful search is making an informed choice of sources to search and avoiding reliance on any single information source.

THE RESEARCH LITERATURE

It is important to be aware of the full range of literature available to support research and practice. The word 'evidence' is widely used to describe the information on which clinical decisions should be based. This evidence comes from a variety of sources (Ehrlich-Jones *et al.* 2008). In the following, we describe some key forms of 'evidence'.

Journals and journal articles

Journals and journal articles inevitably come to mind when we think about the 'research literature'. Journals not only contain research, but also opinion, editorials, letters, case studies and reports. All contribute evidence to support practice and research. However, background questions such as general information on a disease or condition may best be answered from a textbook. Knowledge in journal articles tends to be specialised rather than general. Most key health and social care databases offer increasing numbers of articles electronically as full text (either the complete article as it appears in the print version of the journal or the full version of an article in an Internet-only journal).

Books

While books are not always sufficiently up to date to support research, they can provide useful background information to assist in developing a research question. Electronic library catalogues feature in most health libraries, and these enable relevant books to be identified. Increasingly, libraries offer some textbooks as e-books, with the convenience of being able to read the book via mobile devices such as tablet computers and e-book readers.

Reports

Some research findings are published as reports. Research reports may yield useful information such as statistics and cost data and thus complement information from journals. Bear in mind that some research that has not been successful in getting published in a journal may be issued as a report as a 'last resort' and as many reports may not have undergone a peer review process, quality may be variable. Reports are not included in many of the major databases such as MEDLINE. However, reports can be identified using specialist databases such as the Health Management Information Consortium (HMIC) database or by searching appropriate Internet sites.

Theses

Theses are usually the end product of research degrees at master's or doctoral level. They provide an extensive record of the student's research project and

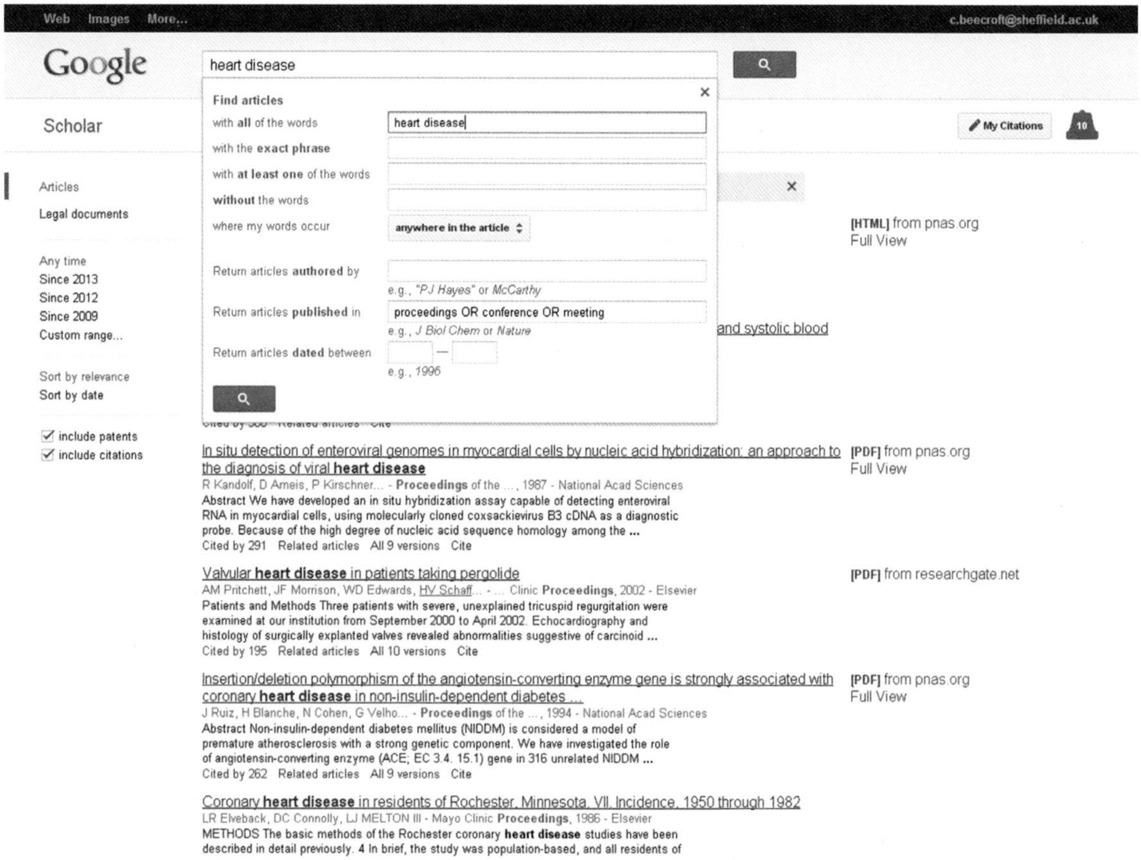

Figure 7.1 Searching Google Scholar for conference proceedings

are therefore considerably longer than most journal articles. To identify relevant theses, major databases and specialised sources such as *dissertation abstracts* (an electronic database of abstracts for theses) and *index to theses* need to be searched. Most university libraries hold collections of theses by their own students and so are a good place to look.

Conference proceedings

Papers presented by speakers at a conference are often collated and published in print or electronic form as 'conference proceedings'. This allows those not attending the conference to read through papers that were presented. Conferences are frequently used as a forum for presenting the results of ongoing or recently completed research and so can provide up-to-date information if proceedings are published soon after the conference has ended. Conference proceedings are often referenced in the major databases (such as MEDLINE and CINAHL). To locate the proceedings of a particular conference, try searching the Internet to see if the conference has a website, as proceedings are sometimes published in this way. Alternatively, you can search Google Scholar (http://scholar.google.co.uk) using the 'advanced search' option and adding a search for 'proceedings OR conference OR meeting' to the 'published in' field, along with your search terms (see Figure 7.1).

Increasingly, conferences have an official Twitter hashtag (for instance, the RCN International Nursing Research conference in 2013 used the hashtag #INRC13). Hashtags are used by conference staff

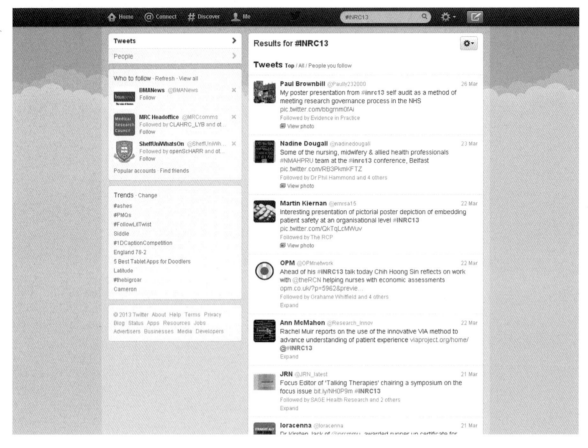

Figure 7.2 Example of use of a hashtag on Twitter during a conference

and delegates to tweet information on the conference presentations. These can be an excellent source of information, links and debate, so it is worth searching for the hashtag of a conference that you are unable to attend. Alternatively, you might search a conference hashtag relating to a past conference to see if it reveals useful information. See Figure 7.2 for an example of conference tweets.

Government circulars

Circulars are published by governmental departments, groups and committees. Such documents are usually available via the relevant governmental website, such as the UK Government's publications site (www.gov.uk/government/publications).

Grey literature

'Grey literature' describes literature, ranging from pamphlets and leaflets to governmental or health service documents, which is often not collected by libraries and is frequently not referenced in electronic databases (Conn *et al.* 2003). The key characteristic of this literature is that it can be difficult to track down. However, the Internet makes grey literature easier to identify and obtain. Specialist databases, such as HMIC (available via NHS Evidence) and OpenGrey (the System for Information on Grey Literature in Europe) (http://www.opengrey.eu/), offer access to grey literature. Other wikis and Internet sites include the Ontario Public Health Libraries Association's Online Database of Public Health Grey Literature (http://ophla.pbworks.com/Public-Health-Grey-Literature-Database%3A-Overview) and the Canadian Agency for Drugs and Technologies in Health (CADTH)'s Grey Matters tool (http://www.cadth.ca/en/resources/finding-evidence-is/grey-matters), although currency of some grey literature resources is not always reliable and updating may be sporadic. Local health library staff are able to identify resources to locate grey literature.

ACCESSING THE LITERATURE

The Internet has resulted in major changes, not only to how the literature is accessed but also where it can be accessed from, be that in the workplace, at home or on mobile devices such as tablets and smartphones (Anderson 2013). Many resources discussed earlier can be accessed in electronic format. Clearly, information technology skills are important for searching the literature, so both traditional and modern methods will be examined.

Finding a library

Most health organisations maintain their own libraries, and additionally, many negotiate 'access agreements' with local libraries to complement their own resources. However, certain services, such as borrowing materials or photocopying, may only be available on a fee-paying basis. If you are unsure which services are available locally, enquire at the nearest hospital-based library. Training in the use of electronic resources is usually provided, as hands-on practical sessions or e-learning resources or on a one-to-one basis.

Some resources may not be available via a local library. In going further afield, three things should be considered:

- Are you certain that the resources you are seeking are not available locally or via the Internet?
- How feasible is it to travel to use the library?
- How can you make best use of libraries that are not nearby?

National/international electronic resources

Many health-care systems support access to major electronic databases, journals and books. For example, NHS Evidence (www.evidence.nhs.uk) offers access to various databases for staff in the NHS. Some nursing organisations provide access to databases and/or electronic journals. For instance, the Royal College of Nursing provides its members with electronic access to a collection of nursing and health-related journals. International databases that may be accessible via the Internet include:

- AMED: an allied and complementary medicine database compiled by the British Library, covering many journals that are not indexed in other health-related databases.
- CINAHL: the Cumulative Index to Nursing and Allied Health Literature has references to almost all English-language journals in the nursing and allied health literature, plus conference proceedings and reports. It is the most comprehensive nursing database.
- MEDLINE: a major medical database of more than 16 million records, with references from more than 3900 journals, covering a broad and expanding range of medical specialties. It includes some references to conference proceedings.
- EMBASE: similar to MEDLINE but with an emphasis on drugs and pharmacology. It has references from more than 3500 journals and includes some references to books and conference proceedings.
- PsycINFO: this specialised database covers psychology and allied fields. It contains references from more than 1900 journals plus books, reports, etc.

In addition, the following Web-based databases are free to access:

- Social Care Online (http://www.scie-socialcareonline.org.uk/): this database abstracts social work and social care literature. It contains references to books, journal articles, government reports, etc. covering English-language publications in the United Kingdom, North America and beyond.

- PubMed (http://www.ncbi.nlm.nih.gov/pubmed/): is produced in the United States by the National Library of Medicine and is a search interface to several databases, including MEDLINE. Although PubMed has powerful searching facilities, it is often easier to use locally available commercial versions of MEDLINE (e.g. via NHS Evidence), particularly if you require links to full-text journals.
- Cochrane Library (http://www.thecochranelibrary.com): is a collection of databases that can be searched simultaneously and is an essential resource for information on the effectiveness and cost-effectiveness of health-care interventions. More details about the Cochrane library follow later in this chapter.
- OpenGrey (http://www.opengrey.eu/): is a European database of grey literature. It is an excellent starting point when searching for Europe-specific grey literature.
- Google Scholar (http://scholar.google.co.uk): is an Internet search engine for academic-related content such as journal articles, book chapters and conference proceedings. It provides more focused results than the general Google search engine. It offers additional features such as citation searching (searching for articles that reference a particular individual article), ready-formatted citations that can be cut and pasted into a bibliography and links to full text where available.

Information about access to other databases, e-journals and e-books can be obtained from a local health library.

Reflection activity

Ask yourself, do I have a key information resource to which I turn again and again? If so, why do I use this? Is it effective? Does it help me to make best use of my time? Are there other resources I might also explore?

Many electronic resources, such as PubMed and Google Scholar, can be used effectively using mobile devices such as smartphones and tablet computers.

PLANNING A LITERATURE SEARCH

Planning a literature search strategy in advance is vital as it can save much time and effort and will dramatically improve the quality of your search results.

The importance of the focused search question

A focused search question is critical when searching the literature (Cleary-Holdforth & Leufer 2008). If the question is not sufficiently focused, you will find yourself wrestling with large sets of mostly irrelevant search results. A focused question helps to ensure that your search is sufficiently narrow and accurate and that you can manage the volume of literature rather than drowning in it (McKibbon & Marks 2001).

The anatomy of a question

It may be helpful to develop a focused question using one of the available models (see PICO or SPICE in the following). These will assist you in planning the search strategy.

PICO

The PICO model is an acronym made up as follows (Glasper & Rees 2012):

- **P**atient/problem (e.g. chronic constipation)
- **I**ntervention/exposure (e.g. fibre supplements)
- **C**omparison (e.g. no fibre supplements)
- **O**utcome (e.g. relief from/reduction of constipation)

PICO works well for questions about health-care interventions. Once the four elements to the question are identified, a list is compiled of all the words and phrases needed to search for each PICO element. Remember to think of synonyms, alternative spellings and plurals. Google is a helpful tool for this task.

Box 7.1 Illustration of the PICO model

Patient/problem	Intervention/exposure	Comparison	Outcome
Chronic constipation	Fibre supplement(s)	Placebo	Relief
	Ispaghula		Relieved
			Reduce
			Reduced

Box 7.2 Illustration of the SPICE model

Setting	Perspective	Intervention	Comparison	Evaluation
Hospital(s)	Hospital nurses	Suicide prevention education	No education	Attitudes
Clinic(s)	Hospital-based nurses	Suicide education		Knowledge
Inpatient	Clinic nurses			Understanding

Box 7.1 provides an illustration of the PICO model. Within the context of systematic reviews, where you also need to identify the types of study required to answer the review question, you will frequently see PICO become PICOS where the additional **S** is used to designate **S**tudy design (see Chapter 25).

There will be many additional terms, so Box 7.1 is a simplified version. Under the 'comparison' heading, the term 'placebo' (i.e. fibre supplements are being compared with no treatment) is provided as a suggestion. The 'comparison' element of PICO is sometimes implicit, and it may be possible to obtain a good set of results by simply identifying the other elements and then combining them using Boolean operators (AND/OR/NOT), of which more later.

SPICE

The SPICE model (Booth 2004) is a useful alternative to the PICO model for questions that relate to qualitative methodologies or the social sciences. Using a similar format to PICO, the SPICE model breaks a search question down into the following:

- **S**etting (e.g. hospital based)
- **P**erspective (e.g. hospital nurses)
- **I**ntervention (e.g. suicide prevention education)
- **C**omparison (e.g. before education intervention)
- **E**valuation (e.g. attitudes to suicide, understanding of suicide prevention)

As Box 7.2 illustrates, it is not necessary to identify terms for all aspects of the SPICE model to

RESEARCH EXAMPLE

7.1 A MEDLINE Abstract

Authors

Chan SW, Chien WT, Tso S

Institution

Nethersole School of Nursing, Chinese University of Hong Kong

Title

Evaluating nurses' knowledge, attitude and competency after an education programme on suicide prevention

Source

Nurse Education Today **29**(7): 763–769; (Oct 2009)

Abstract

The aim of this study was to evaluate an education programme on suicide prevention for nurses working in general hospitals. A mixed method design that included a single group pretest–posttest analysis and focus group interviews was used. A convenience sample of 54 registered nurses was recruited from the medical and surgical units of two regional general hospitals. An 18-hour education programme on suicide prevention based on reflective learning principles was provided to the participants. The outcome measures used included participants' attitudes towards, knowledge of, competence in and stress levels arising from suicide prevention and management. Eighteen participants joined the focus group interviews. There were statistically significant positive changes in the pre- and posttest measures of participants' attitudes and competence levels. Qualitative data showed that participants had applied the new knowledge they acquired in clinical practice. They perceived themselves as being more aware of the problem of suicide and more competent in managing suicide risk. Participants highlighted certain barriers that exist to providing optimal care, including inadequate manpower, lack of support from senior staff and a lack of guidelines. Ongoing education may be necessary to expedite changes. The education programme provided can be delivered to other health-care professional groups and the results further evaluated.

produce a useful list of terms and a search strategy. In this example, combining terms from the 'S', 'P' and 'I' sections may be sufficient to find relevant articles. Adding additional terms from the 'E' section might help to identify papers that investigate the impacts of suicide prevention education. A search using terms related to just the 'S', 'P' and 'I' sections retrieves the article from MEDLINE shown in Research Example 7.1. Developing your search strategy using these models helps to produce a more relevant set of results. Once the PICO or SPICE model has been developed, each element is searched separately, and then search statements are combined to produce a smaller set of results using Boolean operators.

Boolean operators

Boolean operators are simply the words 'AND', 'OR' and 'NOT' that are used to combine search concepts. Box 7.3 shows how they work with the example given earlier. When using the 'OR' operator, you are asking the database to identify papers that feature either of the terms you have searched. In the previous example Box (7.1), the 'Intervention' element retrieves papers that contain the phrase

Box 7.3 Example of Boolean operators

Patient/problem		Intervention/ exposure		Comparison		Outcome
Chronic constipation		Fibre supplement(s)		Placebo		Relief
		OR				OR
	AND	Ispaghula	AND		AND	Relieve
						OR
						Reduce
						OR
						Reduced

Reflection activity

Use the PICO or SPICE model to make a list of search terms for a research question, remembering to think of synonyms and alternative spellings for each term and how you might use wildcards and truncation with some of your terms to ensure the most efficient and effective search.

'fibre supplement(s)' or the phrase 'ispaghula', as both could be relevant. Similarly for the 'Outcome', 'relief' as well as 'relieved' are used to ensure that all variations around the concept of relief are searched; combining these with OR ensures that all your listed terms are searched.

When combining across PICO elements, the 'AND' operator is used. When combining the Patient and Intervention columns, we are instructing the database to find papers featuring the terms 'chronic constipation' AND 'fibre supplement(s)' OR 'ispaghula husk' within the same paper.

SEARCHING THE LITERATURE

Electronic searching

Although databases differ in terms of interfaces and search terminologies, many techniques are common to different databases. Once you have mastered these techniques for one database, it will be easier to use other ones.

Free-text searching

Most databases allow you to type in words and phrases and search for references that feature those terms in the title, abstract, authors, journal name, etc. This is known as 'free-text' searching. This is how most people instinctively search databases, but it has its drawbacks. As mentioned earlier, you need to think of all the synonyms and alternative spellings for each term to be sure not to miss anything important. 'Truncation' is a technique that saves time when typing in variations of a word. Most databases allow you to enter a truncation mark (often a * or $) after a word stem (the first few letters of a word) in order to

RESEARCH EXAMPLE

7.2 A Retrieval Error from MEDLINE

Roerig JL, Steffen KJ, Mitchell JE, Zuncker C (2010) Laxative abuse: epidemiology, diagnosis and management. *Drugs* **70**(12): 1487–1503.

Laxatives have been used for health purposes for over 2000 years, and for much of that time, abuse or misuse of laxatives has occurred. Individuals who abuse laxatives can generally be categorised as falling into one of four groups. By far the largest group is made up of individuals suffering from an eating disorder such as anorexia or bulimia nervosa. The prevalence of laxative abuse has been reported to range from approximately 10 to 60% of individuals in this group. The second group consists of individuals who are generally middle aged or older who begin using laxatives when constipated but continue to overuse them. This pattern may be promulgated on certain beliefs that daily bowel movements are necessary for good health. The third group includes individuals engaged in certain types of athletic training, including sports with set weight limits. The fourth group contains surreptitious laxative abusers who use the drugs to cause factitious diarrhoea and may have a factitious disorder. Normal bowel function consists of the absorption of nutrients, electrolytes and water from the gut. Most nutrients are absorbed in the small intestine, while the large bowel absorbs primarily water. There are several types of laxatives available, including stimulant agents, saline and osmotic products, bulking agents and surfactants. The most frequently abused group of laxatives are of the stimulant class. This may be related to the quick action of stimulants, particularly in individuals with eating disorders as they may erroneously believe that they can avoid the absorption of calories via the resulting diarrhoea. Medical problems associated with laxative abuse include electrolyte and acid/base changes that can involve the renal and cardiovascular systems and may become life threatening. The renin–aldosterone system becomes activated due to the loss of fluid, which leads to oedema and acute weight gain when the laxative is discontinued. This can result in reinforcing further laxative abuse when a patient feels bloated and has gained weight. Treatment begins with a high level of suspicion, particularly when a patient presents with alternating diarrhoea and constipation as well as other gastrointestinal complaints. Checking serum electrolytes and the acid/base status can identify individuals who may need medical stabilisation and confirm the severity of the abuse. The first step in treating laxative misuse once it is identified is to determine what may be promoting the behaviour, such as an eating disorder or use based on misinformation regarding what constitutes a healthy bowel habit. The first intervention would be to stop the stimulant laxatives and replace them with fibre/osmotic supplements utilised to establish normal bowel movements. Education and further treatment may be required to maintain a healthy bowel programme. In the case of an eating disorder, referral for psychiatric treatment is essential to lessen the reliance on laxatives as a method to alter weight and shape.

search for all variations of that word. For instance, if you want to search for:

- prevent
- prevents
- prevention
- preventative

you can simply enter Prevent* (or Prevent$ depending on the database) to find all the above words. However, 'free-text' searches will often generate numerous results that make a fleeting reference to the search term but are not fundamentally about that subject. Research Example 7.2, found by searching MEDLINE for the free-text terms 'constipation' and 'fibre supplements', illustrates this. Although both terms are mentioned in the abstract, this paper is not about these subjects but nevertheless does still contain these terms.

Subject headings

Due to the limitations of free-text searching, it may be helpful to search for subject headings that relate to the topic. Subject headings are standardised terms used to describe the content of an article. They enable searchers to avoid typing multiple terms for the same subject, as a single subject heading is assigned to replace them all. For instance, for a free-text search for papers about 'ispaghula' (a laxative), you would need to enter all of the following terms (and possibly others):

- Ispaghula
- Psyllium
- Ispaghule
- Plantago seed

However, indexers may assign a single subject heading 'psyllium' to describe all papers about this subject, regardless of the exact terminology used by the authors of each paper. Once a paper has been assigned a list of subject headings, the terms that describe the main concepts of the paper are highlighted as 'major subject headings'. Several subject heading systems are used by health-related databases so your search strategy will need to be amended slightly for each database. Each database will include different subject areas and clinical specialisms and therefore needs to use a different array of terminology. The most well known is Medical Subject Headings (MeSH), used by the US National Library of Medicine for the MEDLINE database and by the Cochrane Library.

Limiting searches

Once you have completed initial free-text and subject heading searches, you may wish to limit your results set further. Typical limits include the following:

- Age: to restrict the search to patients within certain age groups

> **Reflection activity**
>
> Using the PICO or SPICE examples you identified in the previous reflection activity, plan an electronic search strategy to access the literature you will require to address your research question. How will you narrow down your search in order to ensure that it is manageable and that you access appropriate literature?

- Language: to confine the search to publications in a specified language
- Date range: to identify papers that have been published in the past few years, or if historical articles are required
- Full text: to limit the search to papers available in full to print or download

Limits make the results set more focused and smaller. They should be used with caution to ensure that relevant material is not missed; this is especially important for systematic reviews where a missed study can have significant effects on overall review results.

Manual searching

Some techniques used for manual searching of the literature are mentioned earlier in this chapter. These are particularly useful when searching for grey literature that is often not indexed in the major electronic databases. For more on supplementary searching, see Papaioannou *et al.* (2010).

Journal indexes

Many journals produce an annual printed index to help users find the articles they need. This is published either as a separate volume or in the last issue of a volume or year. The index usually enables the reader to look up articles by a particular author or that contain a specific keyword. These indexes are useful if you wish to browse a key journal in the subject area but do not want to go through each table of contents individually.

Reference lists

It is useful to search through the list of references of relevant articles that you have found. When a useful reference has been identified, it is worth trying to retrieve the reference from databases you have already searched to identify why it was not found by your search strategy. This will allow you to read the abstract for the paper and decide whether the paper is worth obtaining.

Tables of contents

For journals that do not produce an annual index, you can browse tables of contents, which are often available via the journal websites. This can be a lengthy process so you will need to target key journals in your subject area and read through the titles in the table of contents of each issue to find relevant articles.

Further help with literature searching

Literature searching is an important skill to develop. This chapter has introduced key concepts. However, you may need to seek further assistance from your local health library or research support facility. In the United Kingdom, for example, regional Research Design Services (RDS) for the National Institute for Health Research (NIHR) (www.nihr.ac.uk/) provide a range of services to NHS staff who are applying for research funding, including support for literature searching. Your local research and development office/team will be able to provide information about available support.

SPECIALIST INFORMATION SOURCES

'Digested' forms of evidence: reviews and syntheses

With a wealth of literature available, it is often difficult and time consuming to wade through the vast quantities of studies published. One approach is to limit the search to a particular type of study design (Littleton *et al.* 2004; Flemming & Briggs 2007). However, even within a single study design, studies will vary considerably in quality, due to such factors as poor resourcing, inappropriate methodology, etc. The need to provide health-care professionals with reliable evidence on which to base decisions has led to the increasing importance of published reviews (Docherty 2003). Reviews bring together and 'digest' the body of research on a subject and identify common themes or patterns of effect in the results, enabling the reviewer to draw conclusions for their proposed research question. Broadly speaking, there are two types of review, 'traditional' and 'systematic'. Traditional reviews take many forms, but they are usually highly selective in the literature they include. For instance, in a literature review, a reviewer may include only papers published in the past year or in certain key journals. Reviews such as this can be useful for keeping up to date and managing the volume of literature in a subject area; however, they are susceptible to bias.

Systematic reviews are the focus of Chapter 25. They are the 'gold standard' method for reviewing the literature on effectiveness in health care. They bring the same rigour that characterises primary research to the review process, leaving a reproducible audit trail of methods. Systematic reviews are often characterised by 'meta-analysis': a combination of statistical techniques enabling the reviewer to produce an overall estimate of the results of individual studies. A systematic review will typically include details of included and excluded studies that may be useful to your own research question.

Cochrane Library

The Cochrane Library is produced by the Cochrane Collaboration, an international organisation comprising numerous subject-specific groups conducting systematic reviews in their topic areas. The Cochrane Library comprises seven different databases. The most prominent of these is the Cochrane Database of Systematic Reviews (CDSR), which contains reviews undertaken by the Cochrane Collaboration. Other databases include the Cochrane Central Register of Controlled Trials containing randomised controlled trials used in Cochrane systematic reviews. This database is considered the single best source of information on controlled trials of quality. The Cochrane Library also includes the database of appraised reviews *not* produced by the Cochrane Collaboration, the Database of Abstracts of Reviews of Effects (DARE).

Evidence-based journals

Some journals are devoted to summarising research findings. The BMJ Publishing Group numbers three such titles, *Evidence-Based Medicine, Evidence-Based Mental Health* and *Evidence-Based Nursing.* The last of these produces short podcasts of its digests, providing a useful alternative means of accessing these resources. Similarly, the Cochrane Collaboration produces short podcasts digesting key reviews (www.cochrane.org/podcasts). These digests of systematic reviews, reviews and meta-analysis make research findings even more accessible. Another journal of potential interest to nurses is *Worldviews on Evidence-Based Nursing*.

Web 2.0 technologies

Increasingly, social media technologies are used to disseminate research. In addition to podcasts mentioned earlier, blogging (the practice of keeping an openly accessible online log or diary that is regularly updated) is becoming popular. An example is the 'Nursing Research: Show me the evidence!' blog from St Joseph's Hospital, California, used by nurses to communicate their research activity (www.evidencebasednursing.blogspot.com/) and the Social Sciences in Nursing research blog (http://blog.ssnr.org.uk/), which focuses on the social sciences in nursing research. The micro-blogging site Twitter (www.twitter.com) is increasingly used by journals to promote research articles, so consider following the twitter accounts for key journals in your research area.

Evidence summaries

Clinical knowledge summaries (http://cks.nice.org.uk/) is a service delivered via the NHS Evidence service. It summarises evidence on the effectiveness of health-care interventions, providing guidance on diagnosis and management and offering printable leaflets that practitioners can pass on to their patients. Arranged alphabetically by a clinical specialty (e.g. 'child health'), it enables practitioners to easily identify up-to-date evidence. Similar resources are available via the Internet, such as the via TRIP Database (www.tripdatabase.com).

WRITING A LITERATURE REVIEW

Once the literature search is completed and papers are identified to answer the search question, you are ready to start your literature review. There are three key stages:

- *Sorting the 'wheat from the chaff'* – this involves examining retrieved papers critically to decide whether they meet the criteria for the review and whether they really help to answer the question. Chapter 8 considers this in more detail.
- *Identifying key points, results and things* – this involves interpreting research findings and applying them to your question (see Greenhalgh 2010).
- *Writing up your findings* – this involves using a structured approach. It may be helpful to look at examples of reviews to identify different ways of presenting the results.

MANAGING REFERENCES

Recording and managing your search results

When your electronic and manual searches are completed, you will need to document your search strategies. Outlining search strategies demonstrates the quality and efficacy of your search effort. Also, it may later be necessary to update searches or to rerun them. Searches can be recorded manually (by printing out the search strategies) or electronically. Many

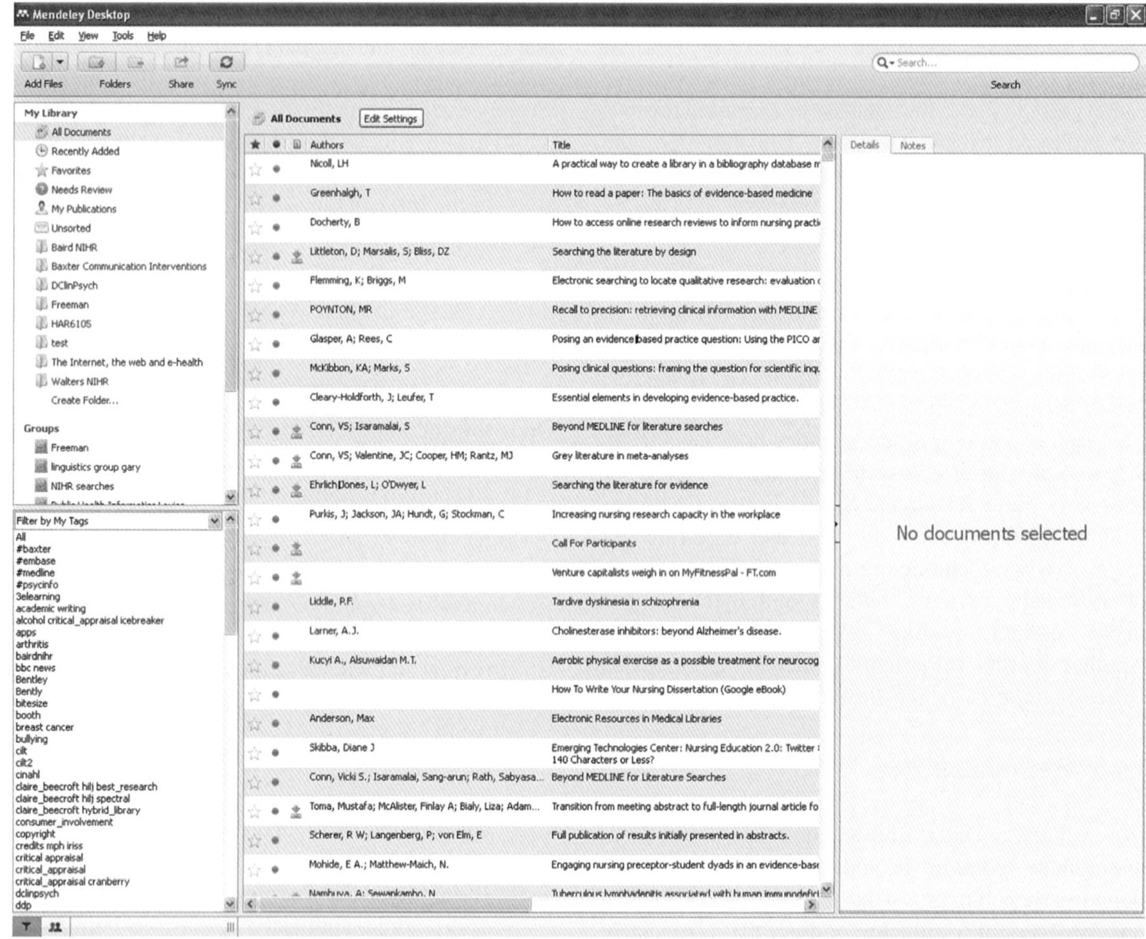

Figure 7.3 Screenshot of Mendeley reference management tool

bibliographic databases permit users to store search strategies for later recall. This is particularly useful if you need to conduct the searches again or modify them, saving you the time-consuming task of retyping the search terms. The databases that have been used should also be documented, with the dates on which they were searched. The 'tagging' function of many reference management tools can facilitate this process and make searching your reference management database easy and quick. For instance, a set of references retrieved from the CINAHL database could be 'tagged' with the name of the database and the date, allowing the database to be searched using these tags at a later date.

Consideration should also be given to using a system to manage your references as you obtain them (Nicoll 2003) as this will help when you are obtaining copies of papers and appraising them. It will also prove valuable when you write up your work and need to produce bibliographies, etc.

Electronic reference management software

Several software packages are available to help manage references. Popular commercial examples include Reference Manager and Endnote, but other products are available to download free of charge from the Internet, the most prominent being

Box 7.4 A manual index card

Author(s):	**Smith A, Jones B**
Title:	Manual reference cards versus reference management software: a review of the literature
Source:	*International Journal of Reference Management*
Year:	2014
Volume:	52
Part:	3
Pages:	79–93
Notes:	Mentioned in footnote 2 (please note this example is a fictional reference)

Mendeley (www.mendeley.com). Most reference management software allows you to produce bibliographies in various formats very efficiently. Many interact with word-processing software to enable references to be inserted directly into the text, saving time and improving the accuracy of referencing. References can be individually annotated and keywords identified as they are imported into the software. This allows subgroups of different records to be kept within the database.

Figure 7.3 shows a screenshot for the Internet reference management software tool Mendeley. Individual references are displayed in the main section of the screen, with tags appearing on the left; these are clickable, allowing speedy access to specific groups of references.

Manual methods

Manual methods of organising references can have advantages. They are often cheaper, may be easier to manage and do not require special training. However, they will typically be more time consuming. One method is to maintain a simple card index. A manual handwritten index card might look like Box 7.4. Whichever method you choose, you should get into the habit of recording references as soon as you identify them. This will help to prevent references 'slipping through the net' and becoming lost, thus saving much hard work at the conclusion of your project.

CONCLUSION

This chapter has examined the importance of focusing a search question and planning the search. It has outlined the various methods of searching and using the literature. Here are some key points to remember:

- Focus your question and plan your search strategy. Make notes and do not be tempted to go straight to the computer to start searching.
- Get to know your local health library and the librarians who work there. They are an invaluable resource and can save you much time and effort.
- Familiarise yourself with the resources that are most relevant to you by using them regularly for current-awareness purposes.
- Practice your searching as frequently as you can in order to hone your skills.

The skills of searching and accessing the literature are not just useful for research; they will support you throughout your professional career. Taking the time to gain these skills will yield great rewards both immediately and for years to come.

References

Anderson M (2013) Electronic resources in medical libraries. In: Peters T, Bell L (eds) *The Handheld Library: mobile technology and the librarian.* Santa Barbara, CA, Libraries Unlimited, pp 119–131.

Booth A (2004) Formulating answerable questions. In: Booth A, Brice A (eds) *Evidence Based Practice for Information Professionals: a handbook.* London, Facet Publishing, pp 61–70.

Cleary-Holdforth J, Leufer T (2008) Essential elements in developing evidence-based practice. *Nursing Standard* **23**(2): 42–46.

Conn VS, Isaramalai S, Rath S, Jantarakupt P, Wadhawan R, Dash Y (2003) Beyond MEDLINE for literature searches. *Journal of Nursing Scholarship* **35**(2): 177–182.

Docherty B (2003) How to access online research reviews to inform nursing practice. *Professional Nurse* **19**(1): 53–55.

Ehrlich-Jones L, O'Dwyer L, Stevens K (2008) Searching the literature for evidence. *Rehabilitation Nursing* **33**(4): 163–169.

Flemming K, Briggs M (2007) Electronic searching to locate qualitative research: evaluation of three strategies. *Journal of Advanced Nursing* **57**(1): 95–100.

Glasper A, Rees C (2012) Posing an evidence-based practice question: using the PICO and SPICE models. In: Glasper A, Rees C (eds) *How to Write Your Nursing Dissertation.* Oxford, Wiley Blackwell, pp 86–92.

Greenhalgh T (2010) *How to Read a Paper: the basics of evidence-based medicine,* 4th edition. Oxford, Wiley-Blackwell.

Littleton D, Marsalis S, Bliss D (2004) Searching the literature by design. *Western Journal of Nursing Research* **26**: 891–908.

McKibbon K, Marks S (2001) Posing clinical questions: framing the question for scientific inquiry. *AACN Clinical Issues, Advanced Critical Care* **12**(4): 477–481.

Nicoll L (2003) A practical way to create a library in a bibliography database manager: using electronic sources to make it easy. *Computers Informatics Nursing* **21**(1): 48–54.

Papaioannou D, Sutton A, Carroll C, Booth A, Wong R (2010) Literature searching for social science systematic reviews: consideration of a range of search techniques. *Health Information and Libraries Journal* **27**(2): 114–122.

Skibba DJ (2008) Emerging Technologies Center: Nursing Education 2.0: Twitter & Tweets. Can you post a nugget of knowledge in 140 characters or less? *Nursing Education Perspectives* **29**(2): 110–112.

Further reading

Aveyard H (2010) *Doing a Literature Review in Health and Social Care.* Maidenhead, Open University Press.

Booth A, Papaioannou D, Sutton A (2011) *Systematic Approaches to a Successful Literature Review.* London, SAGE.

De Brún C, Pearce-Smith N (2009) *Searching Skills Toolkit: finding the evidence.* Chichester, Wiley-Blackwell.

Guyatt G, Drummond R (eds) (2008) *Users' Guides to the Medical Literature: essentials of evidence-based clinical practice.* Chicago, AMA Press.

Hart C (2001) *Doing a Literature Search: a comprehensive guide for the social sciences.* London, SAGE.

Katcher BS (2006). *Medline: a guide to effective searching in PubMed and other interfaces.* San Francisco, Ashbury.

Ridley D (2012) *The Literature Review: a step-by-step guide for students.* London, SAGE.

CHAPTER 8

Critical Appraisal of the Evidence

Angie Rees, Claire Beecroft and Andrew Booth

Key points

- Critical appraisal is needed by researchers and practitioners to assess the validity of a research study or group of studies and whether their results can be applied to a particular situation or setting.
- Three concepts are of key importance to critical appraisal: validity, reliability and applicability.
- Checklists are available to assist with critical appraisal of both quantitative and qualitative researches and for systematic reviews.
- Ready-made critically appraised products are now available in some areas and in evidence-based health-care journals.

INTRODUCTION

Critical appraisal focuses on the practical application of research, whether it be in applying the findings of research to clinical practice or in establishing an evidence base to which our own research will add a distinctive contribution. Critical appraisal skills enable us to assess whether an individual study has particular value for us. Equally, they help us to reconcile dissonant, even conflicting, messages from different research studies. For example, one study conducted in a very selective population may show that a treatment works. A similar study in a general population may show less favourable results. Critical appraisal helps us to understand reasons for such differences and to decide which study, if any, we will use to inform our practice. Critical appraisal is equally valuable whether we have to start from scratch ourselves in assessing a research study for a new treatment or whether we wish to interpret the appraisals of others in the form of systematic literature reviews, guidelines or critically appraised topics (CATS) (Guyatt *et al.* 2000).

For a profession with a justifiable reputation for challenging 'nursing ritual', critical appraisal is a key skill. Critical appraisal of relevant research helps us to recognise ineffective procedures and to avoid an unquestioning adoption of new technologies or innovations. For example, after critically appraising

The Research Process in Nursing, Seventh Edition. Edited by Kate Gerrish and Judith Lathlean.

Companion Website: www.wiley.com/go/gerrish/research

Reflection activity

Think of a journal article about a published research study that you have read recently. How did you judge whether the study was relevant to your area of practice and how did you appraise the quality of the research that had been undertaken?

evidence supporting vitamin C in the healing of pressure sores, a dietician and information specialist were able to challenge textbook recommendations based on a 20-year-old flawed study. They were thus able to 'encourage disinvestment from an ineffective, although non-harmful, treatment in favour of spending resources on treatments for which there is at least sufficient proof of benefit' (North & Booth 1999: 243).

WHAT IS CRITICAL APPRAISAL?

Critical appraisal is 'the process of carefully and systematically examining research to judge its trustworthiness, and its value and relevance in a particular context' (Burls 2009). This definition emphasises not only the process of examining and evaluating research evidence but also questioning its applicability in a given context. This combination of skills and knowledge, while recognising the values and preferences of the individual patient, constitutes evidence-based practice – the framework within which critical appraisal sits.

A key principle of critical appraisal is that a good study usually provides enough information to help a researcher to judge that it *is* a good study. Unfortunately, the reverse is not necessarily true – the Introduction, Methods, Results and Discussion (IMRAD) structure used to present published research may make research appear superficially plausible. To help 'scratch beneath the surface', you typically use a published checklist. Many such checklists exist for different audiences or different types of study. However, checklists should focus on the actual quality of the methods and not merely on how well the study is reported. Avoid checklists that focus on factors that are external to the study itself such as 'Have you heard of the author? What qualifications do the authors have? Is the journal peer-reviewed?' The study should speak for itself! A useful critical appraisal checklist focuses on the validity, reliability and applicability of a study. These three associated concepts are central to all critical appraisal, regardless of whether the research being appraised is quantitative or qualitative or whether it is a primary study (e.g. a randomised controlled trial) or a secondary study (e.g. a systematic review). Each concept will be considered in turn.

Validity (are the results of the study valid?)

Suppose that you were to stand in the work area with a clipboard. What effect might this have on patients or colleagues? Given that even the smallest observational study can, like a pebble in a lake, disturb the 'real world', what might we expect if we design a large and complex experimental study? Clearly, we want limitations arising from our chosen research method to be outweighed by the 'trueness' of the findings. If we suspect that the picture obtained by the research no longer relates to the 'world' that we are investigating, then the study is invalid. The researchers may have based their study on flawed assumptions, there may be some inherent weakness in the study design they have chosen (bias), or they may have failed to take into account an important complicating factor (confounding).

Reliability (what are the results?)

All research results are subject to the possible effects of chance. When we measure outcomes, we want to be sure that the results are reliable. If we were to measure the same outcomes repeatedly, would we still obtain the same results? Statistical measures allow us to interpret whether the results fall within the bounds of reasonable expectation. Finally, when the variability of results from repeated measurements is taken into account, we want to be able to judge whether we would make the same decision based on the best possible result as we would when faced with the worst possible result.

Once we have established that the results are reliable, we want to ascertain whether an effect is meaningful – is it large enough to be clinically significant? For example, a study may demonstrate a change of five points on a pain scale. However, you may know from experience that a change of less than 10 points makes no difference at all to how a patient is feeling. A change of 5 points may be ***statistically significant***, but a change of 10 points or more is ***clinically significant***.

Applicability (will the results help locally?)

If the study is well designed and shows a reliable enough result, we need to consider its implications for both current clinical practice and for future research. It is helpful to separate the strength of the evidence (in terms of validity and reliability) from the strength of recommendations or action (in terms of applicability). Most practitioners will broadly agree whether a study has been designed well or a result is meaningful. However, when they come to determining whether the results can be applied locally, they will take into account available resources, the skills of involved staff and local policies and politics.

THE NEED FOR CRITICAL APPRAISAL

Critical appraisal is important for several reasons. First, the sheer volume of information available, in printed form or via the Web, means that any aspiring researcher needs to filter out unreliable lower-quality studies. Second, even the best journals can publish poor or misleading information. Even where information is of good quality, delays of up to 10 years may occur before research findings become standard practice in textbooks (Antman *et al.* 1992).

Researchers need to judge whether the study design used to conduct research makes the findings either potentially useful or unusable. If an inferior study design has been used, you may be able to examine the same research question with a more robust design. If a robust design has been used and the findings are still open to doubt, you may wish to repeat the study with a larger sample size. Finally, if the research has been conducted well and has conclusive results, you are free to concentrate on other aspects that need to be researched.

Any research study is prone to two potential flaws – bias and confounding:

> Bias is defined as a tendency which prevents unprejudiced consideration of a question. Panucci and Wilkins (2010: 21)

For example, when patients self-report whether they have given up smoking, some may convey a more positive image than is truthful. Whereas self-report is open to bias, biochemical confirmation of nicotine in their blood or saliva would be a more objective (less biased) way of establishing the facts. Confounding is where you cannot ascertain whether an effect is caused by the variable you are interested in or by another variable. For example, a study may demonstrate a link between alcohol consumption and lung cancer. However, alcohol consumption is commonly associated with smoking. Smoking is therefore a potential confounder for your study. Ideally, a researcher identifies potential confounders before they begin and then adjusts their results accordingly in the analysis. Common confounding variables are age, sex, ethnicity and co-morbidity.

Reflection activity

If a journal article is 'peer-reviewed', surely that means that it is 'good enough'. Think about how critical appraisal might add another dimension to your understanding and use of research.

VALIDITY OF RESEARCH DESIGNS

An optimal research design minimises bias and anticipates confounding. The researcher, therefore, has the responsibility to choose the best research design to

Box 8.1 The hierarchy of evidence

1. Systematic reviews and meta-analyses
2. Well-designed randomised trials
3. Well-designed trials without randomisation (e.g. single-group pre-post, cohort, time-series or matched case-controlled studies)
4. Well-designed non-experimental studies from more than one centre
5. Opinions of respected authorities based on clinical evidence, descriptive studies or reports of expert committees

answer the question that they are asking, as far as it is practicable (Bowling 2009). For example, if a researcher believes that keeping pigeons causes bird fanciers' lung, it is not ethical to randomise subjects to keep pigeons or not within a randomised controlled trial. The strongest available design would be an observational study that simply observes what the population chooses to do. A researcher selects the most appropriate research design from within a so-called hierarchy of evidence (Sackett 1986) (see Box 8.1).

This hierarchical approach has several limitations. By emphasising the study design over the features of an individual study, it gives the false impression that a poor randomised trial is better than a good observational study. Nor can it handle conflict between the findings of several observational studies and a single randomised controlled trial or a situation where randomised controlled trials are split in favour of and against the same intervention. It is more important to trade off the strength of a paper's findings against the weaknesses of its methodology than slavishly follow a hierarchy of evidence (Edwards *et al.* 1998). Alternatives to Sackett's hierarchy are being developed to take into account some of these limitations (Evans 2003).

HOW TO APPRAISE QUANTITATIVE RESEARCH STUDIES

As a researcher, you will encounter many checklists that claim to be useful when appraising different types of quantitative study. A useful checklist will only include criteria that are relevant for a given paper. For example, a clinical trial should demonstrate that it has avoided selection and observer bias and that the large majority of subjects (80% or more) are accounted for by the results. We also want to ensure that the outcomes chosen measure the right thing over the right time period. Finally, quantitative studies need large enough numbers of patients to avoid being wrong because of the random play of chance. In summary, for a quantitative paper to provide strong evidence, it must be high quality, valid and well powered.

For an individual researcher, checklists provide a framework for analysing a published article. Similarly, for the reviewer producing a systematic review or a clinical guideline, a checklist provides a standardised, explicit tool for consistently examining all articles being considered. Two main sources for checklists are the Critical Appraisal Skills Programme and the influential Users' Guides to the Medical Literature (Box 8.2).

Getting started

While every quantitative article is different, LoBiondo-Wood and Haber (2013) suggest that critical reading falls into four stages:

- *Preliminary understanding* – skimming or quickly reading to gain familiarity with the content and layout of the paper
- *Comprehensive understanding* – increasing understanding of concepts and research terms

Box 8.2 Sources of critical appraisal checklists

Critical Appraisal Skills Programme: www.casp-uk.net
Evidence Based Medicine Toolkit: www.ebm.med.ualberta.ca
Centre for Evidence-Based Medicine EBM Tools: www.cebm.net
Users' Guides to Evidence-Based Practice: http://www.cche.net/usersguides/main.asp
Guyatt G, Rennie D, Meade M, Cook D (eds) (2008) *Users' Guides to the Medical Literature: a manual for evidence-based clinical practice*, 2nd edition. Ontario, McGraw-Hill Professional.
Guyatt G, Rennie D, Meade M, Cook D (eds) (2008) *Users' Guides to the Medical Literature: essentials of evidence-based clinical practice*, 2nd edition. Ontario, McGraw-Hill Professional.

- *Analysis understanding* – breaking the study into parts and seeking to understand each part
- *Synthesis understanding* – pulling the above steps together to make a (new) whole, making sense of it and explaining relationships

Experience confirms that several practical strategies prove useful when appraising a research article. First, briefly read the abstract. Increasingly, articles use a structured abstract to make it easier to identify the study design, the participants and the intervention being studied. Pay particular attention to the main outcome measures – most studies contain multiple measurements, but you should isolate the outcome measures of importance. If the study is a randomised controlled trial, you should look for a table describing the baseline characteristics. This enables you to assess whether the experimental and controlled groups are similar at the beginning of the study. Having established a 'level playing field', you can look for a detailed description of the study design. While the Introduction, Discussion and Conclusions may inform an understanding of the issue, it is the Methods section that enables you to decide whether or not it is a good study. The Methods and Results sections should command most attention. Increasingly, randomised controlled trials present a flowchart that shows how withdrawals and dropouts are handled within the study – an outcome of the CONSORT agreement among journal editors (Begg *et al.* 1996) that dictates clearer standards of trial reporting. You should also focus on results that are considered significant (i.e. that have a p value of 0.05 or less) as these are where the research has demonstrated a measurable (and possibly important) difference.

Examples of published checklists include those for randomised controlled trials (Box 8.3), those for surveys (Box 8.4) and those for observational and epidemiological studies. Research Example 8.1 gives a sample critical appraisal of a survey.

HOW TO APPRAISE QUALITATIVE RESEARCH STUDIES

While critical appraisal of quantitative research studies is relatively well established and uncontroversial, appraisal of qualitative studies is less widely accepted. Appraisal of qualitative research can be more difficult, with even experienced researchers lacking confidence in their appraisal skills (Jeanfreau & Jack 2010). In addition, tools used for data collection (such as interviews and focus groups) seem more prone to the influence and bias of the observer. Indeed, some argue that such research does not seek a result that is replicable, and hence generalisable, but rather to provide a valid observation of an individual phenomenon.

Research into the use of checklists in appraising qualitative research suggests that it is neither desirable nor practical to select a single instrument or tool (Barbour 2001). With so many different approaches to qualitative research, one checklist might privilege, for example, grounded theory, while another might

Box 8.3 Questions for critical appraisal of a randomised controlled trial

A. Are the results valid?

1 Did the study address a clearly focused issue?
Are you able to describe the study participants, the intervention under study, the outcomes being measured and the comparison(s) being made?
2 Was the assignment of subjects to treatments randomised?
3 Were all the subjects who entered the trial properly accounted for at its conclusion?
4 Blinding: Were the subjects, workers and study personnel 'blind to the treatment'?
5 Were the groups similar at the start of the trial?
6 Aside from the experimental intervention, were the groups treated equally?

B. What are the results?

7 How large was the difference between the two groups? (Consider what outcomes were recorded and how the differences between the groups were expressed.)
8 How precise was the estimate of the treatment effects? (Hint: Look for confidence intervals.)

C. Will the results help locally?

9 Can the results be applied to your work? (How different are the subjects in the study to the population you are interested in?)
10 Were all the important outcomes considered? (Would you make a different decision if other important outcomes had been included?)
11 Are the benefits worth the harms and costs?

Box 8.4 Questions for critical appraisal of a survey

A. Are the results valid?

1 Objectives and hypotheses
- Are the objectives of the study clearly stated?

2 Design
- Is the study design suitable for the objectives?
- Who/what was studied?
- Was this the right sample to answer the objectives?
- Did the subject represent the full spectrum of the population of interest?
- Is the study large enough to achieve its objectives? Have sample size estimates been performed?
- Were all subjects accounted for?
- Were all appropriate outcomes considered?
- Has ethical approval been obtained if appropriate?
- What measures were made to contact non-responders?
- What was the response rate?

3 Measurement and observation
- Is it clear what was measured, how it was measured and what the outcomes were?
- Are the measurements valid?

- Are the measurements reliable?
- Are the measurements reproducible?

B. What are the results?

4 Presentation of results
- Are the basic data adequately described?
- Are the results presented clearly, objectively and in sufficient detail to enable readers to make their own judgement?
- Are the results internally consistent, that is, do the numbers add up properly?

5 Analysis
- Are the data suitable for analysis? Are the methods appropriate to the data? Are any statistics correctly performed and interpreted?

C. Will the results help locally?

6 Discussion
- Are the results discussed in relation to existing knowledge on the subject and study objectives?
- Is the discussion biased?
- Can the results be generalised?

7 Interpretation
- Are the authors' conclusions justified by the data? Does this paper help me answer my problem?

8 Implementation
- Can any necessary change be implemented in practice? What are the enablers/barriers to implementation?

RESEARCH EXAMPLE

8.1 Sample Critical Appraisal of a Survey

Question: What are the determinants or predictors of successful transition from being a nursing student to a registered nurse?

Phillips C, Esterman A, Smith C, Kenny A (2012) Predictors of successful transition to registered nurse. *Journal of Advanced Nursing* **69**(6): 1314–1322.

Aim

The objective of the research was to try to identify those factors that determine a successful progression for being an undergraduate student to a registered nurse and to identify if any paid work undertaken pre-registration impacted on transition.

Design and Setting

A descriptive questionnaire survey was conducted online with newly graduated nurses throughout the study setting (Australia). The **setting may be different** to our own in a variety of ways including teaching methods and employment market, **limiting the applicability** of the research.

Methods

A survey was developed from one used in an earlier study. The questionnaire was delivered online. Focus groups were used extensively during the design and testing of the survey. The survey was validated using a test–retest study. There is **reason to believe** that the survey has been **designed with care** and with effort made to test its **validity and robustness**.

Results

395 registered nurses completed the questionnaire. They were recruited over a 4-month period. All newly qualified registered nurses in their first year of practice who graduated in 2010 were targeted via the national registration body, health departments and nursing unions. Adverts for the study appeared in nursing journals with a link to the questionnaire. There is **reason to believe** that the sample is representative and has been identified **comprehensively** and with **minimal bias**.

Over half the students that completed the questionnaire had worked in a health setting in their final year of study. Transition scores were higher for students who worked (in any setting) compared with students who did not work. However, post-registration institutional work factors appeared to be stronger predictors of successful transition than pre-registration employment.

Conclusions

The results show that while pre-registration employment is **beneficial**, experience gained in the first year of post-registration employment is a **better predictor** of successful transition to registered nurse status.

be more appropriate for ethnographic studies. Nevertheless, qualitative research should still demonstrate:

- a clear aim for the project
- an appropriate methodology
- justification for the sampling strategy, that is, who was and who was not included

In addition, qualitative research should be reflexive on the possible effect that the relationship between researchers and participants might have had upon interpretation of the phenomenon. Ironically, given general mistrust of subjectivity in qualitative research, approaches to handling bias in quantitative research appear crude and formulaic by comparison.

While much is made of differences between quantitative and qualitative research, both should essentially pose and answer the same three questions:

- What is the message?
- Can I believe it?
- Can I generalise?

The recent growth in the so-called mixed methods research has made it more necessary to establish a common approach between both types of research (Gilbert 2006).

While it is clear that qualitative research has an important and expanding role within nursing research, the researcher should be aware that there remains much opposition to criteria-based approaches to appraisal. In an attempt to sidestep such objections, Dixon-Woods and colleagues (2004) have proposed a minimal set of prompts that have been designed to stimulate appraisal of different dimensions of qualitative research but are explicitly methodology neutral. They argue that any approaches to critical appraisal of qualitative studies should recognise the importance of distinctive study designs and theoretical perspectives within qualitative research. They conclude that any such approach should distinguish fatal flaws from minor errors. They further assert that:

> the more important and interesting aspects of qualitative research may remain very difficult to measure

Box 8.5 Critical appraisal checklist for a qualitative research article

A. Are the results of the study valid?

1 Was there a clear statement of the aims of the research?
Why is it important?

2 Is a qualitative method appropriate?

3 Sampling strategy
[Includes selection and purpose of sample, who was selected and why, how they were selected and why, whether the sample size is justified and why some participants may have chosen not to take part]
Was the sampling strategy appropriate to address the aims?

4 Data collection
[Includes whether it is clear why the setting was chosen, how the data were collected and why (e.g. focus group, structured interview etc.), how the data were recorded and why (e.g. tape recording, note-taking, etc.) and if the methods were modified during the process and why]
Were the data collected in a way that addresses the research issue?

5 Data analysis
[Includes a description of the analysis, how categories and themes were derived from the data, whether the findings have been evaluated for credibility and whether we can be confident that data have not been overlooked]
Was the data analysis sufficiently rigorous?

6 Research partnership relations
[Includes whether the researchers examined their own role, the setting in which data were collected and how the research was explained to participants]
Has the relationship between researchers and participants been adequately considered?

B. What are the results?

7 Findings
Is there a clear statement of the findings?

8 Justification of data interpretation
[Includes whether sufficient data are presented to sustain the findings and how the data used in the paper were selected from the original sample]
Do the researchers indicate the links between the data presented and their own findings on what the data contain?

C. Will the results help locally?

9 Transferability
Are the findings of this study transferable to a wider population?

10 Relevance and usefulness
[Includes whether the research is important and relevant in addressing the research aim, in contributing new insights and in suggesting implications for research, policy and practice]
Are the findings of this relevant and important to your patients or problems?

11 Eliciting your patient's preferences and values
Do you and your patient have a clear assessment of their values and preferences?

12 Meeting your patient's preferences and values
Are they met by this regimen and its consequences?

RESEARCH EXAMPLE

8.2 Sample Critical Appraisal of a Qualitative Research Study

Question: What are the decision-making processes used by nurses undertaking intravenous (IV) drug administration?

Dougherty L, Sque M, Rob C (2011) Decision-making processes used by nurses during intravenous drug preparation and administration. *Journal of Advanced Nursing* **68**(6): 1302–1311.

Design and Setting

Qualitative design uses participant observation and face-to-face interviews. The study took place in a single setting of a specialist cancer hospital. The qualitative design is **appropriate to answer the question** as it represents the first two phases of a research design incorporating three different qualitative data gathering methods: focus groups, observation and interviews. This design **presents the opportunity** to collect **'real-life' data** (in the observation phase) as well as **participant-reported data** (in the interview phase). This may **highlight differences** between how nurses perceive their practice and how it actually happens day to day.

Participants

20 nurses were observed in the clinical setting undertaking the preparation and administration of intravenous drugs. Afterwards, they were interviewed about their approach. This is quite a **small sample size** and a very **specific, localised** setting. This may affect the **applicability** of the research.

Methods

The first two phases of the study reported here used focus groups with a small group of 14 nurses and observation of nurses conducting IV treatment with patients. The **focus groups** were used to help the researchers **determine what constituted 'novice' and 'experienced'** IV administration, and the **observation stage** allowed the researchers to **'immerse' themselves in the ward environment** and observe the IV administration process first hand. The **methods are consistent** with the process of observational research and are **appropriate** for addressing questions regarding decision-making processes.

Main Findings

The study had three phases overall: focus groups, observation and interviews. This paper is concerned only with the observation and interview data. Themes derived from the data were:
Interruptions
Identification/knowledge of patient
Routinised behaviour
Prevention of errors

Key finding: Nurses did not always check patient's identity prior to administration of IV drugs. This was due to nurses feeling they knew the patient well and found it unnecessary.

Conclusions

The findings revealed the decision-making processes used by nurses during IV administration. Recommendations included recognising that the reasons for practitioner non-compliance with guidelines around patient checking are complex and often to do with building relationships/

trust with patients. Health-care professionals wishing to apply the findings of this research to their own practice would want to consider the **small sample size** and the fact that **all observations were recorded by just one researcher**. Also, the **behaviour** of the participants may have been **influenced** by the fact that **the researcher was (in most cases) their superior** and had **written the guidelines and policies that they were meant to be adhering to.**

> except through the subjective judgement of experienced qualitative researchers. Dixon-Woods *et al.* (2004: 225)

Box 8.5 and Research Example 8.2 show examples of how a qualitative research article might be appraised.

HOW TO APPRAISE SYSTEMATIC REVIEWS, PRACTICE GUIDELINES AND ECONOMIC ANALYSIS

So far, we have focused on single research studies, either quantitative or qualitative. However, basing research plans on the results of a single research study in isolation may prove misleading. As a researcher, you need to examine the entire body of evidence as captured by a systematic review (overview); typically, this provides a rigorous summary of all the research evidence that relates to a specific question (Engberg 2008).

Systematic reviews make strenuous attempts to overcome possible biases (see Chapter 25). They follow a rigorous methodology of search, retrieval, appraisal, data extraction, data synthesis and interpretation. To protect against possible bias explicit, preset inclusion criteria are used in selecting studies for inclusion. Similar protections are used when producing clinical guidelines. Much time and resources are expended in assuring the quality of the process by using more than one reviewer to independently select studies and by recording explicit details of methods used at every stage.

Systematic reviews focus on high-quality primary research reports in attempting to summarise research-based knowledge on a topic. Nevertheless, not every systematic review is of high quality, and critical appraisal remains essential. Box 8.6 gives guidelines on appraising a review article.

Systematic reviews are one type of research synthesis; other examples include practice guidelines and economic evaluations. These integrative studies frequently draw upon the results of systematic reviews and so share common principles for critical appraisal. Economic evaluations compare costs and consequences of different strategies, with consequences and the values attached to them frequently being generated from systematic reviews.

APPLYING THE RESULTS OF CRITICAL APPRAISAL

Reading, appraising and applying the results from research articles is a time-consuming concern. While the evidence-based health-care movement originally aspired for all practitioners to locate and appraise their own evidence, the development of numerous 'ready-to-use' critical appraisal tools has brought about the lowering of this bar (Guyatt *et al.* 2000). Now proponents suggest all practitioners should learn the skills of critical appraisal primarily to enable them to use other people's products of critical appraisal with confidence. Such products fall into one of two categories: article-based and topic-based. Article-based critical appraisal is represented by a plethora of evidence-based journals such as *Evidence-Based Nursing* and *Evidence-Based Medicine*. These summarise current journal articles in single-page summaries that present the main methodological features of each study and appraise them for likely quality. Each summary is arranged under an indicative title that captures the study's

Box 8.6 How to critically appraise review articles

A. Are the results of this systematic review valid?
1 Is this a systematic review of randomised trials?
2 Does the systematic review include a description of the strategies used to find all relevant trials?
3 Does the systematic review include a description of how the validity of individual studies was assessed?
4 Were the results consistent from study to study?
5 Were individual patient data or aggregate data used in the analysis?

B. What are the results?
1 How large was the treatment effect?
2 How precise is the estimate of treatment effect?

C. Will the results help locally?
1 Are my patients so different from those in the study that the results do not apply?
2 Is the treatment feasible in our setting?
3 Were all clinically important outcomes (harms as well as benefits) considered?
4 What are my patient's values and preferences for both the outcome we are trying to prevent and the side effects that may arise?

principal result in a clinically relevant 'bottom line'. Similarly, databases such as those from the NIHR Centre for Reviews and Dissemination at the University of York (http://www.york.ac.uk/inst/crd) provide free Internet access to article-based summaries of particular types of research synthesis, notably systematic reviews (the Database of Abstracts of Reviews of Effects (DARE)) and economic evaluations (the NHS Economic Evaluations Database (NHS EED)).

Topic-based critical appraisal is question driven, rather than literature driven. Important questions from clinical practice are identified, and specialist staff or volunteer clinicians search for answers from the research literature. Results identified from the literature are summarised and presented in a concise and meaningful summary, for example, as a CAT. Alternatively, this process may contribute to some wider publishing enterprise such as the evidence database, *Clinical Evidence* published by BMJ Publishing Group, or results posted on a website as with the Manchester-based *BestBETS* initiative (http://www.bestbets.org). Concern has been expressed over the quality of CATS – not with regard to appraisal, which is largely found to be satisfactory, but because search procedures have frequently failed to identify the most relevant items to address the clinical question (Coomarasamy *et al.* 2001). Clearly, the value of appraisal depends on first finding the most appropriate research study.

Successful application of appraisal results also assumes that the study population is similar enough to the local population. Questions such as those listed below are key when deciding whether we need to replicate research carried out elsewhere or simply to extrapolate findings from already existing research:

- Can I apply results from a study that only includes patients between 70 and 80 years old to those in the 65–70 age group?
- What about relatively fit and 'biologically young' 81-year-olds?
- Can the results of studies conducted in Edmonton, Alberta, be extrapolated to Edmonton, North London?
- Are rural practices in Finland different to those in Wales?

Reflection activity

Choose a piece of published research relevant to your area of practice, read it and reflect on its quality and usefulness. Now, identify an appropriate checklist from the resources in Box 8.2 and have a go at appraising it in a more structured way. Do you feel differently about the research paper? Has your opinion of it changed?

For the researcher, the value of pre-appraised products is twofold. Firstly, they provide a quality-fortified environment for assessing key research studies that contribute to knowledge within a particular topic area (e.g. hospital infection or hand-washing). Secondly, and more importantly, studies critically appraised by experienced researchers provide a useful benchmark against which you, as a less-experienced researcher, can chart your progress as you become more aware of methodological issues.

CONCLUSION

This chapter demonstrates the importance of critical appraisal. Researchers can use it as a quality control tool to assess individual studies. Alternatively, when reviewing multiple studies, it provides a standardised approach for producing systematic reviews and clinical guidelines. The key concepts of validity, reliability and applicability have been emphasised together with the usefulness of a checklist-led approach. Notwithstanding essential differences between quantitative and qualitative research, this chapter demonstrates the value of a common approach. Above all, the take-home message in critical appraisal is not simply a pure academic skill – it is an ongoing strategy to help you in your continuing clinical and research career.

References

Antman EM, Lau J, Kupelnick B, Mosteller F, Chalmers TC (1992) A comparison of results of meta-analysis of randomised controlled trials and the recommendations of experts. *Journal of the American Medical Association* **268**: 240–248.

Barbour RS (2001) Checklists for improving rigour in qualitative research: a case of the tail wagging the dog? *BMJ (Clinical research ed.)* **322**: 1115–1117.

Begg C, Cho M, Eastwood S, Horton R, Moher D, Olkin I, Pitkin R, Rennie D, Schulz KF, Simel D, Stroup DF (1996) Improving the quality of reporting of randomized controlled trials. The CONSORT statement. *Journal of the American Medical Association* **276**: 637–639.

Bowling A (2009) The principles of research. In: Bowling A (ed) *Research Methods in Health*. Maidenhead, Open University Press, pp 144–182.

Burls A (2009) *What Is Critical Appraisal?* Hayward Medical Communications. http://www.medicine.ox.ac.uk/bandolier/painres/download/whatis/what_is_critical_appraisal.pdf (accessed on 1 September 2014).

Coomarasamy A, Latthe P, Papaioannou S, Publicover M, Gee H, Khan KS (2001) Critical appraisal in clinical practice: sometimes irrelevant, occasionally invalid. *Journal of the Royal Society of Medicine* **94**: 573–577.

Dixon-Woods M, Shaw RL, Agarwal S, Smith JA (2004) The problem of appraising qualitative research. *Quality and Safety in Health Care* **13**: 223–225.

Edwards AG, Russell IT, Stott NC (1998) Signal versus noise in the evidence base for medicine: an alternative to hierarchies of evidence? *Family Practice* **15**: 319–322.

Engberg S (2008) Systematic reviews and meta-analysis: studies of studies. *Journal of Wound, Ostomy & Continence Nursing* **35**(3): 258–265.

Evans D (2003) Hierarchy of evidence: a framework for ranking evidence evaluating healthcare interventions. *Journal of Clinical Nursing* **12**(1): 77–84.

Gilbert T (2006) Mixed methods and mixed methodologies: the practical, the technical and the political. *Journal of Research in Nursing* **11**(3): 205–217.

Guyatt GH, Meade MO, Jaeschke RZ, Cook DJ, Haynes RB (2000) Practitioners of evidence-based care. Not all clinicians need to appraise evidence from scratch but all need some skills. *BMJ (Clinical research ed.)* **320**: 954–955.

Jeanfreau SG, Jack L (2010) Appraising qualitative research in health education: guidelines for public health educators. *Health Promotion Practice* **11**(4): 612–617.

LoBiondo-Wood G, Haber J (2013) Integrating research, evidence-based practice and quality improvement processes. In: LoBiondo-Wood G, Haber J (eds) *Nursing Research: methods and critical appraisal for evidence based practice*, 8th edition. St Louis, Elsevier Mosby, pp 5–24.

North G, Booth A (1999) Why appraise the evidence? A case study of vitamin C and the healing of pressure sores. *Journal of Human Nutrition and Dietetics* **12**: 237–244.

Panucci CJ, Wilkins EG (2010) Identifying and avoiding bias in research. *Plastic and Reconstructive Surgery* **126**(2): 619–625.

Sackett DL (1986) Rules of evidence and clinical recommendations on the use of antithrombotic agents. *Archives of Internal Medicine* **146**: 464–465.

Further reading

Ajetunmobi O (2014) *Making Sense of Critical Appraisal*, 2nd edition. London, Arnold.

Cullum N (2000) Evaluation of studies of treatment or prevention interventions (editorial). *Evidence-Based Nursing* **3**: 100–102.

Cullum N (2001) Evaluation of studies of treatment or prevention interventions. Part 2: applying the results of studies to your patients. *Evidence-Based Nursing* **4**: 7–8.

Cutcliffe J, Ward M (2007) *Critiquing Nursing Research*, 2nd edition. London, Quay Books.

Dixon-Woods M, Booth A, Sutton AJ (2007) Synthesising qualitative research: a review. *Qualitative Research* **7**: 375–422.

Greenhalgh T (2010) *How to Read a Paper: the basics of evidence based medicine*, 4th edition. Oxford, Wiley-Blackwell.

Satherley P, Allen D, Lyne P (2007) Supporting evidence-based service delivery and organisation: a comparison of an emergent realistic appraisal technique with a standard qualitative critical appraisal tool. *International Journal of Evidence-Based Healthcare* **5**(4): 477–486.

Websites

http://www.bestbets.org – This provides appraisal tool checklists to use online or download together with concise summaries of evidence on a range of clinical topics.

www.casp-uk.net – The Critical Appraisal Skills Programme provides resources and learning opportunities to support critical skills development.

www.cebm.net – The Centre for Evidence-Based Medicine provides a range of tools to promote evidence-based practice, including finding the evidence and critical appraisal.

www.sign.ac.uk/methodology/checklists.html – The Scottish Intercollegiate Guidelines Network (SIGN) provides a number of resources to support critical appraisal of different research designs.

www.tripdatabase.com – The Turning Research into Practice (TRIP) database provides a tool for identifying high-quality clinical research evidence.

CHAPTER 9 Preparing a Research Proposal

Julie Taylor

Key points

- A research proposal helps researchers to clarify their intentions and communicate these to funding bodies and committees granting ethical or research governance approval.
- A research proposal should present a reasoned argument about the need for the study, provide explicit details on how it will be carried out and clearly state the deliverables.
- A proposal should include a clear statement of the rationale for the study, the research question, the details of the methods to be used, the resources required and the methods of dissemination.
- Research methods should be appropriate to the research question(s), costed appropriately and undertaken by people who demonstrate the potential to deliver.
- The format of a research proposal will vary depending on the target audience, but all share common features.

INTRODUCTION

One of the most rewarding tasks in a researcher's life is writing a successful research proposal. It is also a task that can be the most frustrating, because writing a proposal is always time consuming and if written to seek funding to support the proposed study, it may not always be successful. However, there are a number of key principles that can be applied to preparing a research proposal and a few tactics that can increase the success rate. This chapter provides an overview of how to construct a robust research proposal, whether this is for an education programme or as an application for funding. It will address the main points that are needed in the proposal and also how to meet the requirements of the intended audience.

Research proposals are written for a number of reasons. These include:

- for a dissertation towards the end of a period of study (e.g. a master's degree)
- to undertake doctoral studies

The Research Process in Nursing, Seventh Edition. Edited by Kate Gerrish and Judith Lathlean.

Companion Website: www.wiley.com/go/gerrish/research

- to respond to a specific research or development tender
- to answer a competitive grant application call
- to seek funding for your own research idea
- to obtain research governance and research ethics approval

Although the reasons for writing a research proposal may vary, the components of a successful proposal are the same whatever the purpose. All research proposals need to be able to meet a few essential criteria; it is just a matter of scale or emphasis.

Once a proposal has been written, it will generally be subject to some form of review, for example, by supervisors or examiners, members of an independent scientific review panel or ethics committee or reviewers acting on behalf of a funding agency. Reviewers will make decisions about the quality of the proposal and in cases where funding is being sought make recommendations about whether or not the proposal should be funded.

So why may a research proposal be rejected? The main reasons are:

- poorly phrased research question
- flawed research design
- no articulation with the aims of the funder/programme/university/supervisor
- the research has been done before
- no evidence that the applicant(s) has the skills or potential to be able to deliver the work
- overambitious in terms of timescale, expected outcomes or funds
- under-ambitious for the amount of money or 'reward' being asked for
- did not respond to feedback given at an earlier stage

Even when a proposal is judged to be of a high quality, it may still be rejected because there is limited funding available and it did not score as highly as others.

Paying careful consideration to the above points when developing a proposal will enhance the likelihood of success.

IDENTIFYING A RESEARCH IDEA

One might think that identifying a research idea is easy. However, the feasibility, practicality and usefulness of ideas are another matter. Key questions to consider are the following:

- Is my idea something that can be researched?
- Is it something that could be made into a proposal?
- Is it something I could do in the time that is available?
- If I need to apply for external funding, is it an idea that would appeal to the funding body?
- If I am undertaking an education programme, is my idea likely to appeal to a potential supervisor? This is especially important with PhD proposals.

Some universities produce a list of topics or research questions that supervisors are interested in, and students may select to develop into their own project. This can be especially useful when students have to complete a research project in a relatively short period of time and can provide a close match between the student's and the supervisor's interests. Alternatively, hospitals and primary care organisations may identify research areas that merit investigation. Selecting a topic that is of interest to the organisation in which you work and which is of interest to the managers may help in securing support for the study and in disseminating the findings.

As discussed in Chapter 2, there are many sources of research questions; however, in a practice-based profession such as nursing, clinical practice is an important source of ideas. We talk a lot about evidence-based practice, but it is equally as important that nursing research is informed by practice. So what do nurses and midwives need to know that would make the patient experience better? Are there perceived gaps in knowledge that practitioners want to know about or problems they think they have to deal with unnecessarily? What do patients and carers require to be done?

> **Reflection activity**
>
> Think about your own area of practice. What do you need to know more about to improve the care provided to patients? How might these ideas be developed into a research project?

IDENTIFYING SOURCES OF FUNDING

If your research proposal is for an education programme, for example, a postgraduate qualification, funding may not be an issue, although you might want to seek funding to support some parts, for example, transcribing interview tapes. However, for most people engaged in research identifying, a source of funding is essential. With increasing financial pressures on health-care organisations and universities, the luxuries of researching a project as part of the job, just for personal satisfaction, are largely gone. Researchers need to ensure that the full costs of their proposed project are covered including, in many instances, overheads specified by their employing organisation.

Securing funding can be difficult; the requirements of funding bodies are stringent, and they will only fund applications of high quality. If this is the first time a researcher has sought funding, it is advisable to start with a relatively small and less competitive funding body, but it will still have to be a high-quality application to stand a chance of success. It is good practice to identify potential funding bodies from the outset and tailor the proposal to meet their requirements. Funding bodies are usually very clear about what they will and will not fund. There is no point submitting a proposal on educational methods for student nurses, however good it is, to a funder who is only concerned with funding clinical trials for interventions on neuromuscular disease!

It is therefore important to seek out information on possible funding bodies in order to ascertain whether your interests match those of the funder. Most organisations funding research display details on their website of the topic areas they are interested in funding together with details of projects they have funded before. There is usually a contact name, and it is often worth discussing your research interests with this person. Do you know anyone who has had success with this funder before? If so, talk to them. Do you know someone who sits on the scientific panel that will review proposals? If so, get in touch.

In the United Kingdom, there are small charities, local health service grants, professional awards, etc. that do not receive enough applications of sufficient quality each year. The funding from a particular organisation may not be much, but it may be possible to approach them to support a particular part of a project (e.g. a systematic review of the literature) and to apply to another organisation to support a different component (e.g. data collection and analysis). Additionally, two or three small-scale projects on related aspects of the same topic can be very convincing when it comes to putting in a PhD proposal or a larger grant application to pursue the topic further, especially if the findings have been published. So targeting a particular funder from the very beginning is a good strategy.

THE RESEARCH PROPOSAL

Whatever the purpose of the proposal, the main topics that need to be covered will probably be dictated by the university or funding body. These generally fall under the same main headings.

Title and summary

Research projects become known by their title, so it is important to provide a brief but accurate summary of the project. An acronym may be helpful as long as it is not too contrived. The title should give a clear indication of the purpose of the study, and it can be helpful to indicate the methodology used, for example, 'survey', 'randomised controlled trial' and 'evaluation'. For example, the titles for three recently funded proposals from the Chief Scientist Office (Scotland) (2013) are given below:

- Maternity-related outcomes in women with a diagnosis of a non-affective psychotic disorder: A data linkage study in two Scottish cohorts
- Men, masculinities, deprivation and sexual health: A qualitative study
- Geographical differences in the uptake of colorectal and breast cancer screening in Scotland

These titles all give enough information to describe the study and provide an indication of how they will be approached. And importantly, they are short and readable.

The summary that follows the title often has a specified word limit or number of characters (e.g. 150 words), so it is important to be succinct in order to ensure that all key areas relating to the proposal are covered. The summary should normally be written for a lay audience and provide an accessible overview of the focus of the study, how it will be undertaken and what the intended outcomes will be. Although the title and summary are usually written last of all, they are the first things that the reviewers will read and therefore give a strong indication of the quality of the proposal.

Background and justification of the study

Explaining why the proposed research study is important is absolutely pivotal. From my experience of reviewing proposals, it is often the flimsiest part of a proposal. There is often a misconception that the background literature can be reviewed as part of the actual study, either during the first few months of the PhD study or by a research assistant employed on a funded project.

Although an in-depth consideration of the known evidence base on the topic is usually included as part of an actual study, a research proposal needs to provide a strong case for the intended research that draws upon relevant literature. It is therefore paramount to undertake a review of key literature on the topic in order to be able to demonstrate that the proposed study is needed because there is a gap in knowledge. Chapters 7 and 8 will be particularly useful in helping to set this out clearly.

Proposals are usually sent out to reviewers who are experts in the topic area. So if I am making an argument that child neglect is under-researched on a particular aspect, I can be sure that the proposal will be sent to someone in the child protection field. I need to convince the reviewer that I have a good understanding of the main literature on the topic. In preparing the proposal, it is essential that, as a nurse, I do not restrict my initial review solely to nursing journals. The two articles on child neglect, for example, that appeared in the *Journal of Advanced Nursing* or *Journal of Clinical Nursing* this year may have been excellent, but these are not the key journals for child neglect research. So assume that the proposal will be sent to the lead researchers on this topic (who may not be nurses) and write the proposal to persuade them of the need for the research. Knowing who the lead researchers are in a field is crucial, and including their work is obvious (but oft forgotten). Venture beyond nursing journals to really contribute to nursing research.

As well as being thoroughly steeped in the literature and contemporary debates on a topic, it is also worthwhile considering the likely impact of the research on health-care policy and/or practice. Moreover, simple statistics can be used to provide a convincing argument for the research, for example, the percentage of the population who experience a particular health problem, the incidence of hospital acquired infection among a patient population or the ratio of the number of qualified to unqualified staff in a particular health-care setting.

So let us say we want to undertake a small-scale local study of student nurses' understanding of drug calculations. In order to provide a convincing case for the proposed research, we can explain how many drug errors occur each year at a local and national level; we could project the costs of these errors to the health service, to the legal system and to the trade unions, as well as the emotional impact on the nurse or the patient if errors occur. We can locate the argument in the topical patient safety agenda and expose numerous benefits on a range of levels for undertaking this research. A small-scale study cannot possibly solve all the problems, but we could make links between our small local project and the much wider political agenda. We could demonstrate that the proposed study could lead to a better understanding of the risks and to identifying potential interventions to be tested in subsequent work that may ultimately save money.

Box 9.1 identifies 10 key points that should be considered when preparing the background and rationale sections of a research proposal.

Box 9.1 Background and rationale

- Refer to key literature in the field (and if you or one of the team has written this, so much the better!).
- Make clear linkages between different theories and models.
- Summarise the main methods and findings in the field.
- Leave an impression of thoroughness and mastery on the topic.
- Succinctly describe what is already known.
- Expose the gaps in the evidence.
- Make a strong argument as to the benefits to practice, to policy and to the mission and aims of the funding body.
- Highlight the value to the health service, to users and carers and to practitioners.
- Point out the consequences of not doing this research.
- Locate the arguments in current and forthcoming priorities and concerns.
- Summarise the potential pathways to impact from the research.

Reflection activity

A number of journals publish research protocols that have been submitted by researchers while their study is underway. Reading such articles can help you to develop a better understanding of the core components of a research proposal. However, not all components of the proposal may be published (e.g. the costings), or the protocol may have been edited to comply with the journal guidelines. Use the Internet or your local library to identify a published research protocol on a topic of interest to you (Chapter 7 may be helpful in guiding your search). Having read the protocol, to what extent have the key points identified in Box 9.1 relating to the background and rationale been addressed. What other information do you require to judge whether this is a worthwhile study to undertake?

Research question and aims

The research question is arguably the most important part of a research proposal and requires careful consideration. It is important to keep the question(s) simple and concise. Ideally, the background discussion will have led directly to the question, demonstrating a lack in current knowledge and why this is a worthwhile area of study. It is also acceptable to have more than one research question, although the design will need to demonstrate that these can all be answered.

Rather than research questions, or indeed in addition to these, you may prefer to describe the aims and objectives. This is a matter of style, but it may be a requirement of the target audience for the proposal. The same principles apply: research aims and objectives need to be clear and precise. Clearly articulating a research question/aim that comes directly from what has been found missing in the literature review and can be investigated is crucial.

The design (or plan of investigation)

At this point in the proposal, the study area should be clear; a good case will have been made for it; and there is a well-constructed question that clearly states the focus of the proposed study. The design of the study (sometimes referred to as a plan of investigation) should then follow. Chapter 2 provides an overview of the main issues to consider in designing a research study. This includes identifying a suitable research methodology (quantitative or qualitative), the methods of data collection and analysis and an appropriate sample. It is essential that the research methodology is selected to address the research question rather than the other way round. A researcher may have a personal preference for undertaking qualitative research, but it is wholly inappropriate to use a qualitative approach to investigate a research topic that requires a quantitative design, for example, investigating the effectiveness of a particular intervention. Use quantitative methods to answer quantitative questions and qualitative methods to answer qualitative questions. Mixed methods may be helpful if the research question has elements of both approaches (see Chapter 27 for more detail on this approach).

The research design should:

- demonstrate clearly how the research questions will be answered
- describe and justify the proposed sample
- explain how the research participants will be identified, approached and recruited to the study
- provide a robust account of how data will be collected and analysed

Chapter 13 provides an overview of factors that should be considered in identifying the sample for both quantitative and qualitative studies. In quantitative studies, for example, a clinical trial, power calculations may be undertaken to ascertain the correct sample size, but if power calculations are inappropriate, then it is still important to justify the proposed sample size in some other way. The advice of a statistician can be usefully sought at this stage.

Although it can be against the ethos of qualitative research to specify a precise sample size in advance, some indication of the number of research participants will need to be provided. This is in order to demonstrate that sufficient data will be collected to answer the research question and that the proposed data collection and ensuing analysis are feasible within the timescale of the study and funding available.

An account should also be provided of the proposed methods of data collection, justifying their inclusion and explaining how they will be carried out. For example, in undertaking a survey, it will be important to state whether an existing validated questionnaire will be used and, if so, to justify its appropriateness for the proposed study. Alternatively, if a new questionnaire is to be developed for the project, an explanation needs to be provided as to how it will be developed, piloted and validated. Likewise, in an interview-based qualitative study, the choice of methods needs to be justified and an explanation provided as to how the interviews will be conducted, including venue, means of recording, etc. Of course, collecting primary data may not be appropriate for the proposed study. Great use can be made of existing reliable datasets and undertaking a secondary analysis of these or of undertaking systematic reviews and other methodical analyses of policies, guidelines or scientific literature. The justification of the method, whatever that is, is the key component.

This section of the proposal also needs to take account of how data will be analysed, by whom, using which methods and at what point in the timeline. It is important to provide as much clarity as possible. It is not sufficient to say that data will be analysed using SPSS v22. What tests will be undertaken using SPSS? Is the appropriateness of such tests demonstrated? Chapters 35 and 36 introduce the reader to statistical analysis; however, it can be useful to involve a statistician at this point to help write this section of the proposal. Clarity regarding the analytic methods used for qualitative research is also required. It is not enough to suggest that themes will be derived from the transcripts. How will this happen? Using what tools and techniques? The analytic methods need to be clearly described and reference made to appropriate frameworks for analysis. Chapter 34 provides an overview of different approaches to qualitative data analysis.

The plan of investigation should clearly demonstrate that every part of the research process has been carefully thought through. Box 9.2 provides 10 areas that should be considered.

Box 9.2 The plan of investigation

- Will the methods answer the questions?
- Is the sample size defined?
- Is access to the population clear (and even agreed)?
- How will participants be recruited and incentivised?
- How will you deal with gatekeepers?
- How will the data collection be undertaken, and by whom?
- What tools will be used for data collection?
- Are there examples of these tools (e.g. questionnaire, interview schedule)?
- Is the timeline clear and feasible?
- How will the data be analysed? By whom? When?
- What feedback will be given to participants and funders and at what stages?
- What are the likely outputs of the research?

Reflection activity

Use the 12 areas that need to be considered in a plan of investigation listed in Box 9.2 to appraise the published research protocol you have identified in the previous reflection activity. To what extent have each of these points been addressed? What information is missing or needs to be developed further? What other information do you require to judge whether this is a robust study?

The research team and project management

If writing a proposal for an education programme, the research 'team' will comprise primarily the student. However, when applying for research governance and ethical approval, the proposal will need to include details of the student's supervisor as approval bodies consider the supervisor (as the more experienced researcher) to have overall responsibility for the research project. Chapter 10 provides guidance on identifying an appropriate supervisor.

If funding is being sought for the proposal, the composition of the research team will be crucial. The lead applicant (usually known as the chief investigator or principal investigator (PI)) should have the experience, reputation and previous research success to give the proposal stature. Of course, everyone has to be PI for a first time, but the PI should still have a reasonable publication record in the field, and if they do not have a track record of successful grant capture, there should be more senior people on the team who can offer support. Crucially, the composition of the research team needs to convince the funder of the experience and expertise to deliver the grant successfully. Usually, this means that one or two people have had previous successes, preferably with the same funder or at least a similar one. The best way to get this experience is to be a co-applicant on some proposals first. Funders are cautious and will be more inclined to fund studies undertaken by people who they consider are most likely to deliver.

The members of the team should provide complementary expertise. The curriculum vitae of each team member (which usually have to be provided as part of the submission) should demonstrate the range of experience in both the topic area and the proposed methods. There should be no glaring gaps in the expertise of the team. If the team (or some combinations within the team) have worked together before, so much the better.

Approaching senior people (who you want to be part of the research team) can be daunting. However, if it is a good research idea and a well-formed proposal, they may well be willing to participate. With a large team, it is important to gain agreement before submission on exactly what and how much everyone will be doing. The PI will have overall responsibility for the management of the project, but individual duties, tasks and areas of responsibility should all be articulated. Contracts of employment should be agreed with relevant human resource departments before commencement, as should agreement about office space and equipment. If there are likely to be issues relating to intellectual property rights (IPR), these should be discussed with the research contracts team at the researcher's place of employment.

Ethical considerations

A research proposal needs to include an account of the main ethical issues associated with undertaking the project and explain how these will be addressed. In the United Kingdom, it is almost certain that ethical approval will be required from either the National Research Ethics Service (NRES) or from another appropriate body (e.g. the university research ethics committee). Chapter 3 introduces the reader to the main ethical issues that need to be considered in developing a proposal, and Chapter 11 outlines the mechanisms required to gain ethical approval for health research in the United Kingdom. The application form for seeking approval from a NHS Research Ethics Committee is extensive, and there are potential benefits to starting to complete the application alongside developing the research proposal. The questions asked on the ethics application form may help the researcher select scientifically sound as well as ethically appropriate methods. The ethical application can then be held on file and submitted once funding has been secured.

Value for money

Reviewers of funded research proposals are always asked to consider whether a study represents good value for money and will weigh up the costs of the study against the likely outputs. Contrary to popular opinion, this is not only whether people have asked for too much but also if they have asked for too little!

All costs will need to be justified, and fortunately, universities and NHS Research Departments provide help with this aspect. Indeed, proposals normally have to be signed off by an appropriate finance officer prior to submission to a funding body.

Salaried time is usually the largest expense incurred. Is the research assistant employed at the appropriate rate? Costs may have been kept low, but the study may require someone on a higher salary scale because of the nature of the work. Employing someone full-time for 2 years to undertake 10 interviews and a focus group is unlikely to be seen as good value. Conversely, is the proposal realistic in how much time is likely to be needed? Are the associated travel, consumables and equipment fully costed? Table 9.1 identifies the main points that need to be considered when costing a research proposal.

Dissemination and knowledge exchange

The dissemination plan requires careful consideration in order to demonstrate to the reviewers how the research team plan to share their findings with research participants and potential users of the research. Funders are increasingly looking for innovative and targeted means of dissemination that take account of practitioners, academics, patients and carers, policymakers and the public. As outlined in Chapter 37, although journal articles and conference presentations are common forms of dissemination, researchers would do well to consider other avenues. For example, research websites, 'good practice' leaflets or stakeholder events are worth considering. Funders

Table 9.1 Preparing the budget

Description	Explanation	Justification
Human resource	Salary costs of those employed; the time of those who are applicants if this is allowable; on-costs (national insurance, superannuation). The finance office will help, but it is the applicant's job to estimate as accurately as possible how much time everyone is going to spend on the study. This section should also include administrative or secretarial support.	What exactly will people be doing with that time? Does the study really need an administrator as well as two research nurses? Highlight the exact scope of work for each person.
Data collection	The costs that will be incurred by the study, such as travel expenses, meeting venues, catering costs for steering group members, participant incentive vouchers, equipment, postage, photocopying, etc.	Check what is allowed. Do not ask for equipment that is provided as standard in your place of work.
Data processing	There may be costs associated with entering data into SPSS or transcribing costs.	Do not double count: these may be covered under human resource.
Dissemination and knowledge exchange	Include the costs of stakeholder events, booklet production, conference attendance, etc.	Check what is allowed. Many funders will not support conference attendance, but they might support the costs of open-access publishing.
Miscellaneous	Will there be a cost for interlibrary loans or books? What printing, consumables and product development costs will be incurred?	Think through every stage of the research, and if it is going to cost something, put it in.
Overheads	There is always a cost for lighting, heating, office space, insurances, etc. Do you have permission to waive this if the funder does not pay?	In UK universities, the use of 'full economic costing' (FeC) means that 'overheads' is no longer in common usage. Some funders have agreed to pay up to 80% of the costs of a study to cover the 'actual' costs of research. It is complicated, but the finance office will help. You need to check what the funder will cover.

increasingly are giving high weightings to a dissemination plan as they seek assurance that the studies they fund have the potential for wide impact. The Research Excellence Framework in the United Kingdom and its equivalent in a number of countries are measuring the impact of research undertaken in universities – the influence the research has had beyond academia. This could be in policy, economics, culture, society more generally and so forth. An integrated knowledge exchange plan articulated at the beginning of a proposal – and costed appropriately – is likely to attract more funding points than one that sees dissemination as something that is added at the end.

Reflection activity

Review the published research protocol you identified in the previous reflection activity. To what extent have the researchers outlined a dissemination plan? Are the people who might use the findings (e.g. practitioners, managers, patients) likely to be made aware of the research? How might the researchers further develop their dissemination plan to maximise awareness of their findings?

User involvement

The time has gone (thankfully) when research was undertaken on patients or other service users, and they were then possibly told about what was found at the very end. As Chapter 5 has demonstrated, patients/service users and carers should be involved in every part of a study. A well-constructed proposal will demonstrate how public engagement has informed the development of the proposal and how they will be involved in the study itself. There is a fine line between tokenism and active participation. Reviewers will be seeking evidence that where claims are made for user involvement, it is meaningful and has been articulated clearly.

SUBMISSION REQUIREMENTS

Before spending hours writing a proposal, it is important to check the requirements of the funding body. When does the proposal have to be submitted, by which date, electronically or in hard copy or both, how many copies, and whose signatures need to be secured? These small bureaucratic details can be enormously time consuming and can unravel everything right at the end. It is worth trying to get everything into place as early as possible. The rules for each submission will be slightly different, but one thing is certain: if the deadline is 12 noon on Tuesday, then it must not be 4 pm Wednesday! If the proposal can be a maximum of 8 pages in font size 12, then 10 pages in font size 6 will be discarded. Whereas it might be possible to adjust the margin width, most reviewers do not want to read a tightly condensed proposal with a magnifying glass! If not specified in the submission requirement, use a plain font (e.g. Arial or Verdana) and a font size of at least 10.

Even with excellent organisational skills, collating signatures can be a challenging undertaking. For larger grants, it is not unusual to require all the applicants' signatures and those of their respective line managers. This is not too problematic, but then you may also need the signature of the research sponsor (usually the head of the research services department in your organisation) who will not sign until she/he has read and understood the full proposal, the financial manager (who will not sign until all costings have been approved), the head of the NHS research and development office (who may not sign until the others have signed) and possibly various other people as well. It is worth alerting such individuals to the timescales and proposal development as early as possible, finding out what they will require to be in place before they sign and checking when and where they will be available. This all needs to be completed before final copies of the proposal are made and posted.

Most successful researchers will have had problems at this stage: mine include having to drive the submission over to another city at 4 am to deliver by hand or racing around in a taxi to gather disparate signatures from across the region because I overlooked the fact that every applicant had to complete an individual equal opportunities form. So the key message is to check the rules of submission and do not wait until the last minute. If you have not followed the rules exactly, you will be giving the supervisor/committee/funder the message that you are not reliable or careful and that you cannot follow instructions. This is not a message likely to help you on your way to success. Box 9.3 suggests 10 points to consider before submission for a grant application for funding.

MAXIMISING SUCCESS

Even experienced researchers are not always successful in seeking funding for their proposals. Having a proposal turned down after all the hard work that has gone into the development is very disappointing and frustrating. It can be very difficult to pick yourself up when this happens, and the temptation is to discard the proposal. But while there are lots of reasons why proposals are not accepted, very few proposals are worth discarding altogether. It is always worth taking some time to reflect on the reasons why it was turned down and then trying again in a modified way, possibly with an application to a different funding body. It is a

Box 9.3 Checklist for final submission

- Date and time of submission.
- Number of copies required and in which format – paper or electronic.
- All signatures have been obtained.
- Costings have been signed off by the relevant department(s).
- All applicant CVs are complete and in the required format.
- All additional forms required from the applicants have been completed and signed.
- Word limits have been checked for each section (if applicable).
- Font sizes and types and line spacing have been adhered to, and the proposal is easy to read.
- Accompanying letter written by principal investigator (either introducing the study or responding to earlier feedback).
- Arrangements for posting/courier/hand delivery are in place.

fact of life that more proposals will be rejected than are ever accepted. The acceptance rates of the larger research councils run at about 25%, and this is probably average for many other funders. This means that for every four proposals written by an experienced researcher, three are likely to be rejected. For novice researchers, this rate is likely to be higher, so the effort–reward ratio in proposal writing is fairly imbalanced. However, the satisfaction that comes from having a grant accepted is perhaps worth the disappointments.

Proposals may not be rejected outright, and the reviewer may provide guidance on how the proposal might be further developed. Because of the personal investment that has gone into developing the research proposal, it may be tempting to ignore the advice and stick to the original ideas. This kind of behaviour rarely pays off, and on the whole, it is well worth responding to feed back from reviewers – even if you submit to a different funder. A proposal submitted after a response to feedback will almost certainly be enhanced. Of course, there may be some aspects of disagreement, or it may appear that the reviewer had not fully understood some aspects of the proposal. Clarifying these points in a revised proposal and sending an accompanying letter in which you indicate that you have given careful consideration to the reviewer's comments and explaining why you may not have addressed some of the concerns will often satisfy the funding body.

CONCLUSION

This chapter has charted the journey through writing a research proposal. The overall message is that the proposal needs to be written clearly, fit for purpose, robust and explicit. While there is no easy way of preparing a proposal, there are various strategies that can be employed to increase the quality of the proposal. Working with more experienced researchers is an extremely useful way to begin. Although some of the bureaucratic detail required can be off-putting, there should be people available to help with this side, and engaging them from the beginning will maximise success. Resilience is key and to learn through the process – even when a proposal is turned down for funding.

Well-constructed proposals using appropriate methods for the research question are generally successful. We owe it to our professional identity and reputation to make sure nurses submit high-quality, appropriately argued, well-constructed research proposals. If nursing is to truly make a difference to clinical practice, then rigorous research proposals that extend our knowledge and evidence base are essential.

References

Chief Scientist Office (2013) *Outputs*. NHS Scotland. http://www.cso.scot.nhs.uk/outputs/ (accessed 26 March 2014).

Further reading

Aldridge J, Derrington A (2012) *The Research Funding Toolkit: how to plan and write successful grant applications*. Los Angeles, SAGE.

Denicolo P, Becker L (2012) *Developing Research Proposals (success in research)*. Los Angeles, SAGE.

Denscombe M (2012) *Research Proposals: a practical guide*. Maidenhead, Open University Press.

Evans C (2013) *How to Write a Research Proposal (a learning booklet)*. APA, e-book Amazon Kindle. ASIN B00B6RLUSC (accessed 9 September 2014).

Offredy M, Vickers P (2010) *Developing a Healthcare Research Proposal: an interactive student guide*. Chichester, Wiley-Blackwell.

Phillips EM, Pugh DS (2010) *How to Get a PhD*, 5th edition. Buckingham, Open University Press.

Trowler P (2012) *Writing Doctoral Project Proposals: higher education research*. APA, e-book Amazon Kindle. ASIN B008UYT5V7 (accessed 9 September 2014).

Websites

http://www.rdinfo.org.uk/Welcome.aspx – R&D funding provides an overview of all stages of the research process, with useful sections on writing a successful proposal. You will need to register (free) to use the site.

http://www.esrc.ac.uk/funding-and-guidance/applicants/how-to.aspx – The Economic and Social Research Council (ESRC) offers useful advice on writing a good proposal.

http://www.mrc.ac.uk/documents/pdf/guidance-for-applicants-and-award-holders/ – The Medical Research Council (MRC) applicant handbook provides detailed advice on how to apply for an MRC grant, information that is useful more broadly.

http://grants.nih.gov/grants/funding/424/index.htm – The main health funder in the United States offers very detailed help and guidance. Download some example proposals to see a commentary on how it all fits together.

CHAPTER 10 Planning and Managing a Research Project

Carol A. Haigh

Key points

- Various resources are available to enable the research student to identify and find funding for their study.
- Academic support is crucial to the success of the research study. Students need to be aware of:
    - how to choose a supervisor
    - what to expect from a supervisor
    - what a supervisor will expect from the research student
- Sources of emotional and peer support need to be identified and used appropriately.

INTRODUCTION

For many research students, finding funding for their studies is the first hurdle they have to overcome for their educational advancement. Students need to be aware of how to identify and secure various sources of funding. However, funding is only one aspect of the support necessary to undertake a research study. The supervisor–student role is crucial to the successful completion of a research dissertation or thesis and cannot be taken for granted. Both supervisor and student need to understand how to get the most out of the supervisor–student relationship by being clear from the outset about expectations, roles and responsibilities. This chapter offers practical advice on how to identify and secure the necessary funding resources and ensure appropriate supervisory, peer and emotional support to ensure success.

IDENTIFYING AND FINDING FUNDING

One of the first challenges facing the research student is how to fund their study. Some employers are open to the idea of supporting students to undergraduate level; however, support for higher levels of study can

The Research Process in Nursing, Seventh Edition. Edited by Kate Gerrish and Judith Lathlean.

Companion Website: www.wiley.com/go/gerrish/research

be harder to obtain. There are several funding bodies that provide financial support for individuals' undertaking advanced study. Some of these may be disease specific such as the Parkinson's Disease Society, which will provide scholarships for nurses undertaking higher-level studies in Parkinson's disease, and there are other similar schemes run by medical charities and professional organisations such as the Royal College of Nursing.

One way of finding funding opportunities is to sign up for e-mail alerts from funding databases such as Postgraduate Studentships (http://www.postgraduatestudentships.co.uk/?gclid=COTxwon21rgCFSGWtAodWhoANQ), which provides scholarship information for researchers in the field of health and social care. Other professional groups or disciplines, such as the Economic and Social Research Council (http://www.esrc.ac.uk/funding-and-guidance/postgraduates) for social policy research, offer similar schemes. Many universities subscribe to the ResearchResearch website (http://www.researchresearch.com), which allows you to search for funding by discipline, by country and by programme/level. There are a number of other such sites, and inserting the search term 'research student funding' into any Internet search engine will bring them up. In addition, UK research scholarships for master's, doctoral and postdoctoral studies are offered by the seven Research Councils, all of whom offer doctoral and postdoctoral fellowships in their associated disciplines, and by the National Institute for Health Research.

For UK students wishing to study overseas or for international students wishing to study in the United Kingdom, there are a number of fellowships run by organisations such as the British Council (http://www.britishcouncil.org/higher-education/uk-students-abroad/funding-grants-and-scholarships) or the Fulbright Commission (http://www.fulbright.co.uk). UK universities occasionally offer scholarships for overseas students, and these are advertised in the UK press and on websites such as the previously mentioned Postgraduate Studentships.

Be aware that if you are planning to apply for a scholarship or funding for training from a specific funding body, timelines are usually quite tight. If you have already selected the institution in which you plan to study and especially if you already have a

Reflection activity

Why is seeking financial support for postgraduate research activity becoming increasingly important? Use the Internet to identify some funding bodies that might be approached to fund the type of research you are interested in undertaking. What can you learn about the process of applying for funding from the details provided on the websites?

contact in that institution, it might be a good idea to involve the programme leader or your potential doctoral supervisor in any scholarly funding bid. Not only will this give you the advantage of having an experienced mentor to help with the bid, but it will indicate to funding bodies that you have identified a research mentor and a host organisation in which to carry out your research activity. Indeed, some funders expect the application to come from the supervisor rather than the student, so you need to be clear about who can actually apply before you start. Competition for studentships and fellowships is fierce, so you need a well-crafted project that makes a clear contribution to your discipline.

ACADEMIC AND PRACTICAL SUPPORT

Most students, at any academic level, find the thought of completing the dissertation or thesis a challenging one. A suitable supervisor and a clear understanding of the roles and expectations of both parties in the supervisory relationship can go some way to making the preparation and production of a dissertation or thesis achievable and fulfilling.

How to choose a supervisor

The relationship between a research student and their supervisor is one that develops over time as the student progresses through the different levels of academic study. The roles of both student and supervisor change over time; as the student acquires more knowledge, they will require different things from their supervisor, and the supervisor, in turn, has different expectations of the student (Ward 2013). It is appropriate at this point to explore what these needs and expectations are before examining the student–supervisor relationship in greater detail.

Undergraduate supervision

Generally, at undergraduate level, the relationship is very much that of a student and teacher. The student is starting out on the research path and can be seen as a novice seeking support and direction from a more experienced colleague. At this stage, the student is often allocated a supervisor and expected to make contact with them.

The main advantage of this approach is that the student, who may have little or no insight into the practicalities of the research process, is spared the stress of selecting someone to support them by an educationalist that has a good overview of the research skills and interests of the university staff and can match students up with supervisors who will be best placed to help them through the process. The two main disadvantages are, first, that students may be allocated a supervisor based upon their research topic rather than their approach. This may result in the student being supervised by a subject specialist who may have little expertise in the chosen research methodology. It is unfortunate when this scenario occurs because undergraduate research is often designed to introduce the student to research methods and processes that can be used in a wider context than in a confined, specific disciplinary field. It can also present a challenge if the student is choosing to explore a methodology that is not widely used in their specific field. For example, person-centred disciplines such as counselling tend to used person-centred research methods, so the student who wishes to undertake a randomised controlled trial in that area may struggle to find a supervisor with the relevant experience.

In addition, undergraduate students are usually only allocated one person to supervise their study, and this can present difficulties if the relationship is not an amiable one. Undergraduate students are generally unaware that they have any influence in the selection of supervisors; it is not inappropriate for students to approach academic staff with supervision requests, although it is sensible to select such staff on their suitability rather than their personality. If a student wants to change supervisors, they should negotiate this with the undergraduate research tutor who may be able to help. It is never in the student's interest to simply disregard their supervisor, no matter how difficult the relationship or the synchronisation of diaries for tutorial time.

Postgraduate supervision

As with undergraduate research, there is some element of pedagogy in the student–supervisor relationship at postgraduate level. In the United Kingdom, the impact that the research governance system had on timescales for research approval led to universities making changes to undergraduate dissertations such that master's level may be the first time the student has attempted a research project. So there needs to be a strong element of educational input from the supervisor. However, at postgraduate level, particularly in the health-care professions, a degree of professional expertise can be assumed, and it is therefore, potentially, more useful to the student to have a supervisor with research rather than clinical expertise.

The relationship between doctoral student and supervisor is different from any other supervision relationship to which the student may have been exposed. The pedagogy of undergraduate and master's level supervision is subsumed by a partnership approach to project management in which it is as acceptable to challenge as to be challenged by your supervisor.

TYPES OF SUPERVISOR

Work carried out by Trocchia and Berkowitz (1999) suggests that there are four main categories of supervisor and supervision:

1 Nurturing – In this relationship, the student obtains a great deal of help and support from

their supervisor and other members of the faculty. Supervision tends to be formal and directive.

2 Top-down – Similar to the formal nurturing role with the exception that the student is expected to show more signs of independent self-management.
3 Near peers – This model is best suited to those students who value a high degree of independence in the direction of their study but who appreciate having access to their supervisor within a relationship of collegial equality.
4 Platonistic – Can be summed up in the phrase 'go away, do something, come back when it's good'. Students who benefit most from a platonistic supervisor are those who are extremely self-motivated and individualistic.

It can be seen that different supervision styles are appropriate at different academic levels and for different study styles; Meyer-Parsons (2011) argues that such categories are still relevant for today's research student. A supervisor's supervision style is something a student may wish to consider when selecting an academic mentor to support them through their research process. Standards for postgraduate student supervision in the United Kingdom are outlined by the Quality Assurance Agency for Higher Education (2012), and most universities base their own guidelines and regulations upon them across all of the academic levels.

SUPERVISION SELECTION CRITERIA

At postgraduate and doctoral level, students will find that they have some input into the make-up of the supervisory team. Ellis (2006) and Lee (2008) have suggested the following criteria that students should consider when selecting a supervisor:

- Find a supervisor who is knowledgeable in their field. Whether methodologically focused or subject specific, it is not inappropriate to expect potential supervisors to be fully conversant with the topic or methods to be used.
- Expect to have or find a supervisor who understands the nature of master's or doctoral work. Any supervisor involved should be familiar with the standards expected of students studying at these specific levels.
- The potential supervisor should have enough time for meetings. Sometimes, this can only be assessed once the student–supervisor relationship has been established, but a simple rule of thumb is that students should expect to have at least an undisturbed hour of their supervisor's time.
- Find someone with whom you can get on. For doctoral students, the relationship with their supervisor will last at least 3 years and even longer for part-time students, so it is important that the association is founded upon mutual regard. Life can be very difficult for both student and supervisor if that regard is absent.

THE RESPONSIBILITIES OF THE SUPERVISOR

As has already been emphasised, the relationship between supervisor and doctoral student is very different from other supervisory relationships. For the relationship to be a success, the expectations of both parties should be made clear at the start.

At the earliest point of the relationship, negotiation is of key importance. A wise supervisor will use initial meetings to ensure that supervision arrangements and the role of progress meetings are clear and agreed. At undergraduate and master's level, when students are working to a strict time schedule, the supervisor may expect such meetings to be regularly scheduled. However, doctoral students have the luxury of more time for the completion of their study, so some supervisors may be more flexible and less prescriptive about contact (Phillips & Pugh 2010).

In the early stages of research, particularly at undergraduate but often at higher levels as well, the student can feel as if they are drifting because they may have an idea of what they wish to study, but not concrete plans as to how to collect information. In these cases, the supervisor may be able to assist in the planning and operation of a realistic plan of research and provide guidance about literature.

Although, at undergraduate and at master's level, the dissertation is the end point of a programme of study – the task that draws all previous work into a coherent whole – one of the defining characteristics of doctoral study is the expectation that the candidate will develop and enhance research skills throughout the process. To this end, a good supervisor will provide an example of good research and academic conduct, arrange instruction in research techniques and supplementary classes as required and support access to doctoral training programmes on offer. They can also encourage integration with the wider academic community via conferences and seminars.

One of the biggest challenges for students who are undertaking health-care research is the requirement to obtain ethical approval from an ethics review committee, and, in the United Kingdom, this is further complicated by the need to obtain research governance approval as well. All students will be expected to obtain ethical approval for their study from the university; however, students whose research includes patients recruited via the NHS will also need approval from an NHS Research Ethics Committee. At this point, supervisors and students should also discuss the personal safety of the student throughout the research process and to delineate lone-worker policies or strategies, if appropriate. Students should expect help with ethical approval, risk assessment and governance forms and for supervisors to attend research ethics committee meetings. Ethics committees appreciate it when supervisors attend to support their students, as do most students. Chapter 11 provides more detail of the processes involved in securing ethical approval.

Supervisors have a significant role to play in monitoring the standard of the work produced and the student's progress. This includes ensuring that the appropriate documents and milestones are met in order for the student to progress. At doctoral level, the supervisor has a responsibility to make sure that the student understands the nature and process of thesis examination; for many students, this can include setting up practice viva voce events. The thought of the viva is one that many doctoral students dread. The challenges of the examination can to some extent be obviated by careful selection of examiners, and the supervisor has a key role in this respect. The recruitment of and liaison with examiners is the sole responsibility of the supervisor, as is approving submission of the finished thesis. Students should be aware that, even though the supervisor approves the thesis for submission, final approval of the thesis is a matter for the examiners and not the supervisor.

What supervisors should do to keep students happy

While the practical element of the supervisory role clearly helps to facilitate the student's progress, there are several things that a supervisor can do to promote peace of mind in their supervisees:

Set clear goals. The first meeting of any supervisory relationship is the most crucial since it is the one at which the tone and direction of all future meetings will be set. Clear outlines of the roles, requirements and expectations can be discussed and agreed by all parties. It is crucial that the student is clear on what is expected of them and what they can expect of the supervisor if the relationship is to flourish.

Be prepared for supervisory meetings. Supervisor and students should view supervision sessions with the same degree of importance. For the supervisor, this means ensuring that work that the student has submitted for the session has been read thoroughly and critiqued and, if necessary, feedback prepared. It is also a good idea to review the notes made at the previous meeting to ensure that there are no outstanding tasks for the supervisor to complete before the next meeting.

Answer e-mails. One of the biggest criticisms levelled at supervisors by their students is the dilatory nature of e-mail response. Even a simple response acknowledging receipt of the student's work and providing a timetable for a more detailed response will help to make the student happy.

Be available to attend seminars, local research ethics committees, etc. to support the student. One of the crucial sources of support that a supervisor can offer is to be present at some of the presentations or professional encounters that students will undertake at various stages of their programme of study. It can be very comforting to a student to have their supervisor present when they give their first conference presentation, for example, if only to field some of the challenging questions that are often posed to novices on the conference circuit (Haigh 2007).

It is also very important that the supervisor makes every effort to attend the local research ethics committee with the student. Although generally ethics committees are sympathetic to student research, especially at undergraduate and postgraduate levels, doctoral students are regarded as researchers first and students second. Having their supervisor with them can provide much needed confidence and support and also shows the ethics committee that the student is adequately supervised.

Be there at all of the important milestone events – especially the viva. As a student progresses through postgraduate and doctoral studies, there are various points of assessment that require the reassuring presence of the supervisor. Different educational institutions manage these in different ways, but the one event that the supervisor must not miss is the PhD viva. Although the supervisor is not often permitted to participate in the viva process, merely having them in the room, taking notes on the proceedings, is a source of tremendous support for the student.

In summary, whether at undergraduate, postgraduate or doctoral level, the supervisor is there to help support and guide the student to a greater or lesser degree. The relationship develops and changes across the academic levels, but students should remember that a fundamental part of the supervisor's role is to support them throughout the process.

Reflection activity

Why is it important for a student to have a clear idea of what the role of the supervisor will be throughout the research project? Educational institutions often provide guidance for supervisors on fulfilling their role. Locate any guidance produced by your own organisation in order to gain an understanding of the support you might expect from your supervisor. Use this guidance to identify any issues you want to discuss with your supervisor.

THE RESPONSIBILITIES OF THE STUDENT

The previous section clearly delineates the responsibilities of the supervisor. However, it must be acknowledged that the supervisor–supervisee relationship is two-way with the student having a significant part to play. It may seem self-evident to suggest that the student should undertake to study conscientiously and at a level appropriate to the research degree. However, this is a fundamental student responsibility. It is not appropriate for the student to interpret the supervisory relationship as one in which they only do what the supervisor suggests or, an even worse-case scenario, they expect the supervisor to do the majority of the work.

It is incumbent on the student to seek the advice and constructive criticism of the supervisor. In many cases, with the exception of doctoral study, the supervisor is involved in marking the finished work, and it is therefore sensible to listen to the suggestions they make. Having said that, it is also important to remember that it is *your* study, so do not allow your supervisor to sidetrack your project if you do not feel it is an appropriate or fruitful direction in which to go.

It is in the student's best interest to attend regular supervisory meetings. This can be difficult if the study is being undertaken on a part-time basis, especially as many health-care students have to fit their studies around the demands of the clinical environment. If it has been difficult to make contact with supervisors or keep appointments and some time has elapsed since the last meeting, students sometimes feel reluctant to make contact. However, most supervisors will be pleased to hear from their student no matter how much time has gone by and will understand the pressures inherent in balancing study with clinical practice. It is important that students do not lose contact with supervisors or allow themselves to 'drift' simply because they are too embarrassed to get in touch. At all levels of study, there is an obligation on the student to undertake to submit their finished dissertation or thesis within the scheduled registration period, and doctoral students will be expected to attend research training provided by the supervisor or the research institute – regular contact with supervisor(s) will facilitate this.

Every university has a number of milestones within the dissertation/thesis route that are designed to assess progress. These milestones tend to be more formalised at the doctoral level. The doctoral student will be expected to work with the supervisor to meet all important milestones, producing any written work expected to deadline and to a suitable standard. Participation in formal progression meetings is another useful source of support, since they often provide an opportunity for a student's work to be scrutinised by people who are external to the supervisory team. This brings the advantage of a new perspective to the work.

The opportunity to integrate with the wider academic community is one that is more likely to be offered to postgraduate and doctoral students than to undergraduates. However, most undergraduate students can expect to be called upon to undertake presentations to their peers at some point in their programme of study. Although this can seem daunting, and even experienced presenters often find it easier to present to strangers rather than peers, it is an important skill to acquire. Research that is not promulgated is pointless, and so developing confidence in presenting your own work is essential.

Many master's students are encouraged by their supervisors to turn their dissertations into conference presentations or published papers. This is an excellent thing to do. Such presentations, developed and produced by the student, are sometimes reviewed and edited by the supervisor. If that is the case, then it is not inappropriate for the supervisor to be credited as a co-author. Authorship, order of authors and potential publications should be discussed very early on in the writing process.

At doctoral level, there is an absolute expectation that the candidate will publish, if not during, then very soon after the completion of their work. In this instance, the supervisor will expect to be credited as a co-author. Students are strongly encouraged to publish their work only with the prior knowledge of their supervisor, since more than their own reputation may be at stake. Conference presentations, particularly at the national and international level, are key to the doctoral student's development, and the supervisor can signpost ones that will be useful to the student. The doctoral student, particularly in the latter stages of their study, will be on the lookout for suitable examiners, and such conferences are often a good way of getting a feel for work of those people who may be potential assessors.

What students should do to keep supervisors happy

So far, this chapter has focused on practical support within the supervisory relationship. However, the key to a successful supervisor–supervisee relationship, as with any other, is understanding the things that can be done to ensure the co-operation and regard of the other party. To ensure that students make the most of their supervisor's time and expertise, the following strategies are recommended:

Do not expect supervisors to comment on written work that they have not seen in advance. Nothing can annoy a supervisor more than if the student arrives for a supervision session equipped with their latest draft chapter (or even the entire first draft of their thesis) expecting the supervisor to read it and comment on the content intelligently while the student sits expectantly at their side. Likewise, if the focus of the supervision session is to be your latest 20,000 word literature review, sending it to your supervisor at 3.30 on a Friday afternoon does not mean you can expect them to have reviewed it by 10.30 on Monday morning.

Make proper appointments. One of the difficulties inherent for most supervisors when supervising work colleagues or full-time students who work on campus is the informal 'pop-in'. Slipping into your supervisor's office to say 'hello' and leaving 2 h later having discussed your latest data collection problems is likely to become irksome to your supervisor sooner rather than later. It is always advisable to make a follow-up appointment at the end of each scheduled supervision session. If you do not need it, you can cancel it at a later date, whereas trying to make an appointment at short notice can be troublesome.

Bring an agenda. One of the expectations of undertaking a dissertation or thesis is that the student will develop or enhance their organisational skills. Whether working at undergraduate level, when you want your supervision to be direct and to the point, or at master's or doctoral level where supervision may be more discursive, bringing an agenda to meetings will ensure that you cover all the points on which you want an opinion and thus derive maximum benefit from the encounter.

Be prepared for constructive criticism. It can be quite difficult, as you nurture your thesis to its conclusion, to expose it to scrutiny and criticism. However, your supervisor will comment on both the strengths and the weaknesses of your work, and you should expect such criticism to be constructive. Your supervisor will probably expect you to take their criticism into account. It is not compulsory, but if the criticism is constructive and you chose not to address it, you should have a strong rationale for your decision.

Keep in touch. It can be easy to lose regular contact with your supervisor and difficult it is to re-establish that contact as time goes by. Most supervisors see maintaining contact as a student responsibility and so would be unlikely to chase up communication defaulters. However, they will value the occasional e-mail to reassure them that your work is continuing.

Do not demand or agree to unrealistic deadlines. Many students, especially at the earlier stages of their academic career, find setting goals or deadlines to be met before the next supervision meeting gives structure and focus to their work. However, if having agreed deadlines with the supervisor the student is regularly unable to meet them, the supervisor may begin to question the student's commitment to study.

Keep comprehensive records. Some supervisors are very efficient in the record they keep of supervision sessions, others less so. It is always in the student's best interests to keep records of the discussion and goal setting that occurs in the supervisory session. Sharing and agreeing these records with the supervisor will help to facilitate the relationship.

Reflection activity

Think further about your responsibilities as a student in need of supervision. Make notes about the actions you should take to ensure that you develop a good working relationship with your supervisor. Are there any areas that you will need to work on? For example, if you tend to leave things to the last minute, how will you ensure that your supervisor has sufficient time to review your work? You can use your notes as a basis for discussion with your supervisor.

In summary, the student must be aware that the supervision process is a collaborative one. The amount of power and autonomy the individual has within the relationship varies across academic levels, but students should remember that a fundamental part of the success of supervisory support is their participation in the process (Abiddin *et al.* 2011).

SOURCES OF EMOTIONAL AND PEER SUPPORT

Your supervisor is there to offer academic advice and support. Boucher and Smyth (2004) have suggested that it is possible for a satisfactory supervisory relationship to be maintained between two people who are also friends. In contrast, Sullivan and Ogloff (1998) have warned that the supervisor's objectivity may be jeopardised if a more personal relationship is in existence, and Lee (2009) cautions that boundaries may become blurred to the detriment of both the supervisory and the personal relationship. However, the nature of the PhD relationship has changed to reflect contemporary institutional values, and there is no 'one-size-fits-all' approach (Hemer 2012). For the supervisory relationship to serve the student's best interests, it is wise to ensure that boundaries are clear and to seek emotional support from other sources.

Personal tutors

Many universities insist on students having a personal tutor. This person is generally external to any academic supervision team, acts in a pastoral role and is usually concerned with the student's welfare. Very often, the personal tutor role is a loose and casual one, and students only seek out their tutor when in the throes of a personal crisis. The uptake of, and satisfaction with, the personal tutor role is enhanced when regular meetings are formally scheduled and the student and tutor work to develop a relationship early on in the education process (Abiddin *et al.* 2011).

Family, friends and other students

There is no doubt that undertaking a dissertation or thesis can impact significantly upon family life. Your family and friends will have to become accustomed to your long periods of absence as you write up your research. However, they can also be a good source of emotional support and may be counted upon to act as passive listeners when things go wrong. They can also help to counteract 'writing-up syndrome' by encouraging you to take a break from the computer.

Sheridan (2011) drawing upon Thomas (2002) noted that the 'family' played a significant role in undergraduate student retention, citing the support offered as a major factor contributing to completion of a programme of study. She also acknowledged that the identity of the 'family' changed to include other students on the programme who provided support. Lack of peer support can be an issue for part-time students who may lose out on this camaraderie and/or doctoral students who very often work in isolation: these students should be encouraged to make an extra effort to connect with their peers.

External support mechanisms

Although friends, family and other students can provide valuable emotional support, it is also a good idea to seek support from people who are external to the educational institution. This is especially true at doctoral level when conversation with other doctoral students allows for comparison of supervisory styles, institutional expectations and a sharing of concerns and worries. There are a number of doctoral student support networks around the United Kingdom; some are organised by universities, while others such as the PhD Forum (http://www.findaphd.com/student/forum.asp) are hosted by other organisations, in this case a commercial website. These networks attempt to provide an arena for doctoral students to exchange experiences. In addition, conferences may host events that are explicitly aimed at research students, and it is often worth making an effort to attend these events.

Online communities and social network sites

One of the difficulties that practitioners face is finding enough time to attend support events in the 'real' or 'offline' world. This is why online communities and social networking sites can be a useful source of support. An 'asynchronous discussion board', which is a site where messages are posted but interaction does not take place in real time, can allow students to post their concerns at any time of day or night. An added advantage of using international rather than national or university-specific discussion groups is that as the Internet transcends geographical boundaries, there is always likely to be someone online to talk to you. The use of social media as a method of support for doctoral students is growing with online chats or 'tweetups' on Twitter (a microblogging site that allows the posting of messages of up to 140 characters) such as #PhDchat providing a quick and easy online support mechanism.

Research students may find blogging a cathartic and useful way of seeking emotional support from others. Blog is a portmanteau word that is a contraction of the term 'Web log'. A blog is a website that has regular entries of commentary that can be read and commented on by others. There are student blogs for all academic levels on the Internet and can reassure students that they are not alone in their experiences.

Reflection activity

Why can it be beneficial to seek support in addition to that provided by your supervisor when undertaking a research project? Identify the various support mechanisms that you could draw upon. Possible sources of support may come from the university where you are studying, the organisation where you work if you are a part-time student, your local community and further afield.

Finally, social networking sites such as Facebook can be attractive to students. Social networking sites are places where users can join networks organised by workplace, university and location to connect and interact with other people. People can add friends and send them messages and update their personal profile to notify friends about themselves. However, some social networking sites are banned in certain countries, and so this option may not be so useful to some international students.

CONCLUSION

This chapter has signposted some of the sources that are available to students for funding of their research activities. Nurses and other health professionals have not had a tradition of seeking funding from external bodies other than their employing institution or from their personal finances. However, an awareness of alternate sources of funding can be beneficial.

The main focus of this chapter, however, has been the roles and responsibilities inherent in the supervisor–supervisee relationship, the nature and style of supervision and the strategies for emotional and peer support. Research students have varying degrees of autonomy in the supervisory relationship, and they should exercise this autonomy if they are to get maximum benefit from the experience.

References

Abiddin NZ, Ismail A, Ismail A (2011) Effective supervisory approach in enhancing postgraduate research studies. *International Journal of Humanities and Social Science* **1**(2): 206–217.

Boucher C, Smyth A (2004) Up close and personal: reflections on our experience of supervising research candidates who are using personal reflective techniques. *Reflective Practice* **5**(3): 345–356.

Ellis L (2006) The Professional Doctorate for nurses in Australia: findings of a scoping exercise. *Nurse Education Today* **26**(6): 484–493.

Haigh C (2007) Peacocks and jellyfish; steps and strategies for successful conference chairing. *Nurse Education Today* **27**: 91–94.

Hemer S (2012) Informality, power and relationships in postgraduate supervision: supervising PhD candidates over coffee. *Higher Education Research & Development* **31**(6): 827–839.

Lee NJ (2008) *Achieving Your Professional Doctorate: a handbook*. Buckingham, McGraw Hill.

Lee NJ (2009) *Achieving Your Professional Doctorate: a handbook*. Buckingham, McGraw Hill.

Meyer-Parsons B (2011) *Exploding Heads, Doing School and Intangible Work: an ethnographic case study of first year education doctoral students becoming education researchers*. PhD Dissertation, Fort Collins, Colorado State University. Available at: http://digitool.library.colostate.edu/exlibris/dtl/d3_1/apache_media/L2V4bGlicmlzL2R0bC9kM18xL2FwYWNoZV9tZWRpYS8xODI3NjY=.pdf (accessed 29 August 2014).

Phillips EM, Pugh DS (2010) *How to Get a PhD*, 5th edition. Maidenhead, Open University Press.

Quality Assurance Agency for Higher Education (2012) *UK Quality Code for Higher Education Part B: assuring and enhancing academic quality Chapter B11: research degrees*. Available at: http://www.qaa.ac.uk/Publications/InformationAndGuidance/Documents/Quality-Code-Chapter-B11.pdf (accessed 29 August 2014).

Sheridan V (2011) A holistic approach to international students, institutional habitus and academic literacies in an Irish third level institution. *Higher Education* **62**(2): 129–140.

Sullivan L, Ogloff J (1998) Appropriate supervisor graduate student relationships. *Ethics and Behavior* **8**(3): 229–248.

Thomas L (2002) Student retention in higher education: the role of institutional habitus. *Journal of Education Policy* **17**(4): 423–442.

Trocchia PJ, Berkowitz D (1999) Getting doctored: a proposed model of marketing doctoral student socialization. *European Journal of Marketing* **33**(7/8): 746–759.

Ward AE (2013) Empirical study of the important elements in the researcher development journey. *Knowledge Management and E-Learning* **5**(1): 42–55.

Websites

http://www.findaphd.com – Find A PhD is a guide to current postgraduate research and PhD studentships. The website lists details of graduate research programmes from universities throughout the United Kingdom, Europe and further afield.

http://www.britishcouncil.org – The British Council provides information on educational opportunities, including master's and PhD studies in UK universities and internationally.

http://www.fulbright.co.uk – The Fulbright Commission offers awards and advice for study, research, lecturing or professional development in any academic field.

http://www.rcn.org.uk/development/researchanddevelopment – The Royal College of Nursing Research and Development Co-ordinating Centre provides information on a doctoral student network and scholarly awards.

http://www.rdinfo.org.uk – RDinfo provides information on research funding and training events for health researchers.

http://www.researchresearch.com – ResearchResearch offers a research funding alert service and regular news bulletins of research opportunities.

CHAPTER 11 Gaining Access to the Research Site

Leslie Gelling

Key points

- All research involving human participants requires a favourable ethical review by an appropriate Research Ethics Committee (REC).
- Research involving NHS patients requires the opinion of an NHS REC.
- In addition to obtaining a favourable ethical opinion, researchers are usually required to obtain local governance approval from research sites. Research undertaken in the NHS requires governance approval from an NHS R&D department before the research can begin.
- Researchers should pay particular attention to issues around informed consent and participants' safety.
- Seeking the required approvals to access the research site can be complex and time-consuming so adequate time should be allowed to plan the research and to prepare the necessary applications.
- Researchers should treat seeking the required approvals as an integral and useful stage in the planning and conduct of their research project.

INTRODUCTION

Requirements for the ethical and governance review of research are constantly being revised and updated to meet changing legal and policy requirements. Since the publication of the sixth edition of *The Research Process in Nursing*, there have been changes to the processes for seeking permissions and approvals to access research sites. Seeking the necessary access approvals for research can be complex and time-consuming but is always required for research involving human participants. This chapter provides a practical overview of the approvals required to access research sites, drawing on the author's experience as a researcher, as the Chair of an NHS Research Ethics Committee (REC) and as the Chair of a University Faculty Research Ethics Panel. Although the specific details of the approval process are pertinent to the United Kingdom, the principles are applicable to other countries.

The Research Process in Nursing, Seventh Edition. Edited by Kate Gerrish and Judith Lathlean.

Companion Website: www.wiley.com/go/gerrish/research

THE NEED FOR REGULATION OF RESEARCH

In recent years, researchers have been expected to adhere to a range of regulations, guidance and codes of practice when undertaking research. Most professional bodies and research organisations have published their own guidance, including the Royal College of Nursing (2011a, b), the Medical Research Council (2012) and the British Psychological Society (2009). The problem with these and other guidelines is that they are not mandatory and can sometimes offer conflicting advice. Researchers are also expected to comply with the principles of the World Medical Association's *Declaration of Helsinki*, first published in 1964. There have been multiple revisions, most recently in 2013, but again the Declaration is not compulsory and there has been much discussion about how the Declaration should be used in different forms of research and in a climate very different to that in which the Declaration was first published (Goodyear *et al.* 2008). Despite the differences of opinion, the *Declaration of Helsinki* remains the foundation upon which ethical practice in all biomedical research, including nursing research, involving human participants is performed.

What is clear is that these various guidelines and codes of practice have repeatedly failed to halt unethical research in the past (Beecher 1966; Pappworth 1967) or more recently (Smith 2006; Saunders & Savulescu 2008; Wells & Farthing 2008). Repeated high-profile incidences of unethical and potentially harmful research, including the retention of children's organs without informed consent at Alder Hey Children's Hospital, resulted in the Department of Health publishing their *Research Governance Framework for Health and Social Care* in 2001, which was revised and updated in 2005 (Department of Health 2005). This Framework clarified the roles of all those involved in health and social care research and added the requirement that researchers seek local NHS approval in addition to seeking an ethical opinion. Researchers are now required to undertake this dual review process before they are able to access research sites or to begin their research.

Not all research requires the same approvals for research ethics or research governance. In 2012, the NHS and the National Research Ethics Service (NRES), which is responsible for the ethical review of research in the NHS, decreed that research involving NHS staff no longer required ethical review by an NHS REC, but this does not mean that ethical review is not required. Some research might need ethical review from a REC outside the NHS. For example, student research projects that involve NHS staff generally require the student to seek research ethics approval from their University Research Ethics Committee (UREC) and research governance approval from the research site.

The United Kingdom has had a system for ethical review in place since the 1970s, but it is only more recently that ethical review has been regulated by law. *The EU Clinical Trials Directive 2001/20/EC* and the Directive's implementation into UK law through *the Medicines for Human Use (Clinical Trials) Regulations* have placed particular legal requirements on RECs, not least the obligation that they make their final opinion available within 60 days of a valid application being submitted. In addition to dealing with practical matters related to the management and organisation of RECs, the *Directive* also outlined the important points to be considered during the process of ethical review. The *Directive* was written primarily to harmonise the management of clinical trials across the EU, and its implementation by member states, including the United Kingdom, has undoubtedly improved the processes of ethical review for both RECs and researchers. Although the *Directive* relates only to clinical trials, there have been advantages for researchers undertaking other forms of research in health and social care. For examples, the 60-day rule has been applied to all research reviewed by NHS RECs in the United Kingdom and not just to clinical trials.

Past failures by researchers to comply with ethical guidelines and codes of practice have resulted in an increasing reliance on the law to provide a structure to the context within which research is undertaken. In addition to the *EU Clinical Trials Directive*, researchers are also now required to comply with a number of legal requirements when seeking approvals to access research sites (see Box 11.1).

Box 11.1 Research ethics and the law

The Children Act 1989
The Data Protection Act 1998
EU Clinical Trials Directive 2001/20/EC
The Human Tissue Act 2004
The Medicines for Human Use (Clinical Trials) Regulations 2004
The Mental Capacity Act 2005

During the process of ethical review, a REC will need to be convinced that all data and personal information will be handled in compliance with the *Data Protection Act 1998*, that the collection and storage of human tissue samples complies with the requirements of the *Human Tissue Act 2004* and that the acquisition of informed consent always complies with the requirements of the *Mental Capacity Act 2005*. This is further complicated because the law can be different in separate parts of the United Kingdom. For example, in Scotland, the *Children (Scotland) Act 1995* and the *Adults with Incapacity (Scotland) Act 2000* take precedence over the above Acts of Parliament.

Recent changes to the law have placed greater emphasis on the need for researchers to act always in a manner deemed acceptable by society and the wider scientific community. RECs, both within and outside the NHS, and R&D departments play important roles in helping to ensure that researchers comply with the law, act always in an ethical manner and do not put research participants or themselves in positions of unacceptable risk while undertaking scientifically rigorous research that will contribute to knowledge. Ultimately, the aim is to generate high-quality evidence to inform clinical practice, an aim shared by researchers, by RECs and by R&D departments. Evidence would suggest that researchers have repeatedly failed to always act in an ethical manner so it is through a meticulous and rigorous dual review process that society can have confidence in the safety and value of nursing, health and social care research.

RESEARCH ETHICS

All research involving human participants requires ethical review by an appropriate REC. Research involving NHS patients always requires the opinion of an NHS REC. Although NHS RECs will give an opinion on any health and social care research placed before them, there are also RECs outside the NHS, including URECs, RECs in social care organisations (e.g. Cambridgeshire County Council) and independent RECs. These non-NHS RECs undertake important work and make a significant contribution to supporting health and social care research in the United Kingdom. The remainder of this chapter focuses on ethical review by NHS RECs, but it is usually possible to find information about other forms of REC on university and organisation websites. Although the organisation, management and membership of different RECs may vary, the principles underpinning ethical review are constant. This is demonstrated by the membership and work of the Association of Research Ethics Committees (AREC). Members are drawn from all of the aforementioned RECs with the shared aim of protecting research participants from inappropriately risky or unethical research while also encouraging research of high quality.

The remit of RECs

NHS RECs (from here on known as RECs) will consider all research involving the NHS or research requiring review by an NHS REC in order to comply with the law. This includes research that needs to meet the requirements of the *Medicines for Human Use (Clinical Trials) Regulations 2004*, the *Mental Capacity Act 2005* and the *Human Tissue Act 2004*. In addition, RECs will review any human research study submitted to it from any source related to health and social care.

RECs have evolved over time, but it remains their principal objective to protect potential and actual research participants from harm associated with research (Gelling 1999). RECs do not attempt to eliminate all risk, but they do try to balance risks against possible benefits. All research involves risk, whether physical, emotional, social or economic. Additionally, much research involves a high degree of uncertainty about possible side effects or as yet unknown consequences of participating in research. RECs will want to be reassured that the risks are not excessive and do not exceed the possible benefits. As importantly, RECs will want to feel confident that research participants are made aware of the risks to which they might be exposing themselves, including the degree of unknown risk, before and during the research.

In addition to protecting research participants, RECs will also be keen to protect others, including researchers, from possible risks associated with a research project. For example, if researchers plan to visit participants in their own homes, the REC will want to be reassured that all reasonable steps will be taken to protect researchers from possible harm. Many research groups have lone worker policies and details should be provided to the REC reviewing the research.

RECs will also want to know that appropriate indemnity arrangements are in place should anything go wrong. For student research projects, indemnity is usually arranged through their university. For all other research, indemnity is usually arranged through the chief investigator's employer. In all instances where the application for ethical approval is being made to an NHS REC, the sponsor will sign to confirm that appropriate indemnity arrangements are in place. Other RECs, including URECs, will also want to be sure that such arrangements are in place.

Reflection activity

When thinking about your research, to what risks might the participants in your study be exposed? Are there any risks to you in undertaking the research? What actions can you take to minimise the risk for participants and yourself? If you are not planning your own research, read a published research paper and identify the risks that participants and/or the researchers may have been exposed to during the course of the research.

Ethical review in the United Kingdom

While there has been a formal research ethics system operating in the United Kingdom for many years, they only acquired legal status in 2004 as a result of *the EU Clinical Trials Directive 2001/20/EC* and the Directive's implementation into UK law through *the Medicines for Human Use (Clinical Trials) Regulations*. As a result of this legislation, it became a requirement to obtain a favourable ethical opinion for all clinical trials of medicinal products. In addition to the 60-day rule highlighted earlier, it also became a requirement that researchers need to only seek the opinion of a single REC, regardless of the number of sites involved in the research.

The ethical review of research came under the control of a single authority known as the UK Ethics Committee Authority (UKECA), headed by the Secretary of State for Health. The day-to-day management and governance of all NHS RECs came under the control of the Central Office for Research Ethics Committees (COREC), established by the Department of Health in 2000. In 2007, COREC was replaced by the NRES, then part of the National Patient Safety Agency (NPSA). In 2011, with the closure of the NPSA, responsibility for NRES and the co-ordination of ethical review of research in the United Kingdom was taken over by the Health Research Authority (HRA). All REC members are now recruited through a transparent process and appointed for a fixed time, usually a maximum of 10 years, by the HRA.

Since its establishment, one of the main objectives for NRES has been to standardise the process for seeking the opinion of RECs in the United Kingdom. In the past, each REC had its own application processes, their own ways of working and their own application forms. This made the process of seeking an ethical opinion hugely time-consuming, especially with multi-site studies. The processes have now been standardised, and all RECs adhere to *The Governance Arrangements for Research Ethics Committees* (Department of Health 2012) and work within a single set of standard operating procedures. This process of standardisation means that all applications submitted in the United Kingdom, to whichever REC, should be treated and reviewed in a similar manner.

The most important change to the process for ethical review has been the introduction of the single standard application process and application form called the Integrated Research Application System (IRAS). Launched in 2008, IRAS in an online application system that enables researchers to input information once for the majority of possible approvals required to access research sites, including research ethics, NHS research governance, Medicines and Healthcare Products Regulatory Agency (MHRA) and others. Described as an intelligent form, it begins with a number of filter questions that determine which questions the researchers will need to answer and unnecessary questions do not appear. It is important that researchers get the filter questions correct to ensure that the REC is provided with all the information required to form an opinion about the research. The IRAS form has made it easier for researchers to seek the approvals required before they can begin their research.

Applying for an ethical opinion

The first point to consider is whether it is necessary to seek an ethical opinion at all. RECs will offer an opinion on all research submitted to them, but their opinion is not required if the project is audit or service evaluation. NRES offers a useful document that differentiates between these three forms of investigation (National Research Ethics Service 2008). There are also online decision tools available to help researchers determine if their project is research (http://www.hra-decisiontools.org.uk/research/) and whether research ethics approval is required (http://www.hra-decisiontools.org.uk/ethics/). It is important that researchers do not describe their research as anything other than research in an attempt to avoid the need to seek the opinion of a REC. Deliberately avoiding the opinion of a REC in this way would be considered a form of research misconduct and could result in serious repercussions for the researcher.

An important early consideration is to determine which REC an application should be submitted to. There are approximately 80 NHS RECs in the United Kingdom, and many have particular expertise in the review of different types of research so it is important that applications for ethical approval are submitted to a REC able to undertake the review. Box 11.2 highlights some of the types of research requiring review by specialist RECs. The NRES Central Allocation System (CAS) will help researchers identify an appropriate REC for their application. If an application is submitted to a REC that cannot undertake its review, there may be a considerable delay for the researcher and unnecessary work for the REC. For

Box 11.2 Types of research requiring review by specialised RECs

Clinical trials of medicinal products
Medical devices
Research involving prisoners
Adults with incapacity
Children and young people
Human tissue and samples

many types of research, the application will be submitted to the most geographically convenient REC.

Applicants are required to submit three sets of paperwork, the protocol, the application form and additional papers, including participation information sheets and consent forms. It is the author's experience that fewer than 10% of projects receive an unfavourable opinion because of ethical issues and only 14% have an uninterrupted passage through the review process (National Research Ethics Service 2007). Of the remaining applications, a small number will have minor ethical problems, but nearly all will display flaws in the paperwork. It is essential therefore that great care is taken in the preparation of the application form and accompanying papers. If there are inconsistencies between the application form and the protocol, or if the application is full of spelling and grammatical errors, the REC will seek clarification and amendment before an application can proceed to a favourable opinion. It is also important that all required documents are submitted with the necessary signatures.

Despite many improvements to the application form, completion can appear a burdensome task, not least because few researchers use the form sufficiently frequently to become comfortable with it. The time required to complete the application form should not be underestimated. The perceived burden can be somewhat eased if researchers make themselves aware of the ethical requirements and expectations of RECs from the outset. This allows for 'built-in' rather than 'bolt-on' ethics and increases the likelihood of smooth passage through the review process. In addition to reading the guidance made available on the NRES website, researchers might consider attending a REC meeting as an observer, enabling them to gain insight into how the REC works, how it deals with applications and the key points the REC is likely to consider when reviewing an application.

The application form should be completed in lay language, making it accessible to all members of the REC. Challenging technical text copied verbatim from the protocol may leave REC members unable to understand the research and unable to reach an informed opinion. This is particularly important for the free-text responses that describe the research questions and objectives, scientific justification and methods. To further ensure clarity, it is recommended that every effort is made to attend the REC meeting to discuss the project with the committee. By attending the meeting, the applicant is able to clarify misunderstandings and to answer the REC's questions. This can help ease the progress of the application through the review process.

The Patient Information Sheet (PIS) is often the document most rigorously scrutinised by the REC and also the one most frequently requiring modification following review. There should be no conflicting information between the PIS and the application form. Such inconsistency is surprisingly frequent and makes it hard for the REC to reach an informed opinion, especially if the researcher is not available to provide clarity. Researchers should note that many REC members start their review by reading the PIS because this is the document most likely to provide a clear introduction to the proposed research.

When appropriate, the PIS template on the NRES website should be used. NRES suggests a two-part PIS, with part 1 providing general information about the research and part 2 providing more detailed information about specific points. The templates also provide a list of questions that might be included in both parts of the PIS (see Box 11.3). These can be amended according to the nature of the research; it may not be appropriate to use all the headings in the template, and it may be helpful to add additional headings. Reordering the questions can also be useful if this helps potential participants to understand the research. Many applicants stick rigidly to the format in the NRES template with the result that the PIS is difficult to read and the information provided can appear muddled.

The PIS should be tailored for the intended audience. Research participants are often members of the public so paperwork should be written at an appropriate level (Franck & Winter 2004), remembering that the average reading age in the United Kingdom is somewhere between 9 and 12 years old. It should be remembered that participants with long-term conditions will become familiar with some of the medical terminology but complex terminology should still be fully explained. Patients and representative groups are often happy to review copies of PIS and other documents during preparation, and it is usually apparent to the REC where this knowledgeable input has been provided.

Box 11.3 Design of participant information sheets

Part 1

Study title
Invitation paragraph
What is the purpose of the study?
Why have I been chosen?
Do I have to take part?
What will happen to me if I take part?
Expenses and payments
What will I have to do?
What is the drug, device or procedure that is being tested?
What are the alternatives for diagnosis or treatment?
What are the possible disadvantages and risks of taking part?
What are the side effects of any treatment received when taking part?
What are the possible benefits of taking part?
What happens when the research study stops?
What if there is a problem?
Will my participation in the study be kept confidential?

Part 2

What will happen if I don't want to carry on with the study?
What if there is a problem?
Will my taking part in the study be kept confidential?
Involvement of the General Practitioner/Family Doctor
What will happen to any samples I give?
Will any genetic tests be done?
What will happen to the results of the research study?
Who is organising and funding the research?
Who has reviewed the study?
Further information and contact details

The ethical review process

REC members are volunteers who take pride in their work and the service they offer to researchers. RECs have both lay and professional members, covering many disciplines including pharmacists, statisticians, nurses and medical practitioners. Professional members are expected to consider matters pertinent to their expertise. For example, the pharmacist will scrutinise more closely the responses to questions about any investigational medicinal products, and the statistician will focus most closely on the responses to questions about the planned sample size and data analysis. Despite their particular expertise, professionals are not polymaths so you should assume that every REC member possesses only lay understanding for the majority of the areas covered on the form.

After submitting your application, the REC Coordinator will check that all the necessary information, papers and signatures have been provided and, if they have been, the application will be deemed

Reflection activity

Think about a research study you are planning to undertake. List the key pieces of information you will need to include in the participant information sheet. If you are not planning to undertake research, read a published research paper and identify the information that you think the researcher(s) should have included in a participant information sheet for their study.

valid and added to the agenda for the review at the next meeting. All members of the REC will review all the applications, usually about six applications, receiving them about 10 days before the meeting. Two members of the committee are usually nominated to act as lead reviewers for each new application. It is the lead reviewer's role to undertake a thorough review and to lead the discussion of the application during the meeting.

The researchers will have been invited to attend the meeting at which their application will be reviewed and, as noted earlier, it is essential that they make every effort to attend if they can. It is not uncommon for a REC to misunderstand an element of a research project so it can help if the researcher is present to clarify any uncertainties and to answer any other questions. Researchers should remember that REC members are faced with up to six new applications and protocols at each meeting so it can be difficult to have a comprehensive understanding of each one.

Following discussion, the committee will form an opinion of the research. The options available to them are as follows:

- *Favourable opinion.* In this instance, the REC is completely satisfied with all parts of the research. The researcher will be informed and their research can begin.
- *Favourable opinion with conditions.* The committee will use this opinion if the researcher is able to make a simple change or clarify a minor point. Once the condition(s) of the opinion has been met, the favourable opinion will be confirmed.
- *Provisional favourable opinion.* This opinion is offered if the committee needs revisions to documentation or needs matters clarifying. The researcher usually responds by dealing with each of the matters raised by the committee. If all the matters raised by the committee are dealt with to the REC's satisfaction, then a favourable opinion will be confirmed and the research can begin. If the committee is not satisfied, then an unfavourable opinion can be issued. The researcher's response is usually dealt with by the Chair or by a subcommittee as soon as it is received.
- *Unfavourable opinion.* Although uncommon, a small number of unfavourable opinions are given and usually result from a significant flaw within the application requiring a major revision and resubmission of the application.
- *No opinion.* The committee uses this opinion when it believes that it has not been provided with sufficient information to form an opinion.

Once an application has been validated, the REC is required to inform the researcher of their final opinion within 60 days. A written summary of the REC's opinion is sent to applicants within 10 working days of the review meeting. If a provisional opinion is granted, all required points of clarification and suggested amendments will be listed in the REC's post-review letter. The 60-day clock stops after the REC has informed the researchers of their opinion if a response is required from the researcher. This ensures that a researcher who is slow to respond to the REC's post-review letter does not cause the review clock to tick over 60 days. Once the REC receives the researcher's response, the clock starts ticking again. Although the REC has 60 days to inform the researcher of its opinion, it usually takes considerably less time than this. Modifications to documents should be tracked and version numbers updated. When the response is received, the Chair or a subcommittee usually reviews changes and offers a final opinion. Concerns with the modifications can be raised, but the REC cannot raise new concerns at this time, unless they arise from a lack of clarity in the new information.

An unfavourable opinion is uncommon and can be appealed to another REC, who will receive the original paperwork. When reviewing an appealed application, REC members do not feel bound by the preceding opinion and it is not uncommon for opinions to be reversed. If a rejection is upheld, advice may be given about how the project could be redesigned to enable a future application to be more successful.

It is important that researchers remember the need to continue their communication with the REC after the initial opinion. For example, annual reports should be submitted to the REC using the template available on the NRES website, and the REC should also be invited to review and approve protocol amendments. If a researcher fails to communicate with the REC, the committee may consider withdrawing their favourable opinion.

Reflection activity

Why is it important that researchers attend the ethical review meeting to discuss their research with the REC? Make notes on how you might prepare to attend the meeting. Remember that students undertaking research generally find it helpful if their supervisor accompanies them to the committee meeting.

R&D APPROVAL

In addition to obtaining a favourable ethical opinion from an appropriate REC, all researchers wishing to undertake research in the NHS must also obtain research governance approval from the site where the research will be conducted. The *Research Governance Framework for Health and Social Care* sets out the principles, requirements and standards for the conduct of high-quality research (Department of Health 2005). The Framework also defines the mechanisms to deliver these and describes the monitoring and assessment arrangements. The Framework also offers clear definitions of the responsibilities of researchers, sponsors, funders, hosts and all NHS employees.

In addition to seeking research ethics approval, the IRAS application form can be used to seek multiple approvals (see Box 11.4), including research governance approval. Researchers are required to submit a Site-Specific Information (SSI) form directly to the relevant NHS R&D office for each of the sites where the research will be conducted. This form combines the information needed for Site-Specific Assessment (SSA), where required, and local R&D approval. SSA involves an assessment of the suitability of each research site to be involved in the research. The R&D office will also wish to review the study-wide form, generated through the IRAS application, and other documents, including PIS, consent forms and any letters or questionnaires to be used.

Box 11.4 Multiple approvals using the IRAS application form

Administration of Radioactive Substances Advisory Committee (ARSAC)
Gene Therapy Advisory Committee (GTAC)
Medicines and Healthcare Products Regulatory Agency (MHRA)
Ministry of Justice (including research involving prisoners)
NHS Research Offices
NRES Research Ethics Committees
Patient Information Advisory Group (PIAG)

In November 2008, the National Institute for Health Research (NIHR) Coordinated System for gaining NHS Permission (NIHR CSP) was introduced for NIHR Clinical Research Network Portfolio studies. Portfolio studies are those that meet eligibility criteria set by the NIHR Clinical Research Network Coordinating Centre (CRNCC), for example, studies funded by the NIHR, research councils and national charities where grants are awarded through open competition and subject to rigorous independent scientific review. This system should streamline the process by which NHS organisations provide permission, research governance approval for new research, and should reduce duplication in NHS review processes. NIHR CSP has a single entry point, using IRAS, so that researchers will be able to apply for permission from all NHS sites in England through a single gateway. It is important to remember that this process can only be used by those whose research fits within the NIHR Clinical Research Network Portfolio. Research outside this portfolio will still need to apply to individual NHS organisations.

Researchers might also need to seek a research passport if they are entering a research site where they are not already employed. Research passports should be available to NHS, to university and to other researchers working in partnership with the NIHR, but other researchers will need to seek advice about honorary contracts from local NHS organisations.

INFORMAL ACCESS TO RESEARCH SITES

While there are formal approval processes to be negotiated before research can commence, it is also advisable that researchers ensure that they have informal approval to access research sites. Once a favourable ethical opinion and research governance approval have been gained, researchers will still encounter numerous 'gatekeepers' who can control access to participants or data. In the vast majority of cases, these gatekeepers are willing to facilitate research, but it helps this process if researchers approach appropriate individuals during the early stages of the project so that they can build up a rapport. Gatekeepers might include:

- *ward sisters or managers.* Ward sisters and managers, or their deputies, are responsible for the day-to-day management of many clinical settings. It can be extremely difficult to undertake research in these settings without the support of these gatekeepers. If the research involves interviewing nursing staff, the scheduling of interviews could be much easier with the ward manager's support.
- *Caldicott Guardians.* Since 2001, and in response to the Caldicott Committee's report (Department of Health 1997), each NHS organisation has appointed a Caldicott Guardian, usually a senior manager, who is responsible for the safekeeping of patient records, to ensure their rights are protected and to oversee how the staff use personal information. Research requiring access to patient information may need the approval of the Caldicott Guardian.
- *patient support groups.* Research frequently focuses on patients in particular groups so it can help if the appropriate patient group supports a research project. They can facilitate recruitment and even encourage patients to participate. One of the biggest ways that patient groups can help researchers is in the preparation of the PIS. As noted earlier, RECs will spend considerable time reviewing this paperwork, and they can be much improved if they are developed with the support of those representing the target patient groups.

It is important that negotiations with gatekeepers happen as early in the research planning as possible. It is also not uncommon for these individuals and groups to suggest useful changes to the planned research. If these negotiations are left until after the formal approvals are gained, then it is more difficult and time-consuming to make any amendments that might be necessary because they will need to be approved by both the REC and R&D departments before they can be implemented.

Reflection activity

Who are the gatekeepers with whom you will have to negotiate access to the research participants and/or the data that you will need for your research? Outline how you will identify the individuals concerned and plan how you will approach them. If you are not planning a research study yourself, select a published research paper and identify the gatekeepers that you would need to approach if you were to replicate the research locally.

BUILDING THE APPROVAL PROCESS INTO RESEARCH PLANNING

Criticising the approval processes has become a popular pastime for many researchers in recent years (Robinson *et al.* 2007). As a result, researchers have treated seeking the required approvals as hurdles to be leaped or barriers to be knocked down before their research can begin. This attitude fails to appreciate the great value that can result from using these necessary processes as an integral part of the research process. Navigating one's way through the appropriate approval processes is also an important part of the learning experience for research students.

The remit of RECs is to maximise benefit and minimise risk while protecting the rights of participants (Gelling 1999). These objectives are best achieved through mutual respect between researchers, RECs and others involved in the approval processes. Within this relationship, an application receives constructive criticism and advice, in a timely manner, before the research is able to proceed. It is also important that the work of researchers is treated with due respect. A view that RECs are intent on obstructing research is misguided, compromises such relationships and achieves nothing. It is similarly misguided for those involved in the approval process to treat every researcher as if they were planning to cause harm to research participants in order to advance their research careers. Seeking approvals is an important part of the research process and has much to contribute to the development of new knowledge if there is mutual respect between all those involved.

Many researchers refine their research project as a direct result of planning applications for a research ethics opinion and approval from an R&D department. This process helps to ensure that research combines ethical standards with the most rigorous science in a way that is most likely to result in meaningful evidence to guide practice.

Consideration of science and ethics

There has been much discussion, sometimes heated, relating to the review of science by RECs. Some have argued that RECs should only consider matters relating to ethics and should leave the scientific review to others (Dawson & Yentis 2007). RECs, however, will argue that ethical review without consideration of the science would be incomplete and inadequate. This is based on the notion that bad science is bad ethics. In many instances, a REC is able to feel confident in the science because the research had already undergone adequate scientific peer review prior to submission to the REC. Scientific reviews are frequently undertaken before seeking an ethical opinion as part of the process of applying for research funding or are required by universities, NHS or other organisations. When scientific review has been undertaken, the REC will need to focus very little of its attention on the science and can concentrate on matters related directly to ethics. If a review has not been undertaken, or if the REC deems the review to be inadequate, then the REC will feel obliged to consider the science. In many instances, this would result in the researcher being asked to have a scientific review undertaken before the REC can form an opinion. It is worth noting that a REC is keen to see an independent external review of the science rather than a review undertaken in the same organisation or the same department. This contributes to ensuring transparency for all those involved in the research process.

Planning the application

There is considerable advice available to those planning applications for an ethical opinion or research governance approval. In addition to the guidance available on the NRES and IRAS websites, advice can be sought from the NRES helpline and from REC Chairs and Co-ordinators. R&D departments also offer advice during the preparation phase of a research project. Both RECs and R&D departments are keen to promote high-quality research, and it can save much wasted time, for both researchers and the reviewing bodies, if advice is sought as early as possible. Approval processes for health and social care research have undergone considerable change in recent years, and it is likely that changes will continue to be implemented so it is advisable to seek advice when preparing an application.

CONCLUSION

The key to navigating successfully through the approval processes and gaining access to the research site is planning and allowing sufficient time to prepare application forms and accompanying paperwork. Often, it is not major ethical concerns that delay approvals but poorly prepared and inadequately thought through application forms and supporting paperwork. Researchers would be advised to treat seeking the required approvals as an integral and useful part of the research process and to use this process to help refine their research project.

Much of what have been described in this chapter has related directly to the approvals required for research being conducted in the United Kingdom. Although different countries will adopt different approaches to the approvals required before research can begin, they will also have much in common. They will all want to be reassured that the risks to research participants and researchers are minimised, that all participants are able to freely give informed consent and that the proposed research has value.

References

Beecher H (1966) Ethics and clinical research. *New England Journal of Medicine* **274**: 1354–1360.

British Psychological Society (2009) *Code of Ethics and Conduct: guidance published by the ethics committee of the British Psychological Society*. Leicester, BPS.

Dawson AJ, Yentis SM (2007) Contesting the science/ethics distinction in the review of clinical research. *Journal of Medical Ethics* **33**(3): 165–167.

Department of Health (1997) *The Caldicott Committee: report of the review of patient-identifiable information*. London, Department of Health.

Department of Health (2005) *Research Governance Framework for Health and Social Care*. London, Department of Health.

Department of Health (2012) *Governance Arrangements for NHS Research Ethics Committees: a harmonised edition*. London, Department of Health.

Franck L, Winter I (2004) Research participant information sheets are difficult to read. *Bulletin of Medical Ethics* **195**: 13–16.

Gelling L (1999) Role of the research ethics committee. *Nurse Education Today* **19**: 564–569.

Goodyear MDE, Eckenwiler LA, Ells C (2008) Fresh thinking about the Declaration of Helsinki. *British Medical Journal* **337**: 1067–1068.

Medical Research Council (2012) *Good Research Practice: principles and guidelines*. London, MRC.

National Research Ethics Service (2007) *Cambridgeshire 4 Research Ethics Committee Annual Report*. Cambridge, NRES.

National Research Ethics Service (2008) *Defining Research*. London, National Patient Safety Agency.

Pappworth MH (1967) *Human Guinea Pigs*. Boston, Beacon Press.

Robinson L, Murdoch-Eaton D, Carter Y (2007) NHS research ethics committees. *British Medical Journal* **335**(7609): 6.

Royal College of Nursing (2011a) *Informed Consent in Health and Social Care Research: RCN guidance for nurses*. London, Royal College of Nursing.

Royal College of Nursing (2011b) *Research Ethics: RCN guidance for nurses*. London, Royal College of Nursing.

Saunders R, Savulescu J (2008) Research ethics and lessons from Hwanggate: what can we learn from the Korean cloning fraud? *Journal of Medic Ethics* **34**(3): 214–221.

Smith R (2006) Research misconduct: the poisoning of the well. *Journal of the Royal Society of Medicine* **99**(5): 232–237.

Wells F, Farthing M (2008) *Fraud and Misconduct in Biomedical Research.* London, Royal Society of Medicine.

Further reading

Beauchamp TL, Childress JF (2009) *Principles of Biomedical Ethics.* Oxford, Oxford University Press.

Long A, Johnson M (2006) *Research Ethics in the Real World: issues and solutions for health and social care.* London, Churchill Livingstone.

Manson NC, O'Neill O (2007) *Rethinking Informed Consent in Bioethics.* Cambridge, Cambridge University Press.

Websites

www.arec.org.uk – The Association of Research Ethics Committees (AREC) is an independent organisation for members and administrators from Research Ethics Committees, including NHS, university and other committees. Their website includes information about courses and conferences for those interested in research ethics and those involved in ethical review.

www.myresearchproject.org.uk – The Integrated Research Application System (IRAS) allows access to registration and use of the IRAS form.

www.mrc.ac.uk – The Medical Research Council (MRC) provides information about the many activities of the MREC, including guidance on matters relating to research ethics.

www.rdforum.nhs.uk – The National Health Service (NHS) R&D Forum is a network for those involved in planning and managing research in health and social care.

www.nres.nhs.uk – The National Research Ethics Service (NRES) provides a wealth of information and guidance on matters relating to research ethics and seeking ethical opinion.

http://www.wma.net/en/30publications/10policies/b3/ – The Declaration of Helsinki includes a full version of the Seoul 2008 revision of the Declaration of Helsinki.

http://www.ushmm.org/information/exhibitions/online-features/special-focus/doctors-trial/nuremberg-code – The Nuremberg Code provides a full version of the Nuremberg Code.

Royal College of Nursing (RCN) guidance on research ethics intended for nurses and others involved in research *http://www.rcn.org.uk/__data/assets/pdf_file/0007/388591/003138.pdf* and informed consent http://www.rcn.org.uk/__data/assets/pdf_file/0010/78607/002267.pdf.

SECTION 3

Choosing the Right Approach

This section forms the heart of this book, as research approaches in nursing are many and diverse, and it is important to understand the range of approaches available before choosing a specific one to answer a particular question.

The section begins with a theoretical chapter, Chapter 12, tackling the two broad approaches available to the nurse researcher. This chapter considers the philosophical underpinning of the qualitative and quantitative paradigms in research and emphasises the necessity to engage in the complex debates raised in the extensive literature on this subject. Both approaches, however, are valid for nursing research, and the perspective adopted should be guided by the nature of the questions to be answered.

Chapter 13 has been written by new authors to this edition and stands alone as an essential pre-requisite to any research design, be it qualitative or quantitative. Sampling procedures are well established for many methodologies, and this chapter discusses a variety of the most common sampling strategies used in nursing research, with appropriate examples from the literature. Sampling cannot be considered separately from issues of research design, as it will determine the resources required and therefore the feasibility of the project.

Chapters 14–17 introduce the major approaches used in qualitative research: grounded theory, ethnography, phenomenology and narrative research. These chapters introduce the characteristics of each of these research approaches, provide an overview of the methods of data collection and analysis and consider the strengths and limitations in order to help the researcher decide which approach might be best suited to their research questions.

The focus of Section 3 then moves on to the major quantitative approaches and a series of chapters that deal with mixed methods. Chapter 18 introduces experimental design, and Chapter 19 surveys. Both these approaches have a long and well-established history in medical and social sciences, and both are also widely used in nursing research. These chapters discuss the strengths and weaknesses of the methodologies, and highlight examples from the nursing literature where they have been used to good effect. Chapter 18 includes a critical discussion of the randomised controlled trial and its place as the 'gold standard' of medical research evidence. Chapter 19 includes a short section on epidemiology – a well-established research tradition that has perhaps been overlooked in nursing research.

The Research Process in Nursing, Seventh Edition. Edited by Kate Gerrish and Judith Lathlean.

Companion Website: www.wiley.com/go/gerrish/research

There follow eight chapters in this section each examining a very specific approaches used in nursing research. Three chapters, Chapters 22 (Evaluation), 24 (Practitioner Research) and 27 (Mixed Methods), have been written by new authors, providing a fresh perspective to these important methodologies in nursing research.

The Delphi approach (Chapter 20), case study research (Chapter 21), evaluation research (Chapter 22), action research (Chapter 23) and systematic reviews (Chapter 25) are well-used methodologies, and these chapters have been updated accordingly. The increasing need for guidance on research undertaken by, and for, practitioners has been addressed in Chapter 24, where those who are engaged in health care practice are encouraged to undertake in systematic and rigorous research that arises directly from their everyday experience. Chapter 26, on the developing methodology of realist synthesis, complements Chapter 25 on the more established discipline of systematic reviews. Realist synthesis is particularly appropriate for assessing the impact of complex interventions in their context and for developing theory. Last in this section, Chapter 27 discusses mixed methods, combining qualitative and quantitative approaches in the same research project.

CHAPTER 12

The Quantitative–Qualitative Continuum

Annie Topping

Key points

- Qualitative and quantitative researches have different characteristics and emerged from different scientific traditions and forms of knowledge.
- Quantitative research methods assume that the world is stable and predictable, and phenomena can be measured empirically. The positivist tradition of quantitative research derives from the biomedical sciences.
- Qualitative research methods take an interpretivist perspective, emphasising meaning and the understanding of human actions and behaviour. The tradition of qualitative research comes from the social sciences.
- Both approaches are appropriate for nursing research; the choice of methodology and methods depends on the nature of the research question.
- A useful strategy is to consider research as a continuum rather than two contrasting polarisations with mixed methods linking approaches.

INTRODUCTION

The differences and relative merits of quantitative and qualitative research have for some time been represented as an intellectual battleground with researchers aligned to a particular camp. Recently, those differences have become less divided with a middle ground emerging and this is particularly marked in nursing. Today, there is a growing consensus that the use of a range of approaches strengthens, rather than divides, enquiry. Researchers, irrespective of their personal preferences or familiarity with particular ways of approaching researchable questions or problems, have a shared purpose to create new knowledge. Quality in research is about using the most appropriate approach and methods for the specific investigation, and researchers should use a systematic, rigorous and transparent approach for exploring, discovering, confirming and understanding (Teddie & Tashakkori 2009). Underlying the practice of research and its findings are fundamental

The Research Process in Nursing, Seventh Edition. Edited by Kate Gerrish and Judith Lathlean.

Companion Website: www.wiley.com/go/gerrish/research

questions about the nature of knowledge, termed epistemology, and what is understood as reality. The debates surrounding those questions have over time moved from two dichotomised poles to a continuum.

THE CHARACTERISTICS OF QUANTITATIVE AND QUALITATIVE RESEARCH

Philosophically, quantitative research is underpinned by a tradition that proposes scientific truths or laws exist; this is called *positivism*. These truths emerge from what can be observed and measured and can be studied as objects. Methods that minimise bias are used in quantitative research, so that greater confidence can be given to any findings. This approach is often referred to as the *scientific* or *empirical method*.

In contrast, qualitative research fits more neatly within an *interpretivist* tradition based on assumptions that in order to make sense of the world, human behaviour should be interpreted by taking account of interactions between people. So research that seeks to understand human behaviour, and the social processes that we engage in, must employ approaches and techniques that allow interpretation in natural settings. This interpretative stance goes further, as qualitative methodologies also strive to emphasise that there is no single interpretation, truth or meaning but recognise that just as human beings are different, so are the societies and cultures in which they live their lives. Box 12.1 sets out the different qualities and characteristics that have been used to describe the two approaches. These are purposefully presented to emphasise the differences, and you may not always be able to recognise all these characteristics in any single report of a quantitative or qualitative study.

Box 12.1 Characteristics of quantitative and qualitative research

Quantitative research	Qualitative research
Hard science	Soft science
Objective	Subjective
Political	Value-free
Reductionist	Holistic
Logico-deductive	Dialectic, inductive, speculative
Cause and effect relationships	Meaning
Tests theory	Develops, advances and reinterprets theory
Control	Shared interpretation
Instruments as data collection tools	Listening and talking, observation as ways of gathering data
Basic unit of analysis: numbers	Basic unit of analysis: words
Statistical analysis	Interpretation
Generalisation	Uniqueness/transferability

Sources: Burns *et al.* (2012) and Silverman (2011, 2013).

INFLUENCES AND CONTRIBUTIONS TO THE DEVELOPMENT OF NURSING RESEARCH

Nursing has a shared history and mutual dependency with a number of disciplines. Biomedicine, like modern nursing, has its roots in the 19th century. This was a period of accelerated social upheaval and industrialisation, scientific breakthroughs and technological innovations and challenges to previously held notions of illness. The earlier premise that illness was caused by an imbalance, a loss of harmony between the individual and the environment, was questioned, and more rational, objectively based approaches were adopted. During the same time period, modern nursing began to emerge under the leadership of such figures as Florence Nightingale and Mrs Bedford Fenwick.

What is now described as *reductionism* emerged as a way for studying the causes and treatment of disease(s). This approach allows disease to be objectified and the experience of ill health to be reduced to the signs and symptoms that allow it to be classified and diagnosed, and the response, if any, to treatments can be monitored. This view of illness as an object inevitably distances the doctor or nurse, encouraging detachment from the influencing effects of subjectivity. This way of problematising illness can be seen in medical practice where routine assessment, involving taking a patient's history to establish diagnosis, might more correctly be described as an illness history.

Objectification and distancing are ingrained in the scientific tradition through separation of the research participant from the investigator. Separating the researcher from the context in which the research is undertaken provides a sense of security that the researcher cannot influence the research findings. This image of research performed by objective scientists is enduring, but many commentators question the notion of neutrality and argue that knowledge is rarely 'disinterested' (Foucault 1973; Annandale 1998).

The study of societies, their members and the ways in which they are organised is the focus of disciplines such as sociology and anthropology that start from an acceptance that people are different from objects. Objects do not have thought or consciousness; do not reason, think or reflect; and therefore are qualitatively different from people. Importantly, objects, unlike people, do not have free will or choice. For that reason, the ways in which a researcher might study and understand objects will, by necessity, be different from the approaches used to understand human society or indeed nursing. This argument becomes quite complex when applied to health care, where people become patients. In so doing, they can be viewed both objectively as malfunctioning machines and subjectively as individuals interacting with others and systems designed to support their illness. This complexity of the subjective person and objective body can be aligned philosophically to interpretivism and positivism, respectively. This reinforces why both qualitative and quantitative approaches make important contributions to creating knowledge to inform practice (O'Cathain *et al.* 2008).

EMPIRICISM AND THE SCIENTIFIC METHOD

The research methods used in modern science have their origins in the philosophical movements of the 16th and 17th centuries when a logical approach to developing knowledge emerged as an approach for examining problems. The scientific method is based on three principles: scepticism, determinism and empiricism. First, anything, irrespective of its origin or authority, is open to analysis and doubt and thus is susceptible to *scepticism*. Second, regular laws and rules of causation determine all things – known as *determinism*. Lastly, *empiricism* asserts that enquiry or problem-solving such as research should be undertaken through observation and verification. The adoption of the scientific method produced a developmental shift in thinking from previously held explanations and encouraged a way of looking at the natural world that was freed from mystery and superstition and clouded by religious explanations (Shipman 1997). The scientific method became a formula for the production of knowledge and as

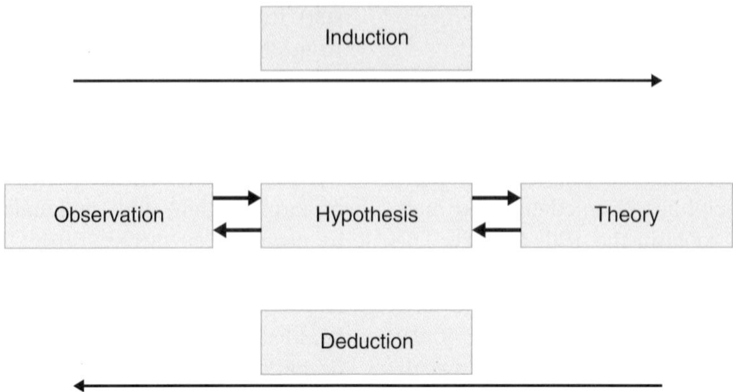

Figure 12.1 The scientific method

Figure 12.1 shows is based on the two processes of *induction* and *deduction*.

The scientific method has become part of how we understand events around us and how information is presented and used to formulate policy. For many, the first encounter with science was at school, learning how to undertake and report a simple experiment. This no doubt involved a number of tasks that required accurate description, reliable measurement and diligent recording of observations about what occurred – all in order to help understanding of whatever was being investigated. From that first exposure to the scientific method, schoolchildren are taught to describe the equipment used, how to undertake a test and record any deviations from the approved recipe, what they used to measure any reaction or outcome, and to document the results. These skills form the basis of *observation*, *description* and *measurement* that underlie much of the conduct of science. By using this approach, findings can be translated into explanations. These explanations are often expressed as *hypotheses* or *theories* that are themselves amenable to testing. This progression from observation to statement of a relationship between different observations (*hypotheses*) to *theory* and ultimately generalisation is termed *induction*. So theories derived through the process of induction move from the particular to the general and provide an organising system for what are essentially conjectures based on observation (Polgar & Thomas 2008).

Reflection activity

Given that knowledge is provisional and many aspects of care are uncertain, what impact might scientific uncertainty have on professional practice?

An essential feature of any scientific theory is the account of how the theory works and its potential to predict. These predictions enable the researcher to *deduce* causal relationships, expressed through theory but testable through controlled observation. The results of testing (*experimentation*) will produce data that can be translated into findings that may be consistent with the predictions expressed in the original hypothesis. This verifies or provides support for the theory. Alternatively, results may fail to support the hypothesis and contradict the theory. Ultimately, the volume of conflicting evidence may swell to such proportions that the original theory is discarded. Scientific theories are not absolute truths, only provisional, therefore open to modification or indeed dispute (Popper 1972, 2002).

It might be helpful to illustrate the scientific method with an example. Imagine you are working on a surgical ward where patients are admitted for elective surgery. You observe that patients who have received preoperative physical assessment and preparation experience less distress and post-operative pain than those who did not attend assessment. You also observe that the unprepared patients require more analgesia and appear to mobilise more slowly. You develop a theory that suggests a relationship between information and post-operative outcomes. In fact, two seminal studies undertaken by the nurse researchers Hayward and Boore in the 1970s did just that (Hayward & Boore 1994). These studies demonstrated a relationship between information and the level of pain experienced by patients recovering from surgery. You could ask whether the relationship between information and pain was an existing theory that Boore and Hayward sought to test using hypothetico-deductive reasoning or whether the theory emerged from them observing patients who received preoperative information. Probably, the initial idea came from the latter, but the former approach was used to demonstrate the relationship. As discussed in Chapter 2, preliminary research ideas often come from observation, but prior to designing a study, they are clarified through appraisal of the literature, so that what is already known is examined first. This allows existing understandings to be refined and avoids ill-thought through research being conducted.

Research studies are like building blocks with different studies constructing the body of knowledge. Patient education has, and continues to have, attention from nurse researchers. A more recent example is a study by O'Connor *et al.* (2010) examining the information needs of individuals with rectal cancer. They found that patients felt relatively well informed about the disease and its treatment but had unmet needs associated with tests and investigations. The deductive approach was in this case tested through using a questionnaire. The researchers also used semi-structured interviews to find out more about the information needs of this group of patients and to give more depth to their findings. In effect, they used an inductive approach to enhance their original assumptions.

In deductive research, the theory normally directs design and drives interpretation. In inductively driven inquiry, theory may provide the 'lens' through which the phenomena are viewed (e.g. feminism) or to justify the methodological approach chosen (Sandelowski 1993). This lens is identifiable as the theoretical framework that informed a research design or the interpretation of the findings provided. Explicit reference to the theoretical basis of the research can help the reader to navigate the interpretation offered. It can also provoke criticism when the theoretical framework itself appears to create a tension within the work, particularly if it appears incongruent with the research approach. For example, Patricia Benner's (1984) influential work 'Novice to Expert' that explored how nurses' competence developed through experience received some criticism on these grounds (Cash 1995), albeit firmly rebutted by the author (Benner 1996). A further consideration concerns the role of theory in research. If data are collected in the absence of an organising framework or theory, it could attract criticism that the researcher is merely confirming their own biases (Grbich 1999); alternatively, too much emphasis on theory may undermine the accessibility of the findings to others (Smith *et al.* 2011).

QUANTITATIVE RESEARCH

Quantitative research is a broad umbrella term for research that uses methods that collect evidence that can be transformed into numerical data and are based upon a *positivist* position. Usually, the numerical data produced can be statistically manipulated in order to confirm or refute the original hypotheses or research question. The findings can then be used to make predictions or indicate trends. Formal, objective and systematic processes are used to explain causal relationships between events or things (variables). Underpinning quantitative research is the principle that the world is stable and predictable and the quantitative researcher, by controlling external influences, can seek to minimise bias that might otherwise explain the findings. The ultimate aim is for the researcher and the consumer of the researcher to be assured that any results are *valid* and *reliable*. Classical experimental design is one such method, but surveys, analysis of official statistics and structured or non-participant observation are all quantitative methods (Silverman 2011). The use of quantitative research methods is illustrated in the study undertaken by Alhalaiqa *et al.* (2012) described in Box 12.1. Here, the research team tested an individualised intervention (adherence therapy). They identified the variable most likely to be influenced by the intervention (blood pressure) that was amenable to measurement and easily represented as numerical data.

From this example, you can see how in quantitative research the focus of study has to be broken down, reduced, into those component parts that can be readily defined and measurable. This provides greater assurance to the researcher and the reader that the results are the product of consistent reproducible measurement. The accuracy of the instruments used to measure whatever is under investigation, and their ability to consistently reproduce results, is fundamental to undertaking quantitative research. It also allows other researchers to replicate the study and therefore compare, confirm and question existing findings. One problem with dependency on measurement is that the theoretical premise or model has to be definable, there needs to be technology available to consistently reproduce the measurement and those involved in data collection have to be able to perform the measurement reliably. Yet no matter how well designed or how diligently the study is executed, it can still be reliable but not valid. In other words, the research may measure something but not necessarily what was under investigation. This is why it is often more challenging to establish with any confidence that the findings represent facts, or truths, about something than to construct an approach to measure it, or some part of it.

Another feature of quantitative research is that it aspires to objectivity and therefore different approaches are used to keep participants at a distance

RESEARCH EXAMPLE

12.1 A Quantitative Research Study

Alhalaiqa F, Deane KHO, Clark A, Gray R (2012) Adherence therapy for medication non-compliant patients with hypertension: a randomised controlled trial. *Journal of Human Hypertension* 26: 117–126.

This study compared adherence therapy (AT) with treatment as usual (TAU) in reducing blood pressure (BP) in people who failed to adhere to prescribed medication. Individualised consultation approaches have been strongly advocated by authorities such as the World Health Organization based on the notion that involving people by exploring their beliefs and preferences about illness and treatment and providing tailored information produces better adherence. The assumption is that patients' beliefs influence their compliance with treatments. AT is a patient-centred intervention involving generation of discrepancy (the gap between what a patient says is important and what they do) with their beliefs about their illness. AT was delivered over seven weekly 20 min long consultations. Patient beliefs were identified from an assessment and then tested through a three-step process (consultation) involving rating the conviction, providing evidence to support or refute the belief and then a clinician rechecking the strength of belief. Each consultation was standardised and participants were expected to undertake 'homework' that was used on the basis for the next meeting.

A parallel group single-blind randomised controlled trial was carried out in three outpatient clinics. This involved 136 hypertensive patients with a baseline mean systolic BP of 164.5 mm Hg over diastolic BP of 102.2 mm Hg; 68 received AT and 60 TAU. The main outcome was systolic BP at 11 weeks' follow-up. AT reduced systolic BP (−23.11 mm Hg) and diastolic BP (−15.18 mm Hg). Also, adherence with medication measured by pill counting was improved in the AT group by 37%. No adverse events were reported. This study suggests that AT leads to a clinically important reduction in BP.

Reflection activity

Think about the ways used in Alhalaiqa *et al.*'s study (Research Example 12.1) to reduce bias. Why was reducing bias important in this study? What else might the researchers have done to reduce bias?

from the researcher. Detachment is used as a strategy to reduce bias and minimise any involvement that might contaminate the results or influence outcomes. There are several ways to increase detachment, for example, randomisation of participants ensures that the researcher remains unaware (blind) to which subjects receive an intervention or which do not by referring to all participants by a coded descriptor, thus protecting anonymity and separating those delivering an intervention from those responsible for collecting data. In Research Example 12.1, in Alhalaiqa *et al.* (2012), a researcher recruited participants and used an online randomisation service to allocate participants to the intervention or normal care; nurses recorded the participants' BP and undertook the pill count but were unaware of which group a participant had been allocated to so removing the danger of bias.

QUALITATIVE RESEARCH

Qualitative research methods are used across a range of disciplines such as the social sciences, management and nursing and are beginning to be used more frequently in the traditional health sciences. Defining what is qualitative research is made more difficult by the absence of a common, unified set of techniques, philosophies or underpinning perspectives (Mason 2002). Qualitative researchers use an array of concepts and terminology that may appear contrary to ideas of 'good research' encountered in quantitative research (Smith *et al.* 2011). This can be particularly confusing to the novice researcher who not only has to contend with the challenge to previously held notions of what is robust research but also has to acquire what at times appears to be a new language. An analogy might be attempting to cook from a recipe where all the ingredients and terms used for techniques such as sieving, mixing, beating and combining were unfamiliar or in a different language. This would inevitably make you feel uncertain about what you had to use, how to use it and what the final product might be like. To manage the uncertainty, the cook has to interpret to make sense of the recipe. This is not dissimilar to processes involved in qualitative research. Ethnography, phenomenology, grounded theory, narrative and case study are just some of the methodologies that are part of the cluster of approaches that can be considered qualitative, although studies without a specific qualitative methodological label are also published. Some of these different approaches will be examined in more detail in subsequent chapters. Research Example 12.2 presents a summary of a qualitative study using a particular methodological approach – grounded theory – to explore why people with a diagnosis of malignant melanoma delayed seeking attention.

Qualitative research offers flexibility and takes account of complexity, detail and context (Mason 2002). The subjectivity associated with using an approach where the researcher and the research are closely intertwined has its problems. In order to address this, reflexivity (critical self-reflection on the research process and interpretation of data) is an important part of the qualitative researcher's toolkit (Schwandt 1997). Reflexivity has some similarities with reflective practice. In qualitative research, acknowledgement of the influence, and hence scrutiny, of the researcher is often subject to the same level of critical examination as the research itself (Carolan 2003). For this reason, qualitative researchers write field notes in which they describe what was seen, said and done when undertaking the research as well as memos outlining their interpretation of the meaning associated with what they observe. These notes and memos often become data.

This emphasis on involvement and analytical detachment can seem paradoxical. The research approach encourages involvement, as the researcher

RESEARCH EXAMPLE

12.2 A Qualitative Research Study

Topping A, Nkosana-Nyawata I, Heyman B (2013) 'I am not someone who gets skin cancer': risk, time and malignant melanoma. *Health, Risk and Society* 15(6–7): 596–614.

This grounded theory study explored the temporal aspects of 'delay' and risk from the perspectives of patients diagnosed with a cutaneous malignant melanoma. Thirty-nine patients with lesions >76 mm Breslow thickness and six patients with lesions <76 mm thickness provided accounts of their journey to diagnosis. Data were collected from in-depth, audio-recorded interviews covering demographic information, journey to presentation, reflections on actions and/or inaction and risk, lifestyle and risk and personal learning. Data were analysed using a constant comparative method that involved open, axial and selective coding. This article focused on the issues of time and risk in order to understand delay in seeking attention for a 'suspicious' lesion.

The findings suggest that the frame of reference of time lapse is influenced by normalisation of symptoms, possibly reinforced by adherence with health promotion advice giving false reassurance; prioritisation of other life concerns; and in some cases refuting of the persons' concerns by health professionals.

frequently designs the study and collects, interprets and reports the data themselves. They can influence and exert a bias on all stages of the research process. Yet the researcher(s), even though the report may be written in an engaging style, more often than not using first person pronouns, employs several devices to assure the reader that the study is trustworthy. For example, in Research Example 12.2, Topping *et al.* (2013) use the pronoun 'we' to signal to the reader the subjectivity of the interpretation yet provide a transparent description of how the research was conducted, which of the research team undertook specific activities and how the findings were created and corroborated. Readers can judge the authenticity of the findings by reviewing the selected extracts of interview data in the report to confirm the interpretation.

Data collection is reliant upon using approaches that are sensitive to the social context in which the data are produced. Qualitative studies often lack standardisation as too rigid or unsympathetic an approach might reduce the authenticity of the data. Semi- or unstructured interviewing and participant observation are commonly used methods of data collection and are often used in combination, recorded on audio or video tapes or in field notes and then transcribed and transformed into words for analysis. Qualitative analysis commonly involves breaking the data up and coding the different segments. Increasingly, researchers use software packages to assist in managing data. Irrespective of whether the researcher uses paper based or electronic software for data handling, analysis involves a process of breaking down, coding, reordering and reconstituting in order to describe, explain or generate theory.

Reflection activity

Read Research Example 12.2 in which the researchers use a qualitative approach (grounded theory) to gain insight into why people with a diagnosis of malignant melanoma delayed seeking medical attention. Why do you think the researchers chose a qualitative research approach to investigate this topic?

CRITICAL ACCOUNTS OF RESEARCH EPISTEMOLOGY

Numerous commentators have offered critical accounts of the epistemology, methodologies and methods used in the name of research. Criticism is not necessarily negative, and debate could be viewed as an indicator of a healthy discipline and quality of its practitioners. Much of the criticism centres on the rigour employed to manufacture results and the questionable disinterest of research and researchers. Two arguments that cast doubt on the validity of many of the assumptions associated with scientific enquiry are those offered by Popper (1972, 2002) and Kuhn (1972). Popper's argument is philosophical and focuses on the provisional nature of any knowledge or truth. He maintains that researchers should seek to refute hypotheses rather than set out to prove them. In contrast, Kuhn focuses on the culture of research communities and how these could be viewed as self-maintaining and constraining. He describes this as a paradigm that fixes thinking and limits alternative ways to look at problems. An example from history is how orthodox understanding of infection transmission contrived to delay publication of alternative viewpoints but was ultimately overturned when the weight of opinion swung in favour of germ theory. This change took time before final adoption, despite the efforts of the Austrian obstetrician Semmelweis (1818–1865). He encountered bitter resistance and was incarcerated in a mental institution when he tried to disseminate his evidence about the positive benefits of hand washing. This *paradigm shift* ultimately led to the introduction of routine hand washing in health care – something that remains a pressing compliance concern today.

So how do these two critiques relate to nursing research? Firstly, think of nursing as a culture with its own orthodoxy. One of the enduring narratives in the nursing literature surrounds the concept of caring. Considerable effort has been exerted in defining caring, understanding it better through research and theorising about the significance of caring to the experience of nursing and being nursed. Recently, caring in nursing has been much debated as a consequence of failings in care coming to light (Francis 2013). Secondly, for the purpose of this discussion, accept as given that caring is a paradigmatic framework for nursing, an explanation of the contribution of nursing and, by extension, a way of interpreting what is done in nursing. In effect, the way caring is theorised prescribes the way(s) in which research is undertaken to understand it. Using a Kuhnian analysis, the volume of effort invested in understanding caring and its elevation as the primary contribution of nursing to care delivery provides an explanation for why qualitative research approaches have been adopted more readily in nursing research (Ramprogus 2002) compared with other health professional disciplines.

A different but associated criticism of research about the discipline of nursing is that it has failed to make visible the caring work done by nurses (Maben 2008). As a result, the efforts of nurses and the consequences of 'caring for' work done by nurses on health and patient outcomes go unrecognised (Enns & Gregory 2006). Applying a Popperian analysis, the research activity seeking to uncover caring should focus on critical appraisal of caring as the essential concept of nursing. In effect, this would challenge the hypothesis or at least encourage critical analysis of any understandings that emerge. Numerous arguments have been put forward to explain why particular methods used to demonstrate the concept are insufficiently sensitive and inappropriate to capture the nature of phenomenon or when there is a lack of criticism of the underlying assumptions (Nelson & McGillon 2004). Kuhn might contend that it is only when there is enough substance to cast doubt that competing sets of assumptions emerge and a paradigm shift occurs. This is when a discipline alters the way it understands problems. Nursing's contribution has undergone a recent reorientation with the attention given to nurses' work across the globe. The research focus has shifted toward the organisational constraints that impact on care delivery (Weinberg 2003) and identification on the outcomes of nursing that can be measured (Griffiths 2008; Aiken *et al.* 2014). This has transformed understanding of the contribution of nurses to patient safety and quality care. Interestingly, the focus on outcomes has driven a shift toward quantitative methods.

BLENDING QUANTITATIVE AND QUALITATIVE APPROACHES

A solution offered as an alternative to using one or other research approach is to blend qualitative and quantitative approaches through the use of mixed or combined methods (Brannen 2005; Teddlie & Tashakkori 2009). Chapter 27 deals with this issue in more depth. The advantage of blending approaches is the added value that complementary approaches offer, particularly if the relative weaknesses of one are offset by another. The use of a number of methods within a research design is termed *triangulation*. The term has traditionally been used to refer to the procedures used to pinpoint a particular geographic position by taking measurements from three or more points. In research, it is used to describe a way that different types of data are obtained from participants and used to corroborate findings (Denzin 1989).

There is a difference between using a number of methods to provide convergent views yet still provide a coherent account and an approach where a range of data collection strategies are used to provide a more complete but layered analysis. According to Denzin (1989), triangulation in research can take a number of forms – data, investigator, theory and method. Data triangulation involves using a number of different data sources that can shed light on a particular phenomenon. That said, Hammersley and Atkinson (2007) warn that using multiple data sources may not always confirm inferences but make differences more blatant and act as a further check to credibility. Theoretical triangulation encourages the use of competing theory to compare and contrast interpretations of data. By this means, theory can be advanced and revised. Methodological triangulation can be within methods where compatible data collection methods such as participant observation, qualitative interviewing and field notes are used. Alternatively, dissimilar data collection strategies from different research traditions may be used to illuminate the same phenomenon such as using a structured questionnaire with focus group interviews.

Criticisms of mixed methods include concerns about philosophical incongruity between the position of positivism, with its emphasis on objective truth, and the interpretative traditions that make no claims to any single reality (Brannen 2005). Another criticism is mixed methods merely compound sources of error (Armitage & Hodgson 2004) inherent in the strategies employed. Lastly, there is the issue of how quality should be judged, particularly if competing research traditions are used in the same study (Creswell & Tashakkori 2007).

Reflection activity

What are the benefits and limitations involved in using a mixed methods approach for a research project? You may find it helpful to read Chapter 27 after you have undertaken this activity.

JUDGING THE QUALITY OF QUANTITATIVE AND QUALITATIVE RESEARCH

Judgement invariably involves comparison. In order to compare one thing with another, an individual will use some form of criteria. In quantitative research, the criteria are normally the concepts of reliability and validity, but these are considered inappropriate to judge qualitative research (Mays & Pope 2000). Lincoln and Guba (1985, 1989) offer a different set of criteria for judging qualitative research that are based on the concept of trustworthiness or authenticity (see Box 12.2). This alternative position for judging quality becomes more difficult with mixed methods research. However, various approaches have been suggested for assessing mixed methods research. For example, Teddlie and Tashakkori (2009) emphasise the adequacy of coverage of the research question, quality of each method, assessment of integration and coherence of inferences. O'Cathain *et al.* (2008) developed a series of questions in the form of a checklist providing technical guidance to judge mixed methods studies (see Box 12.3).

Box 12.2 Comparison of the criteria used to judge the trustworthiness of a study

Quantitative research	Qualitative research Trustworthiness criteria (Lincoln & Guba 1985)
Internal validity – extent to which what is observed truly represents the variable under investigation	Credibility – fit between participant's views and researcher's representation of them
External validity – extent that the results of a study can be generalised to other contexts and populations	Transferability – relates to the adequacy of the description to judge similarity to other situations so findings might be transferred
Reliability – refers to the consistency and accuracy of the data collection approach or instrument	Dependability – relates to transparency of the research process and decision trail
Objectivity	Confirmability – establishing that data, findings and interpretation are clearly linked

Box 12.3 Checklist for assessing the quality of mixed methods studies

1 Has the justification for using a mixed methods approach to the research question been described?
2 Are the design, purpose, priority and sequence of methods described?
3 Is each method described adequately in terms of sampling, data collection and analysis?
4 Where integration has occurred, how has it occurred and who has participated in it?
5 Is there any description of the limitations of one method associated with the presence of the other approach(es)?
6 Have any insights gained from mixing or integrating methods been presented?

Based on O'Cathain *et al.* (2008) The quality of mixed methods studies in health service research *Journal of Health Services Research Policy* 13(2): 92–98.

CONCLUSION

This chapter has examined key assumptions underpinning the research process. An attempt has been made to move attention away from irreconcilable differences between quantitative and qualitative researches to the strengths and weaknesses of different approaches whether used separately or in combination. Subsequent chapters will emphasise that the purpose of research is to adopt the right tools for the task in hand. Just as a driver faced with a punctured tyre would select the appropriate equipment and most effective way to approach the task, the same principles apply to research problems. It would be naïve not to recognise that a researcher experienced in the use of a particular methodology or method, or holding a particular set of beliefs about the world, would be more inclined to explore research problems amenable to their preferred approach(es) just as a chef will return to tried and tested recipes. Research includes a broad constituency of competing perspectives, assumptions, methodologies and methods. All approaches can be criticised or found insufficient and rightly so. Healthy constructive criticism should be encouraged. This chapter has sought to emphasise that research problems or the pursuit of answers, however incomplete, should drive approaches not vice versa.

References

Aiken LH, Sloane DM, Bruyneel L, Van den Heede K, Griffiths P, Busse R, Diomidous M, Kinnunen J, Kozka M, Lesaffre E, McHugh MD, Moreno-Casbas MT, Rafferty AM, Schwendimann R, Scott AP, Tishelman C, van Achterbery T, Sermeus W (2014) Nurse staffing and education and hospital mortality in nine European countries: a retrospective observational study. *The Lancet* **383**: 1824–1830.

Alhalaiqa F, Deane KHO, Nawafleh AH, Clark A, Gray R (2012) Adherence therapy for medication non-compliant patients with hypertension: a randomised controlled trial. *Journal of Human Hypertension* **26**: 117–126.

Annandale E (1998) *The Sociology of Health and Medicine*. Cambridge, Polity Press.

Armitage G, Hodgson I (2004) Using ethnography (or qualitative methods) to investigate drug errors: a critique of a published study. *NT Research* **9**: 379–387.

Benner P (1984) *Novice to Expert*. Menlo-Park, Addison-Wesley.

Benner P (1996) A response by P Benner to K Cash, Benner and expertise in nursing: a critique. *International Journal of Nursing Studies* **33**: 669–674.

Brannen J (2005) *Mixed methods research: a discussion paper*. ESRC National Centre for Research Methods NCRM Methods Review Papers download http://eprints.ncrm.ac.uk/89/1/MethodsReviewPaperNCRM-005.pdf (accessed on 2 September 2014).

Burns N, Groves SK, Gray J (2012) *The Practice of Nursing Research: Appraisal, Synthesis and Generation of Evidence*, 7th edition. Philadelphia, WB Saunders.

Carolan M (2003) Reflexivity: a personal journey during data collection. *Nurse Researcher* **10**(3): 7–14.

Cash K (1995) Benner and expertise in nursing: a critique. *International Journal of Nursing Studies* **32**: 527–534.

Creswell JW, Tashakkori A (2007) Editorial: developing publishable mixed methods manuscripts. *Journal of Mixed Methods Research* **1**(2): 107–110.

Denzin N (1989) *The Research Act: A Theoretical Introduction to Sociological Methods,* 3rd edition. Englewood Cliffs, Prentice Hall.

Enns C, Gregory D (2006) Lamentation and loss: expressions of caring by contemporary surgical nurses. *Journal of Advanced Nursing* **58**(4): 339–347.

Foucault M (1973) *The Birth of the Clinic*. London, Tavistock.

Francis R (2013) *Report of the Mid Staffordshire NHS Foundation Trust Public Inquiry Executive Summary*. London, The Stationery Office HC 947.

Grbich C (1999) *Qualitative Research in Health*. London, Sage.

Griffiths P (2008) The art of losing….? A response to the question 'is caring a lost art?' *International Journal of Nursing Studies* **45**: 329–332.

Hammersley M, Atkinson P (2007) *Ethnography Principles in Practice*, 3rd edition. London, Taylor & Francis.

Hayward J, Boore JRP (1994) *Research Classics from the Royal College of Nursing Vol 1. Information: a prescription against pain and Prescription for recovery*. Harrow, Scutari.

Kuhn TS (1972) *The Structure of Scientific Revolutions,* 2nd edition. Chicago, University of Chicago.

Lincoln Y, Guba E (1985) *Naturalistic Inquiry*. Thousand Oaks, Sage.

Lincoln Y, Guba E (1989) *Fourth Generation Evaluation*. Thousand Oaks, Sage.

Maben J (2008) Editorial debate the art of caring: invisible and subordinated? A response to Juliet Corbin: 'Is caring a lost art in nursing?' *International Journal of Nursing Studies* **45**: 335–338.

Mason J (2002) *Qualitative Researching*, 2nd edition. London, Sage.

Mays N, Pope C (2000) Assessing quality in qualitative research. *British Medical Journal* **320**: 50–52.

Nelson S, McGillon M (2004) Expertise or performance? Questioning the rhetoric of contemporary use of narrative use in nursing. *Journal of Advanced Nursing* **47**: 631–638.

O'Cathain A, Murphy E, Nicholl J (2008) The quality of mixed methods studies in health service research. *Journal of Health Services Research Policy* **13**(2): 92–98.

O'Connor G, Coates V, O'Neill S (2010) Exploring the information needs of patients with cancer of the rectum. *European Journal of Oncology Nursing* **14**: 271–277.

Polgar S, Thomas SA (2008) *Introduction to Research in the Health Sciences*, 5th edition. Edinburgh, Churchill Livingstone.

Popper K (1972) *Conjectures and Refutations*, 4th edition. London, Routledge & Kegan Paul.

Popper K (2002) *The Logic of Scientific Discovery*. London, Routledge.

Ramprogus V (2002) Eliciting nursing knowledge from practice: the dualism of nursing. *Nurse Researcher* **10**(1): 52–64.

Sandelowski M (1993) Rigor or rigor mortis: the problem of rigor in qualitative research. *Advances Nursing Science* **16**(2): 1–8.

Schwandt TA (1997) *Qualitative Inquiry: A Dictionary of Terms*. Thousand Oaks, Sage.

Shipman M (1997) *The Limitations of Social Research*, 4th edition. London, Longman.

Silverman D (2011) *Doing Qualitative Research: A Practical Handbook*, 3rd edition. London, Sage.

Silverman D (2013) *Very Short, Fairly Interesting Book about Qualitative Research*, 2nd edition. London, Sage.

Smith J, Bekker H, Chester F (2011) Theoretical versus pragmatic design in qualitative research. *Nurse Researcher* **18**(2): 39–51.

Teddlie C, Tashakkori A (2009) *Foundations of Mixed Methods Research: Integrating Quantitative and Qualitative Approaches in the Social and Behavioural Sciences*. Thousand Oaks, Sage.

Topping A, Nkosana-Nyawata I, Heyman B (2013) 'I am not someone who gets skin cancer': risk, time and malignant melanoma. *Health, Risk & Society* **15**(6–7): 596–614.

Weinberg DB (2003) *Code Green*. New York, Cornell University Press.

Websites

http://www.qualitative-research.net/fqs/fqs-eng.htm – Qualitative Social Research is an online peer-reviewed multilingual journal for qualitative research.

http://onlineqda.hud.ac.uk/index.php – Online QDA is a set of training support materials that address common problems (both early and advanced) of using Qualitative Data Analysis (QDA) methods and selected Computer-Assisted Qualitative Data AnalysiS (CAQDAS) packages.

http://www.nova.edu/ssss/QR/web.html – The Qualitative Report is an online journal dedicated to qualitative research.

http://www.data-archive.ac.uk/ – ESDS Qualidata is a specialist service of the ESDS led by the UK Data Archive (UKDA) at the University of Essex. The service provides access and support for a range of social science qualitative datasets, promoting and facilitating increased and more effective use of data in research, learning and teaching.

http://www.ncrm.ac.uk/ – ESRC National Centre for Research Methods (NCRM) is a network of research groups, each conducting research and training in an area of social science research methods.

CHAPTER 13

Sampling

Katherine Hunt and Judith Lathlean

Key points

- Sampling methods are adopted to ensure the best possible chance of generating reliable knowledge that is applicable to a wider population.
- Approaches vary across quantitative and qualitative research, according to the context and research design, but there are common principles that can be applied.
- Sample selection and size affect the validity of the research and so should be achieved with maximum rigour.

INTRODUCTION

Sampling is an essential part of all research endeavours as it is not usually possible (except perhaps where a national census is being undertaken) to include the whole of a population in a research study. Sampling also ensures that the research is manageable and feasible, within time and resource constraints. Many of the principles and considerations of sampling cross over both quantitative and qualitative research designs, such as the concept of population and the sampling frame, and these will be considered first. The chapter then focuses on probability sampling, considered the most valid approach in order to achieve statistical generalisation. Non-probability sampling can feature in quantitative research but is characteristic of qualitative approaches, where targeted selection of participants is common.

POPULATIONS AND SAMPLES

When identifying a group of people or units to include in a research study, it is important to understand the difference between the target population and the study population. These are described in the following text.

Target population

This is the entire population of interest. In quantitative research, where the aim is to generalise data collected from a sample to the population from which it was drawn, the target population is the population to whom the results will be applied. In Research Example 13.1, the target population was all residents aged between 65 and 84 years living in four Italian cities. It should

The Research Process in Nursing, Seventh Edition. Edited by Kate Gerrish and Judith Lathlean.

Companion Website: www.wiley.com/go/gerrish/research

RESEARCH EXAMPLE

13.1 Simple Random Sampling

Mureddu GF, Agabiti N, Rizzello V, Forastiere F, Latini R, Cesaroni G, Masson S, Cacciatore G, Colivicchi F, Uguccioni M, Perucci CA, Boccanelli A (2012) Prevalence of preclinical and clinical heart failure in the elderly: a population-based study in Central Italy. *European Journal of Heart Failure* **14**: 718–729.

This cross-sectional study assessed the prevalence of preclinical and clinical heart failure in the population of older people living in central Italy. A simple random sample of 5940 residents aged between 65 and 85 years of age was taken from four cities in the Lazio region. Residents were identified through the Regional Health Registry. In three of the four cities, the entire population of people aged between 65 and 84 was eligible for inclusion in the study. However, in Rome, the largest of the four cities, the population was too big to identify all residents who met the age criteria. The researchers therefore drew up a list of the 74,000 older people living in the 21 neighbourhoods closest to the research centre. Although 5940 residents were randomly selected, more than half were either excluded or declined to participate. The final sample included 2001 older people. Results reported the overall prevalence of heart failure at 6.7%, and this did not differ according to gender. A total of 81.1% of the sample had preclinical heart failure and left ventricular dysfunction increased with age.

be noted in this example that for three of the four cities, everyone aged between 65 and 84 was eligible for inclusion in the study. However, in Rome, the largest of the four cities, the population was too big to identify all residents who met the age criteria, and thus, a manageable number was selected from which to gain a simple random sample.

The concept of target population is also relevant in qualitative research, although the aim is not to generalise to the target population and a different form of non-random sampling is used. This is often referred to as purposive sampling whereby the desire is still to increase understanding of the nature and experience of that population.

Study population

The study or accessible population is a subset of the population from whom the sample is taken – either to maximise efficiency or because it is simply not possible to access the entire target population. In Research Example 13.1, the size of Rome's population meant that it was not feasible to recruit from the target population. It was necessary therefore to identify a study population. This was people aged between 65 and 84 years who lived in 21 neighbourhoods that were close to the cardiology centre. For the other three cities, where the populations were smaller, the sample was drawn directly from the target population, which is the entire city.

Sampling frame

In order to identify a sample in advance, a sampling frame is required. Simply put, a sampling frame is a detailed list of all units, such as people, hospitals or events in a population. Usually, the list relates to the study population rather than the target population. However, a robust study population is one that has similar characteristics to the target population, and if this is not the case, it is more difficult to generalise to the wider population. In Research Example 13.2, the sampling frame was all deaths registered in two English health districts during a given time period. Because all deaths are officially registered, this was in fact the target population, not a study population. This is in contrast to the first research example where the sampling frame was generated from the study population, that is, a list of older people living in the 21 identified neighbourhoods of Rome.

RESEARCH EXAMPLE

13.2 Stratified Sampling

Hunt KJ, Shlomo N, Addington-Hall J (2014) End-of-life care and preferences for place of death among the oldest old: results of a population-based survey using VOICES-Short Form. *Journal of Palliative Medicine* **17**(2): 176–182.

This feasibility post-bereavement survey assessed the quality of care provided in the last 3 days of life from the perspective of bereaved relatives. Two health districts in the south of England formed the setting. The sampling strategy was designed to ensure that deaths included in the sample were representative of all deaths in the two health districts, and so the register of deaths formed the sampling frame. Using all deaths registered in the two health districts between October 2009 and April 2010, a self-weighting, proportionally allocated stratified sample design was employed, using the following strata: primary care team, gender, place of death and primary cause of death. Deaths were sorted according to the variables that defined the strata, and sample selection was carried out using systematic sampling in each stratum after sorting by age at death. A total of 2272 deaths were identified, but the following deaths were then excluded: those registered outside the study dates, deaths in under 18 s, coroner-registered deaths and deaths where the relative lived overseas. Thus, 1422 deaths were included in the survey. The response rate was 33% – 473 bereaved relatives returned questionnaires. The majority of relatives reported that home was the preferred place of death, yet only 13.3% died at home. When rating care in the last 2 days, relatives were more likely to highly rate nursing care, relief of pain and other symptoms, emotional support and privacy if their relative died in their preferred place.

Reflection activity

The idea of a population is important in sampling, but what is the difference between a target population and the actual population identified for a study? In Research Example 13.1, why did the sample generated from three of the cities differ from that relating to Rome? What biases may this have introduced as a result?

TYPES OF SAMPLING

There are two broad categories or types of sampling design in research: probability and non-probability sampling. In quantitative research, where the aim is to recruit a sample that is representative of the target population to permit generalisation, probability samples are favoured. In such sampling techniques, as will be discussed in more depth in the following section, it becomes possible to quantify the risk of bias or error. In qualitative research, where the aim is to target the research on individual 'cases' that are data rich, non-probability samples are predominantly used. However, this is not a hard and fast rule. In reality, and particularly in health research, quantitative studies will frequently opt for convenience samples. This is often a consequence of the nature of the target population or the absence of a sampling frame: for instance, if researchers wanted to examine blood profiles of patients admitted to an emergency department following a stroke, the target population would not be known in advance and the researchers would be forced to recruit people consecutively, as they are admitted. Conversely, qualitative studies increasingly use probabilistic methods of recruitment. This is because they are now often nested within bigger quantitative studies such as randomised controlled trials.

Probability sampling

The fundamental characteristic of probability sampling is the random selection of units from a population. This approach ensures that all members of a target population have a known chance of being selected. For this reason, probability sampling is accepted as the most rigorous type of sampling strategy. In some types of probability sampling, this means that all units of a population have an equal chance of selection, whilst in other probability sampling techniques, units of a population have an unequal chance. Either way, this probability of selection is known in advance and can be quantified. In order to select participants in this way, as previously suggested, a sampling frame is required.

Although probabilistic sampling strategies do not guarantee the generation of a truly representative sample, the random selection of units from a target population means that any differences between the population and the sample are due to chance, except in the presence of sampling error. There are two types of sampling error: *random errors* and *systematic errors*, and both introduce bias. Random errors are common and occur randomly in a sample as a result of under- or over-representation of certain groups. For instance, just by chance, a small sample might not include a sufficiently high proportion of people from minority ethnic groups – this would lead to under-representation of people from those groups in the sample, and the findings would not reflect the views/characteristics of the true population. The likelihood of random errors can usually be reduced by increasing the sample size. Systematic errors, on the other hand, are more difficult to handle because their likelihood cannot be reduced in this way. They usually occur as a result of inconsistencies or errors in the sampling frame. This highlights the importance of an accurate sampling frame: inaccuracies will lead to systematic errors that cannot be corrected through increasing the sample size. For instance, sampling patients discharged from hospital with certain diagnoses relies on the accuracy of discharge codes entered onto the hospital recording system.

Compared to non-probability sampling, probability sampling is more likely to result in a representative sample with reduced sampling errors and bias. In addition, probability sampling removes the potential for researcher bias in the selection of potential participants. There are several types of probability sample: simple random sampling, systematic random sampling, stratified random sampling and multistage/cluster sampling.

Non-probability sampling

Although quantitative study designs commonly apply a probability sampling strategy, a non-probabilistic approach is sometimes taken. This may be because the sampling frame is unknown or this part of the study is exploratory or random sampling would simply be too costly. Nevertheless, in quantitative research, failure to randomly select a sample reduces a study's representativeness and the extent to which generalisations to the target population can be made. Moreover, inferential statistics rely on an assumption that data are generated through random selection, which means that findings from quantitative studies with non-probability samples should be interpreted with caution. Therefore, if the research question necessitates the exploration of relationships between variables or the comparison of groups of people, a probability sample is favoured.

Quota sampling can be mentioned here as a form of non-probability sampling. This is a method of sampling widely used in opinion polls and market research, for example, to gain views on the use of a service or a particular product. It is a form of convenience sampling where the data collector is required to recruit a fairly large number (quota) of people fitting a particular category, for example, males and females over 60 if the views of people over 'retirement' age are sought. Often, the size of the quota in the sample is proportional to the number of people in that category in the target population. Bias can be introduced, however, if data collectors consciously or unconsciously avoid certain types of people such as the homeless, plus it requires a judgement as to whether the person does indeed fall into the 'correct' category, in this example that of age. For the reasons of possible bias and non-randomness, quota sampling is not much used in health services research.

Some authors (e.g. Bryman 2012) also describe convenience sampling and snowball sampling as types of non-probability sampling. Novice researchers and those with limited time and other resources may select an accessible population or setting, which they believe to be typical, rather than select a representative sample. Convenience may be a key feature in this decision, for example, approaching particular participants from a local health facility. In many ways, all researchers use a variant of a convenience sample in the sense that the sample must be accessible to the researcher in some form. However, convenience sampling can lead to significant biases and errors if the sample used is unrepresentative of the target population and should be avoided if possible.

In some respects, snowball sampling is similar to convenience sampling. Here, the researcher asks respondents in a network to identify people who are relevant to a particular topic. It is sometimes used where the sample is difficult to access, for example, Becker's (1963) classic study of marijuana users, in which half of the 50 interviews were with people that had been identified by the initial interviewees. This raises potential problems of representativeness but equally can be an appropriate way of increasing the size and variation within a sample.

Reflection activity

Does quantitative research always have to use probability sampling? If probability sampling is not employed, what are the implications for the generalisability of the study? Is qualitative research always based on non-probability sampling? What effect does this kind of sampling have on the 'validity' of the study? You might need to read more of the chapter to fully answer this question.

APPROACHES TO RANDOM SAMPLING

Simple random sampling

Simple random sampling uses a sampling frame to list all units in a target population and selects a sample of units from that list. This means that all units of the sampling frame have a known and equal chance of selection. For example, we may want to invite all women from one GP practice to join a research study about breast screening. The GP practice register would be used to create the sampling frame, that is, all women aged between 18 and 85 years. Even though the study would recruit a predefined number of women (perhaps 200), all women on that list would be eligible for selection. A total of 200 women would then be selected at random, and all women would have an equal chance of being selected.

There are several methods of selecting a random sample from the sampling frame, such as using a statistical software package or random number tables (found at the back of many statistics textbooks). Random number tables select samples by working either horizontally or vertically through the table. More information on these approaches can be found at www.randomization.com. There are a number of advantages to this sampling approach, namely, that the likelihood of a unit being selected can be quantified, and any differences observed between the population and the sample are due to chance. This, of course, depends on the size of the sample because as sample size increases, so does sample representativeness. Simple random samples are best used in more homogeneous populations where any sample is likely to contain people or units with similar characteristics. Without this homogeneity, rogue samples can be drawn, and systematic or stratified random sampling methods would be more appropriate. The biggest disadvantage to simple random sampling is that, depending on the sampling frame being used, it is time consuming and rather inefficient because all members of a target/study population have to be listed. In cluster sampling, on the other hand, people are grouped into larger units.

Random sampling must not be confused with random allocation. The latter refers to the random assignment of participants to study groups in an experimental study, such as a randomised controlled trial.

Systematic random sampling

Unlike simple random sampling, in systematic sampling, units are selected from a list (generated from the sampling frame) at intervals that are predetermined by the researcher. Ordinarily, this involves selecting every '*n*th' unit (where n is a number) on the list until the desired sample size is reached. Selection of the '*n*th' unit usually depends upon the sampling fraction: the ratio of the required sample size to the size of the population. For instance, if there are 500 units on the list and the required sample size is 50, the sampling fraction would be 10% and selection would be 1 in 10. The starting point for the selection of the first unit is a randomly selected number in the list, between 1 and 10. In this example, every 10th number in the list would be selected until the desired sample size reached – 7, 17, 27, 37 and so forth. A limitation of this approach is that some lists have their own biases that can be transferred into the sample. For instance, every seventh patient in the list may have certain characteristics, such as being admitted to hospital on a Sunday, thereby creating an organisational bias. This means that a systematic random sample can only be truly random if the ordering of units on the sample frame is also random.

Stratified random sampling

As with simple random sampling and systematic sampling, stratified random sampling also requires a sampling frame to list all units in the target population. However, unlike the aforementioned methods, it is helpful in situations where the sampling frame contains highly heterogeneous units, such as where there is considerable variation in age, gender, disease type, etc. This might be a problem if the variable of interest has high variance or, for instance, if disease prevalence is higher in specific demographic groups.

Simply described, stratified random sampling involves dividing all units of a population contained within a sampling frame into strata that are determined by the research question, attributes of interest or important demographic variables. For instance, if body mass index (BMI) is important, it might be necessary to include people from a series of BMI categories, such as those representing underweight, ideal weight, overweight and obese. These categories would form the strata, and then cases would be selected from each stratum in an equal, proportionate or disproportionate manner. In the Research Example 13.2, the researchers wanted to be able to make comparisons between people who died of certain conditions, comparisons between health providers and comparisons between care settings. Therefore, cases were organised according to these strata before a *proportionate stratified sample* from each stratum was drawn. This approach increases the representativeness of the sample so that findings can be generalised to the wider population: if simple random sampling methods are used to select cases, chance may mean that certain groups become over- or under-represented.

In certain instances, it may be necessary to increase representation of particular population groups to facilitate analysis, such as analysis by ethnic origin where the numbers from particular groups may be relatively small. This approach is termed disproportionate stratified sampling and involves increasing the sampling fraction for certain groups. The disadvantage of this approach is that the resulting sample is no longer representative of the target population and the analysis needs to be adjusted to take this over-representation into account.

Importantly, the decision to allocate cases to strata should be based on the research questions and key variables rather than simply due to heterogeneity in the population. Again, this form of sampling can be time consuming and relies on the presence of an accurate sampling frame, and it can be difficult to develop the strata.

Multistage or cluster sampling

The terms multistage and cluster sampling are used interchangeably although there are minor differences between the two. Most noticeably, multistage

RESEARCH EXAMPLE

13.3 Cluster Sampling

Mastersa SH, Bursteina R, Amofahb G, Abaogyec P, Kumara S, Hanlona M (2013) Travel time to maternity care and its effect on utilization in rural Ghana: A multilevel analysis. *Social Science and Medicine* **93**: 147–194.

This retrospective cross-sectional study looked at the impact of distance from the maternity clinic on utilisation of maternity services in Ghana. Because women were nested within households and households were nested within communities, it was very probable that women in the same households would have similar socio-economic characteristics; women in the same communities were likely to share characteristics compared to women from other communities. This necessitated a cluster sampling design, and a two-stage approach to sampling was conducted. In the first stage, 412 geographical clusters were identified by the Ghana Health Service. In the second stage, approximately 30 households from each of the 412 clusters were selected. This resulted in a sample of 11,778 households. Households were then excluded if the mother lived in an urban location, if there were insufficient data about the characteristics of the delivery or if it was unknown where the birth had taken place. These exclusions left a total of 1099 households, 1172 mothers and 1649 births to be included in the study. The study reported that travel time was associated with care facility utilisation, antenatal care visits and in-facility delivery. The quality of maternity care in maternity facilities did not affect service utilisation.

sampling implies, as the name suggests, that there is more than one stage or level of sample. Typically, the first cluster contains larger units than the second cluster and and each subsequent cluster has reducing numbers. Cluster/multistage sampling is used when simple random sampling, systematic sampling or stratified sampling would be too complex and expensive to conduct. If a research question required the selection of a representative sample of nurses working in surgical wards, rather than listing all surgical nurses nationally, it might be more feasible to first, using simple random or stratified sampling techniques, randomly select six large cities, then randomly select three hospitals within each city and then randomly select three surgical wards in each hospital and then all nurses working in those wards. Although this approach is considerably easier than developing a sampling frame comprising all surgical nurses working in a country, it can introduce more sampling error and requires complex statistical techniques because variation needs to be taken into account at each cluster: between-city, between-hospital and between-nurse, for instance.

Reflection activity

We can see there are a number of different kinds of random sampling. What are the factors that determine which might be appropriate for a study? Is the choice of the approach adopted an easy one, or would you need advice from a statistician to select the best method? How would you know what size of sample to achieve? Again, you may need to look at the next section to be sure about how to answer this question.

Furthermore, samples within clusters can be closely related, thus increasing the sampling error – for example, hospitals within a particular city might share certain characteristics. Research Example 13.3 is a study where geographical clusters were used to facilitate appropriate sampling.

CALCULATING SAMPLE SIZE IN QUANTITATIVE RESEARCH

Whilst the rule of thumb that 'bigger is better' does apply to some degree to sample size in quantitative research, the required sample size should be *calculated* during the design and planning of a research study, rather than guessed or calculated retrospectively. There are several reasons why sample size is calculated in quantitative research: for example, a study that is too large may waste valuable resources, whilst a sample size that is too small can be unethical or inappropriate, as it might not be big enough to detect differences. Further, the probability of selecting a non-representative sample is increased if the sample size is small. This is because, as sample size increases, the 'sample mean' becomes closer to the 'population mean'. As a practical example, we may be interested in LDL cholesterol. If a researcher took a sample of people and calculated their mean (average) LDL cholesterol concentration, it may not be the same as the mean LDL cholesterol in the general population. A common cause for such an error is the size of the sample because in a small sample the chance of recruiting people who are different to others in the population is quite high. If the researcher were to recruit another sample of the same size, the mean LDL cholesterol in the sample might again be different to the mean LDL cholesterol in the whole population. However, if the researcher were to identify a bigger sample, the likelihood of only recruiting people who are very different to the general population would reduce. Of course, even in big samples, there is still room for error. It is only through recruiting all people in the population (a census) that the sample mean would be the same as the population mean.

A quantitative research report should outline the required sample size and the way in which it is calculated. The presence of this increases one's confidence in the study's findings for an important reason: it quantifies the likelihood that the results are a chance finding in that sample and not a 'true' finding in the target population. It also describes the power of the study to detect statistically significant differences between groups.

The significance of research findings relates to probability, and probability is simply how we quantify chance. If an event is impossible, then its probability is 0. If an event is certain, its probability is 1. This means that any event that is uncertain, although not impossible, will have a probability between 0 and 1. For brevity, probability is referred to as 'p'. The significance of research findings relate to the probability of detecting a statistically significant effect or difference between study groups in the sample when it does not exist in the target population. This is termed a type I (α) error and in practice means that the researchers will say that the intervention works or that a real difference between groups exists when it does not. In quantitative research, we often set the significance (α) level at 5%. If the α level is set at 5%, a significant result means that we can be 95% confident that a real difference exists in the population and there is a 5% probability that the finding was due to chance alone. In some studies, such as clinical trials of medicines or interventions, the α level can be set more stringently at 1% (a 1% probability that the finding was due to chance alone). A type II (β) error is the opposite: the probability of finding that there is no effect or difference between groups in the sample when, in the population, there is a true effect or difference. The concept of statistical 'power' is used to describe the probability of detecting a real difference that exists in the population.

The required sample size can be calculated using a power analysis (Cohen 1988). As is custom, most studies will use 80% power, which means they will have an 80% probability of detecting a real difference if it exists. Of course, this means there will be a 20% probability of not detecting a real difference. If a power calculation is not conducted, confidence in the findings is reduced because it is unknown whether the sample was too small to detect differences that exist or may detect differences that in fact do not exist in the population. Power analysis requires some information about the expected range of scores (variance or standard deviation) that would be expected within the population being studied. If, for instance, a comparison study wanted to investigate the difference in blood sugar levels between people with diabetes and people without diabetes, the power calculation would be based upon the expected differences in blood sugar levels between the two groups. This information might come from clinical data, previous research or a pilot study. Although there are tools available to help researchers to calculate sample size, often a statistician will conduct the power analysis using the information (expected values and their variance) provided by the researchers. The calculation of sample size also needs to take attrition (people who drop out of a study) into account. This means increasing the sample size beyond that calculated through power analysis.

Generally, when the expected differences between study groups are large, the required sample size is smaller than if expected differences are small. Ultimately, sample sizes aim to ensure that a sample is as representative as it can be whilst minimising sampling error.

SAMPLING IN QUALITATIVE RESEARCH

It has already been pointed out that random sampling can be used within qualitative research, and indeed, Mays and Pope (2006) stated that stratified sampling techniques can be used to ensure that the range of 'cases' chosen are representative of the population to which the researcher wishes to generalise. However, characteristically non-probability sampling is chosen so that individuals, events or settings will be identified that best illuminate the phenomena of interest and provide rich data. It is still important that selection is rigorous, and Mays and Pope (2006) suggested that the following question be asked:

- Does the sample contain the full range of relevant cases or settings so that conceptual rather than statistical generalisations can be made?

Some qualitative researchers argue that selecting a 'sample' is not appropriate since they are doing research in 'naturally occurring' populations or settings (Silverman 2010). Single case studies and 'ethnographic' studies in particular settings can be undertaken. Nevertheless, attention still needs to be paid to the ability to generalise which is theoretical rather than statistical. In the Research Example 13.4, the researchers deliberately targeted three settings in their ethnographic comparative analysis of a single computer decision support system. Their aim was to apply a theoretical perspective, that of normalisation process theory, to understand what was happening in the settings and what were the challenges of implementation of a new system.

Purposive sampling

This is a form of non-probability sampling whereby decisions about the individuals to be included in the sample are taken by the researcher; they are based on

RESEARCH EXAMPLE

13.4 Sampling and Theorisation

Pope C, Halford S, Turnbull J, Prichard J, Calestani M, May C (2013) Using computer decision support systems in NHS emergency and urgent care: ethnographic study using Normalization Process Theory. *BMC Health Services Research* **13**:111. doi:10.1186/1472-6963-13-111.

This was an ethnographic comparative study of a single computer decision support system in three different settings to understand the implementation and everyday use of this technology, which is designed to deal with calls to emergency and urgent care services. The sample comprised three deliberately targeted services – an established 999 ambulance call-handling service, a new single point of access for urgent care and an established general practice out-of-hours service. A theoretical approach known as normalisation process theory (NPT) was used as a framework to enable systematic cross-case analysis and thus to achieve theoretical generalisation from these purposively selected cases.

RESEARCH EXAMPLE

13.5 Purposive Sampling

Bulman C, Lathlean J, Gobbi M (2014) The process of teaching and learning about reflection: research insights from professional nurse education. *Studies in Higher Education* **37**: 1219–1236.

This study investigated the process of reflection in professional nurse education and the part it played in a teaching and learning context. The sample was purposively selected and consisted of different types of units, activities and individuals. Thus, the target university and school were first identified, as was the programme of interest and, within that, a group of related student and teacher participants. Aspects pertinent to the teachers and students were studied such as teaching and learning situations (seminars, tutorials and conversations between participants) and artefacts (programme handbooks and reflective learning contracts (RLCs)). As fieldwork progressed, it became obvious that clinical supervisors were also involved in RLCs, and so they too were recruited and became part of the sample.

various criteria including specialist knowledge of the research topic and about the individuals who are most likely to provide data of sufficient relevance and depth. Thus, in Research Example 13.5, the researchers used an interpretive approach and targeted a sample of lecturers and students, engaged in a post-registration palliative care programme, in order to explore their experiences and use of reflection. It is interesting to note that they referred to 'purposeful' selection in the text (rather than purposive), but the two terms can be used interchangeably to refer to the deliberate targeting of individuals as 'exemplars' of, in this case, individuals who were engaged in a programme of learning.

Patton (2002) suggested that there are a number of different examples of purposive sampling, which include sampling extreme or deviant cases, typical cases, cases that provide maximum variation, confirming and disconfirming cases and cases that are theory based, amongst others. The idea of basing a sample on the ability to theorise is illustrated in Research Example 13.4.

Theoretical sampling

Reference is made in the literature to 'theoretical' sampling. This is where further sampling occurs as a result of data analysis, as opposed to purposive sample that happens prior to data collection. It is also a feature of a study using a grounded theory design (see Chapter 13) whereby data are collected until data 'saturation' has been achieved and no new themes or perspectives are found. It is then assumed that the phenomenon under study has been fully explored. Research Example 13.6 describes an exploration of dental practices in Australia. In doing so, it brings together research that emanated from a randomised controlled trial, whereby random sampling was adopted, followed by a qualitative study that began with a purposive sample and then moved to theoretical sampling.

DECIDING UPON SAMPLE SIZE IN QUALITATIVE RESEARCH

A question that is often posed by novice researchers in particular is, how many participants or 'cases' are required for qualitative research to be 'valid'? The literature sometimes suggests a range or a minimum and maximum number of participants or cases. However, this is not always helpful, as it depends considerably on the type of topic that is being studied, the nature of the research questions, the homogeneity or heterogeneity of the population, the richness

RESEARCH EXAMPLE

13.6 Random, Purposive and Theoretical Sampling

Sbaraini A, Carter SM, Evans RW, Blinkhorn A (2012) Experiences of dental care: what do patients value? *BMC Health Services Research* **12**: 177. doi:10.1186/1472-6963-12-177.

This study was built on a previous randomised controlled trial in private general dental practices in Australia in which the implementation of preventive protocols was the intervention. Twenty-two practices were randomly allocated to either the intervention ($n=12$) or the control group ($n=10$). A total of 847 patients (the initial study population) were recruited (intervention group $n=427$; control group $n=420$). Two dental practices that had offered the preventive care programme agreed to participate in a follow-up qualitative study. The preventive protocols had been successfully implemented in Dental Practice 1, and the programme had been less successful in Dental Practice 2. The qualitative research was designed to explore why these differences may have occurred, primarily from a patient perspective.

A purposive sample of patients ($n=12$), practice staff ($n=5$) and 1 dentist were initially interviewed from Dental Practice 1. Following data collection and analysis using a grounded theory approach, theoretical sampling took place involving the interviewing of patients, dentists and practice staff from Dental Practice 2. In addition, further interviews were held back in Dental Practice 1 in order that the data were fully explored and 'saturated' (see also Sbaraini *et al.* 2011).

of the data when the data collection and analysis are underway and other factors such as feasibility and resources.

Patton (2002) recommended minimum samples to achieve 'reasonable' coverage – a somewhat pragmatic approach. On the other hand, Silverman (2010) suggested that it is possible to derive theory from a fragment of naturally occurring data or one in-depth single case. In practice, most researchers aim for an initial sample that is considered adequate and of sufficient size to provide data that are detailed enough to address their research questions. If, at the point of analysis, the ability to theorise seems limited, they may include other examples to increase the sample size.

Reflection activity

Look at Research Example 13.6. Consider why the researchers' starting point was a randomly selected study, then they moved to a purposive sample and finally they sampled theoretically. In what ways was this process different from or similar to the study illustrated in Research Example 13.5?

CONCLUSION

This chapter has demonstrated that the two main approaches to sampling – probability and non-probability sampling – straddle quantitative and qualitative research designs. Characteristically, though, probability sampling is usually preferred in quantitative research, or the ability to generalise statistically is problematic. Qualitative research tends to adopt methods of sampling whereby the sample is targeted and deliberately selected to provide in-depth and data-rich exemplars of the phenomena that is under exploration. Whichever approach is followed, the technique for sampling should be rigorous, transparent and described accurately in the resulting reporting of the research. Expert advice from statisticians or experienced qualitative researchers should be sought before selecting a sample.

References

Becker HS (1963) *Outsiders: Studies in the Sociology of Deviance*. New York, Free Press.

Bryman A (2012) *Social Research Methods*, 4th edition. Oxford, Oxford University Press.

Bulman C, Lathlean J, Gobbi M (2014) The process of teaching and learning about reflection: research insights from professional nurse education. *Studies in Higher Education* **37**: 1219–1236.

Cohen J (1988) *Statistical Power Analysis for the Behavioural Sciences*, 2nd edition. Lawrence, Erlbaum Associates.

Hunt KJ, Shlomo N, Addington-Hall J (2014) End-of-life care and preferences for place of death among the oldest old: results of a population-based survey using VOICES-Short Form. *Journal of Palliative Medicine* **17**(2): 176–182.

Mastersa SH, Bursteina R, Amofahb G, Abaogyec P, Kumara S, Hanlona M (2013) Travel time to maternity care and its effect on utilization in rural Ghana: a multilevel analysis. *Social Science and Medicine* **93**: 147–194.

Mays N, Pope C (2006) Quality in qualitative health research. In: Pope C, Mays N (eds) *Qualitative Research in Health Care*, 3rd edition. Oxford, Blackwell, pp 82–101.

Mureddu GF, Agabiti N, Rizzello V, Forastiere F, Latini R, Cesaroni G, Masson S, Cacciatore G, Colivicchi F, Uguccioni M, Perucci CA, Boccanelli A (2012) Prevalence of preclinical and clinical heart failure in the elderly. A population-based study in Central Italy. *European Journal of Heart Failure* **14**: 718–729.

Patton MQ (2002) *Qualitative Research and Evaluation Methods*, 3rd edition. Beverly Hills, Sage.

Pope C, Halford S, Turnbull J, Prichard J, Calestani M, May C (2013) Using computer decision support systems in NHS emergency and urgent care: ethnographic study using Normalisation Process Theory. *BMC Health Services Research* **13**: 111. doi:10.1186/1472-6963-13-111.

Sbaraini A, Carter SM, Evans RW, Blinkhorn A (2011) How to do a grounded theory study: a worked example of a study of dental practices. *BMC Medical Research Methodology* **11**: 128. doi:10.1186/1471-2288-11-128.

Sbaraini A, Carter SM, Evans RW, Blinkhorn A (2012) Experiences of dental care: what do patients value? *BMC Health Services Research* **12**: 177. doi:10.1186/1472-6963-12-177.

Silverman D (2010) *Doing Qualitative Research: A Practical Handbook*, 3rd edition. London, Sage.

Websites

www.randomization.com – This site comprises three different types of generator for randomisation, for example, randomising subjects to a single treatment or where subjects are to receive all treatments in random order.

CHAPTER 14

Grounded Theory

Immy Holloway and Kathleen T. Galvin

Key points

- Grounded theory is a research approach that systematically develops theory from the data. The theory is thus grounded in the data collected by the researcher. As well as creating new theory, researchers can also modify and extend existing theories.
- The grounded theory approach or method is most useful when little is known about the area or phenomenon under study or when a new perspective is needed on a familiar situation or setting.
- Key features of grounded theory include interaction of data collection and analysis, theoretical sampling, coding and categorisation of data and a process of constant comparative analysis.
- Researchers using a grounded theory approach need to develop theoretical sensitivity whereby they become attuned to important concepts that arise from the data.
- The analytic process of coding and categorising is facilitated by writing fieldnotes and memos in which the development of ideas and provisional categories or theoretical ideas is recorded. The linking of categories will generate a core category.

INTRODUCTION

Grounded theory is a systematic approach within qualitative research originally developed by Glaser and Strauss (1967). It has its basis in sociology, but the data collection and analysis procedures are also used in other disciplines such as psychology, health care or education. It became popular in nursing in the 1980s and 1990s and is often used now.

Several informative books were written separately by Glaser and Strauss, for instance, *Theoretical Sensitivity* (Glaser 1978) and *Qualitative Analysis for Social Scientists* (Strauss 1987). Strauss then wrote a grounded theory text with Juliet Corbin, a nurse academic, *The Basics of Qualitative Research* (Strauss & Corbin 1990, 1998). Strauss died in 1996, but Corbin subsequently wrote its third edition (2008). Strauss and Corbin (1997) also

The Research Process in Nursing, Seventh Edition. Edited by Kate Gerrish and Judith Lathlean.

Companion Website: www.wiley.com/go/gerrish/research

edited a book demonstrating the use of grounded theory in practice.

Glaser and Strauss used the approach in the health-care field and helped students to apply it, in particular in nursing and in education. One of the early books was the study by Benoliel (1973) on the interaction of nurses with dying patients. Other nurse authors have described the techniques and procedures of grounded theory, such as Schreiber and Stern and their co-writers (2001). An older but useful text for nurses was edited by Chenitz and Swanson in 1986.

In 2006, grounded theory had a new boost with the publication of the guidelines for constructivist grounded theory by Kathy Charmaz (2006). She stresses flexibility and openness for grounded theory rather than a rule-governed rigid approach. The emphasis is also on the way participants construct their social reality on the basis of meanings shared with others. Charmaz has made her approach very clear for beginning researchers. Three texts have recently been published by Stern and Porr (2011), Birks and Mills (2011) and Urquhart (2013), with none taking a new direction but clarifying grounded theory for researchers. Several of these writers label this approach *grounded theory method* (GTM) rather than *grounded theory*. Indeed, Bryant and Charmaz (2007) call the variety of grounded theory approaches 'a family of methods'.

KEY FEATURES OF GROUNDED THEORY

There are many similarities between grounded theory and other qualitative approaches. Grounded theory is, initially at least, inductive. This means that researchers go from the specific and single instances to the general, from data to theory.

There is no hypothesis or theoretical framework prior to data collection in grounded theory. Although researchers have prior ideas that are rooted in their reading or experience, Strauss (1987) stresses that the researcher is not tabula rasa – a blank sheet. This means that researchers need to overcome previous assumptions as the latter might force them into a particular direction and follow preconceived ideas. However, prior experiences or knowledge might become useful sources for the study.

Typical research questions suitable for a grounded theory approach involve interaction and focus on process. Examples might be:

How do the participants make sense of their experience?

How do things change over time in the setting to be studied?

What are the phases or stages of the experience, treatment or condition?

Grounded theory can be distinguished from other qualitative approaches. The main purpose of grounded theory is the generation of concepts and theory from the data. Theory production is possible in other qualitative approaches but is essential in grounded theory; this theory is always rooted in the data. It shows links and relationships between concepts, and the researcher generates explanations, not merely descriptions. The theoretical ideas might be applicable to a variety of similar settings and contexts.

Birks and Mills (2011) summarise the distinctive features of the grounded theory approach:

- The interaction between data collection and analysis
- Theoretical sampling
- Coding and categorising the data
- Constant comparison
- Writing memos
- The generation of a theory grounded in the data

While many other qualitative approaches describe a phenomenon, grounded theorists go further than generating description by producing theory that has explanatory power. Grounded theory, like many other qualitative approaches, focuses on the experience, behaviour and perspectives of participants.

THE RELEVANCE OF GROUNDED THEORY IN NURSING RESEARCH

The findings of grounded theory research in nursing will generally have implications for practice as they identify how participants make sense of their experiences. Life is full of complex transitions, knowledge of which is highly relevant to nursing practice. Becoming a professional with specialist knowledge and skills and undertaking a complex role in a variety of clinical and educational settings is also of interest. There also exist many processes in health care and within nursing practice specifically: assessment for day surgery, discharge from hospital, nurse-led initiatives that impart information and treatments and various models that reflect ways in which aspects of services and care are delivered, to name a few. These are all complex situations where aspects of what goes on and what significance it has are deeply embedded in the everyday world of practice. Becoming a patient or service user, receiving and living with a diagnosis, supporting a loved one through a change in life circumstances, negotiating a path through recovery, debilitating illness or challenging socio-economic conditions are all kinds of journeys that carry significant meaning for people that have not yet been fully explored.

Nurses can take account of the findings of research that describe and explain what happens in such contexts and make use of knowledge about significant stages or important cycles in peoples' experiences. In addition, nurses need evidence that illuminates complex situations and the impact on peoples' lives, such as losing one's health and facing a poor prognosis, becoming ill and undergoing unpleasant treatments, living well with a chronic condition or making a recovery, all examples of poorly understood transitions and implicit processes. In the past, nurse researchers relied on traditional methods of inquiry alone to generate knowledge. They focused on hypothesis testing, using deductive rather than inductive approaches. In the last 40 years, nurses have increasingly utilised qualitative forms of inquiry – these produce rich and deep data; in particular, grounded theory studies have been a major contributor to this field. This long-standing embrace of grounded theory has a number of advantages for nursing, all of which point to the rationale underpinning its frequent use:

- Nurses will be able to understand patients' behaviour and emotions better, and this has implications for professional care and treatment.
- Nurses study interactions between patients and health professionals, and this is important for professional action; solutions to clinical problems might be found more quickly.
- Nurses learn to understand their professional world in more depth when studying the perspectives of their own and other professions as well as students' perspectives. Solutions to clinical problems might be more easily found.
- Through qualitative evaluation, programmes and processes can be improved.
- Nurses have learnt during their education to be structured and systematic in their approach to work; hence, the structured and systematic approach of grounded theory has a particular appeal for them.
- Flexibility and openness is demanded of nurses in clinical practice and nurse educators. Nurses are able to apply these skills to grounded theory.

Holloway (2008) reiterates that much qualitative research, including grounded theory, examines cultural practices and behaviours both of patients and professionals. The illness and suffering of sick people and their perspectives on this can be understood more clearly, and a greater understanding of this will lead to better care. Most of all, however, grounded theory in health care focuses on the way people create meaning in the process of their illness.

Reflection activity

Reflect on your practice and think about examples of where you might use grounded theory. To help you in this reflection activity, think about contexts where you can find distinct stages or phases in patients' journeys or their experience of either treatment or recovery.

SYMBOLIC INTERACTIONISM

Grounded theory originally had its roots in *symbolic interactionism*, a social psychological perspective initially developed by George Herbert Mead in the 1920s and 1930s. He saw the use of symbols in interaction as a major feature of human life (Mead 1934). In Mead's view, individuals develop their own action on the basis of those of others; they take account of each other's behaviour, interpret and respond to it. In the light of change, the meanings are reinterpreted. The emphasis is on the process of interaction between people and the way they understand social roles. The self thus is a social, not merely a psychological, phenomenon. Interactionists contribute to grounded theory the idea that human beings are active agents in their own experience through interpreting this experience and acting according to their interpretations.

Other people affect the development of a person's social self by their expectations and influence. When they start life, human beings develop through interacting with the important people in their lives, significant others. They learn to act according to others' expectations, thereby shaping their own behaviour through the process of socialisation. At a later stage, individuals as members of society analyse the symbols of others, such as language, gestures, mime and appearance, and interpret them. People share the attitudes and responses to particular situations with members of their group. The observation of these interacting roles and responses to each other is a source of data in grounded theory.

Human beings are creative individuals who plan, project and revise their thoughts and behaviour in relation to others within a particular context. Their conduct can only be understood in context. Grounded theory therefore stresses the importance of the context in which people function and share their social world with others.

DATA COLLECTION AND SAMPLING

Researchers use a variety of data sources for grounded theory research. These may be interviews, observation or documents such as patient diaries, letters or professional notes. In-depth and narrative interviews are most useful, though. Unstructured and semi-structured interviews are favoured ways of collecting data, but grounded theorists also stress the value of participant observation.

Data collection and analysis proceed at the same time and interact at each stage. Memos or fieldnotes are written throughout (see later). Researchers decide on the basis of the collection and analysis what data to obtain next. Subsequently, concepts are followed up, and the research becomes progressively focused on particular issues that are important for developing the theoretical ideas. It means that researchers formulate 'working propositions' that they can follow up through further data collection and analysis. In this sense, grounded theory has some deductive elements although it is primarily inductive.

This has implications for sampling. The early sample might include a variety of participants, and concepts emerge from the very beginning. Depending on the findings arising during data collection and analysis, more people may be added to the sample. Others can be interviewed more than once to follow up later findings and to lead to saturation (see later). This means that the number of participants at the beginning might differ from that at the end of the research. For instance, if a researcher finds during early stages that the young feel differently from older people about a particular issue or problem, more young people (or older individuals) can be added to the sample. This is part of theoretical sampling.

Theoretical sampling

The process of theoretical sampling in grounded theory is distinctive from other approaches although other methods also use this type of sampling. Theoretical sampling is guided by concepts and constructs that have significance for the developing theory. At the beginning of the study, initial sampling decisions are made regarding specific individuals or groups of people who have knowledge and information about the area of study. When initial data have been analysed and when theoretical ideas start to emerge, particular concepts arise and are followed up by a choice of

RESEARCH EXAMPLE

14.1 Theoretical Sampling

Monks R, Topping A, Newell R (2013) The dissonant care management of illicit drug users in medical wards, the views of nurses and patients: a grounded theory study. *Journal of Advanced Nursing* **69**: 935–946.

Monks *et al.* (2013) showed how registered nurses manage care to patients with complications of illicit drug use and explored the experiences of the receivers of this care. It had been reported that many nurses had negative feelings towards these patients. The sample consisted of 12 patients and 29 nurses. Particular issues arose from the interviews after data analysis that contributed to the developing categories. This guided the researchers to theoretical sampling. Most nurses in this study had negative feelings towards these patients. The researchers deliberately recruited participants who were known by others to hold more positive attitudes towards these patients.

further participants, events and situations (see Research Example 14.1). The researcher can continue doing this, choosing a variety of settings or a particular age group to extend the conceptualisation. Theoretical sampling continues until the point of saturation and determined by the ideas that arise. Draucker *et al.* (2007) developed a useful theoretical sampling guide.

Unlike other types of sampling, theoretical sampling is not planned from the outset but occurs at a later stage of the research. However, the fact that details of the sample and interview questions are not fully known beforehand may raise challenges during the process of ethical review.

Theoretical sensitivity

Grounded theory needs theoretical sensitivity. Glaser (1978) first employed the term in order to help the researcher develop theory. Theoretical sensitivity means that the researcher becomes aware of important concepts or issues that could be important for the study. There are, however, dangers inherent in having theoretical sensitivity as it might mean reliance on prior assumptions or research developed by others. Sensitivity is rooted in personal and professional experience and in the researcher's reading.

DATA ANALYSIS

Data analysis in grounded theory is iterative and interactive. Iteration means that researchers go backwards and forwards during the course of the research, returning to previous data and the issues contained in them. Constant comparison and theoretical sampling go on throughout the research, and decisions are not made once and for all but are provisional.

Data analysis includes the following procedures:

- Constant comparison
- Coding the data
- Reducing the codes and developing categories
- Linking the categories and finding patterns
- Discovering the core category
- Discovering or building the theory

Constant comparison

Grounded theory is characterised by the *constant comparative method.* Constant comparison means that researchers take a series of iterative steps in which they compare incidents in, and sections of, the data. Researchers not only compare qualitative data from interviews, documents and observations but also related information found in the literature.

Differences and similarities across incidents in the data are explored, and ideas that develop within a category are compared with those that previously emerged in the same category. Through comparison, properties and dimensions (characteristics) of categories can be produced and patterns established that enhance the explanatory power of these categories and help in the development of theory.

Computer software may be used to assist in data analysis. Qualitative software packages, for example, NVivo or ATLAS.ti, are intended for in-depth inductive analysis and allow for theory building models and diagrams. There are limitations to the use of computers, particularly for novice researchers. Where researchers are deeply involved with the participants and need sensitivity, computer analysis might have a distancing effect (Charmaz 2000).

Reflection activity

Examine two or three grounded theory studies from nursing journals and read the methodology section closely. Identify if the researchers undertook further data collection guided by constant comparison, theoretical sampling and theoretical sensitivity.

Coding and categorising

Initially, the data will be coded line by line or sentence by sentence. Coding is the process by which the researcher identifies and names concepts. The first step is *open coding*. This involves breaking down and conceptualising the data and starts as soon as the researcher has collected the first group of data. It includes *in vivo* coding, when the researcher examines phrases that the participants themselves have used. For instance, a patient might say, 'nurses lack time'. 'Lacking time' is then an *in vivo* code. Box 14.1 provides an example of open coding.

The researcher generates a great number of open codes in the first stage of analysis and then has to collapse or reduce them. This process is called categorising. Categories tend to be more abstract than initial codes and group open codes together. Box 14.2 provides an example of a category developed from open coding.

Categories are provisional in that new ideas can be integrated. Also, their characteristics (properties and dimensions) should be uncovered as well as the conditions under which they occur and the consequences that they have. For instance, the analysts might explore the specific conditions and consequences around a category *being in control*. What are the conditions that determine whether patients see themselves as 'in control'? What are the consequences of 'being in control'? Strauss and Corbin (1998: 224) give the properties and dimensions of *the pain experience* as an example; properties refer to intensity, location and duration.

Box 14.1 Open coding

Lines	Codes
1. I did not know what I was doing	1. Being uncertain
2. I felt I was thrown in at the deep end but...	2. Thrown in at the deep end
3. My mentor told me that I was doing it right	3. Being reassured

Box 14.2 Category development

Initial code	Category
Thrown in at the deep end	
Being uncertain	Learning the ropes
Being reassured	

RESEARCH EXAMPLE

14.2 Axial and Selective Coding

Tsonis M, Dougall J, Mandich A, Irwin J (2012) Interrelated processes toward quality of life in survivors of childhood cancer: a grounded theory. *The Qualitative Report* **17**(89): 1–18.

Tsonis and colleagues investigated the quality of life of survivors of childhood cancer. Through a process of open coding, they labelled the initially occurring concepts such as *undergoing treatment* and *cancer diagnosis* and then grouped it into the larger category *past illness experience.* They then related subcategories around this category (axial coding). After doing this with all categories, they searched for one particular category to become the core category and related all other categories to this (selective coding). The central phenomenon, the core category, was *managing lasting impacts and effects.*

Relating categories and linking them with their characteristics and 'subcategories' is important for the emerging theory. Relationships and links are connected with the 'when, where, why, how, and with what consequences an event occurs' (Strauss & Corbin 1998: 22). Strauss and Corbin call this type of categorising *axial coding*. Research Example 14.2 provides an illustration of axial coding. Glaser does not mention this type of coding.

The next stage involves the search for patterns. The constructs developed are major categories formulated by the researchers and rooted in their nursing or academic knowledge. These constructs contain emerging theoretical ideas, and through developing them, researchers reassemble the data. There is no reason why researchers cannot occasionally use the categories that others have discovered. Constant comparison of new data, incidents, codes and categories is needed throughout, but especially at this stage.

The last phase of the analysis is *selective coding*. Selective coding involves integrating and refining the categories and identifying the story line. This means that the theory is starting to emerge; the categories are grouped around a central or core concept – or occasionally concepts – which have explanatory power.

Developing the core category

Through finding relationships between categories, the researcher discovers the core category from the data. Glaser (1978) and Strauss (1987) identify the characteristics for the core category:

- It is a central phenomenon in the research and should be linked to all other categories so that a pattern is established.

RESEARCH EXAMPLE

14.3 Core Category

Machin AI, Machin T, Pearson P (2012) Maintaining equilibrium in professional role identity: a grounded theory study of health visitors' perceptions of their changing professional practice context. *Journal of Advanced Nursing* **68**(7): 1526–1537.

The researchers explored the interaction of health visitors with their changing practice. They interviewed and observed 17 health visitors in two UK community health-care organisations. Their findings showed that establishing equilibrium and consistency in their role identity has priority for them, although other issues were also important. The core category in this research was *professional role identity* to which all other categories were related, which they show in a diagram. Interactions with their professional colleagues affected the equilibrium of this identity, and they showed that they valued autonomy as part of role identity. They focused on professional service provision and resisted the attempts at reducing their roles. (The summary of this research is simplified, and it would be advisable to read it.)

- It should occur frequently in the data.
- It emerges naturally without being forced out by the researcher.
- It should explain variations in the data.
- It is discovered towards the end of the analysis.

The core category is the basic social psychological process involved in the research that occurs over time and explains changes in the participants' behaviour, feelings and thoughts. Research Example 14.3 provides an example of a core category.

Theoretical saturation

Saturation is a particular point in category development. It occurs when no new relevant concepts can be found that are important for the development of the emerging theory. Sampling goes on until categories and their properties and dimensions, as well as the links between the categories, are well established. Researchers should try to establish saturation. When time is limited, researchers may not have sufficient data to reach saturation or may stop without fully analysing the data: this is known as premature closure (Glaser 1978).

Sometimes, it is thought that saturation has taken place when a concept is mentioned frequently and is described in similar ways by a number of people, when the same ideas arise over and over again or when the main concepts have been examined in depth. It is difficult, however, to decide when saturation has occurred. It happens at a different stage in each project and cannot be predicted at the outset.

Reflection activity

Examine a published grounded theory research study and notice how the researcher writes about and describes the process of interaction between data collection and analysis. Consider how the researchers achieved saturation.

THE THEORY

Categories in grounded theory are more abstract than initial codes and assist in building theory. A theory must have 'grab' and 'fit'; it should be recognised by other people working in the field and be grounded in the data. Strauss and Corbin (1998) identify the following characteristics of theory:

- Theory shows systematic relationships between concepts and links between categories.

- Variation should be built into the theory, that is, it should hold true under a number of conditions and circumstances.
- The theory should demonstrate a social and/or psychological process.
- The theoretical findings should be significant and remain important over time.

Glaser and Strauss distinguish between two types of theory, substantive and formal. While substantive theory is derived from the study of a specific context, formal theory is more abstract and conceptual. For instance, a specific theory of negotiating between patients and nurses about pain relief would be substantive theory. A theory about the concept of negotiation in general that can be applied to many different settings and situations becomes formal theory. Most researchers, in particular novices, produce substantive theories that are specific and can be applied to the situation under study or similar settings.

Strauss and Corbin consider the applicability of theoretical ideas to other settings and situations. For instance, the concept of 'transition' or 'status passage' may be applied to a variety of situations, such as 'becoming a mother' or 'seeking a diagnosis'. Indeed, a theory and theoretical ideas can be re-contextualised in a number of situations and verified in a variety of settings.

WRITING MEMOS

Thoughts and ideas need to be recorded throughout in a field diary and memos. Memos are, according to Corbin and Strauss (2008: 117), 'written records of analysis'. They might be physical descriptions of the setting or theoretical ideas. The researcher should date them as well as supply detail.

Memos are meant to help in the development and formation of theory. Initially, they are simple but become progressively more theoretical. In theoretical memos, researchers develop ideas and occasionally working propositions, compare findings and record their thoughts. Strauss (1987) provides examples of different types of memos that might be written. Diagrams may be used in memos to help the researcher capture ideas. They can guide the researcher to base abstract ideas in the reality of the data (Holloway & Wheeler 2010).

THE USE OF LITERATURE IN GROUNDED THEORY

Grounded theory research is generally carried out where little is known about the phenomenon to be studied. Researchers need to identify a gap in knowledge that their research question will address. They should read around the topic as this can generate questions and some initial concepts. Glaser (1998) and Glaser and Holton (2004), however, stated the problems of reviewing the substantive literature at the very beginning. Among others, these are mainly the following:

- Researchers might be influenced by other researchers' ideas, in particular by those of experts in the field.
- Researchers might be affected by irrelevant concepts.
- Researchers might sound 'jargonised' or 'rhetoricalised' by the ideas developed in other studies that might affect the data collection.

Dunne (2011), on the other hand, states that not having a literature review until data collection and analysis is in process is 'unworkable' (p 115) as approval from ethics committees depends on the rationale researchers give for undertaking the study. Dunne also suggests that the advice for use of grounded theory in areas where not much research exists and the lack of at least some prior knowledge of the literature is an inherent contradiction.

Corbin and Strauss (2008) are less extreme in their view than Glaser and state that researchers might become rigid and stifled through reading too much. Of course, there is a need to review the literature on the research topic, but researchers should enter the arena without major preconceptions.

Nurse researchers generally start their research with certain assumptions as they often have some knowledge of the field they wish to explore.

Moreover, their professional experience and reading of the literature can enhance their research as it generates theoretical sensitivity to concepts and issues that are important for the developing theory. Researchers do need to be explicit, however, and uncover their own preconceptions.

As a grounded theory study progresses, categories and theoretical concepts are developed. The literature relating to these concepts, particularly that related to the core category, is reviewed, and a dialogue takes place between the literature and the ideas of the researcher. However, the researcher's data should have priority over those of other studies. Concepts arising from the research can be compared with those emerging from other studies. In this sense, the literature can become a potential source of data. Researchers trawl the literature for confirmation or refutation of their own findings. This interaction and dialogue with the literature, and the debate about it, is integrated into the discussion section of the research report.

THE CHOICE BETWEEN GLASERIAN AND STRAUSSIAN GROUNDED THEORY

Glaser and Strauss started together on the path of developing grounded theory but subsequently diverged from each other. Glaser (1992) criticised Strauss and Corbin (1990), accusing them of distorting the procedures and meaning of the grounded theory approach. A full discussion of the differences between the two perspectives can be found in MacDonald (2001). Glaser and Strauss (and Corbin) differ mainly on the following points.

The research topic

Glaser suggests that researchers approach the topic without preconceptions and have a research interest rather than a research problem. While Strauss and Corbin advise researchers to identify a phenomenon to be studied at the beginning of the study, Glaser claims that this would arise naturally during the process of the research. This has implications for the initial literature review, which would be somewhat more detailed for Strauss and Corbin, while Glaser believes that it might 'contaminate' the participants' data, although he too suggests that the literature should be integrated into the developing concepts and that much general reading should occur before the study starts.

Coding and categorising

Coding is mentioned by both Glaser and Strauss but seems to have slightly different meanings. Although Glaser does not like the term axial coding, his 'theoretical coding' seems very similar to axial coding.

Verification

One of the main factors that distinguish the ideas of Glaser and Strauss is the issue of verification. Strauss and Corbin suggest that working propositions are examined and provisionally tested against new data (as, indeed, the original text by Glaser and Strauss had suggested). Glaser believes that these hypotheses should not be verified or validated at this stage by the researcher and new data should be integrated into the emerging theory. The use of the word verification is not advisable for grounded theory researchers. However, Glaser does not support the view concerning deductive elements in grounded theory. He maintains that it is only inductive.

The process of generating theory

While Strauss and Corbin advocate the building of theory through axial coding, Glaser suggests that the theory will eventually emerge naturally as long as the researcher continuously engages with the data, and they are analysed adequately and in depth. There are also differences of opinion regarding the generalisability of grounded theory. Strauss and Corbin consider that grounded theory is generalisable, whereas Glaser considers this not to be the case.

Which approach?

Both approaches are viable forms of grounded theory research, so researchers have to decide for themselves which one to adopt. The more prescriptive and formulaic approach of Strauss and Corbin (1990, 1998) may be easier for novices, while experienced researchers might find the Glaserian perspective (which he calls 'classic grounded theory') more appropriate. Researchers can modify the approach to fit their own purposes; Charmaz (2008) advises, however, they should be thoroughly familiar with the original approach to justify their modification and deviation from it. She stresses that Strauss was a pragmatist and that grounded theorists should stay pragmatic and not become rigid in their approach. The text by Birks and Mills (2011) relies more on Straussian grounded theory, while Stern and Porr (2011) start from a Glaserian stance.

PROBLEMS AND STRENGTHS OF GROUNDED THEORY

Grounded theory has been criticised for its neglect of social structure and culture and the influence of these on human action and interaction. Researchers who use other qualitative approaches also stress process and human agency rather than society and structure. However, there is no reason why grounded theory cannot be used in the discussion of macro-issues. A number of grounded theory studies have been carried out, some of which do centre on macro-issues such as gender and power, in particular work by feminists. Others, focusing on policy or health education and promotion, cannot help considering structural, cultural and societal factors.

Nevertheless, it should be stressed that most qualitative approaches, including grounded theory, are used for the exploration of micro-issues rather than macro-issues. They are designed to focus on the meanings people give to their experience and behaviour.

Some problems with grounded theory are not connected with style or procedures but with the inexperience of researchers. Many novice researchers end up with a conceptual description rather than a theory. There is nothing wrong with dense, conceptual (sometimes called 'analytic') description but this alone cannot be called grounded theory.

CONCLUSION

Grounded theory is a systematic and processual approach to collecting and analysing data. Good grounded theory produces a theory that has explanatory power or modification of a theory that already exists. Such theory generation is unique within qualitative research.

There are some major elements that are always present in this type of research:

- Data collection and analysis are in constant dialogue and interaction with each other.
- Constant comparison of data occurs throughout the research process.
- Theoretical sampling is used by following up emerging concepts.
- Data are analysed through coding and categorising.
- A core category is developed that forms links between other categories.
- A theory or the theoretical ideas that are generated should always have their basis in the data.

References

Benoliel JQ (1973) *The Nurse and the Dying Patient.* New York, Macmillan.

Birks M, Mills J (2011) *Grounded Theory: a practical guide.* London, Sage.

Bryant A, Charmaz C (eds) (2007) *The SAGE Handbook of Grounded Theory.* London, Sage.

Charmaz K (2000) Grounded theory: objectivist and constructivist methods. In: Denzin NK, Lincoln YS (eds) *Handbook of Qualitative Research,* 2nd edition. Thousand Oaks, Sage, pp 509–536.

Charmaz K (2006) *Constructing Grounded Theory: a practical guide through qualitative analysis.* London, Sage.

Charmaz K (2008) Advancing qualitative research through grounded theory. Paper presented at the 7th Qualitative Research Conference, Bournemouth University, Poole, September.

Chenitz WC, Swanson JM (eds) (1986) *From Practice to Grounded Theory: qualitative research in nursing*. Menlo Park, Addison-Wesley.

Corbin J, Strauss A (2008) *Basics of Qualitative Research: techniques and procedures for developing grounded theory*, 3rd edition. Los Angeles, Sage.

Draucker CB, Martsolf DS, Ross R, Thomas TB (2007) Theoretical sampling and category development in grounded theory. *Qualitative Health Research* **17**(8): 1137–1148.

Dunne C (2011) The place of the literature review in grounded theory research. *International Journal of Research Methodology* **14**(2): 111–124.

Glaser BG (1978) *Theoretical Sensitivity*. Mill Valley, Sociology Press.

Glaser BG (1992) *Basics of Grounded Theory Analysis*. Mill Valley, Sociology Press.

Glaser BG (1998) *Doing Grounded Theory: issues and discussions*. Mill Valley, Sociology Press.

Glaser BG, Holton J (2004) Remodeling grounded theory. *Forum: Qualitative Social Research* **5**(2): urn:nbn:de:0114-fqs040245.

Glaser BG, Strauss AL (1967) *The Discovery of Grounded Theory*. Chicago, Aldine.

Holloway I (2008) *A–Z of Qualitative Research in Healthcare*. Oxford, Blackwell.

Holloway I, Wheeler S (2010) *Qualitative Research in Nursing*, 3rd edition. Oxford, Wiley Blackwell.

MacDonald M (2001) Finding a critical perspective in grounded theory. In: Schreiber RS, Stern PN (eds) *Using Grounded Theory in Nursing*. New York, Springer, pp 113–136.

Machin AI, Machin T, Pearson P (2012) Maintaining equilibrium in professional role identity: a grounded theory study of health visitors' perceptions of their changing professional practice context. *Journal of Advanced Nursing* **68**(7): 1526–1537.

Mead GH (1934) *Mind, Self and Society*. Chicago, University of Chicago Press.

Monks R, Topping A, Newell R (2013) The dissonant care management of illicit drug users in medical wards, the views of nurses and patients: a grounded theory study. *Journal of Advanced Nursing* **69**: 935–946.

Schreiber RS, Stern PN (2001) The 'how to' of grounded theory: avoiding the pitfalls. In: Schreiber RS, Stern PN (eds) *Using Grounded Theory in Nursing*. New York, Springer, pp 55–83.

Stern PN, Porr JP (2011) *Essentials of Accessible Grounded Theory*. Walnut Creek, Left Coast Press.

Strauss AL (1987) *Qualitative Analysis for Social Scientists*. New York, Cambridge University Press.

Strauss AL, Corbin J (1990) *Basics of Qualitative Research: grounded theory procedures and techniques*. Newbury Park, Sage.

Strauss AL, Corbin J (eds) (1997) *Grounded Theory in Practice*. Thousand Oaks, Sage.

Strauss AL, Corbin J (1998) *Basics of Qualitative Research: techniques and procedures for developing grounded theory*, 2nd edition. Thousand Oaks, Sage.

Tsonis M, Dougall J, Mandich A, Irwin J (2012) Interrelated processes toward quality of life in survivors of childhood cancer: a grounded theory. *The Qualitative Report* **17**(89): 1–18.

Urquhart C (2013) *Grounded Theory for Qualitative Research: a practical guide*. London, Sage.

Further reading

Buckley CA, Waring MJ (2013) Using diagrams to support the research process. *Qualitative Research*, January 17, online version http://qrj.sagepub.com/content/early/2013/01/17/1468794112472280 (accessed 1 September 2014).

Charmaz K (2011) A constructivist grounded theory analysis of losing and regaining a valued self. In: Wertz F, Charmaz K, McMullen LM, Josselson R, Anderson R, McSpadden E (eds) *Five Ways of Doing Qualitative Research*. London, Guilford Press, pp 165–204.

Charmaz K, Patterniti DA, Charmaz KG (1998) *Health, Illness and Healing, Society, Social Context and Self: an anthology*. Oxford, Oxford University Press.

Glaser BG (2001) *The Grounded Theory Perspective: conceptualization contrasted with description*. Mill Valley, Sociology Press.

Hall H, Griffiths D, McKenna L (2013) From Darwin to constructivism: the evolution of grounded theory. *Nurse Researcher* **20**(3): 17–21.

Millikin PJ, Schreiber R (2012) Examining the nexus between grounded theory and symbolic interactionism. *International Journal of Qualitative Methods* **11**(5): 683–696.

Morse JM, Stern PN, Corbin J, Charmaz KC, Bowers B, Clarke A (eds) (2009) *Developing Grounded Theory: the second generation*. Walnut Creek, Left Coast Press.

Websites

www.groundedtheory.com – Grounded Theory Institute is dedicated to helping people learn about Glaserian grounded theory (also known as classic or traditional grounded theory).

http://groundedtheoryreview.com – The *Grounded Theory Review* is a free online journal for the promotion of Glaser's classic grounded theory, but it also contains interesting discussions on the approach.

CHAPTER 15

Ethnography

Immy Holloway and Kathleen T. Galvin

Key points

- Ethnography gives a detailed description of a culture or subculture – in nursing, for instance, the study of specific groups or settings.
- Data collection involves immersion in the setting by means of participant observation and interviews with key informants.
- The researcher seeks to uncover the *emic* or 'insider view' of the members of the particular culture being studied.
- 'Thick' description is used to provide a detailed account that makes explicit the patterns of cultural and social relationships and puts them into context.
- Ethnographic data analysis can be carried out in a variety of ways.

INTRODUCTION

Ethnographic research focuses on culture or a social group. It can be seen as a process that includes the methods of research – and a product, which is the written story as the outcome of the research. Researchers study a culture by observing cultural members' behaviours and ask questions about their actions, interactions, experience and feelings. They also write 'an ethnography', a narrative account in which they give a portrayal of the culture they study. Ethnography is both 'doing science' and 'telling stories'.

Ethnography is an umbrella term that encompasses many activities and viewpoints. It is sometimes used synonymously with 'qualitative research' (as in the book by Brewer written in 2000, for instance), but in this chapter, we adopt the original meaning of the term within anthropological/sociological traditions.

The term 'ethnography' means 'writing culture' or 'writing people' and comes from the Greek. The major traits of ethnography include the researcher's first-hand experience of the 'natural setting' that the informants inhabit, the culture or community that is being studied.

The Research Process in Nursing, Seventh Edition. Edited by Kate Gerrish and Judith Lathlean.

Companion Website: www.wiley.com/go/gerrish/research

Ethnographers can utilise both qualitative and quantitative procedures. In this chapter, the qualitative approach will be discussed as this is most often used in nursing. Ethnography is probably the oldest of the research approaches, as even in ancient times travellers to a country other than their own studied and described foreign cultures and wrote about their experiences. Initially, anthropologists explored only foreign cultures, often adopting a colonialist and ethnocentric stance. Today, anthropologists are less ethnocentric, that is, they are less inclined to view other groups from their own (Western) perspective. Ethnographers now also research their own culture and cultural groups.

The Chicago School of Sociology, from 1917 to the early 1940s, influenced later ethnographic methods because its members examined marginal cultures such as ghettos, urban gangs and slums of the city. Researchers subsequently explored their own cultures researching that with which they were already familiar. These studies were carried out by members of many disciplines apart from anthropology, for example, by sociologists, educationists and nurses. Janice Morse, the best-known nurse anthropologist and author of qualitative research texts, has discussed this approach in nursing for several decades. (See the history of ethnographic research in Gobo (2008).)

Like most other qualitative approaches, ethnographic research is inductive, at least initially. This means that it proceeds from the specific to the general and that initially no preconceptions or hypotheses guide the researcher towards the outcomes of the inquiry. In ethnography, as in other forms of qualitative inquiry, the researcher is the main research tool.

Ethnography is distinct from other qualitative approaches in that it generates descriptions of a group in its cultural context and focuses mainly, though not exclusively, on the routine activities and customs in the culture as well as on the location of the people within it.

THE CHARACTERISTICS OF ETHNOGRAPHY

Roper and Shapira state that 'ethnography is a research process of learning *about* people by learning *from* them' (Roper & Shapira 2000: 1).

The main features of ethnography are:

- immersion in a setting and a focus on culture
- the emic (insider's) dimension from the participants, in particular key informants
- 'thick', dense or analytic description

The focus on culture

Fetterman (2010) suggests that the interpretation of a culture (or subculture) is the main aim of ethnography. Culture can be defined as the way of life of a group: the learnt patterns of behaviour that are socially constructed and transmitted. This includes a shared communication system in language, gestures and expressions: the messages that most cultural members understand and recognise. Individuals in a culture often share values and ideas acquired through learning from other members of the group. Learning group values and behaviour is referred to as socialisation. For instance, members of the nursing profession have been socialised into the values and perspectives of their own group through their education and training. The perspectives of the group, the actions and interactions of group members, and the meaning they place on their own and others' behaviour, are legitimate areas of research for the ethnographer. Adopting an ethnographic approach to a familiar culture helps researchers to avoid assumptions about their own cultural group or take its working for granted.

Knowledge that the members of a culture share but do not articulate to each other is referred to as 'tacit knowledge'. Social behaviour and interpretations of the social world are based on this. Ethnographers uncover tacit knowledge and make it explicit. They also reveal some of the hidden meanings in the routines and rituals of a group and place.

Ethnographers have recently changed their perspective from a monolithic understanding of culture where all individuals share values, beliefs and perceptions to a focus on cultural diversity (Holloway & Todres 2003). Rapport and Overing (2000) offer a critique of 20th-century ideas about culture and shared practices:

> … culture as a coherent, bounded, and stable system of shared beliefs and actions has been a powerful

twentieth century idea that has been very difficult to shift …. (Rapport & Overing 2000: 94)

People's understanding and viewpoints depend on their location in the culture (and often on their position of power). They demonstrate how cultural members are located within their setting and how they can only be understood within the specific context. For instance, although nurses and doctors in an orthopaedic department might have certain perceptions in common (particularly about their patients), there are other elements where their beliefs and ways of working are in conflict with each other.

Important research questions are linked to culture or subculture within a health-care setting. For example, a researcher might observe the subculture of nursing students and the culture of a nursing home or a children's hospital.

Emic and etic perspectives

The term *emic* perspective is often used in ethnographic research. Although the concept has a variety of interpretations, in its simplest form, it means 'insider view'. The emic perspective is the perception of those who are members of a particular culture or group, or, in anthropological terms, the 'native' point of view. The linguist Pike coined this phrase, but it was used more extensively and with a different meaning by the anthropologist Harris (1976) and most ethnographers since. Members of a culture have special knowledge of this culture and can share this with the researcher. For instance, nurses in the A&E department know about the special problems facing members of the department, but they would also be able to narrate the dramatic events that might make this type of work exciting.

Insiders give meaning to their experiences and generate knowledge about the reasons for their actions. They know the rules and rituals of their group or subculture. The emic perspective is thus culture specific. Outside observers would find it difficult to gain the same familiarity and intimacy with this setting that insiders do.

In contrast, ethnographers also speak of the *etic* perspective, that is, the view of the outsider who may or may not be a member of the culture being studied. As an example, an A&E nurse might wish to research the culture of A&E departments. In this sense, she or he is a 'native' of the group. Nurses are also researchers, however, and in this particular sense, they are outsiders, and they need to produce scientific knowledge about what they see and hear, which means taking an etic view. Thus, the emic perspective is the subjective view of insiders that has to be retold by the researchers in the account of the research. Indeed, the A&E nurse researchers in the earlier example have to attempt to become 'naïve' observers or interviewers, taking the view of a 'cultural stranger' to the setting. The etic perspective is needed to transform the story into an ethnography with its roots in social science. Harris (1976) explains that etics are scientific transformations of the empirical data by the researchers who adopt an approach to the data that is more theoretical and abstract than that of the insiders.

Thick description

The concept of thick description has its origin in work of the philosopher Ryle and was taken on by the anthropologist Geertz (1973) who applied it to ethnography. He suggests that it is a detailed account that makes explicit the patterns of cultural and social relationships and puts them in context. It is a result of observations and interviews in the field. The notion of thick description is sometimes understood as a detailed description of a culture or group, but this does not suffice. It must be theoretical and analytical in that researchers concern themselves with general patterns and traits of social life, and it gives the reader of the ethnographic text a sense of the emotional experience of the participants in the study. Thick description builds up a clear picture of the individuals and groups in the context of their culture and encompasses their meanings and intentions. On the other hand, thin description is superficial and factual and does not explore the underlying meanings of cultural members (Denzin 1989). It does not lead to a good ethnography.

THE USE OF ETHNOGRAPHY IN NURSING

Many cultures and subcultures exist within nursing. One might think, for instance, of the culture of a hospital or the subculture of an orthopaedic ward. Ethnographic research is therefore helpful in:

- studying cultures, linked to nursing, with their rules and rituals and routine activities – this includes transcultural research, which examines different ethnic groups and their interactions, and meaning creation.
- discovering the 'insider view' of patients and colleagues.
- explaining phenomena related to nursing.
- examining the conflicting perspectives of professionals within the organisational culture.

Nurse researchers contextualise the perspectives, actions and emotions of their patients or colleagues and those of other health professionals through ethnographic methods. They become culture sensitive and learn to identify the influences of the environment on the person. The aim of nurse researchers, however, is different from that of other anthropologists. They do not merely generate knowledge, which is seen as the goal of ethnography (Hammersley & Atkinson 2007), but they also wish to change and improve professional practice through understanding the culture they study.

Leininger (1985) has coined the term 'ethnonursing' to refer to the use of ethnography in nursing. She describes this as an adaptation and extension of ethnography. Ethnonursing, she suggests, is concerned with studying groups and settings linked to nursing but also is specifically about nursing care, produces nursing knowledge and explains or demonstrates nursing phenomena.

Nurse ethnographers do not always investigate their own cultural members. In Britain, nurses care for patients from a variety of ethnic groups and need to be knowledgeable about different cultures. Indeed, all nurses and patients belong to ethnic groups, and sometimes, they come from different countries and have a variety of religions. Awareness of cultural differences is important because both nurses and patients are products of their group. DeSantis (1994) suggested that at least three cultures are involved in nurses' interactions with patients: the nurses' professional culture, the patients' culture and the context in which the interactions take place.

Nurse researchers usually proceed in the following way:

- They describe a problem in the group under study, and through this, they come to understand the causes of the problem and may be able to prevent it.
- They assist patients to identify and report their needs.
- They give information to the readers of their accounts – their colleagues and other health professionals – to effect change in clinical and professional practice.

When undertaking research with colleagues or students, nurse researchers proceed through similar phases. The ultimate goal of their research is to improve professional practice.

Savage (2000) draws certain parallels between ethnography (in particular participant observation) and clinical practice:

- The physical involvement with the setting is common to nursing and research.
- The claims nurses and researchers make about knowledge through experience.
- The assumptions they share as nurses and observers.

Savage suggests that nurses and ethnographers should be concerned with the links between their own experience of the setting and that of their patients. Nurses and researchers also attempt to translate the understanding they gain of patients to others.

Reflection activity

Think about an area of your practice that may be suitable for an ethnographic approach. To help you with this reflection activity, focus on areas of professional practice where there may be a particular culture or a distinctive subcultural group. Write an ethnographic research question about this culture.

RESEARCH EXAMPLE

15.1 Descriptive Ethnography

Williamson S, Twelvetree T, Thompson J, Beaver K (2012) An ethnographic study exploring the role of ward-based advanced nurse practitioners in an acute medical setting. *Journal of Advanced Nursing* **68**(7): 1579–1588.

This ethnographic research was carried out to investigate the role of ward-based advanced nurse practitioners (ANPs) and their impact on care and practice in a teaching hospital in England through observation and interviews. Observation took place in the natural environment of the setting by the researcher shadowing the ANPs on the ward for a considerable length of time, as well as listening and observing their actions and interactions with others on the ward. Also, at the same time, informal interviews generated thoughts from consultants, junior doctors, physiotherapists and clinical pharmacists. More formal interviews were carried out with 5 ANPs, 14 ward nurses and 5 patients. The writers identified the ANPs as 'overarching linchpins' on the ward but also found that these practitioners identified more closely with the medical rather than the nursing staff, while they saw their roles as 'translators' of medical language to nurses and patients. The study in this hospital culture identified the ANP's role as significant for the provision of quality care. It also showed that ANPs are 'more than junior doctor substitutes'.

DESCRIPTIVE AND CRITICAL ETHNOGRAPHY

There are two main approaches to ethnography: descriptive and critical ethnography. Thomas (1993) states the difference:

> Conventional ethnographers study culture for the purpose of describing it; critical ethnographers do so to change it. (Thomas 1993: 4)

It should be noted, however, that most nursing research that is carried out has implications for practice. While descriptive ethnography centres on the description of cultures or groups (see Research Example 15.1), critical ethnography involves the study of macro-social factors such as power and control and examines common-sense assumptions and hidden agendas in this arena (Holloway & Wheeler 2010); it therefore has political elements or focuses on power relationships (see Research Example 15.2). Nurse researchers often use critical ethnography because women form the majority of these professions, and power relations are part of the complex factors influencing interaction between nurses and doctors or nurses and patients. Penney and Wellard (2007) speak of the need to change practice, which is one of the aims of critical ethnography. (See Hardcastle *et al.* (2006) on Carspecken's critical ethnography.)

Whereas the same data collection and analysis procedures are used by ethnographers undertaking descriptive and critical ethnographies, the latter aim to highlight the power dimensions of interaction and are often more reflexive of their own involvement in the research.

SELECTION OF SAMPLE AND SETTING

Ethnographers use purposive or criterion-based sampling; that is, they adopt specific criteria to select their informants and setting such as patients undergoing orthopaedic surgery, children with diabetes, nursing students or a maternity unit. The criteria for sample selection must be explicit and systematic (Hammersley & Atkinson 2007) in order to ensure that participants are representative of the group under study. The participants in ethnographic research are

RESEARCH EXAMPLE

15.2 Critical Ethnography

Livesley J, Long T (2013) Children's experiences as hospital in-patients: voice, competence and work. Messages for nursing from a critical ethnographic study. *International Journal of Nursing Studies* **50**(10): 1292–1303.

The authors worked with a sample of 15 children over two phases in which they researched by observation, interview and other age-appropriate methods such as play or craft activities. Data collection was carried out with one group at home (5–15 years) and with the other group in hospital (5–14 years) and lasted approximately 6 months. One of the major findings was that these children struggled for their competence as human beings to be recognised. The conclusions pointed to the difficulty of hearing children's voices in hospital. When they were heard, they were often seen as challenging. The researchers used critical ethnography specifically to 'transform situations through emancipatory principles' and to show children as competent individuals.

usually called informants because they inform the researcher about issues in their world. Alternative terms include participant, cultural member or key actor. Key informants are those participants whose knowledge of the setting is intimate and long-standing. Patients are often the main informants in nursing ethnography. They tell of their experience and the meanings they attach to it and of the expectations and health beliefs that form part of their perspectives (DeSantis 1994). Informants might be interviewed formally or participate by talking informally about the cultural beliefs and practices as well as ways of communicating. They become active collaborators in the research rather than passive respondents (hence the term 'informant'). Nurses can compare their own interpretations of the group with those of key informants through the process of member checking, whereby they ask informants to check the script and interpretation (Lincoln & Guba 1985).

DATA COLLECTION

Ethnographers have three major strategies for collecting data (Roper & Shapira 2000):

- They observe what is going on in the setting while participating in it.
- They ask informants from the cultural group they are studying about their behaviour, experiences and feelings.
- They study documents about and in the setting in order to familiarise themselves with it.

Observation takes place through engagement and immersion in the setting, interviews are the accounts of the insider experience, and documents are added sources for studying the culture. Indeed, often researchers supplement interviews and observation by audio recording oral histories from the cultural members whose world they study, or they examine photographs or pictures of the group and the setting.

Observing

Participant observation, the type of observation most commonly used, means that the researchers are immersed in the setting and become familiar with it. Prolonged observation produces more in-depth knowledge of a culture. Occasionally, researchers need to withdraw from the setting in order to stand back and take stock. They also need to attempt to put aside their assumptions, come to the setting as 'cultural strangers' and keep an open mind in seeking the emic perspective, the view of the inhabitant of the world they study. Ethnographers observe the setting and situation, the way people act and interact and the use of space and time, but they also observe critical incidents that may occur and the way rules are followed and rituals are carried out.

Spradley (1980: 78), a well-known ethnographer, identifies the dimensions of the social settings that ethnographers study. These include the following:

Space	location of the research
Actor	the people who take part in the setting
Activity	the actions of people
Object	things located in the setting
Act	single actions of participants
Events	what is happening in the setting
Time	sequencing of activities and time frame
Goals	what people aim to do
Feeling	emotions that participants have

The observation setting can be open or closed. Open settings can be highly visible public spaces such as a reception area or a corridor, whereas closed settings have to be more carefully negotiated and could be hospital wards or meeting rooms. In nursing settings, observation is normally overt where the researcher makes explicit their intention to observe the social setting. Covert observation, where participants do not know that they are being observed, is usually seen as unethical. Indeed, participant observation is a challenge to the researcher as ethical issues might become problematic in this type of open setting where the participants' behaviour can be observed throughout. There is a fine line between disclosure for the purpose of the researcher's agenda and confidentiality or anonymity of the participants.

Observations are initially unstructured, although they become progressively more focused as important features emerge that might be of significance for the study. Observations inform the researcher's interviews with key informants. Incidents or issues that are puzzling or problematic are explored with participants.

The ethnographic interview

During and following observations, researchers ask questions about the meaning of behaviour, language and events. This happens initially through informal conversations with participants. There are several consequences of these conversations: researchers familiarise themselves with the arena, bond with participants and acquire cultural knowledge from the informants.

In-depth interviews are commonly used to allow informants the opportunity to explore issues within the culture that they see as important. Although the researcher has an agenda, participants have control within certain boundaries. The researchers follow up the issues and ideas that the informant sees as significant without neglecting their own research agenda. The interviews may be formal or informal, in depth and unstructured or semi-structured (*see* Chapter 28).

Spradley (1979) distinguishes between grand-tour and mini-tour questions. While the former questions are broad, the latter are more specific. An example of a grand-tour question might be: 'Can you describe your life as an orthopaedic nurse?' A mini-tour question might be: 'Tell me about the pain you had after your operation'. Researchers often start an interview with a broad question, and the interview becomes more focused following up participants' answers (see Box 15.1).

These questions are then followed up depending on the participants' answers. If something important emerges, gentle prompts can be used such as 'Can you tell me more about that, please?'

Ethnographers also listen to naturally occurring talk in the setting, for example, people communicating with each other on the ward, in meetings or in the classroom. These conversations may be analysed in the same way as interviews. To make sure that data are not lost, interviewers generally audio-record participants' words, whereas detailed fieldnotes are made of conversations. One critique to note concerns the over-reliance of interviews in ethnographic work at the expense of observation (Atkinson *et al.* 2001). While ethnographers can on occasion use interviews alone, it is desirable to integrate observational fieldwork and interviews. This allows an emphasis on practices and behaviours that elicit cultural insights in deeply contextual ways and helps ensure development of

Box 15.1 Examples of general and focused questions for ethnographic interviews

General question

Tell me about your illness?

Focused questions (following the participants ideas)

What did you feel when you were first diagnosed?
What was your reaction to this?

General question

Can you describe your care and treatment?

Focused questions

Tell me about your experiences of nursing care.
You said that the nurses always make time for patients in spite of having so much work to do, please, can you tell me more about this?

theoretical insights that are in the spirit of the *in depth* afforded by anthropological research.

FIELDWORK AND FIELDNOTES

The field, fieldwork and fieldnotes are well-known concepts used in ethnography. The field is the location in which the research is taking place and in which the researcher has a presence (Gobo 2008). It may be a ward, a hospital or a specific community of people. The term fieldwork refers to the work undertaken in an ethnographic study such as collecting data from various sources. Fieldwork also includes the description and interpretation of cultural behaviour, the meaning people give to their actions and the setting in which the study takes place. This is an ongoing process in the research.

Researchers keep a field journal or diary in which they jot down their thoughts about their experiences and make theoretical comments. These fieldnotes or 'ethnographic record' (Gobo 2008) are used at a later stage to help remember important issues, questions or solutions to problems. They have their basis in the observations and interviews undertaken in the setting. Initially, fieldnotes are only for the eyes of the ethnographer, but ultimately, excerpts are used as data or extended descriptions in ethnographic writing. At first, fieldnotes tend to be simple but become more complex as the study progresses and may become notes about analysis and interpretation.

Spradley (1979) identifies different types of fieldnotes in terms of condensed and extended accounts. Condensed accounts are short descriptions made in the field during data collection, while expanded accounts extend the descriptions and fill in detail. Short fieldnotes are extended as soon as possible after a period of observation or interview if it was not possible to record the full detail during the data collection. Ethnographers also note their own biases, reactions and problems during fieldwork. They may use additional ways to record events and behaviour such as audiotapes, video film or photos, flowcharts and diagrams.

MACRO- AND MICRO-ETHNOGRAPHIES

Spradley (1980) identifies macro- and micro-ethnographies, which can be viewed on a continuum of scale. At one end of this continuum are large-scale studies examining a complex society, one or more communities or social institutions (*macro-ethnography*); at the other are small-scale studies into a single social situation (*micro-ethnography*).

A macro-ethnography examines a large culture with its institutions, communities and value systems.

RESEARCH EXAMPLE

15.3 A Micro-ethnography

Happ MB, Swigart VA, Tate JA, Hoffman LA, Arnold RM (2007) Patient involvement in health-related decisions during prolonged critical illness. *Research in Nursing and Health* **30**: 361–372.

The authors collected data during prolonged mechanical ventilation through observation of the situation and interviews – that is, patterns of communication. Patients participated in decision-making about their care and other critical issues such as artificial feeding and financial and legal issues. This study was restricted to a particular setting, a detailed view of a small unit, namely, a 20-bed ICU and an adjacent unit with 8 beds in which decisions were made about life-supporting treatment and daily care. Although patients were not demanding to be involved in the decision-making processes, there was consistent involvement and shared decision-making in these units through questions and non-verbal and verbal answers of patients.

The study is a micro-ethnography in that it was only conducted in one hospital and two small units. Obviously, the results cannot be generalised to other settings, although some of the ideas can be applied.

In nursing, this might be the wider culture of nursing. Such studies are rarely carried out by a single researcher. Both macro- and micro-ethnographies proceed in similar ways and produce an account of the culture being studied. The type of study depends on the focus of the investigation, the researcher's own interests or those who fund the research.

Novice nurse researchers often choose a micro-ethnography as it makes fewer demands on their time than macro-ethnography and seems more immediately relevant to the world of the nurse. Micro-ethnography focuses on small settings or groups such as a single ward or a group of specialist nurses. Research Example 15.3 provides an example of a micro-ethnography.

Reflection activity

Ethnographic research within nursing has sometimes been criticised for an over-reliance on interviews rather than observations. Read the research examples given in this chapter, and reflect upon the nature of the data collection used. What was the balance between interviews and observations? How were they carried out?

DATA ANALYSIS AND INTERPRETATION

Analysis involves interaction with the data. The data are scanned and organised from the start of the research, and the focus on particular issues becomes clearer as the research progresses. Analysis and interpretation proceed in parallel. The analytic process is not linear but iterative; this means that researchers go back and forth, from the data collection and reading and thinking about them to the analysis. They then return to collecting new data and analysing them. This process continues until the collection and analysis are complete.

The main steps in data analysis include:

- bringing order to the data and organising the material
- reading, rereading and thinking about the data
- coding the data
- summarising and reducing the codes to larger categories
- searching for patterns and regularities in the data, sorting these and recognising themes
- uncovering variations in the data and revealing those cases that do not fit with the rest of the data and accounting for them
- engaging with, and integrating, the related literature

When the audio recordings have been listened to and transcribed and the observation notes ordered, the transcripts of interviews and observation notes are read several times. The researcher thinks about the data and their meaning. The next step is coding, the process of breaking down the data and giving each important section a descriptive label. For instance, the sentence from an informant *I really was sick of all the grand words and could not understand anything that was going on* might be labelled 'feeling frustrated' or 'lack of information', depending on the context. An observation note that reads *The nurse comforted the critically ill patient* could be labelled 'being there'. The names given to codes are determined by the individual researcher.

Once coding has been completed, codes with similar meaning or themes linked to the same area of analysis are grouped together into larger and more abstract categories. For instance, the codes *need for independence, wanting to be in control, reluctance to be helped* and *rejecting care from others* might be reduced to the category *the wish for self-determination* or *being empowered*. Thematically similar sets of categories are grouped together with links and relationships established between them. Broad patterns of thoughts and behaviour emerge at this stage, and major 'constructs' or themes are developed. The ethnographer needs to check that there is a fit between the data and the analytic categories and themes.

While ethnographers sometimes produce theories, they often generate typologies. This means developing a classification system that points to variations in the data. For example, an ethnographer might find two types of nurse in a particular ward, those who take control and make firm decisions and others who generally ask their colleagues and doctors for advice and rarely make difficult decisions. The ethnographer might call these types *decision-makers* and *advice takers*. As in all typologies, these are types at the end of a continuum. At some point on the continuum, these types overlap.

Interpretation of the data or 'going beyond the results' (Roper & Shapira 2000) means that researchers uncover the meaning of the patterns and themes that they developed. It allows them to answer the research question and to reveal elements of the cultural phenomena studied. Interpretation starts in early data collection and proceeds throughout, but data are often reinterpreted at a later stage. While interpreting the data, researchers make inferences and discuss the possible meanings of the data. Interpretation, although linked to the analysis, is more speculative, involving theorising and explaining. Interpretation links the findings of the project, derived from the analysis, to previously established theories through comparing other researchers' work with one's own. At this stage, the research literature related to the themes and patterns will be considered. It might confirm or 'disconfirm', that is, challenge the findings of the study. The researcher discusses this in a critical and analytical way. The processes of analysis and interpretation are stages in which a phenomenon is broken down, divided into its elements and 'reassembled in terms of definitions or explanations that make the phenomenon understandable to outsiders' (LeCompte & Schensul 1999: 5). Thus, researchers build a holistic portrait of a culture from a number of building blocks.

Reflection activity

Read an ethnographic study and notice how the researcher presents the findings. How is the culture portrayed? Can you see a storyline or a distinct picture of the culture?

RELATIONSHIPS AND PROBLEMS IN THE SETTING

Ethnography is an appropriate approach when addressing questions about culture and subcultures or a particular group with common traits. However, problems do exist for nurses who wish to carry out ethnographic research. Ethnography needs prolonged engagement and immersion in the setting under study. Gaining admittance to the group and establishing rapport take time and commitment. Many nurse researchers who study groups other than their own are unable to undertake participant observation over a long period of time such as a year or more. Hence, some nursing ethnographies are not as fully developed as they might be.

Insider researchers also experience problems. They must attempt to see familiar events with new eyes (DeWalt & DeWalt 2010). Nurses who carry out research in their own setting may be seen as health professionals and not as researchers, and this might prevent their colleagues, who are participants in the research, from making themselves explicit. They might have preconceptions and make assumptions about the setting under study and miss nuances or fail to observe important details. Patients, too, might see them as carers who know them well and may be reluctant to disclose their thoughts for fear that this might prejudice their treatment. Nurse ethnographers often experience conflict between their role as researcher and their nursing role. This was demonstrated by Cudmore and Sondermeyer (2007) who reported on the difficulties of doing ethnography in one's own setting. On the other hand, it is easier to gain access and develop rapport with the research participants when being an insider. Holloway and Wheeler (2010) identify a further problem. Nurses have a background in the natural sciences and learn to approach their clinical practice systematically. This means that they might find difficulty in dealing with ambiguity. Social inquiry is always provisional and rarely unambiguous. It is better, however, to admit to uncertainty than to make unwarranted claims about the research. Findings can be reinterpreted at a later stage in the light of reflection or new evidence.

Key informants might have their own preconceptions of the setting and let this guide their own observations or discussions about the culture under study. This means that researchers need to compare the informants' accounts with the observed reality (which is, of course, that of the researcher). There is also the risk that participants might only tell what they think researchers wish to hear. This danger is particularly strong in health care, as patients (and also nursing students) often want to please those who care for them or deal with them in a professional relationship. However, immersion in the culture by the researcher and the prolonged relationship of researcher and informants help to overcome this.

THE ETHNOGRAPHIC REPORT

Ethnography is not only 'analytic' description but also interpretation. Ethnographers describe what they observe and hear while studying cultural members in context; they identify the main features of the group and the setting and uncover relationships between separate and varied data through analysis; they also interpret the findings by asking for meaning and inferring such meaning from the data. It is important that the participants in the study recognise their own social reality and the traits of their culture and group in the final account and also that the readers of the study grasp the perspective of the participants.

The ethnography – the account of an ethnographic study – usually takes the form of a narrative and includes quotes from the interviews of participants and excerpts from fieldnotes that illustrate the descriptions and explanations. Thick description is one of the features of the report. An ethnography should be a clearly written text that engages its readers.

CONCLUSION

Ethnography is the method of choice when the researcher wants to investigate a culture. The complete ethnography paints a detailed, yet holistic, portrait of the culture that has been studied. Ultimately, a nursing ethnography contributes not only to nursing knowledge but also assists in applying that knowledge for the improvement of nursing practice.

Some of the main features of ethnography include the following:

- An ethnography is the description of a culture, a subculture or group.
- The data sources are mainly participant observation by immersion in the setting and interviews with key informants.
- The researcher uncovers the emic view.
- Thick description is used to make the study come alive and to give both an empirical and a theoretical perspective.

References

Atkinson P, Coffey A, Delamont S, Lofland J, Lofland L (2001) *Handbook of Ethnography*. London, Sage.

Brewer JD (2000) *Ethnography.* Buckingham, Open University Press.

Cudmore H, Sondermeyer J (2007) Through the looking glass: being a critical ethnographic researcher in a familiar setting. *Nurse Researcher* **14**(3): 25–35.

Denzin NK (1989) *Interpretive Interactionism.* Newbury Park, Sage.

DeSantis L (1994) Making anthropology clinically relevant to nursing care. *Journal of Advanced Nursing* **20**: 707–715.

DeWalt KM, DeWalt BR (2010) *Participant Observation.* Walnut Creek, Altamira Press.

Fetterman DM (2010) *Ethnography Step By Step*, 3rd edition. Thousand Oaks, Sage.

Geertz C (1973) *The Interpretation of Cultures.* New York, Basic Books.

Gobo G (2008) *Doing Ethnography.* Los Angeles, Sage.

Hammersley M, Atkinson P (2007) *Ethnography: principles in practice*, 3rd edition. London, Routledge.

Happ MB, Swigart VA, Tate JA, Hoffman LA, Arnold RM (2007) Patient involvement in health-related decisions during prolonged critical illness. *Research in Nursing and Health* **30**: 361–372.

Hardcastle M, Usher K, Holmes C (2006) Carspecken's critical qualitative research method: an application to nursing. *Qualitative Health Research* **16**(1): 151–161.

Harris M (1976) History and significance of the emic/etic distinction. *Annual Review of Anthropology* **5**: 329–350.

Holloway I, Todres L (2003) The status of method: flexibility, consistency and coherence. *Qualitative Research* **3**: 345–357.

Holloway I, Wheeler S (2010) *Qualitative Research in Nursing*, 3rd edition. Oxford, Wiley-Blackwell.

LeCompte MD, Schensul JJ (1999) *Analyzing and Interpreting Ethnographic Data.* Walnut Creek, Altamira Press.

Leininger M (ed) (1985) *Qualitative Research Methods in Nursing.* Philadelphia, WB Saunders.

Lincoln YS, Guba EG (1985) *Naturalistic Inquiry.* Newbury Park, Sage.

Livesley J, Long T (2013) Children's experiences as hospital in-patients: voice, competence and work. Messages for nursing from a critical ethnographic study. *International Journal of Nursing Studies* **50**(10): 1292–1303.

Penney W, Wellard SJ (2007) Hearing what older consumers say about participation in their care. *International Journal of Nursing Practice* **13**(1): 61–68.

Rapport N, Overing J (2000) *Social and Cultural Anthropology: the key concepts.* London, Routledge.

Roper JM, Shapira J (2000) *Ethnography in Nursing Research.* Thousand Oaks, Sage.

Savage J (2000) Participant observation: standing in the shoes of others. *Qualitative Health Research* **10**: 324–339.

Spradley JP (1979) *The Ethnographic Interview.* Fort Worth, Harcourt Brace Jovanovich College.

Spradley JP (1980) *Participant Observation.* Fort Worth, Harcourt Brace Jovanovich College.

Thomas J (1993) *Doing Critical Ethnography.* Newbury Park, Sage.

Williamson S, Twelvetree T, Thompson J, Beaver K (2012) An ethnographic study exploring the role of ward-based advanced nurse practitioners in an acute medical setting. *Journal of Advanced Nursing* **68**(7): 1579–1588.

Further reading

Angrosino M (2007) *Doing Ethnographic and Observational Research.* London, Sage.

O'Reilly K (2011) *Ethnographic Methods,* 2nd edition. Abingdon, Routledge.

Savage J (2006) Ethnographic evidence: the value of applied ethnography in health care. *Journal of Research in Nursing* **11**(5): 383–393.

Schensul SL, Schensul JJ, LeCompte MD (1999) *Essential Ethnographic Methods: observations, interviews and questionnaires.* Walnut Creek, Altamira Press.

Website

http://ethnographymatters.net – Ethnography Matters is a blog that provides an opportunity for ethnographers from different disciplines to communicate and gain insight and advice from colleagues.

CHAPTER 16

Phenomenological Research

Kathleen T. Galvin and Immy Holloway

Key points

- The phenomenological researcher uses descriptions and/or interpretations of everyday human experiences (the lifeworld) as sources of qualitative evidence.
- The purpose of phenomenology is to find insights that apply more generally beyond the cases studied.
- Descriptive phenomenology uses 'bracketing' of preconceptions and attempts to arrive at the 'essences' of experienced phenomena.
- Hermeneutic phenomenology uses interpretation and personal or theoretical 'sensitising' to highlight important themes. It seeks to enhance understanding in readers by presenting 'plots' or stories.
- Phenomenology is not a distinct 'technique' but reflects a rich philosophical heritage with many allied phenomenological 'projects'.

INTRODUCTION

Phenomenology as a discrete philosophical research tradition emerged in the early part of the 20th-century. Although Edmund Husserl (1859–1938) is credited as the central founder of this tradition (Spiegelberg 1994), he built on earlier philosophers who wished to describe human experience as the valid starting point of philosophy. This grabbed the attention of researchers who were looking for ways to study human experience on its own terms without reducing it to language that comes from other sciences such as chemistry or physiology. The promise of phenomenology was that human beings could be understood from 'inside' their subjective experience, which could not be adequately replaced by any external analysis or explanation. A view from within a person's perspective is needed for any comprehensive understanding of human behaviour. Phenomenologists thus emphasise the value of describing and interpreting human experience and seek to do this in credible and insightful ways. This chapter will outline the main principles of phenomenology and illustrate some of

The Research Process in Nursing, Seventh Edition. Edited by Kate Gerrish and Judith Lathlean.

Companion Website: www.wiley.com/go/gerrish/research

the practical ways it is used in research. Some illustrations from published studies will be used to demonstrate particular principles or concepts. In some cases, only a brief excerpt of the study will be presented. In other cases, more detail and context will be given in order that readers may get a sense of the research study as a whole.

PURPOSE OF PHENOMENOLOGICAL RESEARCH

Phenomenological research begins with gathering examples of everyday experiences, describing them and reflecting on them. Husserl called these everyday experiences the 'lifeworld', while other phenomenologists have used the term 'lived experience'. So lived experiences such as 'having a baby' or 'the experience of back pain' are chosen as phenomena to be described and studied in depth. The purpose of focusing on such named experiential phenomena is *to find insights that apply more generally beyond the cases that were studied in order to emphasise what we may have in common as human beings.* Husserl called such common themes, 'essences'; they are also known as 'essential structures'. One may find universal 'essences' in nature. For example, gravity can be described as the essence of all falling objects to earth. However, when it comes to human beings, one seldom finds common themes that are universal across all cultures and circumstances. Rather, one finds common themes that are typical within a context such as a particular culture or time in history. The other thing about 'essences' in relation to human experience is that the essential themes relate to other themes, like *in* a story. So when phenomenologists present their findings, they usually express this in such a way as to show how a number of common themes are related. This is referred to as 'the essential structure' of the phenomenon.

Another important concept in phenomenological research is the idea of 'bracketing' in which phenomenological researchers attempt to suspend (or bracket) their preconceptions so that they can approach the phenomenon to be studied with 'fresh eyes'. Husserl called this suspension of preconceptions 'the phenomenological reduction' where a certain open-mindedness is achieved. In such 'openness', something new can be discovered that is not tainted by previous theory or taken-for-granted assumptions. In practical terms, this involves a certain self-discipline similar to true listening in which one lets the information and data 'speak' more fully before imposing one's own understanding or interpretation.

Here is an example of 'bracketing' as an ongoing discipline during the research:

> Imagine an interview situation where something is said which reminds the interviewer of something he or she has read about. He or she then needs to be careful not to influence the interview in the direction of what has been read. Also, when analysing the interview, the researcher needs to be careful not to impose the ideas from his or her reading onto the analysis. This can be done later in a discussion section, but descriptive phenomenology seeks to stay very close to the data when formulating meaningful themes.

Allied with descriptive phenomenological method, Dahlberg *et al.* (2008) have developed a Reflective Lifeworld Approach and have introduced the helpful term 'bridling'. The researcher's previous beliefs, theories and knowledge (pre-understandings) are 'bridled', so that the researcher adopts a careful, controlled, but *open* approach to the phenomenon under study and, rather than rushing in, waits for the phenomenon to show itself. The researcher *slows down* in a mode of reflection, searching for the essence of a phenomenon, offering a description of the essential meanings of the phenomenon that characterise it, paying attention to parts and wholes and clusters of meaning. Here, infinite nuances rather than 'absolutes' are attended to, and the final description illuminates the essence and abstract meaning of the phenomenon along with the constituents of the meaning that characterise the phenomenon. Research Example 16.1 provides insight into how an essential structure is like a story: it has a general plot that brings the essential themes together in an understandable way and at the same time illuminates meaning, in this case, falling ill with diabetes.

RESEARCH EXAMPLE

16.1 Example of an Essential Structure: The Experience of Falling Ill with Diabetes

Johansson K, Ekebergh M, Dahlberg K (2009) A lifeworld phenomenological study of the experience of falling ill with diabetes. *International Journal of Nursing Studies* **46**(2): 193–203.

'To fall ill with diabetes means to abruptly become another person, one with diabetes. As such one becomes involved in a course of events marked by emotional diversity. An initial feeling of bodily imbalance can be (partially) denied or given a natural explanation. If it persists, the feeling gives rise to a suspicion that something is wrong. When the bodily imbalance is verified as an illness, the ill person is thrown between feelings that the situation is inexplicable, unreal, incomprehensible, and on the other hand feelings of relief, which are caused by the bodily imbalance receiving an explanation. The strain of all those contradictory feelings and the bodily imbalance can be hard to embrace and lead to existential chaos and confusion, which means suffering as well as a push towards an understanding of the situation and its gravity.

When the diabetes illness becomes a fact, it can rather soon be acknowledged and eventually accepted. However, the acceptance is possibly an illusory or false reconciliation to be able to go on. There is anyway no choice, if they want to feel well they have to be "adaptable" to their illness, which makes demands that have to be reconciled; demands that must not be allowed to "govern" their lives. *They do not want to become their illness*. Even if they are ill with diabetes they want to continue the same life and be the same persons as before – although they now carry a disease. At the same time a feeling of loss of one's earlier life can manifest itself'. Johansson *et al*. (2009: 199).

USE OF PHENOMENOLOGY IN NURSING

Phenomenological studies have become an increasingly important qualitative approach in nursing. Topics have included the experience of being cared for in a psychiatric setting (Hörberg *et al.* 2012), the experience of surviving out-of-hospital cardiac arrest (Bremer *et al.* 2009), the relatives' experience of recovery of patients who have undergone 'fast track' surgery with early discharge (Norlyk & Martinsen 2013), the experience of falling ill with diabetes (Johansson *et al.* 2009), the experience of older people participating with professionals in meetings about their care (Lindberg 2013) and the experiences of healthcare from the perspective of patients with experience of irritable bowel syndrome (Häkanson *et al.* 2010). By way of illustration, Research Example 16.2 provides a summary of a phenomenological study examining the experience of patients being cared for in a critical care setting and the meanings the intensive care room holds as a place of care (Olausson *et al.* 2013).

This kind of knowledge of 'what it may be like' is particularly helpful in aiding nurses to imagine what the patient is going through. Such understanding can provide a kind of empathy that is an important foundation for making ethical judgements about care. Such kinds and levels of knowledge may also be important in designing nursing education where a grasp of the 'world of the patient' may help to underpin the development of more uniquely tailored, person-centred practice. Such lifeworld-led education may increasingly expand the horizons of evidence-based education to include qualitative evidence about the world from the patient's point of view.

RESEARCH EXAMPLE

16.2 A Reflective Lifeworld Example: The Experience of Being Cared for in a Critical Care Setting

Olausson S, Lindahl B, Ekebergh M (2013) A phenomenological study of experiences of being cared for in a critical care setting: the meanings of the patient room as a place of care. *Intensive and Critical Care Nursing* **29**(4): 234–243.

Consider a patient in an intensive care unit. What kind of struggle does the person endure? What is it like to live and be cared for in a critical care bed space? Is the situation one of security or insecurity, in what ways is it an 'unhomely' place and can this be mediated? What do patients' experiences reveal that is helpful to enhance practice? What do nurses need to understand about the totality of this experience that could help them in their caring tasks? In such a phenomenological study, the authors were able to provide insight into the meaning of intensive care as a place of care and offer insights to these questions. Nine patients were interviewed at a number of points during their recovery from illness and photographs of the room were also used to facilitate description of how patients experienced the room as a place of care. The authors were able to show how the findings revealed the room as a complex liminal place, between life and death, illness and recovery, security and trust, dream states and lucidity. On occasions, it is a life-affirming place, and on other occasions, it is a room resounding with drama and vulnerability. The findings illuminate a number of constituent meanings of the room: a place of vulnerability, a place of in-between; a place of trust and security, a life-affirming place; and a place of tenderness and care, an embodied place. They were also able to articulate the nuances and variance of other meanings that emerged from a 'twilight world' given by the room, what took place there intertwined with the struggle to survive. Here is one of the essential structures, 'A place of in-between' that was formulated on the basis of the interviews. Being in between dream and reality means experiencing a bodily extension to other places and situations. A struggle to be grounded in the room appears in various scenarios – interiors, for example, fittings and equipment are transformed as well as the place itself. 'Every night I woke up at the same time I remember .... Sometimes I was in a sick room, sometimes a fire station and sometimes a flower shop'. The interiors, sounds and encounters with people and occurrences there co-create the dreams and become intertwined with the body. In dreams, the room is constantly in transformation because of the critical illness. Reality and dream are continually *interwoven*. Being in between is sometimes very frightening; the room could be a place of *torture* and death. These experiences are beyond the patient's understanding, both surprising. A window with a view of nature, personal belongings and the presence of next of kin serve as a connection to the room, to reality – a possibility to become grounded. 'I had many weird dreams I would panic ... this room was like a bombed house in the Middle East, broken walls – no door, only a portal here [photo], when I looked out of the window, it made me feel better, I just felt better seeing the greenery'. Different patients may respond to this meaningful structure differently, but the structure helps us to understand these variations in terms of the central issue at stake: the room was at times a place of extreme vulnerability and at times a place of security, for example, 'Sometimes the patients wish to stay in their **dream** rooms, not facing reality. Fantasizing is then a way of gathering vital force and continuing the struggle against the illness'. In articulating this structure, one may see how this could be a plausible transferable theme for other patients as well, where the spaces in which care is delivered take on particular meanings that need some attending to if the space is to be 'a place of care'. It may also be helpful for nurses to understand the transitions that a patient may be experiencing when in such a vulnerable context and engaged in a struggle for survival.

Reflection activity

Think about some practice situations where a deep understanding from the patient's perspective could enhance understanding of the human condition and inform caring practices. These could be situations relevant to a variety of contexts such as 'becoming ill', 'receiving a diagnosis', 'going through a recovery' or 'facing loss' or a dramatic change in life. Having reflected on these situations, in what ways can phenomenology be insightful for practice?

MAIN FEATURES

Phenomenological research as used by nurses is generally divided into two types: descriptive phenomenology and interpretive or hermeneutic phenomenology. Descriptive phenomenology stays close to Husserl and has been translated into an empirical research approach by Amedeo Giorgi, his colleagues and students (Giorgi 1970, 1997; Giorgi & Giorgi 2004). For a specific example of descriptive phenomenology translated to empirical evidence, see Gallegos (2005). Interpretive or hermeneutic phenomenology stays close to Heidegger, Gadamer and Ricoeur, and their philosophical insights are used in various ways to underpin qualitative research. Hermeneutic phenomenologists do not believe that researchers can be very successful in suspending their preconceptions. Rather, they should use their preconceptions positively, making them more explicit so that readers of the research can understand the strengths and limitations of the interpretations that the researcher makes. So, for example, a hermeneutic phenomenologist may use 'feminism' as an interpretive framework and demonstrate how this perspective may throw some new light on the phenomenon studied. Hermeneutic phenomenologists are also very cautious about finding common essences as they wish to emphasise uniqueness and diversity.

In the authors' view, the distinctions between descriptive and hermeneutic phenomenology have been overemphasised. Both these types of phenomenology share the following features: starting from 'lifeworld' descriptions, the use of bracketing' or sensitising as a reflective analytic method and arriving at 'essences' or 'fusion of horizons' to characterise the experienced phenomena.

Starting from 'lifeworld' descriptions

Both descriptive and hermeneutic phenomenologists use the term 'lifeworld' instead of using the traditional term, 'data'. This is because they are not gathering separate pieces of information but rather interrelated themes or stories. Individual experiences are the starting point for enquiry. This approach moves from the specific to the general. In other words, it uses specific examples of concrete, everyday experiences (lifeworld experiences) as a starting point for further analysis and reflection. With insight and reflection, more general insights across cases can then be formulated. So the phenomenological researcher studies 'experiential happenings', and one often finds that fresh insights are 'in the details'. The findings of a good phenomenological study can resonate at a feeling level and richly describe experiences that human beings can either identify with or, alternatively, understand something more about the differences from their own experience.

The use of 'bracketing' or 'sensitising' as a reflective analytic method

Descriptive phenomenology uses the term 'bracketing', while hermeneutic phenomenology is more likely to use the term 'sensitising'. Descriptive phenomenologists do not wish to start out with a hypothesis or pre-conceived idea or theory that they then try to prove or disprove. Rather, they wish to be open-minded about what they may discover and therefore try to suspend preconceptions and theories as much as possible. This attitude has been called the 'phenomenological reduction', whereby fresh meanings can be seen and expressed in language. Both descriptive and hermeneutic phenomenologists would agree that the possibility of 'seeing something' freshly and differently or from a new perspective is a crucial dimension of phenomenology's discovery-oriented approach. But hermeneutic phenomenological researchers may use existing preconceptions as a way of 'sensitising' themselves to what is missing or different. For example, as a researcher, Finlay (Fitzpatrick & Finlay 2008) reflected on her own personal experience of struggling with a severe shoulder injury and how this 'sensitised' her to the impact of pain for patients undergoing the rehabilitation phase following flexor tendon surgery. She notes that such an empathic awareness of 'what it may be like' helped her to 'see' the pain in patients' movements during rehabilitation, something that may have been left implicit without such sensitivity. However, she also acknowledges how important her co-researcher was in helping her to check such personally informed insights against the stories of the participants. Their study is a good illustration of how personal sensitivity can bring 'humanity' to the study, while 'bracketing' can bring a certain discipline and rigour that realises fresh insights beyond the preconceptions of the researchers.

The findings of phenomenological research: essences or 'fusion of horizons'

Descriptive phenomenology uses the term 'essence' or 'essential structure', while hermeneutic phenomenology is more likely to use the term 'fusion of horizons'. Learning about and communicating the meaning and significance of an experienced phenomenon are a qualitative and literary effort. Husserl, in representing the descriptive emphasis, was interested in finding qualitative features that define what a phenomenon is most generally. For example, one defining feature of many different examples of anger may be the quality of wanting to change another person or something in the world. When formulating 'essences' from a number of cases of an experience, one notices and tries to put into words what is common but also what varies or is different between cases studied. So, the findings of phenomenological research should make sense of both the unique details and the commonalities between the experiences studied. This has been referred to as the 'essential structure' of the phenomenon and is expressed in a narrative way that points out how everything fits together. Hermeneutic phenomenologists are also interested in communicating the meaning and significance of experience but express this differently. Meaning is 'pointed out' in multiple ways and relies on personal insight as well as helpful theories that may be relevant. It is less concerned than descriptive phenomenology to come to a specific conclusion and may evoke deeper understandings in a similar manner as that of a good film-maker or novelist who 'paints a picture' from various angles.

This kind of writing requires an artistic capability. Even though the different phases and parts of this writing may not be conclusive, they are aimed at forming a coherent picture so that they can offer the reader a place of 'meeting' and understanding about the topic. Gadamer, a hermeneutic phenomenologist, used the term 'fusion of horizons' to mean how different people's understandings could come together, thus achieving broad shared insights that, nevertheless, tolerate some freedom in how readers interpret the significance of findings for their own lives or situations. By this, he was pointing out that the validity of phenomenological findings are not based on their ability to correspond perfectly to all cases, but rather that they have sufficient coherence to be meaningfully applied in similar situations.

Whether the researcher adopts a descriptive emphasis or a hermeneutic emphasis, we would argue that a coherent phenomenological study would include all three features discussed earlier. Research Example 16.3 outlines a phenomenological research study that shows unique details and commonalties of a complex phenomenon to deepen understanding. We now turn to the more practical details of field work and analytical procedures. We can only be indicative here as the practice of these principles varies. There now exist several established approaches to phenomenological research with various emphases of description or interpretation within the practice of these principles. Finlay (2011) provides a comprehensive and detailed analysis of these distinctions and also offers an important discussion paper concerning phenomenology's research methods (Finlay 2009).

RESEARCH EXAMPLE

16.3 Patients' Experiences of Suffering in Relation to Healthcare Needs

Berglund M, Westin L, Svanstrom R, Sundler AJ (2012) Suffering caused by care: patients' experiences from hospital settings. *International Journal of Qualitative Studies on Health and Well-being* **7**: 1–9.

Phenomenological interviews were carried out with 22 patients where they were asked to describe their experience of illness and difficult situations that arose for them during this time. The following describes the phenomenon as a summary: 'Suffering in relation to healthcare needs entails a suffering where the patient feels distrusted or mistreated. Suffering is experienced when the patients' perspective on illness and health is overlooked. When feeling is ignored or objectified, the patients' autonomy is lessened, which makes them vulnerable and causes them to feel powerless. Healthcare experiences that cause patients to suffer seem to be something one needs to endure without being critical'. In this study, the essential meaning of suffering as the result of healthcare experiences can be understood from its four constituents: to be mistreated, to struggle for one's healthcare needs and autonomy, to feel powerless and to feel fragmented and objectified. The authors then elaborate the phenomenon of suffering through its four constituent parts above; giving detailed examples of what it is like for patients and how each constituent was experienced as a suffering. Through this process, in-depth description of each of these constituents was elaborated upon by drawing on quotations from selected patient interviews to elucidate the themes. The value and relevance of these insights for clinical practice are discussed at the end of the article.

FIELDWORK

It has been suggested that researchers adopting a phenomenological approach should read very little relevant literature about the research topic before starting in order not to be influenced by preconceptions. However, the research questions do need to be informed by what has already been done and what the gaps are. 'Bracketing' is not about pretending that prior knowledge does not exist, but about looking freshly at the area of study, and questioning the assumptions that may be in the literature. So, for example, in a study about the meaning of mobility for rural elders (Todres & Galvin 2012), the authors were aware of the literature and research that referred to 'transport' and 'mobility', relevant policy and different theories and terms such as 'transport needs'. This made the researchers more interested in describing what was occurring without these theoretical ideas, by going back to people's specific experiences and letting the concepts come 'from there'.

The kind of data that need to be gathered in phenomenological studies are from people who can give examples of experiences they have personally lived through. It is thus not enough that they just have general opinions or views about the topic. They must be able and willing to give descriptions of their own personal experiences. So it is often useful as a starting point to ask: 'have you had something like this kind of experience?' Sometimes this is obvious and may not need to be asked, such as in approaching fathers about their experience of becoming a father for the first time. But at other times, it is less obvious such as in a study of the experience of undergoing a liver transplant or living with aphasia following a stroke. This kind of sampling has been called purposive sampling, in that selection of participants is made on the basis of a particular purpose. In the case of phenomenological research, such purpose is that the research participants included in the study can provide good personal accounts of the experience to be studied. It is also important to gather as much relevant context about the person and the experience as possible. This contextual information helps the researcher to not only make sense of the experience but also to help specify the nature of the examples on which the reflections are built.

Phenomenological research can generate valuable transferable insights based on an in-depth analysis of

Box 16.1 Using interviews to obtain 'lifeworld descriptions'

Imagine that we wish to better understand what happens when a patient is given a diagnosis she/he was not expecting. Using a phenomenological approach that focuses on their lifeworld, we would ask patients who have had this experience to describe as fully as possible the story of the happening, the events in sequence, the interactions, the 'before' and 'after' and their thoughts, feelings and actions – all that goes into the meaning of the experience for them. The value of such lifeworld description is that it provides sources of information that may have been unanticipated by both the respondent and researcher. It does not depend on the ability of the respondent to come up with already formulated views or articulate generalisations.

only one case study, but value may be increased by studying a number of cases. Phenomenological research, in the authors' experience, has achieved the most profound insights with in-depth reflections on about 6–12 cases as 'windows' to, and illustrations of, a phenomenon. There is a danger to choosing a sample that is too large. A number of journal reviewers have commented that, in such cases, depth and thoughtfulness in the analysis is sacrificed. One then wonders why an alternative research design was not chosen that is better able to capture the quantitative incidence of themes.

In phenomenological research, cases of relevant experiences have been gathered from written descriptions, autobiographical texts, journals and from dialogues. Most phenomenological studies are, however, interview based. This may be because an in-depth interview is able to focus on the complexity of the experience, as well as provide a clear focus for exploration.

A phenomenological interview, which gathers lifeworld descriptions of experiences, is similar to, but different from, other types of non-structured, open-ended interviews. It begins with a request that an interviewee describe a relevant experience as fully as possible. This request is generally similar for all respondents. Instructions are sometimes given, which may help the respondent to focus on the details of the experience. One can study lived experience in retrospect because it still has meaning for the person even though the event may have taken place a while ago. An account of an experience usually begins with some of the factual details but also includes what they meant to the person, the feelings and attitudes. However, the richness of the account is often better when it is closer to the experience in time. The interviewer then helps the interviewee to 'tell the story' as fully and concretely as possible, eliciting examples of the experience and what it was like for the respondent. The logic of the interview is: 'Have you had this kind of experience, and if so, how did it occur for you and what was it like for you?' The interview is open-ended, but the interviewer at times may become more focused on attempting to clarify in greater depth the nature of the phenomenon being studied. This often requires a sensitivity and timing so that the interviewee feels understood and comfortable about the interaction. Box 16.1 provides an example of an interview designed to obtain a lifeworld description.

Reflection activity

Examine the phenomenological interview questions in Box 16.1. Notice how the questions are designed to give the participants freedom to describe in detail examples from everyday life and to elaborate upon their answers. There is an active seeking of depth by the researcher. Develop and write down three or four interview questions that explore an experience by using the example questions given as a stimulus and guide. This could be everyday experiences, for example, 'feeling angry' or 'feeling comfortable in a work situation'.

ANALYTICAL PROCEDURES

After gathering lifeworld descriptions of personal experiences, each account becomes a 'text' that is ready for the analysis of meanings and for the formulation of these meanings into a coherent story of interrelated themes and insights. The analysis is different from procedures in other qualitative research such as coding or qualitative content analysis. The articulation and clarification of the meanings in the text, both explicit and implicit, require a 'reading' or strategy that entails a back-and-forth movement between particular expressions and details within the text and a sense of the meaning of the text as a whole (see Box 16.2 for an illustration of this process). It is only the whole of the text and its context that can make sense of the details within the text. On the other hand, the details contribute to, and refine, the process of formulating and synthesising meanings into a coherent overall structure as a whole. The danger of computer-aided analysis packages is that they can divert attention in a way that overemphasises a concern with 'parts', and this can obscure an understanding of the text as a whole.

There has been some controversy about how much to use a systematic method of analysis in phenomenology. Giorgi and his colleagues (Giorgi 1985, 2009; Giorgi & Giorgi 2004) have recommended and demonstrated a systematic procedure that includes:

- reading to get a narrative sense of the text as a whole.
- dividing the text into 'meaning units' that discriminate changes in meaning.
- expressing the meanings in more transferable and general ways.
- formulating a narrative structure that highlights and integrates the essential meanings of the experiences across cases.
- illustrating the common themes in greater detail by elaborating further and also by using quotations from research respondents' original descriptions. This phase also indicates some of the different and unique ways that different people 'lived out' the essential meanings of a phenomenon.

Box 16.2 Example of expressing 'meaning units' in more transferable and general ways: these meanings informed the more abstract theme 'Actualization of the trauma: being destroyed by threatening cancer' (Wertz 2011: 137, 139)

Interviewee's narrative	Transferable, more general meaning
The interviewee is a singer. **(One meaning unit divided from the rest of the text)** I froze. I could not breathe, couldn't move and couldn't even blink. I felt like I had just been shot. My gut locked up like I'd been punched in it. My mouth went dry and my fingers, which had been fumbling with a pen, were suddenly cold and numb. Apparently picking up on my shock, the surgeon smiled a little. 'We're going to save your life, though'	As she stops breathing, her life comes to a screeching halt, to a cessation, to a kind of death. She is paralysed and becomes cold and numb. Her strong sense of movement and transcendence, the high velocity engagements of her singing and her more recent efforts to remedy her medical problem all cease. She feels assaulted and the basic qualities in her life – her moisture, her movement, her sentience – cease. In this death-in-life situation, she experiences the doctor responding to her life cessation with counter assurance in the hopeful anticipation that she will not die

RESEARCH EXAMPLE

16.4 Pervasive Life Changes in Exhaustion Disorder

Jingrot M, Rosberg S (2008) Gradual loss of homelikeness in exhaustion disorder. *Qualitative Health Research* **18**(11): 1511–1523.

These researchers conducted a hermeneutic-phenomenological study influenced by the philosopher Hans-Georg Gadamer. Gadamer had written about how illness took one away from the feeling of being at home in one's body and in one's life. The researchers drew on these ideas when interpreting their research data. The phenomenon studied was the lived experience of suffering from exhaustion disorder as medically defined. The study explored the experiences of 11 individuals on sick leave for at least 6 months because of a diagnosis of exhaustion disorder. In open-ended interviews, research informants were asked to describe their experience of the illness and their life situation, work and future. Each interview was transcribed and analysed before the next one was conducted, and the emerging understandings were used to sensitise the dialogue with the remaining research participants. The analysis of the texts involved a variation on the idea that the researchers go back and forth between their sense of the meaning of the text as a whole and an attention to the detailed meanings in the parts of the text. In addition, the concept of 'unhomelikeness' was used to make sense of the findings in an interesting way. By means of this interpretive lens, the researchers were able to identify a gradual process whereby patients experienced an increasing detachment from their body and world. The findings were formulated in terms of five stages of 'unhomelikeness' that progressively characterised the lifeworlds of patients living with exhaustion disorder. These stages included increased bodily preoccupation and withdrawal from 'normal' life, a loss of a sense of continuity (even memory loss), everyday life as weary struggle and a sense of 'uncanniness' in which there was a frightening feeling of detachment from the body and the world. The clinical significance of this study was highlighted: the importance of early interventions designed to help the patient regain a sense of 'homelikeness' in the body and the world through body-awareness exercises and normalising routines.

Other phenomenologists such as Van Manen (1997) take a less systematic approach and are more concerned with the insightful art of writing that is grounded in lifeworld experiences. Van Manen follows some of the thoughts of Gadamer who feels that no method can ensure insight. Insight emerges through the way the researchers interpret the experiences in the act of writing. Narrative writing is used as a method in itself for reflecting further in order to integrate the different strands of meanings that may be implicit in people's descriptions. Van Manen provides some guidance for writing that includes involving the readers by writing in a compelling way, building a plot line with sub-plots, providing enough details and concrete examples to illustrate the themes and offering new insights that come out of the analysis. An illustration of this approach is given in Research Example 16.4, which outlines a hermeneutic phenomenological study exploring the experiences.

As in other forms of qualitative research, the findings of phenomenological research are finally considered in dialogue with the literature and current research in order to offer critique, possible applications and further directions for research.

STRENGTHS AND LIMITATIONS

The central strength of a phenomenological approach is that it provides both philosophical and methodological support in attempting to capture and express

> ### Reflection activity
>
> The overall aim of phenomenological research is to provide a description of the structure and details of a phenomenon, sometimes called an essence and sometimes called essential structure. Look at the research example studies in detail by obtaining the papers and reading the findings sections. Reflect on the descriptions of the phenomenon and notice how they are relevant to a range of individuals and how they point to common and diverse features.

the meaning of significant human experiences in a rigorous manner. When done well, this gives others deeper insight into what an experience or lived situation is like. Such forms of knowledge humanise our understanding, and this may be crucially important as one basis for ethical practice. The narrative product of such studies seeks to express insights in such a way that it may evoke a sense of recognition and understanding in readers. This kind of narrative knowledge is also interpersonal knowledge in that it describes people in situations in holistic and interactive ways, guarding against viewing humans as objects like other objects. This may be why the humanistic school of psychology has adopted phenomenology as one of its core methodological approaches. It is also resonant with some feminist contributions to psychology (Gilligan 1982) and sociology (Oakley 2000).

The central limitations of a phenomenological approach in our view are threefold:

- The use of observation is problematic in phenomenological research. Because phenomenology wants to get the inner perspectives of people from their own point of view, it is reluctant to judge behaviour from an external perspective. Critics of phenomenology have noted that descriptions of the world from an 'insider' perspective may be inadequate as an account of human behaviour. Such critics would say that it is not people themselves that can best explain their behaviour, as their behaviour may be caused by forces that are more appropriately analysed in other ways with reference to social, political or chemical analyses.
- Descriptions of lifeworlds depend on full and rich verbal accounts by people who are articulate. This raises challenges for phenomenological methodology, for example, when studying children. There are some ways forward in this regard, such as using photographs or drawings as prompts for people to talk about a particular topic.
- It can be elitist in that there is an artistic-literary capability required of the researcher when reflecting and writing. The 'method' does not guarantee the quality of the narrative coherence achieved in the writing of the final stages of the research product. This can be said to some degree of all research, but phenomenology is on the literary side of the scientific–literary continuum.

CONCLUSION

Phenomenology is a discrete qualitative research approach that is embedded in the philosophical traditions of the early part of the 20th-century. Phenomenologists emphasise the value of describing and interpreting human experience and seek to do this in credible and insightful ways that apply more generally beyond the particular cases studied. The phenomenological researcher uses descriptions and/or interpretations of everyday human experiences (the lifeworld) as sources of data. When undertaking descriptive phenomenology, the researcher seeks to bracket any preconceptions and attempts to arrive at the essences of experienced phenomena. By contrast, hermeneutic phenomenology uses interpretation and personal or theoretical sensitising to highlight important themes. It seeks to enhance understanding in readers by presenting plots or stories in a narratively coherent way.

ACKNOWLEDGEMENT

The authors would very much like to thank Les Todres for his contributions to the chapter on phenomenology in earlier editions of this book. He has given his permission to use any material that originates from him.

References

Berglund M, Westin L, Svanstrom R, Sundler AJ (2012) Suffering caused by care: patients' experiences from hospital settings. *International Journal of Qualitative Studies on Health and Well-being* **7**: 1–9.

Bremer A, Dahlberg K, Sandman L (2009) To survive out of hospital cardiac arrest: a search for meaning and coherence. *Qualitative Health Research* **19**: 323–338.

Dahlberg K, Dahlberg H, Nyström M (2008) *Reflective Lifeworld Research*, 2nd edition. Lund, Studentlitteratur.

Finlay L (2009) Debating phenomenological research methods. *Phenomenology and Practice* **3**: 6–25.

Finlay L (2011). *Phenomenology for Therapists: researching the lived world*. Chichester, Wiley-Blackwell.

Fitzpatrick N, Finlay L (2008) 'Frustrating disability': the lived experience of coping with the rehabilitation phase following flexor tendon surgery. *International Journal of Qualitative Studies on Health and Well-Being* **3**(3): 132–142.

Gallegos N (2005) Client perspectives on what contributes to symptom relief in psychotherapy: a qualitative outcome study. *Journal of Humanistic Psychology* **45**: 355–382.

Gilligan C (1982) *In a Different Voice: psychological theory and women's development*. Cambridge, Harvard University Press.

Giorgi A (1970) *Psychology as a Human Science: a phenomenologically based approach*. New York, Harper and Row.

Giorgi A (1985) *Phenomenology and Psychological Research*. Pittsburgh, Duquesne University Press.

Giorgi A (1997) The theory, practice and evaluation of the phenomenological method as a qualitative research procedure. *Journal of Phenomenological Psychology* **28**: 235–260.

Giorgi A (2009). *The Descriptive Phenomenological Method in Psychology: a modified Husserlian approach*. Pittsburgh, Duquesne University Press.

Giorgi A, Giorgi B (2004) The descriptive phenomenological psychological method. In: Camic PM, Rhodes JE, Yardley L (eds) *Qualitative Research in Psychology: expanding perspectives in methodology and design*. Washington, DC, American Psychological Association (APA), pp 243–274.

Häkanson C, Sahlberg-Blon E, Ternestedt B-M (2010) Being in the patient position: experiences of health care among people with irritable bowel syndrome. *Qualitative Health Research* **20**(8): 1116–1127.

Hörberg U, Sjögren R, Dahlberg K (2012) To be strategically struggling against resignation: the lived experience of being cared for in forensic psychiatric care. *Issues in Mental Health Nursing* **33**: 743–751.

Jingrot M, Rosberg S (2008) Gradual loss of homelikeness in exhaustion disorder. *Qualitative Health Research* **18**(11): 1511–1523.

Johansson K, Ekebergh M, Dahlberg K (2009) A lifeworld phenomenological study of the experience of falling ill with diabetes. *International Journal of Nursing Studies* **46**(2): 193–203.

Lindberg E (2013) It made me feel human: a phenomenological study of older patients experiences of participating in a team meeting. *International Journal of Qualitative Studies on Health and Well-Being* **8**: 20714. DOI: 10.3402/qhw.v8i0.20714.

Norlyk A, Martinsen B (2013) The extended arm of health professionals? Relatives' experiences of patients' recovery in a fast track programme. *Journal of Advanced Nursing* **69**: 1737–1746.

Oakley A (2000) *Experiments in Knowing: gender and method in the social sciences*. London, Blackwell.

Olausson S, Lindahl B, Ekebergh M (2013) A phenomenological study of experiences of being cared for in a critical care setting: the meanings of the patient room as a place of care. *Intensive and Critical Care Nursing* **29**(4): 234–243.

Spiegelberg H (1994) *The Phenomenological Movement: a historical introduction*, 3rd edition. Dordrecht, Kluwer Academic Publisher.

Todres L, Galvin KT (2012) In the middle of everywhere: a phenomenological study of mobility and dwelling amongst rural elders. *Phenomenology and Practice* **6**(1). Open access publication http://ejournals.library.ualberta.ca/index.php/pandpr/article/view/19854 (accessed 2 September 2014).

Van Manen M (1997) *Researching Lived Experience: human science for an action-sensitive pedagogy*, 2nd edition. London, ON, Althouse Press.

Wertz FJ (2011) A phenomenological psychological approach to trauma and resilience. In: Wertz FJ, Charmaz K, McMullen LM, Josselson R, Anderson R, McSpadden E. *Five Ways of Doing Qualitative Analysis*. London, The Guilford Press, pp 124–164.

Further readings

Galvin KT, Todres L (2013) *Caring and Well-being: a lifeworld approach*. London, Routledge.

Rapport F (2005) Hermeneutic phenomenology: the science of interpretation of texts. In: Holloway I (ed) *Qualitative Research in Healthcare*. Maidenhead, Open University Press, pp 125–246.

Thomas SP, Polio HR (2002) *Listening to Patients: a phenomenological approach to nursing research and practice*. New York, Springer.

Todres L (2002) Humanising forces: phenomenology in science; psychotherapy in technological culture. *Indo-Pacific Journal of Phenomenology* **3**: 1–16.

Todres L (2005) Clarifying the lifeworld: descriptive phenomenology. In: Holloway I (ed) *Qualitative Research in Healthcare*. Maidenhead, Open University Press, pp 104–124.

Todres L (2007) *Embodied Enquiry: phenomenological touchstones for research, psychotherapy and spirituality*. Basingstoke, Palgrave Macmillan.

Websites

http://phenomenology.utk.edu/ – The Center for Applied Phenomenological Research represents a group of scholars from a variety of departments at The University of Tennessee.

http://www.phenomenologyonline.com/ – Phenomenology Online. This site provides public access to articles, monographs and other materials discussing and exemplifying phenomenological research.

CHAPTER 17

Narrative Research

Dawn Freshwater and Immy Holloway

Key points

- Narrative inquiry is a research approach based on stories of experience.
- Data sources might be narrative interviews, oral histories, diaries, autobiographies and visual images.
- Through stories, people give meaning to their experience and shape their identities.
- There are several approaches to analysis in narrative research.
- Storytelling can help ill or vulnerable people, and their careers, to understand their condition and adapt to their situation.

INTRODUCTION

Narratives permeate our everyday lives. Human beings are storytellers and interpret the world to enhance their understanding of it; they define themselves through the stories they tell. The definitions of 'narrative' are diverse; in its simplest form, narrative means a re-creation of experiences and events in people's lives either by themselves or others (in this chapter, the terms story and narrative are used interchangeably). Narratives give meaning to experiences and life course events, and through narrative people make sense of what has happened to them. Narrative researchers view storytelling as a natural way of communicating between people who wish to transmit to others what they live through, think and feel. Indeed, Bruner sees 'no other way of describing "lived time" save in the form of a narrative' (Bruner 2004: 692). The term narrative research is described here as an independent approach within qualitative methods, although other approaches also use narratives, such as ethnography and phenomenology. Narratives are the accounts of people, by people and about people. They describe events and crises referring to people's own and others' behaviour, their motives and feelings as well as interpretations of actions. These stories that are sometimes, though not always, coherent and reflective have the identities of the participants, and their culture is embedded in them. Although the narratives are culture specific

The Research Process in Nursing, Seventh Edition. Edited by Kate Gerrish and Judith Lathlean.

Companion Website: www.wiley.com/go/gerrish/research

and personally unique, universal patterns can be uncovered in the accounts of those who share similar experiences.

There is a long tradition of storytelling in literature, where stories are fictional; linguists and literary theorists expanded on this tradition. The narratives of participants in research, however, are seen as the perspectives on experience and as 'documents of life' (Plummer 2001). They show the participants' 'take' on life events and crises. Narratives have been used in autobiography, life story or oral history in either spoken or written words. In recent decades, narrative works by educationists, such as Labov and Waletzky (1967) and Clandinin and Connelly (2004) (which culminated in the edited text by Clandinin (2007)), have been published. Psychologists such as Polkinghorne (2007), Bruner (1986), and Riessman (1993, 2008) have also been active in doing and writing narrative research. Polkinghorne (2007) states that 'the storying process' is now common in social science, philosophy, history, organisational theory and other areas. In nursing, Sandelowski wrote on narrative in 1991. Since then, Frid *et al.* (2000) have published their article on narrative inquiry in nursing, and articles as well as chapters have appeared in a variety of journals and books. In 2007, Holloway and Freshwater (2007a) wrote a text on narrative research in nursing. This type of research in the caring professions has mostly been based in illness narratives – the stories sick people tell, although stories from nurses and nursing students are also analysed. The sociologist Hydén published a key article on illness narratives in 1997. The foundational text on illness narratives is that of Kleinman (1988). Apart from this definitive text, Mattingly and Garro (2000) as well as Brody (2003) and others have written about illness narratives or stories of sickness. Hurwitz *et al.* (2004) edited a book on narrative research in health and illness among their other writings on narrative. Narrative research as an approach to human inquiry continues to grow and expand its reach and significance (Mosier & Fischer 2010), in methodological developments (Fisher & Freshwater 2014) and in understanding how clinical practice can be improved (Freshwater *et al.* 2014).

Reflection activity

Take some time to reflect on your experience of listening to, telling and reading stories in day-to-day life. What is the difference between a story that you read and one that you are told? How does your experience of reading and listening to stories relate to your experience of taking oral histories as a clinician, a practitioner or an educationalist? Now consider what makes a good research story.

THE NATURE AND PURPOSE OF STORIES

Narratives are stories people tell, usually with a beginning, a middle and an end, though they are not always linear and ordered. They include a plot, a cast of actors, a problem that needs solving or an event that is significant. Emplotment and temporality are central to a story (Ricoeur 1991; Holloway & Freshwater 2007b). Emplotment is an act that links diverse events to form a plot, which generates a coherent story; it is the structure through which sense is made of events and the way in which things and individual identity are connected (Czarniawska 2004; Freshwater & Rolfe 2004). Ryan (1993) points out that emplotment is the real challenge in the story. This links the events into a meaningful sequence and structure. It is natural for the audience or readership to want to create their own emplotment in response to the story. Plot then is a device of narrative. Lee *et al.* (2013), for instance, show in the narratives of older people's transition to residential care that participants' focused on the key plots of power, control and identity.

Greenhalgh and Hurwitz (1998) suggest a difference between a simple story and a plot, taking their suggestion from E.M. Forster's explanation that a simple story continues in a chronology '... and then ... and then...', while the plot suggests 'why'. Plot is the sequential element and the essential structure of narrative (Cortazzi 1993). Plotlines, however, are not always linear; they may be circular and iterative and can be revised or 'edited' in their retelling. Going back and forth is quite common among narrators, but the listener is still left with the essential features of the story. Researchers attempt to find the 'narrative thread' to grasp the whole story and give it coherence. Researchers construct a plot which involve separate events forming a coherent whole.

A narrative is a journey or pathway through time, which is told by its author, who tells the listener what happens on the way. However, narrators do not merely communicate a simple story to the listener; they also clarify and reflect on the past and justify their past behaviour and link the past to their present thinking and actions. Brody (2003) adds to these features of narrative another element: the story has to be special, that is, 'worthy' of narration. It does not rely merely on everyday sequences of events: 'I took the car; I drove to work; I talked to my friends'. Instead, it relies on dramatic and critical events and behaviour, or unusual conditions, such as an illness or an 'epiphany' where some thing or person is illuminated by a sudden insight: 'I was digging in the garden, and all of the sudden, I felt a snap in my back. The pain was excruciating…' 'I had a shock; I found out I had cancer…'.

As already mentioned, the term emplotment describes the way a story is organised. Cortazzi (1993) describes three major elements in a plot:

- Temporality (how time is framed within the story)
- Causation (relationship between events in the story)
- Human interest (how the story interacts with the audience).

Temporality

Temporality is a complex term in philosophy that is about the nature of time (used by Ricoeur (1984) in relation to narrative) and how human beings are bounded by and in time. Sequencing over time and the links between events provide continuity 'this happened and then…'. Everything is seen in relation to everything else. Holloway and Freshwater (2007a) state that the narrative is a journey through time in which narrators share their experience, justify their actions and link the present to the past and the future. The story involves a group of characters who act or who are experiencing the actions of others. Narrators tell personal as well as social/cultural stories, which means that these tales are not only unique to the participants but also present the cultural context in which they are located and thus have commonalities within a particular context. For instance, Price *et al.* (2013) discuss nursing careers, which were temporally and culturally influenced and showed a trajectory.

Temporality implies that the story evolves more or less sequentially (although this could be disputed). It means that there are three linked sequences:

1. When the story is set up and opens up towards the future – the beginning
2. When the story unfolds – the middle
3. When the story is resolved – the end.

The listener can hear that the story has coherence because the narrator links past, present and future.

Causation

A story often contains causal relationships, which the listeners and readers generally perceive, even though it is often assumed by them. The plot includes causality: *why* this happened and *how* this happened. As human beings, we are constructed in such a way that we continually search for the causes of things. Story provides a powerful experience of causation, gratifying this basic need. Porter-Abbott (2002) suggests that:

> 'Narrative itself, simply by the way it distributes events in an orderly, consecutive fashion, very often gives the impression of a sequence of cause and effect'. (Porter-Abbott 2002: 37)

Forster (1927) in his definitive text, *Aspects of the Novel,* gives some practical examples of the way in which readers do not always need causation to be obvious in a text in order to think causally. In other words, human beings have a tendency towards a

Box 17.1 Examples of titles for narrative research

East L, Jackson D, O'Brian L, Peters K (2010) Storytelling: an approach that can help to develop resilience. *Nurse Researcher* **17**(3): 17–25.

Lapurn J, Angus JE, Peter E, Watt-Watson J (2010) Patients' narrative accounts of open-heart surgery and recovery: authorial voice of technology. *Social Science and Medicine* **70**(5): 754–762.

Schick Makaroff KL, Sheilds L, Molzahn A (2013) Stories of chronic kidney disease: listening for the unsayable. *Journal of Advanced Nursing* **69**(12): 2644–2653.

Volante MA (2005) *Biographical Landscapes: nurse' and health visitor narratives*. University of East London, London, PhD thesis.

narrative logic, in which things that follow other things are caused by those things.

Human interest

Human interest is another facet of a story. If no one has an interest in the story, then there is no listener and no narrative. Often, a story of experience includes crises and turning points as well as justification for the storyteller's actions and behaviour that is a response to the interpretation of experience. People do not only develop stories to communicate with others but also to make sense of their own lives and in particular of problematic and tragic circumstances. The title of a narrative account might stimulate interest in the reader. Box 17.1 provides some examples of narrative research.

There are, as already alluded too, many reasons for storytelling, some of which are listed below:

- People try to interpret their experience and make sense of it.
- They communicate with others through stories.
- They organise events and happenings by narrative.
- They justify their own actions and feelings.
- They attribute praise and blame to others and themselves.

(See also Holloway & Freshwater 2007a)

There may be a number of reasons why people wish to tell their stories. Common to all of these is the idea that storytelling provides the narrator with a distance from the (often threatening) experience of vulnerability; in other words, storytelling can be useful as a coping strategy for individuals to manage the psychosocial and emotional aspects of their predicament. Moreover, once the story is in the process of being narrated, it enables the narrator to gain a different perspective on the experience.

Stories therefore can be useful devices for individuals to come to terms with their vulnerability, make sense of their lives and construct their versions of reality and identity through social discourse. According to Ricoeur's (1984) notion of temporality, through storying, people are able to locate their 'now' experience in a context of 'back then' and 'not yet'. For instance, a person might connect an experience in the past with the cause of condition in the 'here and now' or might justify present thought and action, or future behaviour, using a story from the past. Garro (2000) maintains that 'people make sense of the past from the perspective of the present' (Garro 2000: 71); memory helps re-construct past experiences and connects these to the present and to expectations of the future. Fundamental to the process of storying is the imposition of narrative form and sequencing, such that the movement between beginning and end point enacts a relationship to time. Even when storytelling loses its thread and

Reflection activity

Think about a recent conversation in which you were told a story. Having rehearsed the story once again to yourself, give the story a title and ask yourself the following:

How did the story unfold?
In what style was the story narrated?
How was the story organised?
How did you check for authenticity and genuineness?
What were you aware of as you were listening?

the temporal sequencing is disrupted, people still confirm their identity through stories (Holloway & Freshwater 2007b).

Of course, stories are not necessarily factual constructions and are often evaluated for their credibility or authenticity. Researchers usually accept the participants' stories as true, though they know that storytellers sometimes do not remember well, are confused or over-dramatise for effect (Rolfe 2005; Holloway & Freshwater 2007a). Plausibility, of course, does not guarantee authenticity. However, storytellers even when not telling the truth – consciously or not – demonstrate their intentions and motivations as well as give their own understanding of the situation.

NARRATIVE INQUIRY IN NURSING

Narrative as a form of inquiry differs somewhat from other qualitative approaches in that it generates coherent stories rather than 'fractured text' (Riessman 1993). It is important that the researcher listens, does not ask too many intrusive questions and empowers the participants to be in control of their tales. Narratives are sources of data for researchers in many areas of nursing, for instance, stories of caring for patients, of interaction with other professionals and of learning and education. Nursing stories, according to Kelly and Howie (2007), are a means of sharing nursing knowledge and help researchers understand professional practice and the perception of professional roles. Most frequently, however, nurse researchers elicit the stories of patients, and illness narratives – a term made known particularly by Kleinman (1988) – become the focus of their research. Patients tell these stories because they want to make sense of their suffering and share their thoughts and feelings with others. Narrative nursing research is carried out, for example, with care givers (Hennings *et al.* 2013), with older people (Wiles *et al.* 2011), on student learning (Boyd & Mckendry 2012), on the experience of pain (Dysvik *et al.* 2011), on the stories of ill or vulnerable participants such as that by Hydén and Örulv (2009) and in researching mental illness (Fisher & Freshwater 2014). Through listening to stories, nurses are able to gain more understanding of the participants' lives and condition. In the clinical situation, this understanding could improve the care of patients.

ILLNESS NARRATIVES OR STORIES OF SICKNESS

Now, we turn our attention to those stories of sickness and vulnerability, sometimes known as illness narratives. Illness narratives have been told over centuries; nurses have listened to these stories so they can help their patients. Only in recent decades have they become a focus of research. Illness in these stories is perceived as a 'biographical disruption' (Bury 1982), not only as a significant life event but one that might change the identity of the storyteller who often wishes to regain his or her former self and return to normality (see restitution narrative in the following). Frank (1995) discusses stories of sickness in his classic *The Wounded Storyteller*. The three types of narrative that he proposes are 'the restitution narrative', 'the chaos narrative' and 'the quest narrative'. He suggests that these types have fit with the stories people tell, though they often overlap.

The most frequent story type is the *restitution narrative* with the plot stressing a future of normalisation and the regaining of the old identity. The restitution narrative is one that is not only favoured by ill patients but also by health professionals. For acute illness, this is often the general outcome as patients see themselves regaining their health and their former selves, although the chronically ill also wish to reclaim at least some sort of normality. (In relation to this, Frank (1995) also discusses Parsons' concept of 'sick role'.) The *chaos narrative* contains a plot of not getting better. Stories of terminal cancer are chaos narratives, but also, some tales of chronic illness with its ups and downs of suffering and pain can contain disorder, disruption and chaos. Nurses and other health professionals feel impotent in the face of people who tell these types of tales. We found that chaos narratives are the least welcome and not as often used in research. *Quest narratives* contain the missionary spirit of the storyteller who accepts, uses and confronts illness to gain something in the process; often, they wish to be a model or an example to others. Frank claims that quest narratives are the most commonly told in public. He suggests that they often include a call for social action; many of us have heard stories from the media where narrators use their experiences in the health system 'so that this will never happen again', where people showed their scars to give testimony to suffering. Stoicism and heroism are part of the plot. This is shown in particular by Smith and Sparkes (2004) narrative of disabled sportsmen. Terms such as 'battle', 'struggle' and 'victory' are used frequently.

ETHICAL ISSUES IN NARRATIVE RESEARCH

Elliott (2005), in her writings on ethics in narrative research, discusses both ethics and political issues. The ethical dimensions are issues relating to the relationship between the researcher and participant and the impact of the research process on individuals directly involved in the research. The political dimension is defined by the broader implications of research, namely, the impact on society or subgroups in society.

Reflection activity

You are at the beginning of your research study. Consider the steps you should take regarding managing the ethical issues of conducting narrative research. How would you approach gatekeepers to gain permission for your study and explain the approach that you are taking? Consider how you would approach participants. Is there a way in which you can make sure that they cannot be identified either during or after the research when using narrative methods?

In more detail, Elliott (2005) suggests that the researcher enters into a personal and moral relationship with the participants during data collection, analysis and dissemination. She focuses her attention on the full research process – data collection, informed consent, the potential impact of the research encounter on the participant and additionally the implications of using narrative with regard

Reflection activity

Power is a key aspect of any relationship, it is especially difficult to manage the power dynamic within a relationship in which one person is viewed as an authoritative expert, such as a researcher, or is a professional delivering care. All researchers have the opportunity to exercise power, whether this is through the interview process or through the analysis. What are some of the key considerations in regard to the exercise of power when conducting narrative research? What are the sorts of dilemmas that the narrative researcher is faced with when thinking about the power imbalance in the research situation?

to confidentiality and anonymity during analysis and dissemination. The processes can be quite complex. Most ethical issues are similar to those in other forms of qualitative research, though the relationship between researcher and participants is more intimate; hence, the researcher needs to be particularly sensitive and mindful.

COLLECTING AND ANALYSING NARRATIVE DATA

The initial research question (not to be confused with interview question) needs to be broad to fit with a narrative approach. Narrative inquiry has sampling strategies and data sources that are similar to those of other forms of qualitative inquiry such as interviews or diaries, even occasionally visual sources. However, narrative researchers often use fewer questions in their interviews, usually starting with an open and general question about their experience, which elicits a full story. On completion of this, researchers might pursue issues that they do not understand or that are unclear. These questions could enhance the relationship between the researcher and the participant. Starter questions might be general (for instance, tell me about your condition; how did it all start?) and follow-up questions (for instance, what happened then? what about your stay in hospital?). Narrative interviews rely on the stories of participants and not on detailed questions of the researcher.

In narrative inquiry, a number of models of analysis exist and different researchers adopt a particular stance or orientation. There are various ways to analyse narrative data; whatever model researchers choose, they need to be analytic and theoretical and take the stories to a new level as narrative research is more than retelling or even reformulating the participants' tales.

Riessman (2008) describes several models of narrative analysis. *Thematic analysis* focuses on the content of stories, and researchers proceed in the same way as other qualitative researchers do. Braun and Clarke (2006) describe this type of analysis in detail. Researchers organise, label and group related data together in themes and illustrate their accounts with quotes from the participants and short vignettes of the individuals involved. Hence, the researcher centres on 'what' is said. Less attention is given to 'how is the story told', 'who is the narrator' and 'to whom is it addressed'. Accounts of experience first looked at the plot as a whole without breaking the text into its structure. The 'voice' of the narrator is heard throughout. Riessman (2008) states that this type of analysis neglects context when context, knowledge of culture and circumstance are essential for understanding the contents of these stories. Research Example 17.1 gives an example of thematic analysis.

RESEARCH EXAMPLE

17.1 Thematic Analysis

Tighe M, Molassiotis A, Morris J, Richardson J (2011) Coping, meaning and symptom experience: a narrative approach to the overwhelming impacts of breast cancer in the first year following diagnosis. *European Journal of Oncological Nursing* **15**(3): 226–232.

In a British narrative study with 39 women who were newly diagnosed with breast cancer at an oncology centre, a thematic narrative approach to analysis was carried out. The research uncovered how women coped with treatment, their relationships and self-management of symptoms.

The thematic analysis approached the narratives in context and time. The key themes were 'symptom experiences', 'coping and meaning' and 'relationships'. Within these, subthemes were also uncovered.

RESEARCH EXAMPLE

17.2 Example of Structural Analysis

Yelle MT, Stevens PE, Lanuza DM (2013) Waiting narratives of lung transplant candidates. *Nursing Research and Practice* **2013**: Article ID 794698, http://dx.doi.org/10.1155/2013/794698.

Yelle and colleagues examined the experiences of seven lung transplant patients who experienced the scoring system for lung transplants through listening to their stories. A structural analysis of these stories was carried through use of the analytic strategy by Labov and Waletsky (1967).

The authors state that this analysis centres on the event to gain insight into the situation.

They showed that listening to the meaning of people's stories was essential for health-care providers.

Riessman (2008) states that *structural analysis* focuses on the language and analyses how the story is told, not only on the storyline. This type of analysis has its origin in the work of Labov and Waletzky (1967) and resembles conversation analysis because of the emphasis on text. They analyse how language is used in stories. The text is broken down into a variety of elements. In structural analysis, the researcher takes account of the following six major features:

1 *Abstract* – summary, the point of the story.
2 *Orientation* – towards location, characters and time, for instance.
3 *Complicating action* – the plot, which includes crisis point and sequence.
4 *Evaluation* – the narrator takes stock of what has been said.
5 *Resolution* – the outcome of the story.
6 *Coda* – an end to the story, which rounds it off.

In other words, the story is organised into ideas and units, which rely on the spoken narrative and not on its content. This micro-analysis of text seems inappropriate for stories, which, after all, are told as a whole, and the storytellers wish them to be understood as wholes. This type of analysis is not often used in nursing. Research Example 17.2 provides an illustration of structural analysis.

Riessman (2008) discusses three more types of analysis, interactional, dialogic/performance and visual analysis. The first two focus on the interaction of researcher and storyteller and the research situation as a dialogue and seem to be the same as other dialogic research in qualitative inquiry. Visual analysis is based on the non-language-based sources of data such as pictures, photographs, films and other images, which complement the story or the written account. It should be stressed, however, that no definitive type of narrative analysis exists.

Lieblich *et al.* (1998) develop *holistic or holistic-content analysis*. This is possibly the most appropriate way of analysing narrative data as it keeps the 'gestalt' of the story, that is, the researcher considers the whole rather than breaking it down into small parts. Lieblich *et al.* give the steps in analysis as follows:

- Read (or listen) to the story for content many times until you discern a pattern and attempt to find its meaning and examine its context.
- Write down overall impressions as well as unusual elements.
- Find special facets or themes that you wish to follow up.
- Detect the main themes in the story.
- Follow these themes throughout the story, look at the context and determine their importance and look at contradictory features in the story.

Lieblich *et al.* see these as the stages to be followed for each story. However, they do not discuss how to

RESEARCH EXAMPLE

17.3 Example of Holistic Analysis

Beal CC (2013) Keeping the story together: a holistic approach to narrative analysis. *Journal of Research in Nursing* **18**(8): 692–704.

Claudia Beal describes a holistic-content analysis, which was used in a study by Beal *et al.* (2012) about nine women patients' early symptom experience of ischemic stroke. She described how the authors used the ideas of both Polkinghorne (2007) and Lieblich *et al.* (1998) to make sense of the women's stories. The authors placed both plot and temporality at the centre of their analysis. She maintains that the holistic-content approach to analysing narrative data is useful because it considers individual variations in common experiences, identifying similar and dissimilar characteristics while also taking a 'gestalt' view of the phenomenon under investigation.

This article includes relevant references for holistic analysis.

manage a number of stories. Beal (2013) uses holistic-content analysis with a variety of stories, and she compares these for similarities and differences. After analysis, she synthesised the contents of these stories, which had many commonalities but were also unique for each person. Research Example 17.3 presents an example of holistic analysis.

CRITICAL ISSUES IN NARRATIVE INQUIRY

Narrative research has been criticised by several insiders such as Atkinson (1997) and Atkinson and Delamont (2006). These writers suggest a preoccupation of qualitative researchers with narratives and maintain that narrative research is not privileged over other forms of research and it needs analytic rigour. These authors emphasise that narrative research does not consist of the retelling of stories in an uncritical and non-analytic way. Atkinson and Delamont regret that narratives are often used in an unreflective way and not contextualised. Nevertheless, analytic and reflexive narrative research gives voice to people who might not have been heard before and focus on their perspectives.

Storytelling can include imagination or even distortion; thus, storytellers do not always tell the truth. If people tell stories to make sense of their experiences, even unconscious 'untruths' are important as these are based on the tellers' perceptions and upon which they act (it is rare that narrators tell deliberate lies to the researcher). Lorem (2008) suggests that in these stories, individuals reconcile themselves with their experience and justify their own and others' behaviour. What is revealed will include the elements in the story that the narrators wish to show as central to their experience even if it is not factually true. Polkinghorne (2007: 479) maintains that 'storied texts serve as evidence for personal meaning, not for the factual occurrence of the events reported in the stories'. Furthermore, the validity of the research does not depend on the 'truth telling' of the participants but on their perspectives and the credibility of the researcher's account.

The standards for establishing validity and reliability in narrative research are similar to those of other qualitative approaches. Freshwater and Rolfe (2004: 532) identify that these rely on three principal criteria:

1 Detailed writing ('thick description') that makes both the research process and the context of the research transparent.
2 Exposure of the researcher's bias (or 'interest'). The final draft should refer to the way in which the researcher has come to an awareness of the underlying 'plots' in his/her developing narrative.

3 The way in which the professional community view the research (which should also be included in the final write-up). Ideally, this should include reference to peer response to any published work.

The main judgement evaluates its appropriateness, relevance, holism, credibility and readability.

CONCLUSION

The main tenets of narrative research have been outlined in this chapter, such as concepts of narrative, story, plot and emplotment; however, it is acknowledged that the concept of narrative is open to multiple interpretations. Narrative and storytelling are part of human nature; narrative research is closely associated with understanding people's lives rather than abstract principles, and as such, it is aligned with the humanistic perspective in nursing.

References

Atkinson PA (1997) Narrative turn or blind alley? *Qualitative Health Research* **7**(3): 325–344.

Atkinson P, Delamont S (2006) Rescuing narrative from qualitative research. *Narrative Inquiry* **16**(1): 164–172.

Beal CC (2013) Keeping the story together: a holistic approach to narrative analysis. *Journal of Research in Nursing* **18**(8): 692–704.

Beal CC, Stuifbergen A, Volker D (2012) A narrative study of women's early symptom experience of ischemic stroke. *Journal of Cardiovascular Nursing* **27**(3): 240–252.

Boyd V, Mckendry S (2012) Staying the course: examining enablers and barriers to student success with undergraduate nursing programmes. *European Journal for Research on the Education and Learning of Adults* **3**(1): 59–75.

Braun V, Clarke V (2006) Using thematic analysis in psychology. *Qualitative Psychology* **3**(2): 77–101.

Brody H (2003) *Stories of Sickness*, 2nd edition. New York, Oxford University Press.

Bruner J (1986) *Actual Minds, Possible Worlds*. Boston, Harvard University Press.

Bruner J (2004) Life as narrative. *Social Research* **71**(3): 691–710.

Bury M (1982) Chronic illness as biographical disruption. *Sociology of Health and Illness* **4**(2): 167–182.

Clandinin DJ (ed) (2007) *Handbook of Narrative Inquiry: mapping a methodology*. Thousand Oaks, Sage.

Clandinin DJ, Connelly FM (2004) *Narrative Inquiry: experience and story in qualitative research.* San Francisco, Wiley.

Cortazzi M (1993) *Narrative Analysis*. London, Falmer Press.

Czarniawska B (2004) *Narratives in Social Science Research*. London, Sage.

Dysvik E, Somerseth R, Jacobson FF (2011) Living a meaningful life with chronic pain from a nursing perspective: narrative approach to a case story. *International Journal of Nursing Practice* **17**(1): 36–32.

Elliott J (2005) *Using Narrative in Social Research: qualitative and quantitative approaches.* London, Sage.

Fisher P, Freshwater D (2014) Methodology and mental illness: resistance and restorying. *Journal of Psychiatric and Mental Health Nursing* **21**(3): 197–205.

Forster EM (1927) *Aspects of the Novel*. London, Penguin.

Frank AW (1995) *The Wounded Story Teller: body, illness, and ethics*. Chicago, University of Chicago Press.

Freshwater D, Rolfe G (2004) *Deconstructing Evidence Based Practice*. London, Routledge.

Freshwater D, Cahill J, Essen C (2014) Discourses of collaborative failure: identity, role and discourse in an interdisciplinary world. *Nursing Inquiry* **21**(1): 59–68.

Frid I, Őhlén J, Bergbom I (2000) On the use of narratives in nursing research. *Journal of Advanced Nursing* **32**(3): 695–703.

Garro LC (2000) Cultural knowledge as a resource in illness narratives: remembering through accounts of illness. In: Mattingly C, Garro LC (eds) *Narrative and the Cultural Construction of Illness and Healing.* Berkeley, University of California Press, pp. 70–87.

Greenhalgh T, Hurwitz B (1998) Why study narrative? In: Greenhalgh T, Hurwitz B (eds) *Narrative Based Medicine: dialogue and discourse in clinical practice.* London, Routledge, pp. 3–16.

Hennings J, Froggatt K, Payne S (2013) Spouse caregivers of people with advanced dementia in nursing homes: a longitudinal narrative study. *Palliative Medicine,* **27**(7): 683–691.

Holloway I, Freshwater D (2007a) *Narrative Research in Nursing*. Oxford, Blackwell.

Holloway I, Freshwater D (2007b) Storying vulnerability: narrative research in nursing. *Journal of Research in Nursing* **12**(6): 1–9.

Hurwitz B, Greenhalgh T, Skultans V (eds) (2004) *Narrative Research in Health and Illness*. Oxford, Blackwell.

Hydén LC (1997) Illness and narrative. *Sociology of Health and Illness* **49**(1): 48–69.

Hydén LC, Örulv L (2009) Narrative and identity in Alzheimer's disease: a case study. *Journal of Aging Studies* **23**(4): 205–214.

Kelly T, Howie L (2007) Working with stories in nursing research: procedures used in narrative analysis. *International Journal of Mental Health Nursing* **16**(2): 136–144.

Kleinman A (1988) *The Illness Narratives: suffering, healing and the human condition*. New York, Basic Books.

Labov W, Waletzky J (1967) Oral versions of personal experience. In: Helm J (ed) *Essays on the Verbal and Visual Arts*. Seattle, University of Washington Press, pp. 12–44.

Lee V, Simpson J, Froggatt K (2013) A narrative exploration of older people's transitions into residential care. *Aging and Mental Health* **17**(1): 48–56.

Lieblich A, Tuval-Mashiak R, Zilver T (1998) *Narrative Research: reading, analysis and interpretation.* Thousand Oaks, Sage.

Lorem GF (2008) Making sense of stories: the use of patient narratives within mental health care research. *Nursing Philosophy* **9**(1): 62–71.

Mattingly C, Garro LC (2000) *Narrative and the Cultural Construction of Illness and Healing*. London, University of California Press.

Mosier KL, Fischer UM (eds) (2010) *Informed by Knowledge: expert performance in complex situations*. New York, Taylor and Francis.

Plummer K (2001) *Documents of Life 2: an invitation to critical humanism.* London, Sage.

Polkinghorne D (2007) Validity issues in narrative research. *Qualitative Inquiry* **13**(4): 471–486.

Porter-Abbot H (2002) *The Cambridge Introduction to Narrative.* Cambridge, Cambridge University Press.

Price SL, McGillis Hall L, Angus JE, Peter E (2013) Choosing nursing as a career: a narrative analysis of millennial nurses' career choice of virtue. *Nursing Inquiry* **20**(4): 305–316.

Ricoeur P (1984) *Time and Narrative* (Vols. 1–3). Chicago, University of Chicago Press.

Ricoeur P (1991) Life in quest of narrative. In: Wood D (ed) *On Paul Ricoeur: narrative and interpretation.* London, Routledge, pp. 29–33.

Riessman CK (1993) *Narrative Analysis.* Newbury Park, Sage.

Riessman CK (2008) *Narrative Methods for the Human Sciences.* Los Angeles, Sage.

Rolfe G (2005) Evidence, memory and truth: towards a deconstructive validation of reflective practice. In: John C, Freshwater D (eds) *Transforming Nursing through Reflective Practice*, 2nd edition. Oxford, Blackwell, pp. 13–26.

Ryan ML (1993) Narrative in real time: chronicle mimesis and plot in baseball broadcast. *Narrative* **1**(2): 138–155.

Sandelowski M (1991) Telling stories: narrative approaches in qualitative research. *Image, Journal of Nursing Scholarship* **23**(3): 161–168.

Smith B, Sparkes A (2004) Men, sport, and spinal injury: an analysis of metaphors and narrative types. *Disability and Society* **19**(6): 513–626.

Tighe M, Molassiotis A, Morris J, Richardson J (2011) Coping, meaning and symptom experience: a narrative approach to the overwhelming impacts of breast cancer in the first year following diagnosis. *European Journal of Oncological Nursing* **15**(3): 226–232.

Wiles JL, Wild K, Kerse N, Allen RES (2011) Resilience from the point of view of older people: there is still life beyond a funny knee. *Social Science and Medicine* **7**(3): 416–424.

Yelle MT, Stevens PE, Lanuza DM (2013) Waiting narratives of lung transplant candidates. *Nursing Research and Practice* **2013**: Article ID 794698, http://dx.doi.org/10.1155/2013/794698.

Further reading

Andrews M, Squire C, Tamboukou M (2008) *Doing Narrative Research.* Los Angeles, Sage.

Bold C (2012) *Using Narrative in Research.* London, Sage.

Charon R (2006) *Narrative Medicine: honoring the stories of illness.* New York, Oxford University Press.

Gubrium JF, Holstein JA (2009) *Analyzing Narrative Reality.* Thousand Oaks, Sage.

Webster L, Mertova P (2007) *Using Narrative Inquiry as a Research Method: an introduction to using critical event narrative analysis in research on learning and teaching.* London, Routledge.

CHAPTER 18

Experimental Research

Andrea E. Nelson, Jo Dumville and David Torgerson

Key points

- Experimental research makes a useful contribution to nursing research as it is a powerful design able to distinguish between cause and effect.
- There are many different types of experimental design used in health-care research.
- The randomised controlled trial is particularly valued for its ability to test rigorously the effectiveness of treatments and interventions.
- Experimental research seeks to minimise all possible sources of bias and confounding.
- Strengths and weaknesses of the experimental design for different research questions and contexts must be acknowledged.

BACKGROUND

Well-designed and well-executed experimental research can contribute to theoretical understanding and to nursing practice. There are several different types of health-care interventions, including screening, drugs, information giving, education and different ways of delivering care (e.g. walk-in clinics) that are amenable to experimental research as a way of testing their effectiveness. Since the thalidomide disaster, drugs must be evaluated in large randomised controlled trials (RCTs) before they are licensed for use. However, other types of interventions are not routinely evaluated in this way, with some commentators arguing that RCTs are of limited use in evaluating nursing interventions.

EXPERIMENTAL VERSUS OBSERVATIONAL STUDIES

True experimental studies are more powerful than observational studies in determining the cause of an observed outcome. Using an observational design, an association may be found between two variables,

The Research Process in Nursing, Seventh Edition. Edited by Kate Gerrish and Judith Lathlean.

Companion Website: www.wiley.com/go/gerrish/research

Box 18.1 'Surprising' results of treatments

Question	Impact of intervention	Reference
Are occlusive dressings better than gauze-based dressings for surgical and traumatic wounds?	Occlusive dressings were associated with higher total costs and had longer hospital stay than the gauze dressing group. Groups did not differ for complete wound healing, time to wound healing or pain	Ubbink *et al.* (2008)
Do honey-impregnated dressings help the healing of venous ulcers or reduce infection rates?	There was no significant difference in the number of infections or ulcer healing rate between people who had honey dressings and those who had a dressing chosen by their nurse. People treated with honey dressings had more pain and withdrawals	Jull *et al.* (2008)
Does providing an automated external defibrillator (AED) in the home in patients at risk of sudden cardiac arrest reduce deaths?	There was no difference in mortality between patients given an AED for home use and a control group that received CPR training and usual access to emergency services from home	Bardy *et al.* (2008)
Does using larval therapy (maggots) clean sloughy venous ulcers quicker than a hydrogel, and does it lead to quicker healing and reduced infection rates?	Larval therapy reduced time to removal of slough tissue in venous ulcers but had no impact on time to healing when compared with a simple hydrogel dressing	Dumville *et al.* (2009)

but it is difficult to be certain about the direction in which the causal effect is operating. For example, women who give up breastfeeding soon after birth use dummies more often than women who maintain breastfeeding. An RCT of discouraging dummy use found no effect on breastfeeding rates (Kramer *et al.* 2001). In fact, the association between dummy uses was observed because women who were going to give up breastfeeding (for whatever reason) tended to use dummies more. Cessation of breastfeeding led to increased dummy use, not the other way around!

It may be tempting to address questions about the effects of interventions by surveying a large number of people. This approach can also be misleading as the intervention a person receives may be related to another factor. For example, in a study of the impact of support group meetings for people with angina on their quality of life, it may happen that those people who attended the support group report a higher quality of life, but this could be because the most active patients attend the group. Concluding that support groups lead to a higher quality of life, *on the basis on this evidence alone,* would be inappropriate.

Results from observational studies should normally be used to generate further questions for study, rather than to give the definitive answer. Treatments with plausible modes of action, and some limited support through anecdotal evidence may in fact be ineffective or harmful. This means that robust evaluation of interventions sometimes gives 'surprising' results (see Box 18.1).

CHARACTERISTICS OF EXPERIMENTAL DESIGN

In an observational study, the researcher describes a number of variables without changing any of them. Conversely, in an experimental study, the researcher (or someone else, e.g. the government) manipulates some aspect of the phenomenon under study, and researchers then observe what happens.

An experiment is carried out in order to test a hypothesis or research question. An example might be:

> 'Does patient-controlled analgesia (PCA) reduce post-operative pain better than intra-muscular analgesia (IMA)?'

Formally, hypotheses are usually expressed as a statement rather than a question, for example:

> 'PCA is more effective than IMA at reducing pain scores in the 48 hours after major surgery'.

It is important to specify the components of the hypothesis precisely, for example, the population being studied, the variable being changed (the independent variable) and the variable being measured (the dependent variable).

It is common to express the hypothesis as a null hypothesis (Ho), a statement that there is no relationship between the variables under investigation, for example:

> 'There is no difference between IMA and PCA with respect to pain scores in the 48 hours after major surgery'.

Statistical testing is commonly set up with the assumption that the null hypothesis is true until there is enough evidence to reject it (see Chapter 36 for further information on null hypotheses). More recently, there has been a resurgence of interest in statistical methods that do not assume that the null hypothesis holds, for example, Bayesian analysis. These methods are complex and beyond the scope of this book.

In the PCA example, the independent variable is the type of analgesia (IMA, PCA), and the pain score is the dependent variable. Increasingly, the terms participant/population, intervention, comparator and outcomes (PICO) rather than independent and dependent variables are used when reporting experiments. The relationship between these terms can be seen in Box 18.2. PICO helps clinicians frame questions by defining the elements of a patient problem (population), intervention, comparator and outcomes.

Box 18.2 Terms used to describe elements of an experiment

Population	Independent variable	Dependent variable
Population	Intervention	Outcome
For example, people undergoing surgery	For example, analgesia administered via a patient controlled device	For example, pain levels

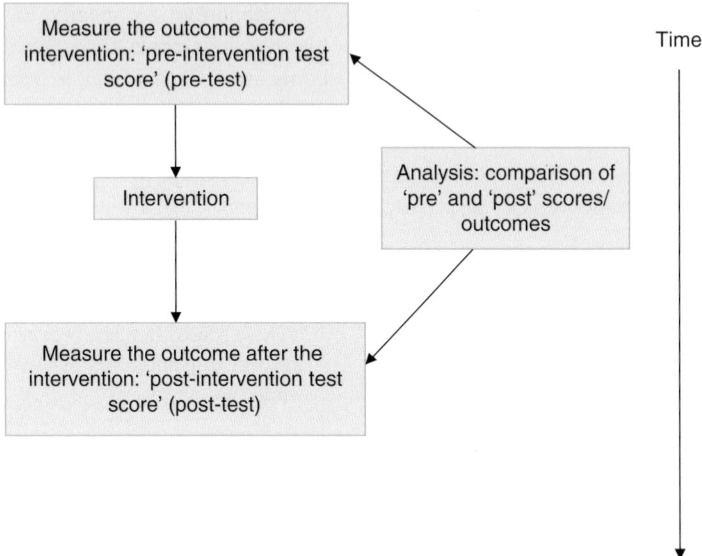

Figure 18.1 Diagrammatic representation of a simple experiment: Pre-/post-test study

As with all research, the characteristics of the study population, the type of interventions used and the outcome(s) of interest must be defined.

PRE-/POST-TEST STUDIES

There are a number of forms of experiment used in health care. The simplest type of experiment uses a pre-/post-test design (before-and-after study). Figure 18.1 shows a representation of this design.

This design reports a change in an outcome following a change in an intervention. It does not, however, allow us to confidently state that the change occurred *because of* the intervention; that is, it does not allow us to ascribe cause and effect. Three reasons that a change in the outcome might not be due to the intervention are temporal effects, testing effects and regression to the mean.

Temporal effects

A change in an outcome over time might be due to changes over time rather than the intervention. In our example, a reduction in pain scores after use of the PCA device might be due to the reduction in pain levels that would be observed anyway in the first few days after surgery.

Testing effects

A change in outcome may occur because the initial measurement highlighted to the participants that they should pay attention to particular phenomena or it showed up deficits in knowledge. These may affect the robustness of pre-/post-test designs, particularly in studies of educational interventions, as the initial testing may affect the outcomes (see Research Example 18.1).

Regression to the mean

Regression to the mean describes a phenomenon that occurs when a variable is measured in a group of people more than once. In our example, the researchers recorded pain scores from a number of people, introduced PCA and recorded pain scores for a second time. In the baseline pain scores, a few people had very high pain scores, a few had low pain scores, and the majority of people had pain scores that

RESEARCH EXAMPLE

18.1 Example of the Possible Testing Effect on Outcome

Jones JE, Nelson EA (1997) Evaluation of an education package in leg ulcer management. *Journal of Wound Care* **6**(7): 342–343.

A before-and-after study to assess the impact of an educational intervention on the knowledge of nurses managing venous ulcers.

Community nurses involved in leg ulcer care attended two study days. At the first day, they attended lectures and workshops and were given an open learning pack and a video on compression bandaging. Between the first and second days, they had a supported visit from a local expert in leg ulcer care to address any issues in practice. At the second day, there were more lectures and workshops. Knowledge on leg ulcer aetiology and management was tested by means of a self-administered questionnaire at the start of the first study day, repeated at the end of the second study day. The number of correct responses was compared. The number of correct responses increased, but this may not have been due to the study day content, as the questionnaire itself may have helped nurses identify gaps in knowledge and prompted further study.

clustered around the average (mean). If the pain scores are measured again, the people with low pain scores will tend to 'regress' upwards towards the mean, and the people with very high pain scores will tend to 'regress' down towards the mean due to measurement error. This phenomenon means that if an intervention is tested on people with a high pain level, then as a group, their pain scores will decrease, whether or not the intervention is actually effective (Bland & Altman 1994).

One approach to addressing the limitations of the pre-/post-test design is to monitor the outcomes over long periods before and after the introduction of the intervention. An alternative is to form a group who are not given the intervention being studied but are still followed. The former is called an interrupted time series, the latter, a controlled trial.

INTERRUPTED TIME SERIES

The stability of the outcome can be assessed both before and after use of the intervention by measuring it several times prior to and after the intervention's introduction. This design might be used when it is impossible to allocate people to different groups, for example, if there are ethical barriers to randomisation or if it is not possible to control the release of the intervention, for example, advice from the government. Dowding *et al.* (2012) used this approach to evaluate the impact of electronic health record implementation on hospital-acquired pressure ulcers and falls in a number of hospitals in the United States.

CONTROLLED BEFORE-AND-AFTER STUDIES

The simplest way to evaluate the effect of an intervention is to administer it to one group and compare this with a similar group who happened not to receive it. Both groups must be similar at baseline, and data collection should have happened contemporaneously, reducing testing and temporal effects. Controlled before-and-after (CBA) studies, sometimes called quasi-experimental studies, are often used in evaluating public health interventions as it is often not possible to allocate people or groups to different interventions. Turner *et al.* (2013) evaluated the impact of the urgent care telephone service (NHS

111) introduced into the NHS in England by comparing four pilot sites where the scheme was introduced with three control sites that continued with the existing service. CBA studies are limited by threats to internal validity such as having similar groups at the baseline for both known and unknown characteristics, as well as problems identifying similar groups and high-quality data.

CONTROLLED TRIALS

In a controlled trial, a group (the control group) is formed to act as a comparison to assess whether changes in outcomes are unrelated to the intervention under study. Outcomes from the intervention group are then compared with outcomes from the control group. The design is similar to that shown in Figure 18.1 but has at least two groups so that you can be confident that any changes in outcome were not due to temporal effects (see Figure 18.2).

If the two groups have different outcomes, it might be concluded that the differences were due to the experimental treatment being given to the first group (i.e. ascribing cause and effect). However, this is only the case *if the groups were similar at the outset.* If people self-selected their treatment group or if clinicians chose treatments, then the groups are likely to be systematically different at the outset due to this bias and therefore likely to have different outcomes regardless of the intervention received. Where people in the different treatment arms of a study have been allocated, such that their chances of experiencing the outcome differ from the very start of the study, there is a 'selection bias', which will potentially influence the findings of the study.

Essentially, controlled trials allocate people to groups so they form similar cohorts (rather than simply observing similar groups as in a CBA study). 'Matching' patients with important characteristics is one approach, for example, medical history, but this can only 'match' for those variables already known to be prognostic, that is, we know that it has an effect on the outcome. There are unknown factors that predict outcomes (such as genetic make-up); hence, 'matched' groups might still be quite different in some important aspects, such as compliance. In order

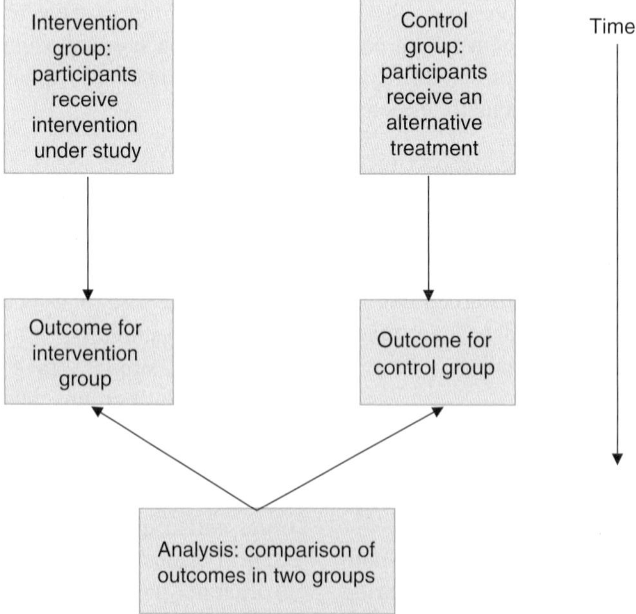

Figure 18.2 Diagrammatic representation of a controlled trial

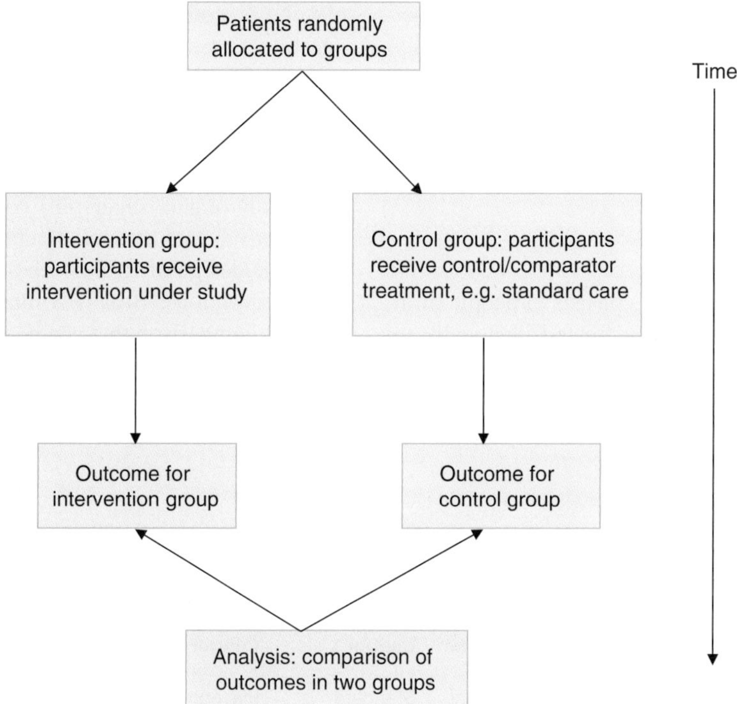

Figure 18.3 Diagrammatic representation of a randomised controlled trial

to address this problem, the most powerful way of allocating people to groups is to allocate them 'randomly'. People are allocated to the groups in a purely random manner, with no way of predicting which group the next person will be allocated to. A controlled trial in which the participants are allocated to the intervention groups at random is an RCT (see Figure 18.3). In a quasi-randomised trial, researchers allocate people using methods that are not strictly random, for example, according to case note number (e.g. odd/even), date of randomisation, week of admission or ward/clinic. Meyer *et al.* (2008), for example, allocated smokers to one of three groups: personalised letters, brief counselling by GP or no intervention. The aim was to assess whether there was any impact on quit rate. Patients were allocated according to the week of visit to GP practice (1/2/3); hence, the three groups may not be completely comparable, as holidays may mean that patients seen in these periods may be different.

THE RCT

In addition to assessing the direction of causal effects and removing temporal effects, the RCT reduces the possibility of selection bias. Most commonly, people are randomised to a treatment group, in which they remain until the end of follow-up: an individually randomised, parallel group trial. Other designs build upon the simple RCT and are described in the following section.

Randomisation

To ensure that selection bias does not take place, the process of random allocation should be concealed from the person(s) recruiting participants into the study if possible. Methods of randomisation, which minimise selection bias, have two components: randomly generated number sequences and blinded (or masked) allocation either via remote telephone/computer randomisation or sealed, sequentially numbered, opaque envelopes. Failure to adequately mask allocation has led, in some studies, to inflated estimates of effectiveness of interventions (Schulz & Grimes 2002).

Comparator/control intervention

The control group in an RCT consists of people from the same population, who are treated identically to the treatment group except they receive a different intervention to that being tested. The choice of a comparison treatment may be 'standard care', a placebo or nothing at all, depending on the clinical question and state of knowledge. A placebo treatment is identical to the active treatment in every respect, except that it does not contain the proposed therapeutic benefit of the active intervention. Placebo controls are easier to develop and use in pharmaceutical trials (e.g. a sugar pill) compared with many nursing trials, but the lack of a placebo does not preclude the design of RCTs with meaningful comparison interventions. Box 18.3 illustrates the different types of comparison that can be used.

If there is an accepted standard of care, then this should be used as the comparison, as failure to use this means the trial cannot be used to determine if a

Box 18.3 Examples of control groups

Population	**Intervention**	**Outcome**	**Control 1**	**Control 2**	**Comment**
Young people with asthma	New low-allergy bedding	Reducing asthma attacks (number and severity)	Standard treatment – old bedding	Placebo – new 'non-allergenic' bedding	If one uses old bedding, then any reduction in asthma attacks may be due to the fact that newer bedding has fewer allergens. If new 'non-allergenic bedding' is used and participants are not told which group they are in, then the control bedding is a placebo.
People with diabetic foot ulcers	Growth factor	Healing foot ulcer	Standard care – for example, semi-occlusive dressings	Placebo – the gel 'vehicle' without the growth factor	If one uses a standard care comparator, then any improvement in healing with the growth factor gel may be due to the gel or growth factor or both.

Reflection activity

Explore the idea of control in an RCT. Which aspects of the study design are important to consider and why?

change in policy from current practice to the new system would be beneficial. For example, an RCT of compression bandages compared a multilayered system with non-compressive technologies for venous ulcers (O'Brien *et al.* 2003). As we already know that compression is better than no compression, this trial simply reaffirms what was already known.

RCTs AND THE REDUCTION OF BIAS

RCTs are designed to reduce an important source of bias – selection bias – where people in the different treatment arms of a study have been selected in some way such that their chances of experiencing the outcome differ from the very start of the study. The results cannot therefore be attributed to the intervention. However, there are other forms of bias that may lead to systematic error in the results of an RCT, and well-designed and well-executed RCTs will seek to minimise these.

Performance bias/confounding

In an RCT, if people are treated in different ways other than the treatment of interest, for example, one group gets an 'active' treatment plus extra attention such as more visits, then that group may fare better because of the effect of the extra 'care' rather than the treatment being evaluated. Where interventions are complex, in that they have more than one component that could contribute to the interventions' effectiveness, researchers should ensure that they have an understanding of the various elements that make up the intervention. For example, in a study comparing cognitive behavioural therapy (CBT) with drugs for depression in primary care, it needs to be recognised that the CBT group would also receive, potentially, increased frequency and duration of contact with health-care professionals. Both may contribute to improvement in depression as well as the CBT. An RCT might take account of this by having a control group in which people received extra attention and contact but not CBT.

Attrition bias

Attrition bias refers to differences between the comparison groups due to the loss of participants from the study. These can be described as withdrawals, dropouts or protocol deviations, and the way in which they are handled has potential for biasing the results of an RCT. This is because the reasons for 'withdrawing' from a trial might be related to the intervention or outcomes.

Having a significant minority of people without any final outcome data can threaten the validity of the results of an RCT as it is not known whether the missing people on the treatments fared well or badly. People who were 'lost to follow-up' should not be ignored in the results and analysis, as this would undermine what was achieved by using randomisation.

Figure 18.4 explains this. Two treatments, A and B, are being evaluated in a trial of 100 people (50 in each group), and in each group, 10% of people are lost to follow-up. The remaining two groups, of 45 people each, may differ in a systematic way, because people leave trials for reasons that may be related to their condition or the treatment: one cannot assume these withdrawals are random events. If one assumes that treatment A was ineffective, then it may be that five people lost to follow-up in that group had not improved and were demoralised, so they did not return for follow-up. By contrast, let us assume that treatment B was mildly effective and the five people lost to follow-up did not return because they had experienced a complete cure. The 45 people remaining in group A would consist of people with mild to moderate disease (the more severe cases dropped out), whereas the people remaining in group B would be people with moderate to severe disease (the least

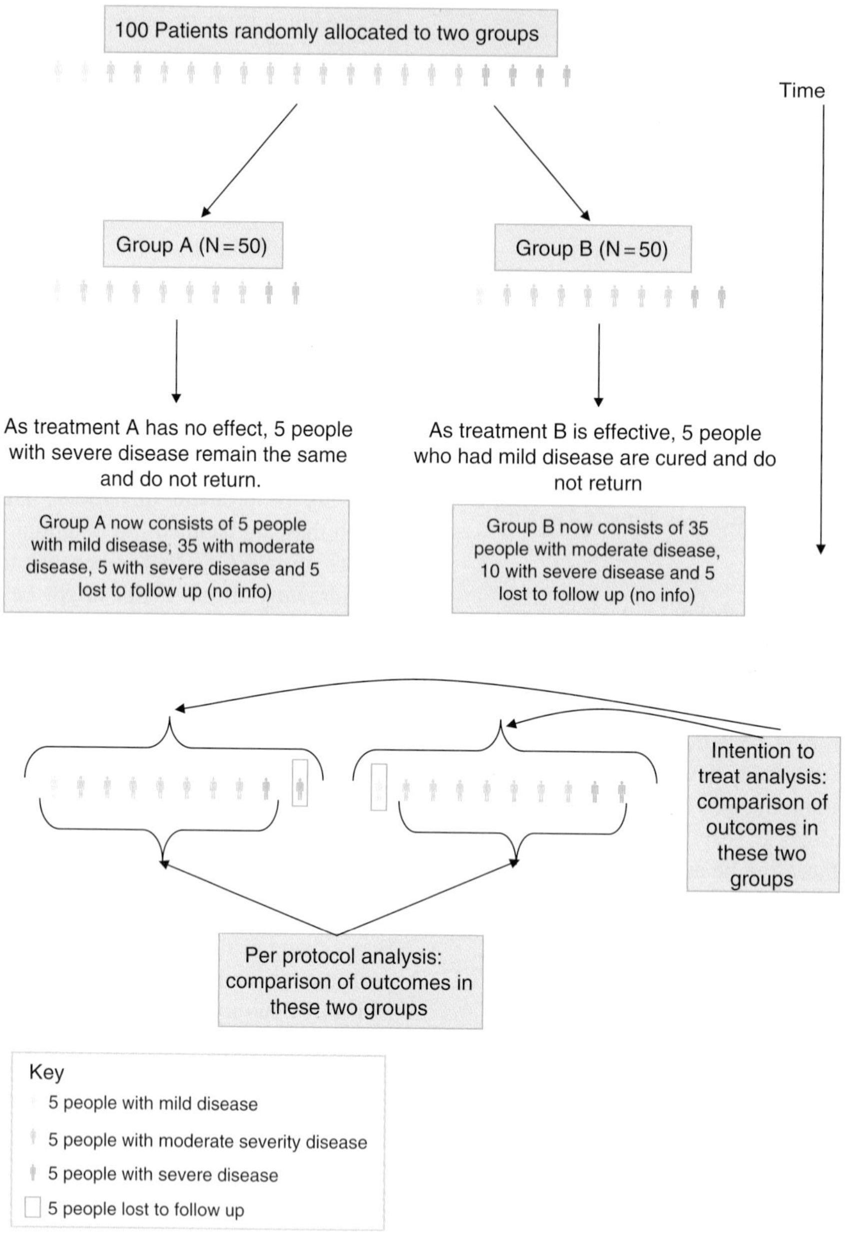

Figure 18.4 Impact of loss to follow-up on results of trials

severe cases having been cured). Making a comparison between the two groups on the basis of the 90 people remaining would not maintain the comparable groups obtained through randomisation and could mislead.

An analysis in which all randomised participants are included, regardless of whether they received the intervention or not or had any follow-up data, is called an 'intention to treat' (ITT) analysis. Analysing data only from those people who received the intervention

RESEARCH EXAMPLE

18.2 An Example of Measurement Bias

Reynolds T, Russell L, Deeth M, Jones H, Birchall L (2004) A randomised controlled trial comparing Drawtex with standard dressings for exuding wounds. *Journal of Wound Care*, **13**(2): 71–74.

In an RCT in wound care, a new dressing was compared to standard care. Both patients and nurses were aware of the allocation. The outcomes were assessed in two ways: by asking the nurse treating the patient if the wound was improving/deteriorating/static and by taking photographs of the wound to be assessed by someone unaware of the dressing being used. When nurses knew which group the patients belonged to, they rated the new dressing as being better than standard care. This apparent benefit associated with the new dressing disappeared when the wounds were assessed by blinded assessors looking at the photographs.

and attended follow-up is called a 'per protocol' analysis, and these tend to be less conservative than an ITT analysis. Note that articles may state that they undertook an ITT analysis, but did not (Hollis & Campbell 1999) so the reader should check the number of people analysed is the same as the number starting the trial.

In order to prevent RCTs being threatened by loss to follow-up, they should be designed and conducted to maximise follow-up. In some studies, for example, cancer RCTs, it may be possible to determine eventual outcomes by 'flagging' patients in national registers.

Measurement bias

Outcome data should be collected in the same way, and with the same rigour, for all the study groups. To facilitate this, where possible, participants, health professionals and outcome assessors may remain unaware of the intervention being received. Such blinding (also called masking) aims to prevent knowledge of the participant's treatment group consciously or unconsciously influencing the measurements made in the study (see Research Example 18.2). Blinding can be especially important if the outcome measure has a subjective aspect to it. Various people may be 'blinded' to the allocation, for example, the person randomising the patients, the patient, the person delivering care, the outcome assessor and the statistician analysing the results. 'Single-blind' studies usually mean that the patient is unaware of the group to which they have been allocated. In 'double-blind' studies, both the patient and their clinician are unaware of treatment allocation. It is always possible to mask allocation and the person conducting the analysis. It is usually possible to mask the person performing the outcome assessment, while it is sometimes possible to mask the patient and their clinician.

Hawthorne effect

Franke and Kaul (1978) described the effect of being observed and studied on workers in the Hawthorne factory. A series of experiments were designed to assess if environmental changes, for example, lighting, improved productivity. It was found that at each change in environment, productivity rose. Strangely, productivity even rose when there was no actual change in environment, as the participants (factory workers) knew they were being studied and the effect of being studied changed their behaviour. The Hawthorne effect emphasises the need for control groups in experimental research.

Reflection activity

What actions can researchers take when conducting an RCT to minimise bias?

OTHER EXPERIMENTAL DESIGNS

Cluster RCTs

In the trials described earlier, individuals were randomised to two or more interventions. An alternative is for natural groups of people (clusters) to be randomised, for example, hospital wards or geographical areas. By allocating a cluster of people to an intervention, it is possible to be more confident that there will be no contamination between groups. For example, if testing the impact of advanced training for nurses to recognise and treat depression in primary care, one could not expect nurses with this additional training not to assess or treat a patient if the trial was designed with individual patient randomisation. One would allocate whole practices to 'advanced nurse training' or not and compare the outcomes across the clusters. The reporting and analysis of cluster RCTs must take into account that people in clusters have shared characteristics and therefore cannot all be regarded as independent from each other.

Factorial RCTs

The majority of RCTs seek to test out the effect of changing just one element of treatment at a time. Factorial trials, by contrast, evaluate the effect of multiple interventions at the same time. These RCTs, therefore, may reflect clinical practice where multiple treatments are introduced, such as wound management or lifestyle changes. For example, with a factorial trial the effects of two wound dressings and two compression bandages for venous leg ulcers can be compared at the same time.

In a '2 by 2' factorial RCT, there are two comparisons of two interventions being made: for example, two bandages and two dressings. Half the people would get dressing 1, and half would get dressing 2; half would get bandage 1 and half would get bandage 2. Figure 18.5 shows a diagram of a factorial trial making this comparison for venous leg ulcers (Nelson *et al.* 2007).

In order to evaluate the two dressings, the healing rates in the columns are compared, and to evaluate the two bandages, the healing rates in the rows are compared. As people were randomly allocated to

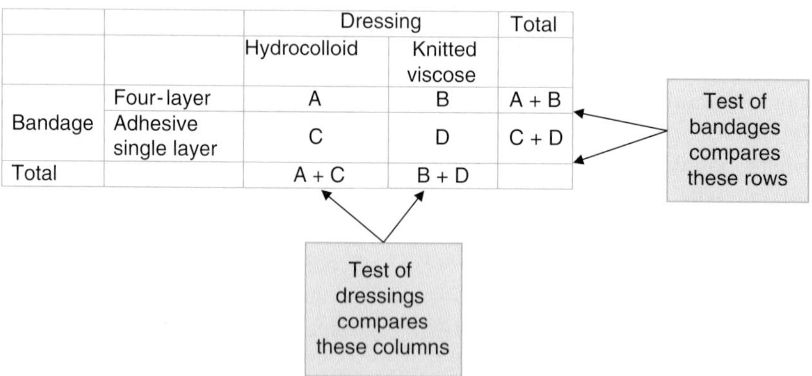

Cell A: patients receive four layer bandage with hydrocolloid dressing
Cell B: patients receive four layer bandage and knitted viscose dressing
Cell C: patients receive adhesive single layer bandage with hydrocolloid dressing
Cell D: patients receive adhesive single layer bandage and knitted viscose dressing

Figure 18.5 A '2 by 2' factorial trial

the dressings and to the bandages, the two-dressing groups are assumed to be balanced for bandages, in the same way that age, sex, ulcer size, etc. are balanced across trial groups by randomisation.

One strength of a factorial trial is that it allows researchers to undertake more than one trial at a time, reducing the cost and increasing efficiency. The sample size needed is usually the same as for a simple trial, so two trials can be completed in the same time and at almost the same cost as a single treatment trial (as long as there is no interaction between treatments). The other advantage of the factorial trial is that it allows determination of whether the interventions being evaluated have a synergistic (additive) or an antagonistic (working against each other) effect.

Crossover trial

One of the reasons control groups are used is to determine whether any change in outcome is part of the pattern of the disease process or whether it is due to the intervention. However, if studying the impact of an intervention in a very stable health condition, that is, one in which there is unlikely to be rapid resolution or deterioration, it is possible to perform *some* evaluations with patients acting as their own control. Essentially, the effect of a treatment is evaluated over a period and then the participant is given an alternative treatment (the crossover). The outcomes at the end of each period are compared for each patient to see whether there is any systematic difference in outcomes. In order to check that any change in outcome is due to the intervention being evaluated rather than temporal changes in outcomes, it is usual to randomise participants to either start on treatment A and crossover to B or start on B and crossover to A (see Figure 18.6). This also allows determination of whether there is an 'order effect' whereby treatment B performs differently if preceded by treatment A than if B is given first. Treatments should not have a prolonged effect, as otherwise their effects may not be seen until the second period of the crossover and therefore the effectiveness would be wrongly attributed to the second treatment used. The analysis of these trials also requires care, as the crossover design needs to be accounted for. Behavioural or educational interventions cannot be evaluated in this way as it is not possible to 'take away' the knowledge or behaviour from the first period.

Single-case experimental design (n of 1 trial)

In the face of incomplete evidence to guide a decision about selecting a treatment for a chronic condition, or if a patient does not get relief from those treatments recommended in guidelines, there is a systematic alternative approach to 'trying things out'. In an 'n of 1' trial, the clinician and patient work together to evaluate which of the treatments result in consistent benefit. As in the crossover trial, the condition of interest should be a relatively stable one, for example, arthritis, so that attributing the effect of the treatment to any improvement or deterioration is a robust conclusion and not undermined by any natural change in the underlying severity of the condition over time. For example, in an 'n of 1' trial of two treatments for osteoarthritic knee pain, the clinician would draw up a randomly selected schedule of options being investigated, for example, a magnetic or heat wrap. The patient would keep a pain and stiffness diary and agree to use one of the treatments for a specified time before swapping to the alternative and then back again, possibly a few times. Evaluating the two treatments over a number of swap-overs allows the researcher to be more confident that any difference in pain or stiffness is due to the treatment rather than temporary changes in arthritis. If a drug is being evaluated in this way, the clinician may even arrange with a pharmacist to supply the preparation in a masked container so that the patient is 'blinded' to the effective treatment. The clinician and patient review the outcomes for the different treatments using the patient's diary, at the end of the trial, and decide on future management. Given the limited number of conditions for which this is relevant and the need for relatively intensive input from the clinician and the patient, this design is not common. This design may be a powerful tool to distinguish between the placebo effect and true effects

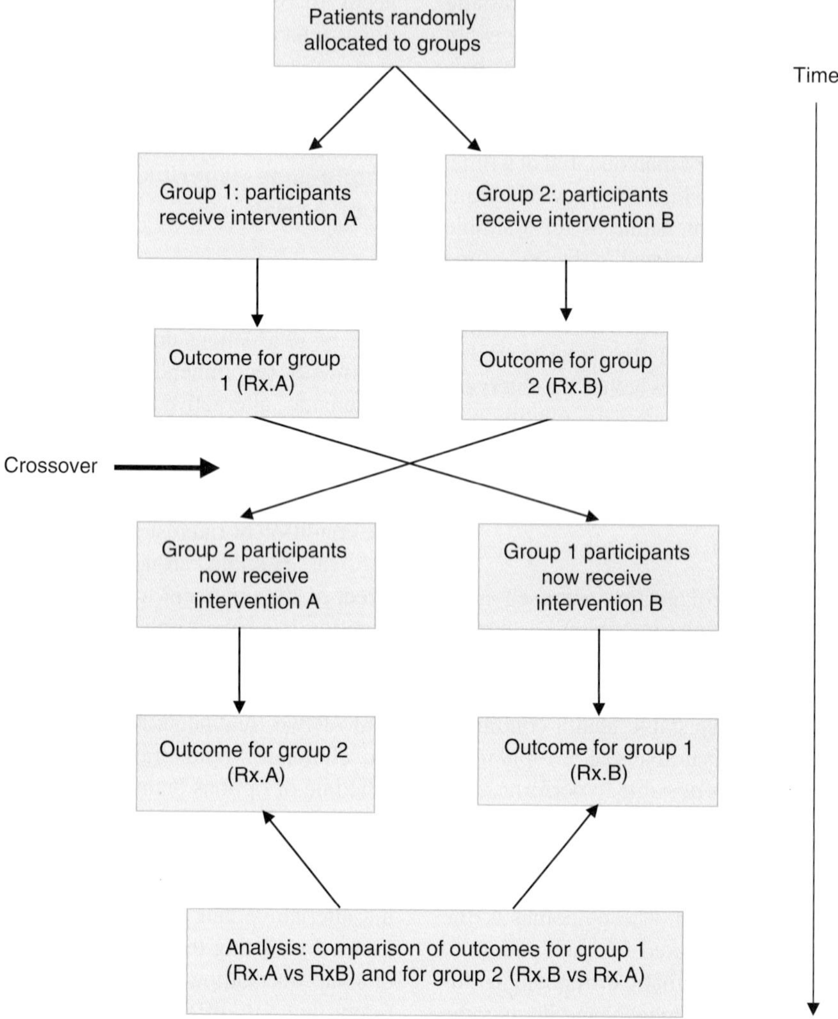

Figure 18.6 A crossover trial

of treatment for individual patients. Dallery *et al.* (2013) provide a useful discussion of the use of single-case experimental design to evaluate novel technology-based health interventions.

REPORTING AND READING RCTs

Given the important role RCTs have in informing clinicians of the effects of interventions, and the number of potential threats to their validity, it is important that researchers report exactly what they did in a trial. This allows readers to decide whether the study results are robust. A statement on the reporting of trials (CONSORT) (http://www.consort-statement.org) describes what researchers should report, and journals are increasingly asking researchers to use the CONSORT 2010 framework to structure their articles on RCTs for publication. Extensions to CONSORT are available for cluster trials, non-inferiority and equivalence trials, herbal medicinal interventions, non-pharmacological treatment interventions, harms and journal and conference abstracts.

Reflection activity

What criteria do you think are important in evaluating the quality of an RCT and why have you selected them? Compare your ideas with those included in a published checklist such as that produced by CASP.

There are a number of critical appraisal checklists and tools available to help the reader determine whether RCTs are valid and reliable (e.g. CASP, www.casp-uk.net).

IMPORTANT CONSIDERATIONS IN USING RCTs

Securing ethical approval

In order to have ethical approval, an RCT must conform to the procedures discussed in Chapters 3 and 1. Participants must usually give their informed consent to be involved in the RCT. However, it is possible, and indeed necessary, to conduct trials in people unable to give consent, for example, in emergency care, but approaches for obtaining consent are governed by individual country arrangements in the United Kingdom, following the EU Clinical Trials Directive and the Mental Capacity Act (2005).

Equipoise

Clinicians recruiting to an RCT must be in collective equipoise, that is, they must believe that the question of whether treatment A or B is better needs to be answered. If there is a clear preference for one intervention over another, then it is not appropriate to conduct an RCT in that area, as researchers would be asking clinicians to administer a treatment that they believed was less beneficial than an alternative.

There is a window of opportunity for RCTs, therefore, in evaluating interventions that clinicians think might be beneficial, before they become convinced that it is better than standard care, when RCTs will not be possible.

Reflection activity

What are the main ethical issues that need to be considered when designing and conducting an RCT?

Complexity and cost

RCTs can be expensive to carry out. The adherence to the legislation that underpins trials (such as the EU Clinical Trials Directive and data protection) and the need for ethical and research governance approval all increase the time it takes to set up a trial. RCTs also require the infrastructure to support randomisation and data collection and management. Trials may be cost-effective, however, if they demonstrate that a treatment is no more effective than standard care or is better at a very high cost and therefore inappropriate for many cases. Health economists study the cost-effectiveness of treatments within RCTs, comparing the cost of a treatment with its benefit to participants, to ensure that limited health-care resources are used most efficiently. They can also assess the likely benefit of trials to determine which should be prioritised so that greater value for money can be obtained.

STRENGTHS AND LIMITATIONS OF RCTs

Strengths

An RCT is the best way to determine, with certainty, whether an intervention works. It controls for those variables we know might influence the outcome, like concordance, age and disease severity, but, crucially, for those factors that affect prognosis, but that are not measurable or are as yet unknown. Results from well-conducted RCTs are the most reliable research source for informing medical practice about the clinical effectiveness of treatments and interventions and as such are regarded as the 'gold standard' for answering questions of effectiveness in evidence-based practice.

Limitations

Poorly designed and conducted RCTs can mislead, as often the sizes of effect we are observing in health care are small, and the potential problems with designing and doing trials well can introduce biases and errors that swamp the treatment effect between groups.

Learning curve for technologies

Designing, implementing and completing an RCT can take a long time – if an intervention is changing, the trial evidence may prove to be irrelevant. It is important to consider when an RCT was conducted if there is likely to be a 'learning curve'. If a trial is done when few people know how to deliver the intervention effectively, then the trial may conclude no benefit when in fact there might be benefit if a trial was done in the middle or top of the learning curve, when more people were using it appropriately, for example, skills like compression therapy or endoscopy.

Explaining the results of trials

Experiments only answer the question of whether something works, not why it does so. For example, a few RCTs of hip-protector pads to prevent fractured hips on falling have found that they do not work and that many people did not wear them. The reasons why the participants did not wear them or why, in those who did fall, the hip protectors did not reduce fracture rates are not explored. Qualitative studies are increasingly nested within RCTs to help explain the findings.

Poor choice of control groups

If a study has stated that it intends to evaluate the effectiveness of a new treatment but compares it against a treatment not in current use, for example, a sub-therapeutic dose of the standard care regimen, then it is likely to conclude that the new therapy was effective even if it offers no benefit over the current best practice.

Surrogate/interim outcomes

Some RCTs may report outcomes that are easier or quicker to assess rather than the actual outcome of interest for patients and clinicians. For example, in an RCT investigating rehabilitation after myocardial infarction, to determine the effect on life expectancy, a long-term follow-up would be needed. In order to avoid having to follow-up participants for decades, researchers might report a surrogate outcome instead, for example, treadmill walking distance. They may assume that improvements in the physiological outcomes will mirror longer life expectancy. Such use of surrogate outcomes relies on their association with the more relevant, patient-oriented outcomes, such as incidence of disease or survival. Surrogate outcomes commonly mislead, and if they are used, there should be clear evidence of their ability to predict long-term outcomes.

Patient-reported outcomes

As well as reporting objective outcomes such as infection rates, wound healing, death, falls, pressure ulcers or resource use (number of GP visits, hospital stay), it is increasingly important for decision-makers to have information on patient perspectives derived not only from single-domain scales (e.g. pain, anxiety) but also from quality of life tools, as they assess the effect of changes in the condition being treated and the impact of the treatment.

CONCLUSION

Given the ever-increasing pressure on health-care systems to make efficient use of the limited resources available, the question of 'what works' needs to be answered by high-quality studies with minimal potential to mislead and thereby waste resources. For evidence of effectiveness, RCTs are often described as 'the gold standard' as they seek to minimise confounding and selection bias that may make the results of other comparative studies unreliable. There are a number of biases that may threaten the results of studies, including RCTs; therefore, decision-makers need to be able to understand how these may threaten the validity of studies and to identify and appraise such studies to inform their decision-making.

References

Bardy GH, Lee KL, Mark DB, Poole JE, Toff WD, Tonkin AM, Smith W, Dorian P, Packer DL, White RD, Longstreth WT, Anderson J, Johnson G, Bischoff E, Yallop JJ, McNulty S, Ray LD, Clapp-Channing NE, Rosenberg Y, Schron EB (2008) Home use of automated external defibrillators for sudden cardiac arrest. *New England Journal of Medicine* **358**: 1793–1804.

Bland JM, Altman DG (1994) Regression towards the mean. *British Medical Journal* **308**: 1499.

Dallery J, Cassidy R, Raiff B (2013) Single-case experimental design to evaluate novel technology-based health interventions. *Journal of Medical Internet Research* **15**(2): e22.

Dowding D, Turley M, Garrido T (2012) The impact of an electronic health record on nurse sensitive patient outcomes: an interrupted time series analysis. *Journal of the American Medical Informatics Association* **19**(4): 615–620.

Dumville J, Worthy G, Bland JM, Cullum N, Dowson C, Iglesias C, Mitchell JL, Nelson EA, Soares M, Torgerson DJ (2009) Larval therapy for leg ulcers (VenUS II): randomised controlled trial. *British Medical Journal* **338**: b773.

Franke RH, Kaul JD (1978) The Hawthorne experiments: first statistical interpretation. *American Sociological Review* **43**: 623–643.

Hollis S, Campbell F (1999) What is meant by intention to treat analysis? Survey of published randomised controlled trials. *British Medical Journal* **319**(7211): 670–674.

Jones JE, Nelson EA (1997) Evaluation of an education package in leg ulcer management. *Journal of Wound Care* **6**: 342–343.

Jull A, Walker N, Parag V, Molan P, Rodgers A (2008) Randomized clinical trial of honey-impregnated dressings for venous leg ulcers. *British Journal of Surgery* **95**: 175–182.

Kramer MS, Barr RG, Dagenis S, Yang H, Jones P, Ciofanis L, Jane F (2001) Pacifier use, early weaning, and cry/fuss behaviour. *Journal of the American Medical Association* **286**: 322–326.

Meyer C, Ulbricht S, Baumeister SE, Schumann A, Ruge J, Bischof G, Rumpf HJ, John U (2008) Proactive interventions for smoking cessation in general medical practice: a quasi-randomized controlled trial to examine the efficacy of computer-tailored letters and physician-delivered brief advice. *Addiction* **103**(2): 294–304.

Nelson EA, Prescott RJ, Harper DR, Gibson B, Brown D, Ruckley C (2007) A factorial, randomized trial of pentoxifylline or placebo, four-layer or single-layer compression, and knitted viscose or hydrocolloid dressings for venous ulcers. *Journal of Vascular Surgery* **45**(1): 134–141.

O'Brien JF, Grace PA, Perry IJ, Hannigan A, Clarke Moloney M, Burke PE (2003) Randomized clinical trial and economic analysis of four-layer compression bandaging for venous ulcers. *British Journal of Surgery* **90**: 794–798.

Reynolds T, Russell L, Deeth M, Jones H, Birchall L (2004) A randomised controlled trial comparing Drawtex with standard dressings for exuding wounds. *Journal of Wound Care* **13**(2): 71–74.

Schulz KF, Grimes DA (2002) Allocation concealment in randomised trials: defending against deciphering. *The Lancet* **359**: 614–618.

Turner J, O'Cathain A, Knowles E, Nicholl J (2013) Impact of the urgent care telephone service NHS 111 pilot sites: a controlled before and after study. *BMJ Open* **3**: e003451.

Ubbink DT, Vermeulen H, Goossens A, Kelner RB, Schreuder SM, Lubbers MJ (2008) Occlusive vs gauze dressings for local wound care in surgical patients: a randomized clinical trial. *Archives of Surgery* **143**: 950–955.

Websites

http://www.casp-uk.net/ – Critical Appraisal Skills Programme, resources to help appraise clinical studies such as trials.

http://www.consort-statement.org – The Consolidate Standard of Reporting Trials provides guidance on how clinical trials should be written up for publication.

http://www.cochrane.org/cochrane-reviews – Cochrane Library, contains databases of systematic reviews and of trial reports.

CHAPTER 19

Surveys

Felicity Hasson, Hugh McKenna and Sinead Keeney

Key points

- Descriptive surveys aim to describe what exists, whereas correlational and comparative surveys investigate and compare the relationship between variables.
- Surveys can capture the time dimension by being retrospective (past behaviour) and prospective (future propensities).
- Longitudinal surveys are conducted to monitor changes across a period of time.
- Data collection methods used in surveys include questionnaires, interviews, observation and analysis of secondary data.
- Epidemiology is a form of survey research that is concerned with how and why diseases and risk factors occur in populations.
- Epidemiological research has a long tradition in medicine but is less commonly applied to nursing.

HISTORICAL DEVELOPMENT OF SURVEY RESEARCH IN HEALTH

It is impossible to determine when the first survey was conducted. Several accounts are given in the Bible, beginning with a census taken after Moses ascended Mount Sinai (Weisberg *et al.* 1996). Later, the Romans carried out censuses to prepare for taxation. The social surveys that were at the heart of the early 20th-century survey movement were also total censuses of the cities studied, merging census data with special surveys of topics, such as housing conditions. In England, 19th-century surveys were conducted by independent individuals and government agencies in attempts to study social conditions and the nature of poverty. For instance, in 1902, Charles Booth conducted his monumental inquiry into the *Labour and Life of the People of London* (1889–1902). In 1912, Bowley undertook a study of working-class conditions. This was published as *Livelihood and Poverty* (Bowley & Burnett-Hurst

The Research Process in Nursing, Seventh Edition. Edited by Kate Gerrish and Judith Lathlean.

Companion Website: www.wiley.com/go/gerrish/research

1915). Bowley's great methodological contribution was his use of statistical sampling, which came to act as a decisive stimulus to social surveys (Moser & Kalton 1971).

At the end of World War I, a new approach was adopted that was different to censuses; it used psychophysical laboratories in which a small number of consumers were brought for standardised product testing (Rossi *et al.* 1983). Market research psychologists introduced the techniques of questioning people on their preferences to a range of issues. The mid-1930s saw an expansion in the use of survey methods in public opinion polling. This was pioneered by George Gallup in America.

At the beginning of the 21st-century, the survey is an established method of social inquiry. Since the time of Booth and Bowley, great changes have occurred in the amount of survey activity and in the interest by the public to this research approach. There have been considerable changes in methods of collecting and storing survey data due specifically to technological developments.

DESCRIPTIVE SURVEYS

The most common objective of survey research is to describe. In descriptive surveys, statistics are collected about a large group: for example, the proportion of men and women who view a television programme or who participated in a health-screening programme. They can be designed to measure events, behaviours and attitudes in a given population or sample of interest. So a descriptive survey is used to obtain information on the current status of phenomena so as to describe *what exists* with respect to variables or conditions (Sim & Wright 2000).

For example, a Gallup Poll conducted during a political election campaign has the purpose of describing the voting intentions of the electorate. Descriptive surveys are based on the assumption that the answer to the research question may exist in the present so the objective is to collect this information in a systematic way. They are indispensable in the early stages of studying a phenomenon (Dublin 1978) because the information gained helps to develop concepts that can then be developed into theories.

Descriptive surveys are also carried out to describe populations, to study associations between variables and to establish trends and possible links between variables. While this is valuable, they cannot provide robust evidence about the direction of cause and effect relationships. Research Example 19.1 provides an example of such a survey.

Descriptive surveys have several advantages, but perhaps, the main one is that they are relatively easy to undertake as they only involve one contact with

RESEARCH EXAMPLE

19.1 A Descriptive Survey

Healy K (2013) A descriptive survey of the information needs of parents of children admitted for same day surgery. *Journal of Paediatric Nursing* **28**: 179–185.

While is it recognised that being admitted and discharged for same-day surgery can evoke feelings of anxiety for parents and children, few research studies have explored the information required to prepare them for this experience. This study used a cross-sectional, descriptive, correlation survey design to establish parents' information needs in relation to the operating room procedures and how this information may best be provided to assist parents and their children who are undergoing same-day surgery. A total of 120 questionnaires were distributed to a convenience sample of parents on admission to the same-day unit. In total, 70.8% (n=85) were retuned. Findings indicated that parents were satisfied with the information currently provided but sought further advice on the waiting times, equipment used, pain relief options and procedures in the recovery room. Gaining insight into parents' information needs can assist them to prepare for new and unfamiliar experiences and also aid the healthcare professional to minimise potential anxiety and stress.

> **Reflection activity**
>
> Why are descriptive surveys important? Consider when this design would be appropriate to use. Identify a research question from your own area practice that could be answered by undertaking a descriptive survey.

the study population. However, there is the potential problem that the respondents give the answers that they believe the researcher wants to hear, rather than their true views. Another disadvantage is that they cannot measure change, so if things change rapidly, the survey information may easily become outdated. To measure change, it is necessary to have at least two observations, that is, at least two cross-sectional studies, at two points in time, on the same population. Furthermore, the results of surveys can be wrong. One of the most famous examples of this was the survey polls that predicted a landslide victory of Thomas E. Dewey over Harry S. Truman in the 1948 presidential elections. Truman won with a two million majority.

CORRELATIONAL AND COMPARATIVE SURVEYS

These types of surveys are devoted to investigating and comparing the relationship between variables. For example, a questionnaire may be administered to a large number of patients to find out whether there is a difference in the self-reported levels of postoperative stress between those who received information and those who did not. In each case, the question is whether there is a relationship between variable X and variable Y. In correlational studies, a researcher can collect demographic details such as age, occupation, gender and educational background and seek to establish links between these and other characteristics of participants such as their beliefs and behaviours (Parahoo 2006). The purpose is often to develop hypotheses and in turn contribute to theory development. It does so from theory-based expectations on how and why variables should be related. Hypotheses could be basic (i.e. relationships exist) or directional (i.e. the relationship is positive or negative). Such surveys only tell us that there is a relationship between the two variables; they do not tell us whether one variable 'caused' the other. Correlational studies have little control over the respondents' environment and thus have difficulty ruling out alternative explanations for causation.

In comparative surveys, data are collected that allow comparisons to be made according to demographic features such as age, gender or class. Therefore, the main purpose of such studies is to compare variables across people, places or time. If changes are surveyed over time, we may need to compare data collected as a baseline with those collected some time later. If we want to know the effects of behaviour such as smoking or drinking, we can compare those who indulge in these practices with those who do not. Such studies can be quantitative, qualitative or both.

Comparative surveys encounter a number of potential limitations including problems in ensuring comparable measures and samples. For example, over 65 countries participate in the World Values Survey (http://www.worldvaluessurvey.org). This involves comparing results across countries. Different sample designs in different countries, different methods of administering surveys, different acceptance of survey research and different levels of interviewer training and technique can cause problems. This can result in design-based measurement errors arising in which the same methods of data collection and the same questions are used in very different cultural contexts.

Prospective and retrospective survey designs

While surveys can capture a snapshot of the attitudes, beliefs and behaviours of individuals and groups in the present, they can also be applied retrospectively and prospectively.

A retrospective design is one in which researchers study a current phenomenon by seeking information from the past. Researchers have to work backwards and search for variables or factors to help shed light on issues. Such a design aims to describe or explain a phenomenon by examining factors with which it was associated. For example, patients' notes hold a considerable amount of information on the treatment and progress of their illness as well as demographic details. These can be used retrospectively to explain phenomena. Most cross-sectional studies are retrospective. This is a relatively inexpensive research method as large numbers of people can be surveyed quickly and data are easily coded (Bowling 2009; Lalkhen & McCluskey 2008).

One of the main drawbacks of retrospective designs is that the researcher relies on existing data that were, most probably, not collected for research purposes and therefore lack the required rigour. Furthermore, many archives that could be of interest to future researchers are being lost. For example, with the closure of many psychiatric hospitals, patients' notes and other materials are being destroyed. Also, descriptions of past behaviour may be highly subjective; records may be incomplete and/or rely on respondents' memories. For instance, respondents may be asked questions about past diet and other lifestyle factors and the potential for selectivity in recollection and recall bias is great. Despite these shortcomings, retrospective studies have been useful in, for example, studying the experiences of hospital care reported by bereaved relatives of patients after a stroke (Young *et al.* 2009).

The prospective survey is one that takes place over the forward passage of time with more than one period of data collection. Such studies attempt to establish the outcome of an event or explore what is likely to happen. For example, nurses may want to know the effects of new practices on patients' behaviour. Researchers using this design can have control over what they want to include in their study and how data are collected. Another example could be noting if and how the lifestyles of newly diagnosed cancer patients change over time. The researcher may compare this group of respondents with another group who do not have the illness (control group). With this design, data are collected at one or multiple points in the future. Such studies require careful definitions of the groups under study and careful selection of variables for measurement.

Prospective surveys can be expensive, take a long time, and need a great amount of administration (e.g. update and trace addresses) and can suffer from high sample attrition through natural loss, geographical mobility or refusals over time. Respondents can also become conditioned to the study and learn the responses that they believe are expected of them. In addition, there can be reactive effects of the research arrangements – the 'Hawthorne effect' as people change simply as a result of being studied (Roethlisberger & Dickson 1939). Chapter 18 has a fuller discussion of this effect in experimental research. There needs to be a clear rationale to support the timing of repeated survey points, retaining the respondents' interests and participation, and employ sensitive instruments with relevant items that will detect change.

Reflection activity

What are the major advantages and disadvantages of prospective and retrospective survey designs?

LONGITUDINAL SURVEYS AND COHORT STUDIES

Longitudinal surveys are normally conducted over a long period of time. Data collection takes place at regular intervals throughout the life of the study. The purpose of this is to monitor changes over time. Such surveys are sometimes referred to as panel studies. The British Household Panel Survey (Research Example 19.2) is a large-scale example of a longitudinal survey. The purpose of this survey is to monitor householders over a long period of time to analyse their responses to changes in the social and economic environment.

The longitudinal survey may be of particular use in nursing research as certain phenomena from these professions lend themselves to being studied over a long period of time. As part of a wider investigation of residential and nursing home care, Bebbington *et al.* (2000) used a longitudinal design to survey 2540 people admitted to care homes at 6, 19, 30 and 42 months after admission. Cowin and Hengstberger-Sims (2006)

RESEARCH EXAMPLE

19.2 British Household Panel Survey

Funded by the Economic and Social Research Council, the British Household Panel Survey began in 1991 and has followed the same group of respondents over the last 24 years. It is one of the longest running panel surveys in the world. The main aim of the survey is to gain insight into social and economic change at the individual and household level. The survey is a resource for a wide range of social science disciplines and supports interdisciplinary research in many subject areas. It is a household-based study interviewing every adult member of a sampled household. It contains representation from different social groups including the elderly. The original panel consisted of 5500 households from 250 areas of Great Britain. This equated to 10,300 individuals. In 1999, 1500 households were added from Scotland and 1500 households were added from Wales. In 2000, a further sample of 2000 households was added from Northern Ireland, enabling a UK-wide research to be conducted.

https://www.iser.essex.ac.uk/bhps

http://ukdataservice.ac.uk/

adopted a similar design to explore graduate nurses' dimensions of nursing self-concept and its relation to graduate nurse retention plans at three points in time throughout their graduate nursing year. It is obvious that in both these cases, the collection of data on one isolated occasion would not be as beneficial as the collection of data at regular intervals over several years.

A cohort study is a form of longitudinal survey that uses a specific group of respondents for the entire study. Cohort studies chart the development of these groups from a particular time point either prospectively or retrospectively. Such studies are concerned with life histories of sections of populations. They provide information on developmental changes across stages of life in any domain including employment, education, housing, family and health.

Cohort studies have been used to study nurses. The most notable of these studies is the Nurses' Health Study (http://www.channing.harvard.edu/nhs/). The original Nurses Cohort Study was established by Dr. Frank Speizer in 1976 and was funded by the National Institutes of Health. The primary idea behind the survey was to investigate the potential long-term consequences of oral contraceptives, diet and lifestyle risk factors. However, this has expanded to produce new insights into cancer prevention, cardiovascular disease, diabetes and many other conditions. Over 170,000 nurses completed baseline questionnaires for this study. Questionnaires are administered to the cohort every 4 years.

One of the main problems of longitudinal and cohort studies is that the respondents may drop out of the study. This is termed 'mortality' or 'attrition' (Rubin & Bellamy 2012). It can affect the success of a cohort study. Researchers can also move on to other roles or jobs and it is not uncommon to find that a succession of researchers have worked on the survey over the years.

Another difficulty with longitudinal studies is the effect of the research on the attitudes and behaviours of the respondents. By their very nature, longitudinal studies could serve to raise the awareness of the respondents and introduce bias. Time and cost are other inevitable considerations with longitudinal studies. In addition, it may be difficult to ensure continuity among respondents. In some cohort studies, the researchers send Christmas cards and birthday cards to respondents to encourage continued participation.

SOURCES OF DATA IN SURVEY RESEARCH

Most people will have encountered a survey at some stage either as a respondent to a postal survey or being approached by a market researcher in a supermarket or on the telephone. Organisations carry out surveys for a wide variety of reasons and results are used for different purposes, from changing policy to making decisions on a marketing strategy. Social researchers regard surveys as a valuable source of data about respondents' attitudes, beliefs, experience and behaviour.

Questionnaires and interviews

Chapters 28 and 30 describe the main data collection tools for surveys in more depth. Here, we will discuss the relative merits of questionnaires and interviews for the purpose of a brief comparison of the two methods. There is no universal agreement among researchers about what should be called a questionnaire. It can mean a document containing a list of questions for respondents to complete on their own (the self-completion questionnaire) or it can mean a set of questions that a researcher reads out to a respondent. For the purposes of this chapter, a questionnaire will be considered to be a list of questions contained in a document that respondents complete themselves.

Questionnaires are usually distributed by post although they can be distributed by hand, for example, to patients or visitors in a hospital. More recently, researchers have been distributing questionnaires by email using a distribution list or by simply asking respondents to complete an online questionnaire (see Schmidt *et al.* 2011).

Generally, questionnaires follow a standardised format in which questions are pre-coded to provide a list of responses for selection by the respondent (tick-box questions). However, open-ended questions can be included with space to allow the respondent to provide a written answer. Questions should be easily comprehensible, as the respondent will not be able to seek clarification. For this reason, a questionnaire is often 'piloted' with a small subsection of the target population to ascertain if it is understandable, valid and acceptable. This may result in changes being made to question content or the length of the questionnaire. For a fuller discussion of questionnaires, turn to Chapter 30.

Face-to-face interviews use a list of questions sometimes called an interview guide. This guide may contain either open or closed questions or a combination of both. There is an important distinction between an interview schedule and an interview guide. An interview schedule uses a set of questions in a predetermined order that is adhered to during the interview. An interview guide is a list of areas to be covered, leaving the exact wording and order of the questions to be determined by the interviewer.

As the name implies, structured interviews tend to use an interview schedule with very explicit questions and leave no room for veering off the topic. Semi-structured interviews use the interview guides referred to previously, and there is room for exploration and for altering the questions based on a respondent's circumstances of replies. In contrast, unstructured interviews are totally open, and the researcher has freedom to explore a range of issues around a general subject area. The Internet also facilitates opportunities to conduct electronic interactive interviews via email or through the use of chat rooms. However, although electronic technologies are convenient and low cost for the researcher, they are still novel and raise many ethical questions.

Within face-to-face interviews, researchers may record responses by pen or directly onto a laptop computer. This approach is generally reserved for structured interviews that include many closed questions. For interviews using more open-ended questions, the interview is usually audio recorded. This recording would subsequently be transcribed as an interview transcript. Generally, data from questionnaires are analysed using computerised database and statistical analysis software such as the Statistical Package for the Social Sciences (SPSS). Chapter 28 provides a more detailed consideration of interviewing.

Self-completion questionnaires and face-to-face interviews are long established methods of data collection and each have their own strengths and weaknesses (see Box 19.1).

Interview schedules are also used for interviews carried out over the telephone. Telephone surveys have similar benefits to face-to-face interviews but also facilitate reaching a much wider population at less cost. Telephone surveys are less popular with social researchers than they are with market and commercial researchers. While they may be less expensive to undertake than face-to-face interviews,

Box 19.1 Face-to-face interviews versus self-completion questionnaires

Face-to-face interviews	Self-completion questionnaires
Costly due to time-intensive nature	Less costly – slower data collection method.
Longer and more complex questions are possible	Limited in length and complexity.
High response rates	Often associated with poor response rates.
Can adapt to include visual materials (e.g. show cards)	Exclude the less literate and those who may have a disability (e.g. dyslexia, blind).
Provide additional opportunities to clarify questions and responses	No opportunity to explain complex instructions, to answer questions or to probe for more detail on open-ended questions.
Interviewee is not anonymous	Respondent cannot be connected to their response. As a result, more honest responses may be provided.
Can be subject to bias – acquiescence and social desirability bias if not carefully recruited	Respondents have more time to weigh the issues carefully before responding – less prone to acquiescence.
Enable interviewer to ensure data are being collected from the correct sample	Researcher cannot ensure the target person completes the questionnaire. For example, a questionnaire aimed at exploring the views of a patient may be completed by a carer.

telephone surveys do not take cognisance of non-verbal cues and surroundings and certain groups may have to be excluded from the survey because they do not have a telephone. The issue of the growing ownership of mobile phones is also creating problems for researchers. Nicolaas (2004) has identified sampling problems in relation to mobile phone users who tend not to be listed in phone directories.

Furthermore, mobile phone numbers cannot be linked to a geographical area and they tend to belong to one individual rather than a household. However, recently, IPSOS MORI (2009) identified that as of August 2007, 87% of people in the United Kingdom owned a mobile phone. Figures from the Mobile Data Association (2008) have also shown that more than 12.3 million people used their mobile phone to access the Internet in the last quarter of 2006. Research has shown that the average number of SMS and MMS messages sent per person per month in the United Kingdom is 200 (Office of Communications 2012). In the United Kingdom, a growing number (12%) of adults live in a home with a mobile phone but with no fixed line (Office of Communications 2008). International figures also reflect the increasing numbers of households that have no landline, but are reliant on mobile phone only. For example, it is estimated that one-fifth of adults in Australia live in mobile-only households (Australian Communications and Media Authority 2011) as do a third of households in the United States (Blumberg & Luke 2012), while mobile phone-only households outnumber those with a landline in nine European countries (Vehovar *et al.* 2012).

This could be viewed as an interesting and important way to reach participants to complete surveys. Organisations such as IPSOS MORI have panels of mobile phone users, in this case 11,000 people willing to take part in surveys via mobile phone. Among the advantages of this method of data collection are wide geographical reach, fast response, wide demographic reach and immediacy.

Reflection activity

What factors should you consider when deciding how you would administer a survey?

Secondary data sources

Gilbert asserted that it is 'a truism of social research that almost all data are seriously under-analysed' (Gilbert 1993: 256). This may be one of the reasons that analysis of secondary data sources is continuing to grow in popularity with social researchers. Secondary analysis of data sources implies that the data are being subjected to further analysis than that for which it was originally collected. There are many sources of data that can be used for secondary analysis. Examples include patient or public records such as medical records, audit data, attendance records, nationally available statistics stored in data banks, government data, academic data and research data collected for other purposes. Hospitals retain patient medical records, attendance records, complaints records and other statistical data on both patients and staff.

Census data is also available for secondary analysis. The National Statistics Office is responsible for UK census data. It can provide access to the UK data bank, and this can provide large amounts of data on many and varied topics across a lengthy period of time. In the United Kingdom, the National Data Archive is located at the University of Essex. It holds mainly UK data but has reciprocal arrangements with other countries for access to their national data. However, the secondary analysis of some of these data may raise ethical questions and may be difficult to access. After all, respondents provide the data for a specific purpose and to use it for another purpose without their consent is potentially problematic.

Observation

Moser and Kalton described observation as 'the classic method of scientific enquiry' (Moser & Kalton 1971: 245). Nonetheless, social researchers use observation relatively infrequently. One type of observation employed in survey research is non-participant observation. Chapter 31 deals in detail with this and other ways of using observation for research purposes.

In terms of practicality and validity, direct observation can have a number of advantages to using a questionnaire or an interview schedule. For example, studies of children may have to rely on observational techniques as children may not be able to verbalise or write down the answer. Responses provided within questionnaires or interviews may also be inaccurate, whereas observation will provide a true picture of the situation, for instance, interview data on how nurses' practice may differ from data collected through observing them working.

Observation also has limitations. Non-participant observation does not allow the researcher to explore peoples' attitudes or perceptions. It is also difficult to ensure representativeness using observational techniques. Furthermore, there are obvious ethical issues relating to seeing unsafe practices while being a non-participant observer.

EPIDEMIOLOGY

Epidemiology is the study of how often diseases occur in different groups of people, why they occur (Coggon *et al.* 1997) and the risk factors for these diseases (Bowling 2009). Historically, the impact of epidemiology on the health of the nation has been far-reaching (Whitehead 2000). There has been a long-standing tradition of epidemiology within healthcare. This is due to the fact that epidemiological research is used to plan and evaluate strategies to prevent illness and as a guide to the management of patients who have already developed a disease (Coggon *et al.* 1997). Epidemiology is concerned with observing, measuring and analysing health-related occurrences in human populations (Trichopoulos 1996). Therefore, it is not only concerned with death, illness and disability but also tries to find ways to improve health states (Bonita *et al.* 2006). As nursing roles become more involved in preventative care and public health, epidemiology will become increasingly appropriate as a research method. There are five main types of epidemiological surveys.

Descriptive study

Descriptive epidemiology describes the health status of a population or characteristics of a number of patients and attempts to find correlations among such characteristics as diet, air quality and occupation. Research Example 19.3 gives an example of such a

RESEARCH EXAMPLE

19.3 Descriptive Epidemiological Survey

Patten SB, Wang JL, Williams JV, Currie S, Beck CA, Maxwell CJ, El-Guebaly N (2006). Descriptive epidemiology of major depression in Canada. *Canadian Journal of Psychiatry* **51**:84–90.

This national study was undertaken as part of the Canadian Community Health Survey: Mental Health and Well-Being to describe the epidemiology of major depression in the Canadian population. One person aged 15 years or over was randomly selected from sampled private households (98% of the population). A response rate of 77% ($n = 36{,}984$) was achieved from the 48,047 households that were approached. The majority of participants were interviewed at their place of residence (86%). Interviews were based on the World Mental Health Composite International Diagnostic Interview. Interviews were undertaken by trained lay interviewers using computer-assisted technology to administer the survey. Results indicate that lifetime prevalence of major depressive episode was 12.2% with 4.8% of the sample reporting past-year episodes. Major depression was more common in women than in men. Married people had the lowest prevalence, but the effect of marital status diminished with age. The results have led to the generation of several hypothesis testing studies and have been used for planning the delivery of services.

study. As alluded to earlier, descriptive studies may be considered weak because they make no attempt to link cause and effect and therefore no causal association can be determined.

Cross-sectional studies

A cross-sectional study measures the prevalence of health outcomes or determinants of health, or both, in a population at a point in time or over a short period (Coggon *et al.* 1997). For example, such designs have been used to explore students' attitude to smoking and smoking behaviour following the implementation of a university smoke-free policy (Chaaya *et al.* 2013). However, associations must be interpreted with caution as bias may arise because of selection into or out of the study population.

Case-controlled studies

A case-controlled study is a retrospective comparison of exposures of persons with disease (cases) with those of persons without the disease (controls). In case-controlled studies, such individuals are selected with and without the particular disease and asked about past exposure. Exposure rates within the two groups are compared. Case-controlled studies offer several advantages in that they are quick and relatively inexpensive to conduct and are suitable for studying multiple exposures and rare diseases. However, case-controlled studies present possible biases such as recall bias and interviewer bias.

Cohort studies

A cohort study is a study in which a healthy group of people are followed over time to measure their exposure to certain conditions or receive a particular treatment and are compared with another group who are not affected by the condition under investigation. As with general cohort studies, they are expensive, time-consuming and logistically difficult; however, the design is less subject to bias because it measures exposure before researchers learn the health outcome. Research Example 19.4 provides an example of an epidemiological cohort study.

RESEARCH EXAMPLE

19.4 Epidemiological Cohort Study

Mehrabadi A, Hutcheon JA, Lee L, Kramer MS, Liston RM, Joesph KS (2013) Epidemiological investigation of a temporal increase in atonic postpartum haemorrhage: a population-based retrospective cohort study. *British Journal of Obstetrics and Gynaecology* **120**(7): 853–862.

Internationally, incidences of postpartum haemorrhage (PPH) and severe PPH have been increasing; however, isolating the cause of the rise is key in developing prevention strategies. A population-based study was undertaken to identify the potential cause of the temporal increase in atonic PPH using data from Canada. The British Columbia Perinatal Data Registry provided information for 371,193 women resident in British Columbia who delivered between 1 April 2001 and 31 March 2010. Findings revealed that there were 372,259 deliveries during this period. However, analysis was restricted to 371,193 deliveries that had complete information for gestational age and birth weight (0.3% missing). The incidence of atonic PPH increased from 4.8% in 2001 to 6.3% in 2009. The rate of atonic PPH with blood transfusion ≥1 unit, PPH with blood transfusion ≥3 units or procedures to control bleeding also increased. It is unclear why atonic PPH and severe atonic PPH have increased. One explanation may be due to improvements in diagnostic or coding practices, which may be responsible for an artificial increase in atonic PPH. The study demonstrates the need for future studies to continue to investigate the risk factors in order to identify and address causes.

Reflection activity

You have been set a task to undertake a survey on patterns of smoking behaviour among adults, what design would you adopt and why?

CONCLUSION

This chapter has set the survey in its historical context and outlined the main types of surveys used within nursing research. The sources of data have been discussed and the pros and cons of self-completion questionnaires, face-to-face interviews and telephone interviews considered. Other methods used within survey research have also been explored including secondary data analysis and observations. Epidemiological research and its applicability to nursing research were also outlined. Due to the fact that nursing's body of knowledge continues to be in the early stage of development, there is every indication that survey research will continue to be popular for some time to come.

References

Australian Communications and Media Authority (2011) *Communications Report, 2010–11 Series. Report 2 Converging communications channels: preferences and behaviours of Australian Communication Users.* Melbourne, Australian Communications and Media Authority.

Bebbington A, Darton R, Netten A (2000) *Longitudinal Study of Elderly People Admitted to Residential and Nursing Homes: 42 months on.* Personal Social Services Research Unit P51, Canterbury, University of Kent at Canterbury.

Blumberg SJ, Luke JV (2012) *Wireless Substitution: early release of estimates from the National Health Interview Survey.* July-December 2011, Atlanta, Centre for Disease Control.

Bonita R, Beaglehole R, Kjellstrom T (2006) *Basic Epidemiology.* 2nd edition. Geneva, World Health Organisation.

Booth C (ed) (1889–1902) *Labour and Life of the People of London (17 volumes)*. London, Macmillan.

Bowley AL, Burnett-Hurst AR (1915) *Livelihood and Poverty: a study in the economic conditions of working-class households in Northampton, Warrington, Stanley and Reading*. London, Bell.

Bowling A (2009) *Research Methods in Health: investigating health and health services*. 3rd edition. Buckingham, Open University Press.

Chaaya M, Alameddine M, Nakkash R, Afifi RA, Khalil J, Nahhas G (2013) Students' attitude and smoking behaviour following the implementation of a university smoke-free policy: a cross sectional study. *BMJ Open* **3**(4): DOI: 10.1136/bmjopen-2012-002100.

Coggon D, Rose G, Barker DJP (1997) *Epidemiology for the Uninitiated*. 4th edition. London, BMJ Publishing.

Cowin LS, Hengstberger-Sims C (2006) New graduate nurse self-concept and retention: a longitudinal survey. *International Journal of Nursing Studies* **43**: 59–70.

Dublin R (1978) *Theory Building*. New York, The Free Press.

Gilbert N (1993) *Researching Social Life*. London, Sage.

Healy K (2013) A descriptive survey of the information needs of parents of children admitted for same day surgery. *Journal of Paediatric Nursing* **28**: 179–185.

IPSOS MORI (2009) *Research via Mobile Phones*. Available at http://www.ipsos-mori.com/researchareas/researchtechniques/datacollection/online/researchviamobilephones.aspx (accessed 1 September 2014).

Lalkhen GA, McCluskey A (2008) Statistics V: introduction to clinical trials and systematic reviews. *Continuing Education in Anaesthesia, Critical Care and Pain* **8**: 143–146.

Mehrabadi A, Hutcheon JA, Lee L, Kramer MS, Liston RM, Joesph KS (2013) Epidemiological investigation of a temporal increase in atonic postpartum haemorrhage: a population-based retrospective cohort study. *British Journal of Obstetrics and Gynaecology* **120**(7): 853–862.

Mobile Data Association (2008) *The Q3 2008 UK Mobile Trends Report*. London, MDA.

Moser C, Kalton G (1971) *Survey Methods in Social Investigation*, London, Heinemann.

Nicolaas G (2004) *Sampling Issues for Telephone Surveys in Scotland, Survey Methods Unit*, National Centre for Social Research. Available at http://www.bioss.ac.uk/people/adam/rsse/2003-2004/presentations/gerry_nicolaas.ppt (accessed 1 September 2014).

Office of Communications (2008) *The Communications Market 2008: nations and regions. English Regions*. England, OFCAM.

Office of Communications (2012) *Communications Markey Report 2012*. United Kingdom, OFCAM.

Parahoo AK (2006) *Nursing Research: principles, process and issues*. 2nd edition. Houndmills, Palgrave Macmillan.

Patten SB, Wang JL, Williams JV, Currie S, Beck CA, Maxwell CJ, El-Guebaly N (2006) Descriptive epidemiology of major depression in Canada. *Canadian Journal of Psychiatry* **51**: 84–90.

Roethlisberger EJ, Dickson WJ (1939) *Management and the Worker*. Cambridge, Harvard University Press.

Rossi P, Wright J, Anderson A (1983) *Handbook of Survey Research*. New York, Academic Press.

Rubin A, Bellamy J (2012) *Practitioner's Guide to Using Research for Evidence-Based Practice*. New Jersey, John Wiley & Sons, Inc.

Schmidt CK, Davis JM, Sanders JL, Chapman LA, Cisco MC, Hady AR (2011) Exploring nursing students' level of preparedness for disaster response. *Nursing Educational Perspectives* **32**: 380–383.

Sim J, Wright C (2000) *Research in Health Care. Concepts, Designs and Methods*. Cheltenham, Stanley Thornes.

Trichopoulos D (1996) The future of epidemiology. *British Medical Journal* **313**: 436–437.

Vehovar V, Slavec A, Berzelak N (2012) Costs and errors in fixed and mobile phone surveys, In Gideon L (ed) *Handbook of Survey Methodology for the Social Sciences*. New York, Springer.

Weisberg H, Krosnick J, Bowen B (1996) *An Introduction to Survey Research, Polling and Data Analysis*. 3rd edition. Thousand Oaks, Sage.

Whitehead D (2000) Is there a place for epidemiology in nursing? *Nursing Standard* **14**(42): 35–38.

Young AJ, Rogers A, Dent L, Addington-Hall JM (2009) Experiences of hospital care reported by bereaved relatives of patients after a stroke: a retrospective survey using the VOICES questionnaire. *Journal of Advanced Nursing* **65**(10): 2161–2174.

Further reading

Alreck PL, Settle RB (2004) *The Survey Research Handbook*. 3rd edition. Boston, McGraw-Hill/Irwin.

Bowling A (2005) Mode of questionnaire administration can have serious effects on data quality *Journal of Public Health* **27**: 281–291.

Bruce N, Pope D, Stanistreet D (2008) *Quantitative Methods for Healthcare: a practical interactive guide to epidemiology and statistics*. London, John Wiley & Sons, Ltd.

Bulmer M, Sturgis PJ, Allum N (2009) *The Secondary Analysis of Survey Data (Sage Benchmarks in Social Research Methods Series).* London, Sage.

Gordon JS, McNew R (2008) Developing the online survey. *Nursing Clinics of North America* **43**: 605–619.

Kelley K, Clark B, Brown V, Sitzia J (2003) Good practice in the conduct and reporting of survey research. *International Journal of Quality Health Care* **15**: 261–266.

Keough, VA, Tanabe P (2011) Survey research: an effective design for conducting nursing research. *Journal of Nursing Regulation* **1**: 37–44.

Lavrakas PJ (ed) (2008) *Encyclopaedia of Survey Research Methods.* Thousand Oaks, Sage.

Merrill R (2010) *Introduction to Epidemiology.* 5th edition. Sudbury Massachusetts, Jones & Bartlett.

Rai D, Lee BK, Dalman C, Golding J, Lewis G, Magnusson C (2013) Parental depression, maternal antidepressant use during pregnancy, and risk of autism spectrum disorders: population based case controlled study. *British Medical Journal* **346**: f2059. DOI: 10.1136/BMJ.f2059.

Ray LM, Parker RA (2005) *Designing and Conducting Survey Research: a comprehensive guide,* 3rd edition. San Francisco, Jossey-Bass.

Scott A (2006) Population based case control studies. *Survey Methodology* **32**: 123–132.

Websites

http://www.worldvaluessurvey.org/ – World Values Survey is designed to provide a comprehensive measurement of all major areas of human concern, from religion to politics to economic and social life.

http://www.socialresearchmethods.net/kb/survey.php – Research Methods Knowledge Base: Survey Research.

CHAPTER

20 The Delphi Technique

Sinead Keeney

Key points

- The Delphi technique is an approach used to gain consensus on a certain issue or set of issues. It is based on the assumption that group opinion is more valid than individual opinion.
- The Delphi technique is a structured process that uses a series of questionnaires to gather information from a panel of experts and is continued until group consensus is reached. The number of rounds depends upon how easily consensus is reached on a topic, the time available and the type of Delphi approach used.
- The Delphi technique has evolved into a number of modifications. Each type of Delphi has the same aim, to gain consensus on the issue at hand, but differs in the process used to reach this consensus.
- Consensus reached using the Delphi technique does not mean that the correct answer has been found, but rather that the experts have come to an agreement on the issue or issues under exploration.

INTRODUCTION

The Delphi technique is a research approach used to gain consensus on a certain issue or set of issues. It is a structured process that uses a series of questionnaires or rounds to gather information and is continued until group consensus is reached (Keeney *et al.* 2010). The name 'Delphi' is derived from the site of legendary Oracle of Delphi (the most important oracle in the classical Greek world) in which anyone could visit the oracle to ask a question and receive an answer.

The main premise of the Delphi technique is based on the assumption that group opinion is more valid than individual opinion. A novel and contemporary way of illustrating this is through the use of 'ask the audience' in the popular game show *Who Wants to Be a Millionaire?* where the audience effectively acts as the 'expert panel', experts in general knowledge,

The Research Process in Nursing, Seventh Edition. Edited by Kate Gerrish and Judith Lathlean.

Companion Website: www.wiley.com/go/gerrish/research

RESEARCH EXAMPLE

20.1 Example of Delphi Study

Jirwe M, Gerrish K, Keeney S, Emami A (2009) Identifying the core components of cultural competence: findings from a Delphi study. *Journal of Clinical Nursing* **18**: 2622–2634.

The aim of this study was to identify the core components of cultural competence from a Swedish perspective. The methodology comprised a four-round modified Delphi technique. The initial round involved individual semi-structured interviews with a purposive sample of 24 experts (8 nurses, 8 researchers, 8 lecturers) who were knowledgeable in multicultural issues. The interviews explored the knowledge, skills and attitudes that formed the components of cultural competence. Content analysis of interview transcripts yielded statements that were developed into a questionnaire. Respondents scored questionnaire items in terms of perceived importance. The consensus level was set at 75%. Statements that reached consensus were removed from questionnaires used in subsequent rounds. Three rounds of questionnaires were distributed in total.

118 out of the 137 questionnaire items reached consensus. These were grouped into five categories: cultural sensitivity; cultural understanding; cultural encounters; understanding of health, ill-health and healthcare; and social and cultural contexts.

Acquisition of the knowledge, skills and attitudes identified should enable nurses to meet the needs of patients from different cultural backgrounds. The components of cultural competence can form the basis of nursing curricula.

and the contestant asks the audience for their opinion on a certain question. The audience is asked to vote on the answer using a keypad and the results displayed in a bar chart format showing where the consensus lies. Obviously, the word 'expert' is used loosely here, but this demonstrates the main premise of the Delphi technique that group opinion is considered more 'valid' and 'reliable' than individual opinion.

The Delphi technique has been used by nurse researchers in a variety of studies over the last three decades. The purpose of these studies has been to identify research priorities for a particular area within nursing (McCance *et al.* 2007; Bäck-Pettersson *et al.* 2008; Blackwood *et al.* 2011), to gain consensus on an issue or set of issues within nursing (Handler *et al.* 2008; Polivka *et al.* 2008; Jirwe *et al.* 2009) or to solve a particular problem (McKeown & Gibson 2007; Chang *et al.* 2010). There have been numerous variations in application, design, administration and analysis of the Delphi technique within these studies that demonstrate the flexibility and diversity of the technique. Research Example 20.1 illustrates the use of the Delphi within a nursing research study.

DEFINING THE DELPHI TECHNIQUE

The original advocates of the Delphi technique, Dalkey and Helmer (1963) defined the Delphi technique as a method used to obtain the most reliable consensus of opinion of a group of experts by a series of intensive questionnaires interspersed with controlled feedback. With increasing usage, other definitions have been put forward. For instance, Reid (1998) described the Delphi as a method for the systematic collection and aggregation of informed judgement from a group of experts on specific questions and issues, whereas Lynn *et al.* (1998) described the Delphi technique as an iterative process designed to combine expert opinion into group consensus. However, common among all definitions is the intention to achieve consensus among a group of

Box 20.1 Characteristics of a classical Delphi

1 The use of a panel of 'experts' for obtaining data
2 Participants do not meet in face-to-face discussions
3 The use of sequential questionnaires and/or interviews
4 The systematic emergence of a concurrence of judgement or opinion
5 The guarantee of anonymity for participants' responses
6 The use of frequency distributions to identify patterns of agreement
7 The use of two or more rounds, between which a summary of the results of the previous round is communicated to and evaluated by panel members

(McKenna 1994a)

experts on a certain issue through using a forecasting process to determine, predict and explore group attitudes, needs and priorities. Box 20.1 sets out the characteristics of the classical Delphi approach.

Reflection activity

What characteristics do you think an expert panel for a Delphi study should have?

THE EXPERT PANEL

The popularity of the Delphi technique has centred upon the fact that it allows the anonymous inclusion of a large number of individuals across diverse locations and expertise and avoids the situation where a specific expert might be anticipated to dominate the consensus process (Keeney *et al.* 2001). It uses a purposive sample of 'experts' rather than a random sample that is representative of the target population. An expert has been defined as an informed individual (McKenna 1994a), a specialist in the field (Goodman 1987; Kennedy 2004) or someone who has knowledge about a specific subject (Green *et al.* 1999; Hsu & Sandford 2007).

Choosing an appropriate expert panel is critical for success (Hung *et al.* 2008). It is the first stage of the Delphi process and regarded as the 'lynchpin of the method' (Green *et al.* 1999). However, the selection of the expert sample raises some methodological concerns. The claim of the Delphi to represent valid expert opinion has been criticised as scientifically untenable and overstated (Strauss & Zeigler 1975). It is not surprising that Goodman (1987) warns about the 'pitfalls of illusory expertise' and the 'potentially misleading title of expert'.

Simply because individuals have knowledge of a particular topic does not necessarily mean that they are appropriate 'experts'. Those who are willing to engage in discussion are more likely to be affected directly by the outcome of the process and are also more likely to become and stay involved in the study. Hence, the commitment of participants is related to their interest and involvement with the issue being addressed. However, respondents must be relatively impartial so that the information obtained reflects current knowledge or perceptions (Goodman 1987; Eberman & Cleary 2011). This balance is difficult to achieve and justify to the consumers of the finished research.

Size of the expert panel

There is little agreement about the size of the expert panel, the relationship of the panel to the larger population of experts and the sampling method used to select such experts (Williams & Webb 1994). Sample size and heterogeneity depend upon the purpose of the project, design selected and time frame for data collection (McKenna 1994a; Green *et al.* 1999). For the conventional Delphi, a heterogeneous sample is used to ensure that the entire spectrum of opinion is determined (Moore 1987; Keeney *et al.* 2010). Sampling different groups of experts such as nurse educators and nurse students may ensure heterogeneity.

There is no agreed optimum expert panel size. Dalkey and Hemler (1963) proposed a minimum number of seven experts, Burns (1998) suggested that there should be 15 in each panel, Alexander and Kroposki (1999) argued for 60, and Akins *et al.* (2005) stated that panels could be any size between 10 and 100. However, panels of between 20 and 50 participants are most frequently recommended (Endacott *et al.* 1999; Keeney *et al.* 2010).

It can be helpful to specify inclusion criteria to create boundaries around an expert panel (Keeney *et al.* 2006). These criteria may include, for example, specific qualifications, number of publications in the area of expertise, geographical location or years of experience in a particular area. Consideration also needs to be given to the workload generated by the various rounds, which has to be balanced with the time available to complete the study. A large panel of experts will require more time to administer the questionnaires and to follow up people who fail to respond than a smaller and more manageable sample.

Reflection activity

Imagine you are planning a Delphi study to identify research priorities in relation to the area of practice in which you work. Who do you consider to be the 'experts' in identifying the research priorities? To what extent is it important to include people who undertake research and/or who use research to inform policy or in their day-to-day practice?

DELPHI ROUNDS

The Delphi technique employs a number of rounds in which questionnaires are sent out until consensus is reached (Beretta 1996; DuPlessis & Human 2007). In each round, a summary of the results of the previous round is included and evaluated by the panel members in order to facilitate the systematic emergence of a concurrence of opinion among the panel of experts (McKenna 1994a). The number of rounds depends upon the time available and whether the first round is intended to generate items to be considered in subsequent rounds or whether the items are identified by the researcher in advance.

The process raises the question of how many rounds it takes to reach consensus. The classical original Delphi used four rounds (Young & Hogben 1978). However, this has been modified by many to suit individual research aims, and in some cases, it has been shortened to two or three rounds (Beech 1997; Keeney *et al.* 2001). It can be difficult to retain a high response rate within a Delphi study that has many rounds. The topic needs to be of great interest to the panel members or they need to be rewarded in other ways.

Round one

Round one of the classical Delphi (see Box 20.1) starts with an open-ended set of questions, thus allowing panel members freedom in their responses. The number of items generated can be extremely large and can lead to a very lengthy second round questionnaire if the researcher opts to include all panel members' round one views. This may put panel members off participating and it can become very difficult to sustain the experts' interest in the study (Green *et al.* 1999).

Traditionally, round one is used to generate ideas and the panel members are asked for their responses to or comments about an issue. There is now some support for revising the approach and providing pre-existing information (e.g. from the literature) for ranking (Tolsgaard *et al.* 2013). However, it must be recognised that this approach could bias the responses or limit the available options. Nonetheless, a clear advantage to commencing the process in this way is that it is more time efficient (Keeney *et al.* 2010).

Subsequent rounds

Subsequent rounds generally take the form of structured questionnaires incorporating feedback to each panel member. The data from each round are analysed and circulated to panel members. In this way, the Delphi allows efficient and rapid collection of expert opinions, while the feedback is controlled (Buck *et al.* 1993; Keeney *et al.* 2010). This process encourages panel members to become more involved and motivated to participate (Walker & Selfe 1996) and can lead to perceptions of ownership and acceptance of the findings (McKenna 1994a).

The Delphi study might encounter problems due to a decline in response rate because, in order to achieve consensus, it is important that those panel members who have agreed to participate stay involved until the process is completed (Keeney *et al.* 2010). However, poor response rates are often a characterisation of the fourth and final round of the Delphi. This could be why many researchers are now stopping at two or three rounds rather than the originally recommended four rounds.

Number of rounds

One of the basic principles underpinning the Delphi technique is to have as many rounds as are required to achieve consensus or until the law of diminishing returns occurs (McKenna 1994a). Provision for feedback and opportunity to revise earlier responses obviously requires that the Delphi has at least two rounds. However, the number of rounds can be a matter of dispute. Although there are no strict guidelines on the correct number of rounds, the number can depend upon the time available and whether the researcher initiated the Delphi sequence with one broad question or with a list of questions or events.

RESPONSE RATES

In general, questionnaire research is notorious for its low response rates. Researchers often have to send out two or three reminder letters to non-responders. With anything up to four rounds of questionnaires, a Delphi study asks much more of respondents than a simple survey and the potential for low response rates increases dramatically.

To enhance response rates in Delphi rounds, it is critical that participants are interested in the topic and feel that they are partners in the study. The researcher should take every opportunity to remind participants that each round is constructed entirely on their responses to previous rounds, encouraging ownership and active participation. This attempt to encourage participants psychologically to sign up to a study is common in longitudinal cohort studies where researchers send regular updating newsletters to participants as well as sometimes birthday or Christmas cards.

McKenna (1994b) suggested that the personal touch could help enhance return rates. Using face-to-face interviews as his first round, he achieved a 100% response rate, which is rare in a Delphi study. Such a relationship is necessary to increase the likelihood of ongoing commitment from the participant. It starts at initial contact where the researcher gains informed consent and explains either in writing or verbally the nature of the research, what the participant's role is and what is required of them. Recruiting letters should include an explanation of the study, anticipated number of rounds, outline of time commitment and a consent form or confirmation of acceptance to take part in the study. The idea behind this is to get the expert panel to sign up to take part in the study before it begins.

The follow-up of non-respondents is essential. Researchers may do this in different ways including sending follow-up letters, a further copy of the questionnaire or a follow-up phone call or email (Keeney *et al.* 2010). Prompt and appropriate feedback can also facilitate a high response rate as it keeps the members of the expert panel on board. Interest will be lost if weeks or even months pass before feedback is received on the previous round.

Reflection activity

How many rounds do you think would be appropriate for your proposed study to identify research priorities for your area of practice, and why? What actions could you take to ensure a high response rate in each round?

MODIFICATIONS OF THE DELPHI TECHNIQUE

Since its inception, the Delphi technique has evolved into a number of modifications. Each type of Delphi has the same aim – to gain consensus on the issue at hand – but differs in the process used to reach this consensus. There are numerous accounts in the literature reporting Delphi studies using these different manifestations, and this is tribute to the flexibility of the method.

At present, there are no formal, universally agreed guidelines on the use of the Delphi, nor does any standardisation of methodology exist (Evans 1997). Consequently, there is flexibility in the design and format of the Delphi, and this often depends on the study's aims and objectives. The most popular formats include the modified Delphi (McKenna 1994b; Rognstad *et al.* 2009), the policy Delphi (Turoff 1970; Franklin & Hart 2007), the decision Delphi (Couper 1984; Tichy 2001), the real-time Delphi (Beretta 1996; Gnatzy *et al.* 2011) and the e-Delphi (Sheikh *et al.* 2008; Pinnock *et al.* 2012). Box 20.2 shows the different forms and main characteristics of these types of Delphi.

The approaches used with a Delphi study may differ. For example, in the traditional design (Linstone 1978), the content for the first round is normally obtained from the literature rather than the qualitative views of participants or from other secondary data. Other variations to the Delphi exist,

Box 20.2 Types of Delphi and main characteristics

Classical Delphi	Uses factual based information to elicit opinion and gain consensus (e.g. first round based in literature in the area) and uses three or more postal rounds
Modified Delphi	Modification usually takes the form of replacing the first postal round with face-to-face interviews, or focus group may use fewer than three postal rounds
Decision Delphi	Same process usually adopted as a classical Delphi focuses on making decisions rather than coming to consensus
Policy Delphi	Uses the opinions of experts to come to consensus and agree future policy on a given topic
Real-time Delphi	Similar process to classical Delphi except that experts may be in the same room and consensus reached in real time rather than by post, sometimes referred to as a consensus conference
e-Delphi	Similar process to the classical Delphi but administered by email or online web survey
Technological Delphi	Similar to the real-time Delphi but using technology such as handheld keypads allowing experts to respond to questions immediately while the technology works out the mean/median and allows instant feedback, allowing experts the chance to revote moving towards consensus in the light of group opinion

for example, Procter and Hunt (1994) sent participant nurses three patient profiles with the remit to identify the care needs of each patient, while Jones *et al.* (1992) involved the use of face-to-face meetings of participants after two initial Delphi rounds.

The lesson here is to acknowledge that modification of the technique without being systematic and rigorous may be problematic. For example, using literature sources as the basis for round one can cause premature closure of ideas and bias the results. Without care, this could result in a self-fulfilling prophecy where participants could be steered to agree on a highly visible issue in the literature. The researcher should allow participants freedom to bring their views to the first round.

TIME FRAME

The time it takes to administer a Delphi study varies considerably and depends on several factors, not least of which the type of Delphi used. Obviously, a real-time Delphi study will be completed in one day, whereas a classical Delphi study could take over six months to complete. The size of expert panel will be a major determining factor in the time frame of the study. The more participants that are in an expert panel, the more views and opinions will be elicited in the first place and the wider the spread of opinion is likely to be. This in turn can lead to a greater number of rounds being needed to reach consensus.

Reflection activity

How long do you think it would take for a classical three-round Delphi to be administrated in order to identify research priorities? Sketch out the timetable from when you first administer the questionnaire until you anticipate having the third round completed. Remember to allow sufficient time to send reminders to participants if you consider this to be important.

ANONYMITY

The intention in a Delphi study is to seek to ensure anonymity whereby panel members are not known to each other. Anonymity provides an equal chance for each panel member to present and react to ideas without being influenced by the identities of other participants (Keeney *et al.* 2006). Reactions are given independently so each opinion carries the same weight and is given equal importance in the analysis. In this way, subject bias is eliminated (Jeffery *et al.* 1995).

This promise of anonymity facilitates respondents to be open about their views on certain issues, which in turn provides insightful data for the researcher. Furthermore, it gives each participant the opportunity to express an opinion to others without feeling pressured by more influential panel members (Couper 1984; Gnatzy *et al.* 2011). It is unclear at present whether respondents in a Delphi process change their opinions on the basis of new information or, despite the protection of anonymity, feel pressurised to conform to the group's view.

However, complete anonymity cannot be guaranteed when using the Delphi technique. Firstly, the researcher knows the panel members and their responses. Secondly, it is often the case that panel members know each other; however, they cannot attribute responses to any one member. McKenna (1994b) coined the term 'quasi-anonymity' for when the respondents may be known to one another, but their judgements and opinions remain anonymous.

GAINING CONSENSUS

The reason for using the Delphi technique is to gain consensus or a judgement among a group of perceived experts on a topic. However, experts can differ and it would be difficult to gain 100% agreement on all issues. Therefore, a key question in any Delphi study is what percentage agreement a researcher would accept as synonymous with consensus. As with most aspects of the Delphi, the literature provides few clear guidelines on what consensus level to set. Loughlin and Moore (1979) suggested

Reflection activity

What consensus level would you use within a Delphi study to identify research priorities in your area of practice and why? How does the consensus level influence the interpretation you can place on the results? What other factors will you need to consider when interpreting the results?

that consensus should be equated with 51% agreement among respondents. Any views that get less than this percentage cut-off point are rejected and not used in subsequent rounds. By contrast, Green *et al.* (1999) employed an 80% consensus level. Establishing the standard is crucial since the level chosen determines what items are discarded or retained as the rounds unfold. It is good practice to establish the consensus level before data collection.

INTERPRETING RESULTS

According to Evans (1997), the terms 'agreement' and 'consensus' are essentially two different ideologies. Is there a difference between the extent to which each participant agrees with the *issue* under consideration and the extent to which participants agree with *each other*? When reporting findings, few studies do so in the context of these different principles. Most researchers report findings on participants' agreement with *each other*. However, the extent to which participants agree with each other does not mean that consensus exists, nor does it mean that the 'correct' answer has been found. This is especially the case when the issues have ethical implications.

Advocates of the Delphi approach would argue that panel members change their minds and move towards consensus because they see that someone else has identified a more relevant issue that they had not thought of. Delphi cynics would assert that panel members are cajoled to change their minds because of a possible mistaken belief that the views expressed by the majority of the panel must be right. The obvious conclusion of this assertion is that strong-willed panel members hold rigidly to their views across rounds and weak-willed panel members alter theirs. If true, this challenges seriously the validity and reliability of Delphi findings.

Therefore, there is a danger of placing too much reliance upon the results without acknowledging the influence of bias and other factors of validity and reliability. Ultimately, there is the possibility of obtaining the 'wrong' answer from the participants. Several strategies can be used to enhance authenticity. For instance, pilot testing could be undertaken, as well as the integration of an additional methodological technique such as focus groups or the comparison with secondary validated data.

SKILLS OF THE RESEARCHER

The success of a Delphi study relies upon the skills of the researcher. These include establishing an administration system and analysing and presenting both qualitative and quantitative data. While these skills are not paid much attention in the literature, their presence is vital for an effective and efficient Delphi study.

Researchers must design their own administrative system to allow for tracking of individual responses for each round, which will enable non-respondents to be traced and targeted. Employing self-administrative questionnaires requires a mail base to be established and physical and financial resources allocated to cover costs of postage, printing, telephone bills and photocopying. Like most research studies, the Delphi study will fail if administrative systems are not in place to ensure that proper processes are followed. Due to the multiple rounds that make up a Delphi study, high-quality administrative systems are crucial for success.

CRITIQUE OF THE TECHNIQUE

There are many advantages to using the Delphi technique but also some limitations, and these should be considered before beginning a study using the

Box 20.3 Advantages and criticisms of the Delphi technique

Advantages	Criticisms
• Versatile technique	• No universally agreed guidelines
• Relatively inexpensive	• Potential for lack of methodological rigour
• Simple technique to use	• True anonymity?
• Confidentiality of responses	• Lack of evidence of reliability and validity
• No geographic restrictions	• No pilot testing reported in the literature
• Protects participants' anonymity	• Lack of consideration of ethical implications
• Avoids 'groupthink'	• Time commitment from participants
• Cost-effective	• Potential for low response rate
• 'Two heads are better than one!'	

Delphi. Box 20.3 summarises the advantages and limitations of the technique.

It should be noted that the existence of consensus from a Delphi study does not mean that the correct answer has been found. There is a danger that the Delphi can lead the researcher to place greater reliance on the results than might otherwise be warranted. In addition, the Delphi has been criticised as a method that forces consensus and is weakened by not allowing participants to discuss issues, providing no opportunity for respondents to elaborate on their views (Walker & Selfe 1996).

ETHICAL CONSIDERATIONS

A Delphi study is subject to the same ethical considerations as any postal survey (see Chapter 19). However, there are some particular ethical issues that merit consideration. The issue of anonymity has been discussed earlier in this chapter, and it has been noted that, despite the researcher's best endeavours, participants may be known to each other, especially when the field from which the experts can be drawn is small. Nevertheless, it is important that the researcher does not disclose the responses from individual respondents to other panel members.

Beretta (1996) has drawn attention to a study by Hitch and Murgatroyd (1983) who maintained telephone contact with respondents while waiting for their questionnaire to be returned. Beretta suggested that this could cause respondents to feel coerced into returning the questionnaire, even though they may wish to withdraw from the study. Care should therefore be taken in following up panel members.

Reflection activity

Assume that you are planning a Delphi study to identify the information technology competences required of clinical nurses in your area of practice. You plan to include university lecturers who teach healthcare information technology, nurse managers and clinical nurses in you locality as the 'experts'. What ethical issues will you need to consider in planning this study and how will you address these concerns?

CONCLUSION

The Delphi technique is a valuable method for achieving consensus on issues where none previously existed. The versatility of the technique lends itself to a wide range of applications and topics within nursing. The benefits of the technique are many including simplicity of use, inexpensive nature, wide geographical reach, confidentiality and quasi-anonymity for expert panel members and ultimately gaining consensus on important issues while avoiding 'groupthink'. However, researchers considering using the technique should contemplate its complexity before use to ensure that they get the best from the technique in attempting to address the research objectives of their study.

References

Alexander J, Kroposki M (1999) Outcomes for community health practice. *Journal of Nursing Administration* **29**: 49–56.

Akins RA, Tolson H, Cole BR (2005) Stability of response characteristics of a Delphi panel: application of bootstrap data expansion. *BMC Medical Research Methodology* **5**: 37.

Bäck-Pettersson S, Hermansson E, Sernert N, Björkelund C (2008) Research priorities in nursing – a Delphi study among Swedish nurses. *Journal of Clinical Nursing* **17**(16): 2221–2231.

Beech BF (1997) Studying the future: a Delphi survey of how multi-disciplinary clinical staff views the likely development of two community mental health centres over the course of the next two years. *Journal of Advanced Nursing* **25**: 331–338.

Beretta R (1996) A critical review of the Delphi Technique. *Nurse Researcher* **3**(4): 79–89.

Blackwood B, Albarran J, Latour J (2011) Research priorities of adult intensive care nurses in 20 European countries: a Delphi study. *Journal of Advanced Nursing* **67**(3): 550–562.

Buck AJ, Gross M, Hakim S, Weinblatt J (1993) Using the Delphi process to analyse social policy implementation: a post hoc case from vocational rehabilitation. *Policy Sciences* **26**(4): 271–288.

Burns FM (1998) Essential components of schizophrenia care: a Delphi approach. *Acta Psychiatrica Scandinavica* **98**: 400–405.

Chang AM, Gardner GE, Duffield C, Ramis MA (2010) A Delphi study to validate an advanced nursing tool. *Australian Journal of Advanced Nursing* 66(10): 2320–2330.

Couper MR (1984) The Delphi technique: characteristics and sequence model. *Advances in Nursing Science* 71: 72–77.

Dalkey N, Helmer O (1963) Delphi technique: characteristics and sequence model to the use of experts. *Management Science* **9**(3): 458–467.

Du Plessis E, Human SP. (2007) The art of the Delphi technique: highlighting its scientific merit. *Health SA Gesondheid* **12**(4): 1–11.

Eberman LE, Cleary MA (2011) Development of a health-illness screening instrument using the Delphi panel technique. *Journal of Athletic Training* **46**(2): 176–184.

Endacott R, Clifford CM, Tripp JH (1999) Can the needs of the critically ill child be identified using scenarios? Experiences of a modified Delphi study. *Journal of Advanced Nursing* 30: 665–676.

Evans C (1997) The use of consensus methods and expert panels in pharmacoeconomic studies: practical applications and methodological shortcomings. *Pharmacoeconomics* **12**(2): 121–129.

Franklin KF, Hart JK (2007) Idea generation and exploration: benefits and limitations of the policy Delphi research method. *Innovative Higher Education* 31: 237–246.

Goodman CM (1987) The Delphi technique: a critique. *Journal of Advanced Nursing* **12**: 729–734.

Gnatzy T, Warth J, von der Gracht H, Darkow IL (2011) Validating an innovative real time Delphi approach: a methodological comparison between real time and conventional Delphi studies. *Technological Forecasting and Change* **78**: 1681–1694.

Green B, Jones M, Hughes D (1999) Applying the Delphi technique in a study of GPs information requirement. *Health and Social Care in the Community* **7**(3): 198–205.

Handler SM, Hanlon JT, Perera S, Roumani YF, Nace DA, Fridsma DB, Saul MI, Castle NG, Studenski S (2008) Consensus list of signals to detect potential adverse drug reactions in nursing homes. *Journal of the American Geriatrics Society* **56**(5): 808–815.

Hitch PJ, Murgatroyd JD (1983) Professional communications in cancer care: a Delphi survey of hospital nurses. *Journal of Advanced Nursing* **8**: 413–422.

Hung HL, Altschuld JW, Lee YF (2008) Methodological and conceptual issues confronting a cross-county Delphi study of educational program evaluation. *Evaluation and Program Planning* **31**: 191–198.

Hsu CC, Sandford BA (2007) The Delphi technique: making sense of consensus. *Practical Assessment, Research and Evaluation* **12**(10) 1–8.

Jeffery G, Hache G, Lehr R (1995) A group based Delphi application: defining rural career counselling needs. *Measurement and Evaluation in Counselling and Development* **28**: 45–60.

Jirwe M, Gerrish K, Keeney S, Emami A (2009) Identifying the core components of cultural competence: findings from a Delphi study. *Journal of Clinical Nursing* **18**: 2622–2634.

Jones J, Sanderson C, Black N (1992) What will happen to the quality of care with fewer junior doctors? A Delphi study of consultant physician's views. *Journal of the Royal College of Physicians* **26**(1): 36–40.

Keeney S, Hasson F, McKenna HP (2001) A critical review of the Delphi technique as a research methodology for nursing. *International Journal of Nursing Studies* **38**: 195–200.

Keeney S. Hasson F, McKenna HP (2006) Consulting the oracle: ten lessons from using the Delphi technique in nursing research. *Journal of Advanced Nursing* **53**(2): 1–8.

Keeney S. Hasson F. McKenna HP (2010) *The Delphi Technique in Nursing and Health Research*. London, Wiley.

Kennedy HP (2004) Enhancing Delphi research: methods and results. *Journal of Advanced Nursing* **45**(5): 504–511.

Linstone HA (1978) The Delphi technique. In: Fowles RB (ed) *Handbook of Futures Research*. Westport, Greenwood, pp. 271–300.

Loughlin KG, Moore LF (1979) Using Delphi to achieve congruent objectives and activities in a paediatrics department. *Journal of Medical Education* **54**(2): 101–106.

Lynn MR, Layman EL, Englebardt SP (1998) Nursing administration research priorities: a national Delphi study. *Journal of Nursing Administration* **28**(5): 7–11.

McCance TV, Fitzsimons D, Keeney S, Hasson F, McKenna HP (2007) Capacity building in nursing and midwifery research and development: an old priority with a new perspective. *Journal of Advanced Nursing* **59**(1): 57–67.

McKeown C, Gibson F (2007) Determining the political influence of nurses who work in the field of hepatitis C: a Delphi survey. *Journal of Clinical Nursing* **16**(7): 1210–1221.

McKenna HP (1994a) The Delphi technique: a worthwhile approach for nursing? *Journal of Advanced Nursing* **19**: 1221–1225.

McKenna HP (1994b) The essential elements of a practitioners' nursing model: a survey of clinical psychiatric nurse managers. *Journal of Advanced Nursing* **19**: 870–877.

Moore CM (1987) *Group Techniques for Idea Building*. Applied Social Research Methods. Newbury Park, Sage.

Pinnock H, Ostrem A, Rodriguez MR, Ryan D, Stallberg B, Thomas M, Tsiligianni I, Williams S, Yusuf O (2012) Prioritising the respiratory research needs of primary care: the International Primary Care Respiratory Group (IPCRG) e-Delphi exercise. *Primary Care Respiratory Journal* **21**(1): 19–27.

Polivka BJ, Stanley SA, Gordon D, Taulbee K, Kieffer G, McCorkle SM (2008) Public health nursing competencies for public health surge experts. *Public Health Nursing* **25**: 159–165.

Procter S, Hunt M (1994) Using the Delphi survey technique to develop a professional definition of nursing for analysing nursing workload. *Journal of Advanced Nursing* **19**: 1003–1014.

Reid N (1998) The Delphi technique: its contribution to the evaluation of professional practice. In: Ellis R (ed) *Professional Competence and Quality Assurance in the Caring Profession*. London, Croom Helm, pp. 223–262.

Rognstad S, Brekke M, Fetveit A, Spigset O, Wyller TB, Straand J (2009) The Norwegian General Practice (NORGEP) criteria for assessing potentially inappropriate prescriptions to elderly patients: a modified Delphi study *Scandinavian Journal of Primary Health Care* **27**(3): 153–159.

Sheikh A, Major P, Holgate ST (2008) Developing consensus on national respiratory research priorities: key findings from the UK Respiratory Research Collaborative's e-Delphi exercise. *Respiratory Medicine* **102**(8): 1089–1092.

Strauss HJ, Ziegler LH (1975) The Delphi technique: an adaptive research tool. *British Journal of Occupational Therapy* **61**: 4153–4156.

Tichy G (2001) The decision Delphi as a tool of technology policy: the Austrian experience. *International Journal of Technology Management* **21**(7/8): 756–766.

Tolsgaard MG, Todsen T, Sorensen JL, Ringsted C, Lorentzen T, Ottesen B, Tabor A. (2013) International multispecialty consensus on how to evaluate ultrasound competence: a Delphi consensus study. *PLoS One* **8**(2): e57687.

Turoff M (1970) The policy Delphi. *Journal of Technological Forecasting and Social Change* **2**: 2.

Walker AM, Selfe J (1996) The Delphi method: a useful tool for the allied health researcher. *British Journal of Therapy and Rehabilitation* **3**(12): 677–681.

Williams PL. Webb C (1994) The Delphi technique: an adaptive research tool. *British Journal of Occupational Therapy* **61**(4): 153–156.

Young WH, Hogben D (1978) An experimental study of the Delphi technique. *Education Research Perspective* 5: 57–62.

Further reading

Keeney S, Hasson F, McKenna HP (2010) *The Delphi Technique in Nursing and Health Research.* London, Wiley.

Linstone HA, Turoff M (2002) *The Delphi Method: Techniques and Applications.* Reading, Addison-Wesley.

Websites

http://is.njit.edu/pubs/delphibook – The Delphi Method: Techniques and Applications, free digital version of Linstone and Turoff's 2002 book on the technique.

http://www.rand.org/topics/delphi-method.html – The RAND Corporation's Delphi website that provides details of the Delphi technique.

CHAPTER 21

Case Study Research

Charlotte Clarke, Jan Reed and Sarah E. Keyes

Key points

- Case study research explores a phenomenon in its context and assumes that this context is of significance to the phenomenon.
- It is a flexible and holistic approach to research design in which data collection is shaped by the boundaries of the case being studied.
- A critical step is to define the case, making sure that it illustrates the issue under investigation.
- Insider knowledge of the context, or at least the ability to access it, is important in shaping the sampling and data collection methods.
- The ability to transfer knowledge beyond the case is important in developing high-quality case study research.

INTRODUCTION

For many practitioners, the idea of case study methodology strikes several chords. As practitioners have become more aware of the importance of taking a holistic and individualised approach to care, a research method that is in tune with these ideas seems a natural fit. Case study methodology has a connection with the ways in which nurses and other healthcare practitioners think about practice, in terms of 'cases' or individual service users. This connection between research and practice is perhaps most clearly demonstrated by the use of the 'case study' in healthcare practice. The medical profession, for example, has a long tradition of using 'cases' as a method of exploring practice, from the case conference, where people gather to assess and plan care, to the case study publication in professional journals, where an example of a patient's history and treatment is presented.

As such, case study research offers a valuable means of exploring a phenomenon in its context and sees that the context is of significance to

The Research Process in Nursing, Seventh Edition. Edited by Kate Gerrish and Judith Lathlean.

Companion Website: www.wiley.com/go/gerrish/research

understanding the phenomenon, a point emphasised in an integrative review of qualitative case study research by Anthony and Jack (2009). Phenomena may be conceptual (such as vulnerability), or about people, or organisations depending on the focus of the research being undertaken. This emphasis on knowing the phenomenon in its context and as it occurs in practice characterises case study research, and even those forms of case study that are single-case clinical trials (e.g. testing within a single individual whether a new medication improves their health) assume the need to understand the impact of the context on the establishment, processes and outcomes of the phenomenon.

Using case studies in research, then, has a resonance with professional practice. It offers the opportunity of learning in a way that pays attention to and respects the individuality and unique nature of service users and services. One example is in the use of case study research to explore the implementation of a nurse practitioner role (Sangster-Gormley 2013) in which the methodology contributed to understanding the diversity of settings and complexity in which nurse practitioners worked. In addition, it is a way of exploring the dimensions of each case in a holistic way, where key factors or variables can be investigated as their relevance becomes evident in each case.

This flexibility and individuality, however, leads to the main difficulties of case study research. Firstly, there is the problem of relevance to other cases, sometimes expressed in other research traditions as 'generalisability'. In other words, there is a question about how the phenomena observed in one case can have any relevance to other cases – after all, if it has no relevance, then the effort to learn has very little benefit for wider practice. As Kozma and Anderson (2002) argue,

> 'In instrumental case studies, the focus of the analysis is on underlying issues, relationships, and causes that may generalise beyond the case. With this type of case study, the focus is not on the uniqueness of a special case but on what can be taken away from it and cases are selected for this purpose. Analysis of instrumental case studies goes beyond the specific case to examine an underlying issue or research question'. Kozma & Anderson 2002: 387)

The second difficulty is one of structure and design, that is, if case studies are too flexible and data can be collected in an ad hoc way as and when it looks interesting or becomes available, then there is a danger of the original questions being lost in a sea of data, producing findings that do not go very far in addressing the issues that gave rise to the study.

Both of these points have been raised in the literature discussing case study research (e.g. see Meyer 2003; Corcoran *et al.* 2004; Anthony & Jack 2009; Yin 2013). Some writers have either dismissed case studies as a useful approach because of perceived methodological limitations or argued that its potential has not been realised because researchers have had only a superficial understanding of the methodology, seeing it simply as a convenient label to describe their small-scale studies. Writers such as McGloin (2008) have exhorted case study researchers to pay more attention to the theoretical and methodological aspects of case studies in order to move beyond these limitations. As Corcoran *et al.* (2004) have argued,

> 'case-study research…. falls short of its promise due to a lack of theorising about the research methodology or an understanding about the methodology' (Corcoran *et al.* 2004: 7)

Anthony and Jack (2009) similarly emphasise the need for methodological clarity across multiple data sources so that the authenticity of the data, and in turn the quality of the research, is optimised. In addition to the need for authenticity, credibility is fundamental to ensuring quality in qualitative research. There are several ways of achieving credibility that are specific to different research philosophies, but as an example in case study research, Houghton *et al.* (2013) emphasise the need for:

- prolonged engagement and persistent observation in the research environment
- multiple methods to allow confirmation and completeness between multiple data sources
- peer debriefing discussion, in particular during data analysis
- member checking allowing participants to read the transcription of their interviews to ensure that these have been accurately recorded and are therefore credible

Further quality measures include ensuring an audit trail and explicit reflexivity to promote dependability and confirmability of data and the use of 'thick description' to enable robust transferability (ensuring that the reader has sufficient information about the 'case' and its context to make a decision about applicability of the findings to other settings (Houghton *et al.* 2013)).

It is useful to outline some of the measures that allow case study research to confidently challenge these criticisms about rigour and ensure high-quality research. In principle, the measures are no different from those needed for high-quality research of any design, namely, that the researcher should:

- have an effective conceptualisation of the issue under study and the research questions. For case study research, this means knowing how to define 'the case', something that is somewhat harder to achieve than may at first appear.
- have a good understanding of the research philosophy that is being used. This will ensure that the data collected 'fits' together; it all contributes to addressing the question and helps to avoid the risk of collecting whatever data is to hand (the magpie effect).
- think through carefully what is being learned from the case study and how this can contribute to learning that is beyond the specific case. For example, case study methods may be best at answering questions about processes, and the notion of a population from which a sample is drawn may be very different to that of other research approaches.

It is important to emphasise that case study research is complex and tackles real-life issues in their full glory in practice. The scale and scope of case studies are very variable, and they can be very substantial multi-site studies. It is certainly not a way of adding gloss to a poor quality and poorly developed research design, whether small or large scale. This chapter includes illustrations from several studies that we have been involved with which use case study approaches, either as part of a larger study or as the primary research design.

DEFINITIONS OF CASE STUDY METHODOLOGY

One of the most commonly quoted definitions of case study methodology is that of Yin (2013) who described the case study as an approach to empirical enquiry that

> 'investigates a contemporary phenomenon (the 'case') in depth and within its real world context, especially when the boundaries between phenomenon and context may not be clearly evident' (Yin 2013: 16)

There are, of course, other definitions, but this one is used frequently, perhaps because it comes from one of the key writers on case studies, whose book, first published in 1984, has become an important resource for researchers. It also points to some of the features of a research question that would make case study methodology appropriate. First, there is the emphasis on the contemporary nature of the phenomenon; second, there is the importance placed on its 'real-life' nature; and finally, and most importantly, there is the idea that a division between setting and phenomenon is difficult to draw: the phenomenon is intimately connected to the context, and to research one without the other would be to produce only a partial account of what is happening. A similar definition is offered by Robson (2011) who defines case study as a strategy for doing research that involves an empirical investigation of a particular contemporary phenomenon within its real-life context using multiple sources of evidence. This points to another dimension, the complexity of real life and the need for multiple sources of data to capture this.

Case study research, then, is about treating the phenomena being researched as a distinct entity or case and exploring it in the context in which it occurs. This, however, does not explain what a case is, or how this can be demarcated, so further clarification is needed. This is quite a difficult move to make, paradoxically, because the links between phenomena and context that are so integral to the justification of using a case study approach make it difficult to put boundaries around a case for the purposes of definition.

One way to approach this is to eschew an overall definition of a case that could be applied across studies and to see this definitional process as one that each researcher needs to engage with – in other words that the definition of a case needs to be thought through carefully in the light of the research goals of the study. For example, if the goal is to understand the experiences of an individual service user, then the case can be defined around that service user – their experiences and thoughts. If the study is about how an organisation responds to change, then the case can be defined as an organisation. This is not to say that the case needs to be defined as an inviolable unit that cannot be thought of in different ways: there may be a utility in breaking down a case into subunits for the purpose of data collection and analysis. A case study of a family, for example, may be broken down at some point into parents and children as subunits, depending on the questions being asked. Matching the boundaries of the case study to the research questions being asked enables the data collection and analysis to be focused and relevant. Defining the case, then, can be seen as a process not reliant on textbook terminology but on the specific aims and focus of the research.

Defining the case depends much on the 'pre-understanding' of the researcher (Gummesson 2000). Meyer (2003) has described this pre-understanding as potentially arising from 'general knowledge such as theories, models and concepts or from specific knowledge of institutional conditions and social patterns' (Meyer 2003: 331). Researchers come to projects from a range of different experiences and debates about the researched topic. Building on 'pre-understanding' leads to the definition of the case and its boundaries, the processes of data collection and the process of data analysis. As Gummesson (2000) has argued, the challenge for researchers is not to split their pre-understanding from their research, but to be 'able to balance on a razor's edge using their pre-understanding without being its slave' (Gummesson 2000: 65). Pre-understandings lead to research aims and questions, which then lead to specific definitions of what a case is for a particular study.

Nurses and other healthcare practitioners have a particular advantage in pre-understanding the issues and contexts they seek to research as they possess considerable 'insider' knowledge from their practice experiences (Reed *et al.* 1996). The challenge lies in using this insider knowledge effectively to shape research questions and design. An example is Lovell (2006), who used his work with people with learning difficulties to identify and explore the issues arising in one specific case.

Much like grounded theory, case study approaches to research may integrate sampling with data collection and with data analysis, each informing the other. For example, the analysis of one piece of data may suggest that the study could be informed by data collected from a different part of an organisation. This allows for structured and defensible flexibility in the research and maximises the ability of the study to respond to the theoretical sensitivity of the researcher.

RESEARCH QUESTIONS

A fundamental part of carrying out a case study is to identify the research questions. This is pertinent, of course, in any study, but because of the individual nature of the case study, the research questions and the ways of answering them are correspondingly individual and need careful thinking through: methodology cannot be simply 'off the peg', that is, standardised and predetermined. Bergen and While (2000) describe how case study method has derived from a wide variety of disciplines, each with their own methodological orientation (e.g. pure science through to sociology) and implications for the research questions asked. Case study methodology can be either quantitative or qualitative, that is, the research questions can be about exploring the case, either in words or numbers. In addition, case studies may have goals or questions that are about describing phenomena or making links (often causal between aspects of phenomena). These different aims give rise to questions as follows:

- How does this family deal with and manage the implications of this family member's health problem?

- How are services for people with this health problem organised?
- How do staff manage appointments in this clinic?
- Has the reorganisation of the system for making appointments reduced non-contact time for the staff?

These questions are a mix of the descriptive, 'what is happening here', and the inferential, 'how are these things linked here?' They will vary according to the research aims and how it is hoped they will inform and contribute to debates about practice, policy or theory. There should be a logical flow from the research question to the selection of the case and the process of data collection and analysis.

Reflection activity

In what ways does case study methodology in nursing research enhance nursing practice? What kind of insight into nursing practice does case study research provide that may be difficult to gain from other research methodologies?

SELECTION OF CASES

Discussions of sampling in case study methodology are somewhat different from those of other research approaches. They go back to the pre-understanding of the researcher and what they want to do with their research and are therefore about how a case can be defined, its constituents and its boundaries. Some approaches, for example, Soft Systems Methodology (SSM) (Checkland & Scholes 1999), can work well with case study methodology, because they have a theoretical framework that is specific about the dimensions of the phenomena being studied. SSM focuses on the communication patterns within and between organisations and provides a framework for identifying what the constituents of a system might be. It is based on the idea that the way to understand organisational activity is to think of it as being part of a communication system, and that exploration should focus on the way that communication happens across the system. SSM has an inherent set of research goals and a way of defining a case as the system of communications between and within organisations. Starting off with one point in the system, the boundaries of the case can be mapped out by asking who communicates with whom at this point. The identification of the sample is shaped by the theory underpinning the study. An example of SSM in a case study design is given in Research Example 21.1.

RESEARCH EXAMPLE

21.1 Using Soft Systems Methodology in Practice Development Research

SClarke CL, Wilcockson J (2001) Professional and organisational learning: analysing the relationship with the development of practice. *Journal of Advanced Nursing* **34**: 264–272.

Clarke CL, Wilcockson J (2002) Seeing need and developing care: exploring knowledge for and from practice. *International Journal of Nursing Studies* 39: 397–406.

The study aimed to understand how developments in practice spread and were sustained within an organisation. Three case study sites were identified as NHS organisations with a good level of practice development. Approximately 15 people in each organisation were interviewed about the ways in which they develop practice and why. The Soft Systems Methodology guided questions about the social and political aspects of practice development as well as organisational structures and allowed theory to be developed and explored with the participants.

Table 21.1 Sampling criteria for case study sites for specialist services and older people survey (Reed *et al.* 2006)

Sampling criteria	Rank
Roles of specialised staff (i.e. whether they are used as advisors to other staff or have a direct role in care provision)	1
How does the service utilise user opinion/feedback/advocacy groups (e.g. in service development or service audit)?	2
Integration and partnership of healthcare organisation activity across the whole system of service provision (i.e. whether the role is restricted to the healthcare organisation or has the potential to impact on other agencies)	3
How the client group has been demarcated (i.e. whether older people are explicitly identified as a group or whether this is subsumed under other headings, such as medical speciality or type of provision)?	4
How the service/post has been developed?	5
How does the service offer services for older people of diverse ethnic backgrounds/or cater for older people of all ethnic backgrounds?	6
Which National Service Framework – Older Person themes and/or standards – does this service contribute to?	7

Where a theoretical framework is not so clear, however, researchers need to think through their definition of the phenomena under study very carefully in order to map out its dimensions. It may be necessary for some preliminary work to be done to make sure that the cases chosen will help to answer the research questions. This issue arose in a study that examined specialist services for older people (Reed *et al.* 2005, 2006, 2007). It began with a national survey to identify the scope and range of specialist services and then explored the processes of development in more detail, focusing on the development of specialist nursing roles. The sampling matrix shown in Table 21.1 was circulated to the research steering group so that the variables identified by the project team could be ranked by steering group members in order of importance to the project aims (the final ranking is given in the right-hand column).

The ranking of the variables was based on the research objectives and was translated into a sampling matrix (Reed *et al.* 1996). Matrix sampling is a process where the key variables of interest in a study are laid out in a matrix form. Possible cases for inclusion in a study are entered into the matrix, so that the characteristics are set out in a way that makes selection processes visible to researchers and readers. This allowed the team to match up case study sites with the research priorities and ensure that there was a range of cases that would explore key issues and reflect the range of models of specialist services that had been developed.

A further concern is whether a sample should be homogeneous or heterogeneous, in other words whether the case study should include similar or dissimilar phenomena. Again, this is a product of the study aims: it may be that a case study will seek out a range of phenomena in order to broaden the understanding of difference, or it may be that a study would select similar examples in order to increase the amount of data available over a narrower range.

This discussion of sampling echoes the earlier discussions about the definitions of a case. Case study approaches can involve 'subunits' where a case may have different components, so a case study of an organisation may involve a number of different departments or partners or clients, which may be chosen because of their similarities or differences. Moving up a level of unit of analysis, the sampling strategy for the study as a whole may involve multiple case study sites, which might, as with case subunits, be selected in order to provide contrasting examples or similar ones.

Box 21.1 Sampling in case study research

Phenomenon under investigation
↓
Identification of characteristics of the phenomenon to create case criteria
↓
Data collection to inform matrix sampling to identify illustrative case(s)
↓
Identification of those with local context knowledge as 'informants'
↓
Identification of sample inclusion/exclusion criteria
↓
Matrix sampling to identify data collection sample

The context dependency of case study research leads to the need for local knowledge to ensure that sampling reflects this context. As a result, sampling in case study research for researchers who are unfamiliar with the area can be particularly complex. One approach that we have developed and used in a number of studies takes a multistage approach to sampling. For example, Box 21.1 illustrates the sampling flow from issue to unit of data collection within a case. Research Examples 21.2 and 21.3 describe studies that illustrate this process in practice.

RESEARCH DESIGN

The idea of flexible sampling is linked to the idea of a responsive and reflexive research design. The design, for example, can have a built-in facility for inductive sampling (where subsequent samples are based on previous analysis of data and intended to allow deeper analysis of the phenomenon), as an initial case study leads to a need to explore the research question with further cases chosen for their utility in exploring key issues. Alternatively, the design can be planned from the outset. Yin (2013) has talked about multiple case studies, where parallel investigations can be carried out, again, either to explore differences or similarities as indicated in the research question.

There are, though, challenges to achieving consistency across multiple case study sites. Research Example 21.4 describes a multinational study into the strategies that older people use to maintain well-being. Appreciative Inquiry gave the research a coherence, which could have been missing given the diversity of the study sites and the differences in background and experience of the researchers. Appreciative Inquiry is an approach to organisational evaluation and learning that begins by identifying and examining examples of successful working and further explores ways of building on these (Reed *et al.* 2002). This allowed the analysis to identify the unique developments in the study sites and the lessons to be learned across sites.

RESEARCH EXAMPLE

21.2 The Healthbridge Evaluation: Selection of In-depth Case Study Sites

This mixed-methods research (Clarke *et al.* 2013) evaluated 40 demonstration sites (22 dementia advisers and 18 peer support networks) that were established as part of the implementation of the National Dementia Strategy for England (DH 2009). In order to identify eight in-depth case study sites for Stage 3 of the Healthbridge Evaluation that were representative of activity within the 40 demonstration sites, the following information was gathered from all 40 sites as part of Stage 2 of the evaluation:

1 Lead and partner organisations in each site
2 The extent to which services were developing:
- Social networks
- Social learning
- Personal value and effectiveness

3 Ways in which these were achieved:
- Helping people access services
- Helping provide information for other people
- Helping people get emotional support from others
- Helping people share information with each other
- Helping people access practical support

4 Whether the service was designed with a focus on a specific group:
people with dementia; carers; professional carers; newly diagnosed; black and ethnic minority communities; younger people with dementia; learning disability; lesbian, gay, bisexual and transgender communities; socio-economically deprived areas; and general public awareness

This information was tabulated and eight in-depth case study sites (four dementia advisers and four peer support networks) were selected that represented a range of activity in relation to the areas listed above.

RESEARCH EXAMPLE

21.3 Case Study Sampling

Clarke CL, Gibb C, Keady J, Luce A, Wilkinson H, Williams L, Cook A (2009) Risk management dilemmas in dementia care: an organisational survey in three UK countries. *International Journal of Older People Nursing* **4**: 89–96.

In a study exploring how people with dementia construct and manage risk, the 56 people with dementia (who were interviewed twice over 2 months) each nominated a family member and a non-family carer for interview. In this way, many case studies were created. However, this high number of cases to explore the issue under investigation posed particular challenges at the point of analysis.

RESEARCH EXAMPLE

21.4 Using Appreciative Inquiry to Guide Data Collection

Reed J, Richardson E, Marais S, Moyle W (2008) Older people maintaining well-being: an International Appreciative Inquiry study. *International Journal of Older People Nursing* **3**: 168–76.

The study used Appreciative Inquiry as the methodological basis for the case studies. Appreciative Inquiry is a 'strengths-based' approach, which begins from an exploration and appreciation of the ways in which participants have acted positively in their lives. These issues play out in different ways across different cultures and countries, as service development has taken place against the background of different policy frameworks. In order to explore these processes, this study identified a number of different international settings, or cases, as follows:

- United Kingdom – welfare state structure and services
- Germany – voluntary sector/Church sector and services
- Australia – private sector and services
- South Africa – limited service development

Appreciative Inquiry focus groups/individual interviews were held in each of these countries. The initial questions were as follows:

- What strategies have you developed to respond to physical challenges? What sort of challenges were these, and did your strategies involve any of the following examples – thinking through strategies, using aids or assistance, changing or reflecting on lifestyles or any other responses?
- What strategies have you developed to respond to psychological challenges? What sort of challenges were these, and did your strategies involve any of the following examples – thinking through strategies, using aids or assistance, changing or reflecting on lifestyles or any other responses?
- What strategies have you developed to respond to social challenges? What sort of challenges were these, and did your strategies involve any of the following examples – thinking through strategies, using aids or assistance, changing or reflecting on lifestyles or any other responses?

The data from each focus group in each case study country was pooled and used to explore different theoretical dimensions, but prior to this the context in each case was described using the Community Capitals Framework (Flora *et al.* 2004). In this way, the diversity of cases and their common themes were identified. The data analysis contributed towards a framework for international service and practice development (Moyle *et al.* 2010).

DATA ANALYSIS

This chapter began by pointing out the criticism levied at case studies regarding the failure of the methodology to reach its potential because of the lack of rigour in analysis. As case studies are so embedded in particular contexts, it is tempting to produce an analysis with only local relevance. There is a huge difference between simply saying 'this is what happened in this case' and extending this to discuss the relevance of the case to broader issues.

There are three approaches that can be taken to consider the way in which case study research can contribute to broader issues. First, a broader perspective needs to be built into the research questions and study design from the outset. Appropriate modelling and theorising of the phenomenon from its conception will ensure that the study is set up to produce data amenable to analysis that can make a wider contribution. For example, the project described in Research Example 21.2 was an evaluation of peer support networks and dementia advisers (as recommended in the National Dementia Strategy for England, Department of Health, 2009) but was designed to also contribute to a knowledge base about the processes of practice and service development. There was learning about the ways in which services develop as well as learning about peer support and information provision (Clarke *et al.* 2013). To achieve this, the research team needed to know how to access local, on-the-ground knowledge to ensure context sensitivity. They also had to be sufficiently aware of the contemporary knowledge base and philosophical options to allow theoretical sensitivity to inform the project development.

Second, having collected the data, there is a need to analyse it in two ways. Initially, the internal patterns in the data must be carefully teased out and confirmed, whether through qualitative or quantitative data analysis methods. This is the level of analysis that is most often described and concerns getting to grips with the detail of the data and organising it in a way that allows those patterns to be described. In the second part of the analysis, which may be concurrent with the first or most often will follow it, the results of the data analysis need to be analysed in relation to the external knowledge base generated by other research and the practice and policy environment. This can be best described as external patterning. In this way, the contribution of the internal data analysis can be explored in relation to the external knowledge environment and the study's contribution to that knowledge base carefully articulated.

Third, there needs to be careful consideration of the transferability of the results of the study from one context to another. This has some similarities to the process of generalising from a sample to a wider population in that the researcher needs to know what characteristics of the sample need to be present in the wider population to legitimately claim that the results can be generalised from one to the other. In case study research, with dependence on context, there needs to be an examination of the factors that reside in the context that can be found in other contexts to which claims of transferability may be made with some credibility. The classic example is a case study of some innovative development that is perceived to have happened 'only because Mary is here', and that if others had a Mary, then they would achieve the same development. It is important to move beyond the 'Mary factor' and analyse just what it is about the way in which Mary works and has been able to work within the organisation that has allowed an innovation to occur. In this way, having examined and analysed data within its context, there is a step required of decontextualising the issue, transferring it to another context and recontextualising it there. In other words, the analysis needs to identify the critical aspects of context that would allow something to be used elsewhere so long as those certain critical aspects of context were (or were not) present.

One important consideration in the analysis of data in multiple case study research is the extent to which data are analysed within or across cases. It may be that the cases have been purposefully selected to reflect different dimensions of the phenomenon. In this situation, analysis across cases is necessary to ensure that all dimensions are taken into account in developing the findings from the data. Cross-case analysis can be used to emphasise commonality or difference between cases. Within-case analysis involves each case being analysed in turn as an interdependent set of data. This will maximise identification of the context-dependent aspects of the phenomenon. For example, Stake (1995) refers to seeking to refine an understanding of an issue by searching for patterns across a number of cases. For most studies, some analysis at both 'within' and 'across case' level is appropriate. In the study of care management conducted by Bergen and While (2000), Yin's (2013) ideas of designating a unit smaller than the case for the purposes of analysis were adopted: the case was care management and the unit of analysis was individual community nurse's practice.

Data analysis in case study research requires attention to the analytical demands of the very wide range of data sources that may be involved. Yin (2013) refers to documentation, archival records, direct observation, participant observation, interviews and physical artefacts as of equal relevance to case study

> ### Reflection activity
>
> What criticisms have been made of case study methodology? How can researchers counter these criticisms when designing case study research?

research. Many of these, such as documentary analysis, are a way of using pre-existing materials as data sources (Reed 1992). While such data has the advantage of being relatively 'untouched' by the research process, as it was written for other reasons, it has been produced for particular audiences, and these need to be borne in mind when analysing these data.

PRESENTATION AND REPORTING

The presentation and reporting of any research study requires consideration of the audience. In case study research, this is coloured by issues such as maintaining confidentiality and the plurality of audiences. As case study research is context dependent, it is necessary to describe organisations and people in considerable detail, and even if anonymity of names is maintained, this level of context description may make it quite easy for people and places to be identified. This should be acknowledged with participants at the start of the research and when seeking informed consent, and it may be necessary for some forms of reporting to obscure the association between place/person and reported detail. This may be most easily achieved through cross-case reporting that does not seek to portray each case individually. On the other hand, people and organisations can become very involved in case study research and naturally wish to see their role profiled appropriately. They may also wish to learn what they can from the work, and in this instance, they may find it helpful to receive the research presented in a way that is very explicit about each case. For example, in one study (Clarke *et al.* 2013), brief reports were written for each case study site that were in addition to the overall (and more public) report of the research in which only the cross-case analysis was presented.

> ### Reflection activity
>
> What ethical issues are researchers likely to encounter when undertaking and reporting case study research? What steps should researchers take to ensure high ethical standards in case study research?

In addition, reporting to people and organisations in a way that is accessible for their practice needs to be complemented by making the findings of the research accessible to the wider academic and practice communities through publication and presentations. To achieve this effectively will require the work to have relevance beyond the local case study sites, as described previously. There also needs to be a level of theoretical analysis in presenting and disseminating the work so it can be transferred to other settings and can enable people to think about their current knowledge and practice.

CONCLUSION

Case study research is unique in the emphases it places on the importance of the context and the impact of the context on the phenomenon under investigation. The design, sampling and data collection methods reflect this emphasis on context dependency. There is, however, a need to analyse the data and articulate the findings in a way that is both respectful of this context and that allows the research to be transferred to other environments. It is a form of research that is attractive to researchers and practitioners alike and that draws on the knowledge base of both.

References

Anthony S, Jack S (2009) Qualitative case study methodology in nursing research: an integrative review. *Journal of Advanced Nursing* **65**(6): 1171–1181.

Bergen A, While A (2000) A case for case study studies: exploring the use of case study design in community nursing research. *Journal of Advanced Nursing* **31**: 926–934.

Checkland P, Scholes J (1999) *Soft Systems Methodology in Action*. Chichester, Wiley.

Clarke CL, Wilcockson J (2001) Professional and organisational learning: analysing the relationship with the development of practice. *Journal of Advanced Nursing* **34**: 264–272.

Clarke CL, Wilcockson J (2002) Seeing need and developing care: exploring knowledge for and from practice. *International Journal of Nursing Studies* **39**: 397–406.

Clarke CL, Gibb C, Keady J, Luce A, Wilkinson H, Williams L, Cook A (2009) Risk management dilemmas in dementia care: an organisational survey in three UK countries. *International Journal of Older People Nursing* **4**: 89–96.

Clarke CL, Keyes SE, Wilkinson H, Alexjuk J, Wilcockson J, Robinson L, Reynolds J, McClelland S, Hodgson P, Corner L, Cattan M (2013) *Healthbridge: The National Evaluation of Peer Support Networks and Dementia Advisers in implementation of the National Dementia Strategy for England*. London, Department of Health.

Corcoran PB, Walker KE, Wals AEJ (2004) Case-studies, make-your-case studies, and case stories: a critique of case-study methodology in sustainability in higher education. *Environmental Education Research* **10**: 17–21.

Department of Health (2009) *Living Well with Dementia: a National Dementia Strategy*. London, Department of Health.

Flora, CB, Flora JL, Fey S (2004) *The Community Capitals Framework. Rural Communities: legacy and change*. 2nd edition. Boulder, CO, Westview Press.

Gummesson E (2000) *Qualitative Methods in Management Research*. 2nd edition. London, Sage.

Houghton C, Casey D, Shaw D, Murphy K (2013) Rigour in qualitative case-study research. *Nurse Researcher* **20**(4): 12–17.

Kozma RB, Anderson RE (2002) Qualitative case studies of innovative pedagogical practices using ICT. *Journal of Computer Assisted Learning* **18**: 387–394.

Lovell A (2006) Daniel's story: self-injury and the case study as method. *British Journal of Nursing* **15**(3): 167–170.

McGloin S (2008) The trustworthiness of case study methodology. *Nurse Researcher* **16**(1): 45–54.

Meyer CB (2003) A case in case study methodology. *Field Methods* **13**: 329–352.

Moyle W, Clarke CL, Gracia N, Reed J, Cook G, Klein B, Marais S, Richardson E (2010) Older people maintaining mental health well-being through resilience: an appreciative inquiry study in four countries. *Journal of Nursing and Healthcare in Chronic Illness* **2**: 113–121.

Reed J (1992) Secondary data in nursing research. *Journal of Advanced Nursing* **7**: 877–883.

Reed J, Procter S, Murray S (1996) A sampling strategy for qualitative research. *Nurse Researcher* **3**(4): 52–68.

Reed J, Pearson P, Douglas B, Swinburne S, Wilding H (2002) Going home from hospital – an appreciative inquiry study. *Health and Social Care and the Community* **10**: 36–45.

Reed J, Watson B, Cook M, Clarke C, Cook G, Inglis P (2005) Developing specialist practice for older people in England: responses to policy initiatives. *Practice Development in Health Care* **4**(4): 192–202.

Reed J, Cook M, Cook G, Inglis P, Clarke C (2006) Specialist services for older people: issues of negative and positive ageism. *Ageing and Society* **26**: 849–865.

Reed J, Inglis P, Cook G, Clarke C, Cook M (2007) Specialist nurses for older people: implications from UK development sites. *Journal of Advanced Nursing* **58**(4): 368–376.

Reed J, Richardson E, Marais S, Moyle W (2008) Older people maintaining well-being: an International Appreciative Inquiry study. *International Journal of Older People Nursing* **3**(1): 68–76.

Robson C (2011) *Real World Research*. 3rd edition. Oxford, Blackwell.

Sangster-Gormley E (2013) How case-study research can help to explain implementation of the nurse practitioner role. *Nurse Researcher* **20**(4): 6–11.

Stake RE (1995) *The Art of Case Study Research*. Thousand Oaks, Sage.

Yin RK (2013) *Case Study Research: design and methods*. 5th edition. Thousand Oaks, Sage.

CHAPTER 22

Evaluation Research

Judith Lathlean

Key points

- Evaluation occurs in everyday life and is especially a feature and an expectation in health and social care.
- Evaluation research takes on a variety of forms, dependent on its purpose and the questions it seeks to answer.
- A range of different approaches are evident including ones that focus on outcomes and others that are equally concerned with process and context.
- Evaluations can be politically driven and are often sensitive. Therefore, they need to be undertaken thoughtfully and in an ethical manner.

INTRODUCTION

Evaluation, or assessing the worth or value of something, is an inescapable feature of everyday life and especially within hospital and health settings. It is linked to a number of imperatives, such as the desire to ensure that health service resources are being used appropriately, that they are value for money and that patients and consumers of services are satisfied with their experiences. It can be undertaken in a number of ways, ranging from 'opinion polls', surveys of various kinds and auditing, through to the use of formal research processes, whether they be quantitative or, increasingly, qualitative. Nevertheless, as judgements are being made, they are not necessarily value-free, and the motivation for conducting an evaluation can be questionable. Thus, caution may be needed when carrying out an evaluation or using the results of one.

WHAT IS EVALUATION RESEARCH?

Some authors suggest that evaluation research is a particular kind of 'applied' research that is concerned with the evaluation of, for example, an intervention, a type of service, a policy initiative or a programme of education. Typical questions asked in this kind of

The Research Process in Nursing, Seventh Edition. Edited by Kate Gerrish and Judith Lathlean.

Companion Website: www.wiley.com/go/gerrish/research

research relate to how effective the programme or intervention has been in achieving its goals. Historically, its methods and terminology have been derived primarily from educational and psychological research (see, e.g. the substantial text by Stufflebeam and Shinkfield (2007)). Within health sciences, it has been associated with positivism and the search for objective assessment, thus lending itself to an experimental (or quasi-experimental) design. Recently, though, evaluation research has become more diverse as evaluators try to answer questions about the processes and not just the outcomes. This has also led to the revival of 'models' of evaluation, such as the logic model of evaluation, once used primarily to evaluate programmes but now applied to a range of innovations, which in turn tends to be more all-encompassing in seeking to understand all aspects of the change (see Box 22.1).

Another framework put forwards to evaluate process is that of critical realism (McEvoy & Richards 2003). This is based on the philosophical assumptions of realism and relativism that stress the need to look at both *context* and *mechanisms* in order to understand outcomes. A critical realist framework is used in two areas of evaluation research: theory-driven programme evaluation and policy evaluation. Marchal *et al.* (2012) provide a useful review of studies in the field of health systems research and address the questions of whether realist evaluation is 'keeping its promise', which is to explain 'how' and 'why' things work. They conclude that while realist evaluation is gaining momentum in research on health systems, more clarity is needed regarding the methodology adopted. (See later section on realist evaluation.)

Other approaches have emerged, and frequently, evaluation studies can be found using a mixed-methods or purely qualitative design. The qualitative evaluation researcher is usually interested in obtaining different views of various stakeholders as to how the subject or topic of study is working, and there is less focus on establishing the relationship between variables as is normally the case for the experimental researcher.

Box 22.1 A logic model to evaluate a programme or intervention

Inputs	Activities/ mechanisms	Outputs	Outcomes/impacts
What resources go into a programme/ intervention?	*What activities does the programme/ intervention involve?*	*What is produced through those activities?*	*What changes or benefits result from the programme/intervention?*
e.g. human, financial, organisational and community resources	e.g. the processes, tools, events, technology and actions that are an intentional part of the programme or implementation	e.g. direct products of programme activities and may include types, levels and targets of services to be delivered by the programme/intervention	*Outcomes* - specific changes in programme/intervention participant's behaviour, knowledge, skills, status and level of functioning; *Impacts* – the fundamental intended or unintended change occurring in organisations, communities or systems as a result of programme activities
Planned work →		Intended results →	

Reflection activity

Politicians, health and social care managers and professionals are inevitably interested in the way resources are used and how satisfied recipients are with services. Is one type of approach to evaluation the best way to address these different issues? What are the merits of the different approaches outlined earlier?

EVALUATION OF SATISFACTION

In its simplest form, evaluation of satisfaction is an attempt to find out people's views of being involved in a service. Patient satisfaction is one of the most widely used outcome indicators or evaluation of the quality of health care, and it can be ascertained by approaches that range from limited and focused surveys to the use of validated instruments, often on bigger scale. For example, many hospitals provide a short patient satisfaction questionnaire, which can be completed following a hospital stay. They typically comprise a few questions. On a larger scale, the NHS patient survey programme systematically gathers the views of patients about the care they have recently received, and these are collated and published online (see www.nhssurveys.org).

There are a number of small-scale studies that use questionnaires to elicit patient views. For example, Sutherland *et al.* (2008) undertook a survey of people with cancer and their friends and families about a cancer education programme. A very much larger national survey was that by Marian *et al.* (2008) that compared the patient satisfaction and side effects of homeopathic treatment versus conventional medicine in Switzerland. Physician and patient questionnaires were used, with 6778 adult patients receiving the questionnaire and 3126 responding (46.1%). Statistically significant differences were found with respect to health status (higher percentage of chronic and severe conditions in the homeopathic group), perception of side effects (higher percentage of reported side effects in the conventional group) and patient satisfaction (higher percentage of satisfied patients in the homeopathic group).

Reflection activity

What kind of strategy could be used to find out about client and consumer satisfaction with services? What biases may be present in patient satisfaction surveys?

There are many scales available to find out patient satisfaction. Indeed, Abusalem *et al.* (2012), in a literature review of surveys to measure patient satisfaction with health care at home, identified no less than 23 dating from 1994 to 2007. Yet few studies have evaluated and further developed psychometrically sound patient satisfaction scales. Thus, researchers looking for a ready-made tool to assess satisfaction should proceed with some caution.

Not all evaluation research concentrates on satisfaction, and there are a number of different approaches with different foci. Sometimes, they are referred to as 'models of evaluation'. These are discussed in the next section.

APPROACHES TO EVALUATION

Evaluation research is undertaken for different reasons, and these reasons are often related to the style or type of design that is chosen. The following are the main types of question that the evaluation seeks to answer:

- What are the outcomes: is the service, programme, innovation achieving its objectives and what are the results?
- What processes are important: what is actually happening and is its operation working as planned?

- What is the relationship between process, outcome and context: are there theoretical ways in which the programme or innovation can be explained?

Evaluation of outcomes

This is a traditional view of evaluation that many (mistakenly) believe is the only valid approach to evaluation. In its pure form, it looks at the extent to which a service (or intervention) has achieved its goals and attempts to use largely quantitative measures. Often, an experimental design is adopted. To guide randomised controlled trials (RCTs), the Medical Research Council (MRC) has issued a framework for the development and evaluation of RCTs for complex interventions to improve health (MRC 2000) (see website details in the following text). The intention of this framework is to provide investigators with guidance in recognising the unique challenges that arise in the evaluation of complex interventions, as well as to suggest some strategies for addressing these issues in the development of their own trials 'by the use of a step-wise [non-linear] approach to the evaluation' (MRC 2000: 1).

An example of research using an experimental design is that of Wilkinson *et al.* (2007) who examined the effectiveness of aromatherapy massage in the management of anxiety and depression in patients with cancer. A sample of 288 cancer patients was randomly allocated to a course of aromatherapy massage (one session for 4 weeks) or usual supportive care alone. The results demonstrated a significant relationship between those receiving aromatherapy and reduced clinical depression/anxiety after 2 weeks. However, this was not sustained nor was there found to be a significant association between the intervention and other symptoms such as pain, insomnia, nausea and vomiting.

Kendrick *et al.* (2005) used a randomised controlled design to compare the treatment of patients with common mental health problems (see Research Example 22.1). It is of interest to note, though, that the reasons why significant differences were not found between two of the experimental groups (those undertaking problem-solving sessions and treatment by community mental health nurses) were not entirely understood within the trial and could only be explored fully by a qualitative study (Simons *et al.* 2008), which ran in tandem with the trial.

Before and after studies also attempt to examine the effect of an intervention. Knowles *et al.* (2013) evaluated the implementation of a bowel management protocol in an intensive care setting, with the intention of finding out about clinical practices and patient outcomes (see Research Example 22.2). Again, as with

RESEARCH EXAMPLE

22.1 Evaluation using a randomised controlled trial

Kendrick T, Simons L, Thompson C, Mynors-Wallis L, Lathlean J, Pickering R, Gerard K (2005) Trial of problem solving by community psychiatric nurses (CPNs) for anxiety, depression and life difficulties among general practice patients (the CPN-GP study). *Journal of Affective Disorders 78*(Suppl. 1): S44.

This study used an experimental deign whereby patients presenting to the general practitioner (GP) with mild to moderate symptoms of anxiety and depression, referred to as common mental health problems, were randomly allocated to three groups: the first comprised problem-solving sessions administered by community psychiatric nurses (CPNs), the second was the usual treatment from CPNs, and the third was referral to the GP only. The trial failed to demonstrate a significant difference between the outcomes (i.e. diminution of symptoms) for patients attending the problem solving and the usual CPN treatment, although both arms of the trial fared better than those attending the GP alone. The reasons for this were later teased out within a qualitative study undertaken by a member of the research team (Simons *et al.* 2008).

RESEARCH EXAMPLE

22.2 Before and After Evaluation

Knowles S, McInnes E, Elliott D, Hardy J, Middleton S (2013) Evaluation of the implementation of a bowel management protocol in intensive care: effect on clinician practices and patient outcomes. *Journal of Clinical Nursing* **23**: 716–730.

The aim of this study was to evaluate the effect of the implementation of a bowel management protocol on the outcomes for intensive care patients, notably the incidence of constipation and diarrhoea, and on clinicians' bowel management practices. The method used was to implement the protocol with education sessions, printed educational materials (fact sheets) and reminders. Retrospective data were then collected from patients' medical record, pre- and post-implementation. Results showed no significant differences in the incidence of constipation and diarrhoea at these two time points. There was a slight (non-significant) increase in bowel assessment on admission by medical officers post-implementation. The researchers hypothesised that the lack of differences may have been due to clinicians' non-adherence to the protocol, but they suggested that further research was needed on clinical decision-making to examine whether this was so and why.

the Kendrick *et al.* study, having found no significant relationship between the implementation and patient symptoms, they could only conjecture why this may be so, suggesting that it could be due to lack of clinician adherence to the protocol.

Thome and Arnardottir (2012) also used a before and after design in a pre- and post-test single group quasi-experimental study, when they investigated the effects of an antenatal family nursing intervention for 39 emotionally distressed women and their partners. Although the conclusion reached was that the intervention (four home visits guided by a nursing model) did reduce the stress of couples, the authors suggested that follow-up studies would be needed in order to understand the course and management of perinatal distress in the longer term. Thus, all of these types of study appear to have limitations, requiring either complementary qualitative studies or follow-up research to be clear about the reasons for the results or the effects over a longer period.

Reflection activity

The study of outcomes is a popular aim within evaluation. Are quantitative approaches the design of choice, and are they sufficient to answer all the questions about outcomes, especially why particular results were found?

Process evaluation

The term 'process evaluation' has been used in different kinds of ways. For example, Oakley *et al.* (2006) used it to overcome the limitations of an RCT that focuses primarily on the outcomes and not the process of implementation. They complemented the randomised intervention of pupil peer-led sex education (RIPPLE) study, which was a systematic review and pilot study in four schools, with questionnaire surveys and focus groups with students and peer educators, teacher interviews and researcher observation. Another study by Hoddinott *et al.* (2012) used process evaluation involving qualitative and quantitative methods to assess the acceptability, feasibility and intervention fidelity of a trial of proactive and reactive telephone support for breastfeeding up to 14 days after hospital discharge for women living in more disadvantaged areas.

Similarly, Kemp *et al.* (2013) used this type of evaluation to investigate how the processes by which prenatal activities, such as sustained home visiting by nurses, achieve effective outcomes in relation to psychosocial support for families in the postnatal period. The conclusion of these three studies was that process evaluation should be integral to the design of many RCTs, especially when evaluating complex interventions.

Process evaluation is not restricted however to being an adjunct to an intervention. Appleton *et al.* (2013) used what they referred to as a 'process evaluation' mixed-methods design to compare health visitor ratings of mother–infant interactions, as observed in laboratory conditions, with ratings gained from a Global Rating Scale (see Research Example 22.3). Another study, using the same design, by Metzelthin *et al.* (2013) employed both quantitative and interview data to examine the extent to which an interdisciplinary care approach for frail older people was being implemented as planned, the aim being to gain insight about health professionals' views and people's experience.

Logic model of evaluation

The logic model of evaluation is another approach that incorporates an examination of process. This stems from original work undertaken in the United States and Canada on the evaluation of educational or policy programmes (see Weiss 1998). It comprises a useful set of steps, which, for a programme evaluation, are illustrated in Box 22.1. They entail gathering data on the inputs, activities, outputs and outcomes or impacts. This rationale can be applied to a number of different situations and research topics. For example, Dykeman *et al.* (2003) developed a 'programme logic model' to measure the processes and outcomes of a nurse-managed community health clinic specifically aimed at looking after the health needs of homeless people. They then used it to inform the way the effectiveness of this service and the clinic was assessed.

MacPhee (2009) constructed a theoretical model from the literature to guide the process of establishing a successful partnership between a school of nursing and nurse leaders from a local hospital. The foci of this pilot and subsequent project were the inputs,

RESEARCH EXAMPLE

22.3 Evaluation of Process Using Mixed Methods

Appleton J, Harris M, Oates J, Kelly C (2013) Evaluating health visitor assessments of mother-infant interactions: a mixed methods study. *International Journal of Nursing Studies* **50**(1): 5–15.

This study sought to examine the processes by which health visitors identify problems in mother–infant relationships in the postnatal period. This two-phase, mixed-methods evaluation study involved video recordings of mother's interaction with her baby for 20 min in an observation laboratory, and then the recorded data were analysed using the Global Ratings Scales (GRS) of mother–infant interaction (phase 1). The second phase comprised 12 health visitor rating and assessing 9 video clips from phase 1, followed by interviews with them about their rationale for their ratings. These ratings were compared with those from the GRS.

Correlations between health visitor ratings and GRS ratings were only statistically significant in four cases. In explaining this, health visitors commented on mother's behaviours or the relationship between mother and baby and often ignored the baby. As a result of the study, the researchers concluded that the frequent lack of attention to the baby's behaviour suggested an area for further training.

activities, outputs and outcomes, and the data gathering and action involved led to practice–academic collaborations, such as educational workshops, affiliated academic positions and joint nursing research. Nevertheless, the conclusion reached by MacPhee was that this kind of change is complex and encompasses components and linkages of the model at different levels.

Some studies using the logic model for evaluation distinguish between short-, medium- and long-term outcomes. For example, Sitaker *et al.* (2008) evaluated a large-scale programme designed to decrease heart disease and stroke, and they identified immediate public awareness of signs and symptoms (short term), then control of blood pressure and cholesterol (medium term) and much later fewer heart disease and stroke events (long term).

Realist evaluation

There has been a growing popularity of an approach called realist evaluation, largely stemming from the work of Pawson and Tilley (1997) and Pawson (2006). They argue that adopting a realist philosophy, which emphasises the mechanisms operating in a particular setting, enables a better understanding of what works and what is the effect of the context. (See Chapter 26 for an explanation of the realist paradigm.) Realist evaluations begin by identifying the underlying assumptions about how an intervention is supposed to work (i.e. the programme theory) and then uses this to guide the actual evaluation. Examples of evaluations following this approach include Clark *et al.* (2007) who discuss a programme of research into secondary prevention programmes for heart disease. Tolson *et al.* (2007) focused on the development of a clinical network in palliative care, and Williams *et al.* (2013) (see Research Example 22.4) used a similar method to study the impact of intermediaries (nurses working to a consultant nurse specialist) on infection control practice.

Subirana *et al.* (2014) made an interesting link between the use of a realist approach and the development of a logic model, of the kind referred to in the previous section and illustrated in Box 22.1.

RESEARCH EXAMPLE

22.4 Realist Evaluation

Williams L, Burton C, Rycroft-Malone J (2013) What works: a realist evaluation case study of intermediaries in infection control practice. *Journal of Advanced Nursing* **69**(4): 915–926.

This study was a single mixed-methods case study of an infection control intermediary programme in one health-care organisation in the United Kingdom. The approach was chosen because it is consistent with realist evaluation that seeks theoretical propositions about what works, for whom and in what contexts. The sample comprised designated intermediary posts, that is, qualified nurses operating under the direction of the consultant nurse for infection control, collaborating with clinical leads and the infection control team to contribute to the prevention and control of health-care-associated infections. Additionally, employees of the chosen NHS organisation with infection control responsibilities were included. Methods used were unstructured observation and focused interviews, based on an interview guide, the content of which was determined by a theoretical framework. This was complemented by review of documentation, such as audit reports, policies and job descriptions.

The main focus of the analysis centred around the mechanisms used by the intermediaries, such as watching practice; giving thoughtful feedback, support and recognition of the patient perspective; practice-based teaching; and building rapport. The researchers claimed that by using a realist evaluation approach, they were able to examine the context and the mechanisms used within that context and relate these to the outcomes.

RESEARCH EXAMPLE

22.5 Linking Realist Evaluation and Logic Modelling

Subirana M, Long A, Greenhalgh J, Firth J (2014) A realist logic model of the links between nurse staffing and the outcomes of nursing. *Journal of Research in Nursing* **19**(1): 8–23.

This study arose from concerns about the problem of nursing staff shortages and nurse retention, primarily within the United States. Its aim was to focus on the potential causal mechanisms between nurse staffing levels and skill mix and issues of patient safety and outcome. It used the principles of realist evaluation and followed a step-by-step process, building a tentative logic model, to show how nurse staffing might influence patient and nursing outcomes. The method adopted differentiated the context for the intervention, its mechanism and outcomes or the context–mechanism–outcome (CMO) configuration. They used data drawn from literature reviews of existing research and from Magnet Hospital studies (Kramer & Schmalenberg 2005) such as nurse staffing levels and nurse experience (C), levels of clinical monitoring and early detection of problems (M) to 'model' the likelihood of specific outcomes, such as prevention of patient death. They concluded that their generation of a logic model, 'based on the interrogation of the evidence base for accounts of how nurse staffing might affect patient outcomes, provides another step to help guide future research (p20)'. Nevertheless, they also point out that the 'difficult to measure' attributes, such as nurse intuition, operation of clinical judgement and missed care, require further exploration.

Reflection activity

The evaluation of process, the use of a logic model of evaluation and realist evaluation have in common the desire to examine the effect of the mechanisms at work in the implementation of a service or intervention. In what clinical and education settings is it likely to be as important to know how an outcome was achieved as what was achieved?

Research Example 22.5 describes how they employed such a strategy to understand ways in which nurse staffing and skill mix may affect patient care, drawing primarily on existing research and data.

Evaluation using case study

Although, as already described, evaluation most typically employs a quantitative or mixed-methods design, some studies use a case study strategy. Elliott *et al.* (2013) (Research Example 22.6) is an example of a national study that adopted a multiple case study methodology over a 2-year period to identify the professional and leadership activities of advanced practitioners. Another study that employed multiple case studies was that of Gerrish *et al.* (2013). This research aimed to develop a framework that could then be used to evaluate the impact of nurse consultants on patient, professional and organisational outcomes and other associated indicators of impact. As with other forms of evaluation, case study approaches tend to focus on context as well as an in-depth study of individual settings or cases.

INSTRUMENTS TO AID EVALUATION

In the quest for ever more rigorous evaluative studies, researchers have concentrated on developing and testing tools and instruments to assess a variety of practice and education situations. Research Example 22.7, a study by Duprez *et al.* (2013),

RESEARCH EXAMPLE

22.6 A Case Study Approach to Evaluation

Elliott N, Higgins A, Begly C, Lalor J, Sheerin F, Coyne, I, Murphy K (2013) The identification of clinical and professional leadership activities of advanced practitioners: findings from the Specialist Clinical and Advanced Practitioner Evaluation study in Ireland. *Journal of Advanced Nursing* **69**(5): 1037–1050.

This was a commissioned national evaluation of advanced practitioners in nursing and midwifery, with the aim of informing policymakers about further developments in Ireland. It used a multiple case study methodology whereby a purposive sample was selected of 23 cases – clinical nurse/midwife specialists and advanced nurse/midwife practitioners – from a total population of 2101 across 28 health service provider sites within each region in Ireland. Methods used to collect data included structured observation (with an observation tool) of the 23 cases, interviews with directors of nursing/midwifery (n=28) and clinical team members (n=41) and scrutiny of on-site written records. The study concluded that hitherto research evidence about advanced practice and leadership had been sparse and that this research, by using a case study approach, contributed empirical evidence on how clinical nurse/midwife specialists and advanced nurse/midwife practitioners 'enact clinical and professional leadership in real-life practice'.

RESEARCH EXAMPLE

22.7 Development of Evaluation Instruments

Duprez V, de Pover M, de Spiegelaere M, Beeckman D (2013) The development and psychometrical evaluation of a set of instruments to evaluate the effectiveness of diabetes patient education. *Journal of Clinical Nursing Studies* **23**: 429–439.

This study had two phases. The first was instrument development by a systematic literature review, focus groups with patients and a testing of content validity in a two-round Delphi procedure with clinical experts. The second phase was the psychometric evaluation of the knowledge, self-management and self-efficacy instruments. A convenience sample of 188 diabetic patients (with just over half having type II diabetes) in two hospitals was involved in the evaluation.

The researchers concluded that the resultant instruments can be used in patient educational settings and research to assess knowledge, self-management and self-efficacy of diabetic patients. Also, the instruments can support the design and evaluation of patient education interventions and health professional training programmes and reduce inconsistencies in information giving.

describes the evaluation of instruments that are designed to look at the effectiveness of education for diabetes patients and concludes that these can be used to benchmark the quality of diabetic education. The aim of the Long *et al.* (2014) study was to assess the core outcomes in graduates, again by undertaking a psychometric evaluation of a nursing knowledge and skills test in a paediatric setting. They conclude that the instrument shows 'encouraging psychometric properties' and that with additional refinements would provide educators and managers with a valid tool for assessing skills and knowledge.

McIlfatrick and Hasson (2013) take a somewhat different tack but still in line with tool development. Their aim was to evaluate what they describe as a holistic assessment tool for palliative care practice, and they used a mixed-methods design, with a combination of the analysis of assessments undertaken using the tool, and focus groups with health professionals. They concluded that a tool can assist the process of assessment but is only an aid when discussing sensitive aspects of care.

USING DIFFERENT METHODS TO EVALUATE

The examples already given show that a range of different methods can and have been employed in studies that are referred to as 'evaluation'. No one design should be preferred although the choice is directly related to the purpose of the research and questions it seeks to answer. It does not have to be an either/or decision as shown by the several examples of mixed-methods design and the emphasis in some on the process of the intervention or programme as much as its outcomes. Furthermore, a whole range of methods of data collection are utilised. Evaluations can be based primarily on one method. For example, a large-scale evaluation of prescribing practices in Ireland by Naughton *et al.* (2013) used multi-site documentation evaluation of 142 patient records and 208 medications prescribed by 25 registered nurse prescribers. Two expert reviewers then rated the decisions found recorded in the documentation using a modified Medication Appropriate Index tool. The conclusions reached indicated a high level of safe and clinically appropriate prescribing decisions, but there was the risk of drug errors. Continuing education and evaluation were therefore recommended.

Another apparently innovative method was that adopted in a study by Mann *et al.* (2014) of the evaluation of a particular approach to the training of nurses who were recruiting to a trial. This training was called 'internal peer review', and the evaluation was based on a literature review of processes used to consent subjects into a trial and the discussion of the actual peer review process. It concluded that nurse-led peer review can provide a forum to share communication strategies.

CONCLUSION

This chapter has shown how there are many different forms of and approaches to evaluation research. It is not the case that one type fits all, and studies can vary in their scale, purpose, design and methods. It may be undertaken by single researchers or large teams. Evaluation research, by the very intention of establishing worth and value, can be political and sensitive. It may be commissioned by powerful administrators and policymakers with the desire to 'prove' the effectiveness or otherwise of an initiative, and therefore, care needs to be taken in its conduct and presentation. Ethical considerations are paramount, even in small-scale, apparently benign endeavours.

References

Abusalem S, Myers J, Aljeesh Y (2012) Patient satisfaction in home health care. *Journal of Clinical Nursing* **22**: 2426–2435.

Appleton J, Harris M, Oates J, Kelly C (2013) Evaluating health visitor assessments of mother-infant interactions: a mixed methods study. *International Journal of Nursing Studies* **50**(1): 5–15.

Clark AM, MacIntyre PD, Cruikshank J (2007) A critical realist approach to understanding and evaluating heart health programmes. *Health: An Interdisciplinary Journal for the Social Study of Health, Illness and Medicine* **11**: 513–539.

Duprez V, de Pover M, de Spiegelaere M, Beeckman D (2013) The development and psychometrical evaluation of a set of instruments to evaluate the effectiveness of diabetes patient education. *Journal of Clinical Nursing Studies* **23**: 429–439.

Dykeman M, MacIntosh J, Seaman P, Davidson P (2003) Development of a program logic model to measure the processes and outcomes of a nurse-managed community health clinic. *Journal of Professional Nursing* **19**(3): 197–203.

Elliott N, Higgins A, Begly C, Lalor J, Sheerin F, Coyne I, Murphy K (2013) The identification of clinical and professional leadership activities of advanced practitioners: findings from the Specialist Clinical and Advanced Practitioner Evaluation study in Ireland. *Journal of Advanced Nursing* **69**(5): 1037–1050.

Gerrish K, McDonnell, Kennedy F (2013) The development of a framework for the evaluating of nurse consultant roles in the UK. *Journal of Advanced Nursing* **69**(10): 2295–2308.

Hoddinott P, Craig K, MacLennan G, Boyers D, Vale L (2012) Process evaluation for the FEeding Support Team (FEST) randomised controlled feasibility trial of proactive and reactive telephone support for breastfeeding women living in disadvantaged areas. *BMJ Open* **2**: e001039.

Kendrick T, Simons L, Thompson C, Mynors-Wallis L, Lathlean J, Pickering R, Gerard K (2005) Trial of problem solving by community psychiatric nurses (CPNs) for anxiety, depression and life difficulties among general practice patients (the CPN-GP study). *Journal of Affective Disorders* **78**(Suppl. 1): S44.

Kemp L, Harris E, McMahon C, Matthey S, Vimpani G, Anderson T, Schmied V, Aslam H (2013) Benefits of psychosocial intervention and continuity of care by child and family health nurses in the pre- and postnatal period: process evaluation. *Journal of Advanced Nursing* **69**(8): 1850–1861.

Knowles S, McInnes E, Elliott D, Hardy J, Middleton S (2013) Evaluation of the implementation of a bowel management protocol in intensive care: effect on clinician practices and patient outcomes. *Journal of Clinical Nursing* **23**: 716–730.

Kramer M, Schmalenberg C (2005) Revising the essentials of magnetism tool: there is more to adequate staffing than numbers. *Journal of Nursing Administration* **35**(4): 188–198.

Long D, Mitchell M, Young J, Rickard C (2014) Assessing core outcomes in graduates: psychometric evaluation of the Paediatric Intensive Care Unit-Nursing Knowledge and Skills Test. *Journal of Advanced Nursing* **70**(3): 698–708.

MacPhee M (2009) Developing a practice-academic partnership logic model. *Nursing Outlook* **57**(3): 143–147.

Mann C, Delgado D, Horwood J (2014) Evaluation of internal peer-review to train nurses recruiting to randomized controlled trial – Internal Peer-review for Recruitment Training in Trials (InterPReTiT). *Journal of Advanced Nursing* **70**(4): 777–790.

Marchal B, van Bell S, van Olmen J, Hoeree T, Kegels G (2012) Is realist evaluation keeping its promise? A review of published empirical studies in the field of health systems research. *Evaluation* **18**: 122–212.

Marian F, Joost K, Saini K, von Ammon K, Thurneysen A, Busato A (2008) Patient satisfaction and side effects in primary care: an observational study comparing homeopathy and conventional medicine. *BMC Complementary and Alternative Medicine* **8**: 52. DOI: 10.1186/1472-6882-8-52.

McEvoy P, Richards D (2003) Critical realism: a way forward for evaluation research in nursing? *Journal of Advanced Nursing* **43**(4): 411–420.

McIlfatrick S, Hasson F (2013) Evaluating an holistic assessment tool for palliative care practice. *Journal of Clinical Nursing* **23**: 1064–1075.

Medical Research Council (MRC) (2000) A framework for development and evaluation of RCTs for complex interventions to improve health. MRC (http://www.mrc.ac.uk, accessed 15 April 2014).

Metzelthin S, Daniels R, van Rossum E, Cox K, Habets H, de Witte L, Kempen G (2013) A nurse-led interdisciplinary primary care approach to prevent disability among community-dwelling frail older people: a large-scale process evaluation. *International Journal of Nursing Studies* **50**(9): 1184–1196.

Naughton C, Drennan J, Hyde A, Allen D, O'Boyle K, Felle P, Butler M (2013) An evaluation of the appropriateness and safety of nurse and midwife prescribing in Ireland. *Journal of Advanced Nursing* **69**(7): 1478–1488.

Oakley A, Strange V, Bonell C, Allen E, Stephenson J, RIPPLE Study Team (2006) Process evaluation in randomised controlled trials of complex interventions. *British Medical Journal* **332**(7538): 413–416.

Pawson R (2006) *Evidence Based Policy: a realist perspective.* London, Sage.

Pawson R, Tilley N (1997) *Realistic Evaluation.* London, Sage.

Simons L, Lathlean J, Squire C (2008) Shifting the focus: sequential methods of analysis with qualitative data. *Qualitative Health Research* **18**(1): 120–132.

Sitaker M, Jernigan J, Ladd S, Patanian M (2008) Adapting logic models over time: the Washington State Health Disease and Stroke Prevention Program experience. *Preventing Chronic Disease* **5**(2): 1–8.

Subirana M, Long A, Greenhalgh J, Firth J (2014) A realist logic model of the links between nurse staffing and the outcomes of nursing. *Journal of Research in Nursing* **19**(1): 8–23.

Sutherland G, Hoey L, White V, Jefford M, Hegarty S (2008) How does a cancer education program impact on people with cancer and their family and friends? *Journal of Cancer Education* **23**: 126–132.

Stufflebeam D, Shinkfield A (2007) *Evaluation Theory, Models and Applications*. San Francisco, Jossey-Bass.

Thome M, Arnardottir S (2012) Evaluation of a family nursing intervention for distressed pregnant women and their partners: a single before and after study. *Journal of Advanced Nursing* **69**(4): 805–816.

Tolson D, McIntosh J, Loftus L, Cormie P (2007) Developing a managed clinical network in palliative care: a realistic evaluation. *International Journal of Nursing Studies* **44**(2): 183–195.

Weiss C (1998) *Evaluation*, 2nd Edition. Upper Saddle River, NJ, Prentice Hall.

Wilkinson SM, Love SB, Westcombe AM, Gambles MA, Burgess CC, Cargill A, Young T, Maher EJ, Ramirez AJ (2007) Effectiveness of aromatherapy massage in the management of anxiety and depression in patients with cancer: a multicenter randomized controlled trial. *Journal of Clinical Oncology* **25**(5): 532–539.

Williams L, Burton C, Rycroft-Malone J (2013) What works: a realist evaluation case study of intermediaries in infection control practice. *Journal of Advanced Nursing* **69**(4): 915–926.

Further reading

Astbury B, Leeuw F (2010) Unpacking black boxes: mechanisms and theory building in evaluation. *American Journal of Evaluation* **31**: 363–381.

Bauman A, Nutbeam D (2013) *Evaluation in a Nutshell: a practical guide to the evaluation of health promotion programs*. Sydney, McGraw-Hill.

Bryman A (2012) *Social Research Methods*. 4th edition. Oxford, Oxford University Press.

Hickey JV, Brosnan CA (2012) *Evaluation of Health Care Quality in Advanced Practice Nursing*. New York, Springer Publishing Company, LLC.

Martin J, McCormack B, Fitzsimons D, Sprig R (2011) Evaluation of a clinical leadership programme for nurse leaders. *Journal of Nursing Management* **20**(1): 72–80.

Websites

http://www.innonet.org/ – The website for the Innovation Network: Transforming Evaluation for Social Change. This contains evaluation tools and resources such as the Logic Model Builder and Evaluation Plan Builder specifically aimed at planning and evaluating programmes.

http://www.nhssurveys.org – A website for NHS trusts and patients who have been asked to complete a questionnaire. This survey coordination centre is run by Picker Institute Europe and coordinates the NHS acute, mental health and primary care patient survey programmes on behalf of the Care Quality Commission.

http://www.york.ac.uk/inst/crd/ – University of York: Centre for Reviews and Dissemination (CRD). CRD is part of the National Institute for Health Research (NIHR) and is a department of the University of York (United Kingdom). It provides research-based information about the effects of health and social care interventions via their databases and undertakes systematic reviews evaluating the research evidence on health and public health questions of national and international importance.

CHAPTER 23

Action Research

Julienne Meyer and Julie Cooper

Key points

- Action research is a research approach that involves interpreting and explaining social situations while implementing a change intervention.
- Action researchers adopt a participatory approach, involving participants in both the change and the research process.
- Both qualitative and quantitative methods of data collection may be employed during the three phases of action research: exploration, intervention and evaluation.
- Action researchers act as agents of change and need skills not only in research but also in change management and reflexivity.
- Although sometimes criticised as unscientific, action research has a real-world focus and directly seeks to improve practice.

PRINCIPLES OF ACTION RESEARCH

Action research is an approach to research rather than a specific method of data collection. The approach involves doing research *with* and *for* people (users and providers of service), in the context of its application, rather than undertaking research *on* them. The action researcher is seen as a facilitator and evaluator of change, whether the focus is on their own practice or the practice of others. Typically, in health and social care settings, action researchers begin by exploring and reflecting on patient and/or client experience and, through a process of feeding back findings to providers of services (formal and informal), go on to identify gaps in care that those engaged in the research would like to improve. Through an ongoing process of consultation and negotiation that gives democratic voice to all participants about the best way forwards, the action researcher then works to support and systematically monitor the process and outcomes of change. An eclectic approach to data collection is taken, using whatever methods best address the

The Research Process in Nursing, Seventh Edition. Edited by Kate Gerrish and Judith Lathlean.

Companion Website: www.wiley.com/go/gerrish/research

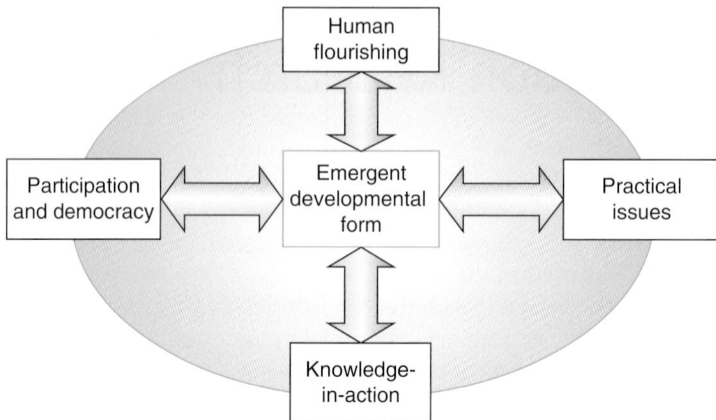

Figure 23.1 Characteristics of action research. Reproduced by permission Sage Publishing from Reason P, Bradbury H (2008) *The Sage Handbook of Action Research Participative Inquiry and Practice,* 2nd edition, London, Sage.

problem being researched, although often action research is written up in its rich contextual detail as a case study.

From case studies of action research, two types of knowledge can be generated – theoretical and practical. In contrast to other forms of research, the action researcher cannot predetermine the nature of the study, as it is dependent on the views and wishes of those with whom they are collaborating. Action researchers thus have to work in a flexible and responsive way to deal with issues as they naturally occur in practice. In so doing, they have to rely as much on their interpersonal skills as their research skills. This requires special thought to be given to how those involved in the research can be protected from harm. Gaining formal ethical approval for the study is not enough. It is important to agree a code of ethical practice at the start of the study that allows participants control over what change happens, how it is researched and how the findings are shared with others.

As nurses, we are particularly attracted to the underlying characteristics of action research (see Figure 23.1), namely, its emergent developmental form, its focus on practical issues, the creation of knowledge in action, its links to participation and democracy and its interest in human flourishing (Reason & Bradbury 2008). Action research typically blurs the boundaries between education, practice and research. If nothing else is gained as a result of the research, at least participants in the study should learn and develop from the process of being actively involved with it. Too much research is built around the researcher as expert with a 'hit-and-run' approach to data collection; at least, this approach aims to give something back (social change), at the same time as contributing to social knowledge.

COMMON MODELS OF WORKING WITH ACTION RESEARCH IN NURSING

Action research is not easily defined, as there are many different models of action research, largely influenced by the level of focus (own practice, collective practice of others, wider political events), degree of participation and vision of knowledge (Whitelaw *et al.* 2003). A systematic review of the uptake and design of action research in published nursing research, 2000–2005, by Munn-Giddings *et al.* (2008) found that 24 different terms were used to define the action research approach including *collaborative action research*, *emancipatory and enhancement action research*, *participatory research* and *evaluative action research*.

Reason and Bradbury (2008) view action research as a 'family of practices of inquiry' and offer the following broad definition:

> 'Action research is a participatory process concerned with developing practical knowing in the pursuit of worthwhile human purposes. It seeks to bring together action and reflection, theory and practice, in participation with others, in the pursuit of practical solutions to issues of pressing concern to people, and more generally the flourishing of individual persons and their communities' (Reason & Bradbury 2008: 4)

They suggest that for some, action research is primarily an individual affair concerned with how practice might be improved. For others, action research is more concerned with organisational development, whereas for a third group, it is more about how imbalances of power in society can be restored so that ordinary people can better manage their everyday lives. They argue that there can never be one 'right way' of doing action research and urge readers to value and embrace its many varied forms (Reason & Bradbury 2008). Soh *et al.* (2011) have suggested that while action research is a promising methodological approach to address clinical practice improvement, action researchers need to focus more on clinical outcomes and not just process and formative evaluation.

Action research is complex and it is not easy to categorise neatly any specific study into a particular type. However, typologies of action research can help us appreciate and articulate the complexity of action research, even if we would be unwise to label and categorise individual studies using them.

In our view, Hart and Bond (1995) provide one of the most accomplished typologies of action research. They suggest that there are seven criteria that not only distinguish action research from other methodologies but that also determine the range of approaches used in action research. They present a typology of action research identifying four basic types: experimental, organisational, professionalising and empowering (see Box 23.1). They suggest that each type embodies a different theoretical perspective on society.

Hart and Bond's (1995) typology provides a useful framework for critiquing individual studies and, in particular, for thinking about how concepts are operationalised, the features of particular settings and the contribution of the people within those settings to solutions.

It is worth noting that, over time, health-related action research appears to have moved away from 'experimental' to more 'empowering' models of research (Whitelaw *et al.* 2003). However, empowering models have to be used with care. Within an emancipatory action research project, practitioners, as co-researchers, need to make a commitment to the project in terms of reflecting on their practice and working towards changing the way they work. This can be very challenging, and researchers should not make the assumption that practitioners will be willing or able to engage at this level. Dewing (2005) found that the emancipatory approach originally used in the Admiral Nursing Competency Project did not suit the context or existing culture and a more participatory approach needed to evolve. Somekh (1994) reiterates this point, arguing that different occupational cultures can affect action research methodology. For this reason, she suggests that action research should be grounded in the values and discourse of the individual or group rather than rigidly adhering to a particular methodological perspective.

ACTION RESEARCH IN HEALTH-CARE PRACTICE

As an increasingly popular method of inquiry, action research is widely used in health care to investigate professional practice and patients' experience (Koshy *et al.* 2011). Action research is particularly useful when:

- no evidence exists to support or refute current practice
- there are poor knowledge, skills and attitudes to carry out evidence-based practice
- gaps have been identified in service provision
- services are underutilised or deemed inappropriate

Box 23.1 Action research typology

	Consensus model of society **Rational social management**		**Conflict model of society** **Structural change**	
Action research type: distinguishing criteria	**Experimental**	**Organisational**	**Professionalising**	**Empowering**
1. Educative base	Re-education	Re-education/ training	Reflective practice	Consciousness raising
	Enhancing social science/ administrative control and social change towards consensus	Enhancing managerial control and organisational change towards consensus	Enhancing professional control and individual's ability to control work situation	Enhancing user control and shifting balance of power; structural change towards pluralism
	Inferring relationship between behaviour and output, identifying causal factors in group dynamics	Overcoming resistance to change/ restructuring balance of power between managers and workers	Empowering professional groups; advocacy on behalf of patients/clients	Empowering oppressed groups
	Social scientific bias/researcher focused	Managerial bias/ client focused	Practitioner focused	User/practitioner focused
2. Individuals in groups	Closed group, controlled, selection made by researcher for purposes of measurement/ inferring relationship between cause and effect	Work groups and/ or minted groups of managers and workers	Professional(s) and/or (interdisciplinary) professional group/negotiated team boundaries	Fluid groupings, self-selecting or natural boundary or open/closed by negotiation
	Fixed membership	Selected membership	Shifting membership	Fluid membership
3. Problem focus	Problem emerges from the interaction of social science theory and social problems	Problem defined by most powerful group; some negotiation with workers	Problem defined by professional group, some negotiation with users	Emerging and negotiated definition of problem by less powerful group(s)

	Problem relevant for social science/ management interests	Problem relevant for management/ social science interests	Problem emerges from professional practice/ experience	Problem emerges from members' practice/ experience
	Success defined in terms of social sciences	Success defined by sponsors	Contested, professionally determined definitions of success	Competing definitions of success accepted and expected
4. Change intervention	Social science, experimental intervention to test theory and/or generate theory	Top-down, directed change towards predetermined aims	Professionally led, predefined, process led	Bottom-up, undetermined, process led
	Problem to be solved in terms of research aims	Problem to be solved in terms of management aims	Problem to be resolved in the interests of research-based practice and professionalisation	Problem to be explored as part of process of change, developing an understanding of meaning of issues in terms of problem and solution
5. Improvement and involvement	Towards controlled outcome and consensual definition of improvement	Towards tangible outcome and consensual definition of improvement	Towards improvement in practice defined by professionals and on behalf of users	Towards negotiated outcomes and pluralist definitions of improvement: account taken of vested interests
6. Cyclic processes	Research components dominant	Action and research components in tension; action dominated	Research and action components in tension, research dominated	Action components dominant
	Identifies causal processes that can be generalised	Identifies causal processes that are specific to problem context and/or can be generalised	Identifies causal processes that are specific to problem acid/or can be generalised	Changes course of events, recognition of multiple influences upon change
	Time limited, task focused	Discrete cycle, rationalist, sequential	Spiral of cycles, opportunistic, dynamic	Open ended, process driven

(*Continued*)

7. Research relationship, degree of collaboration	Experimenter/ respondents	Consultant/ researcher, respondent/ participants	Practitioner or researcher/ collaborators	Practitioner researcher/ co-researchers/ co-change agents
	Outside researcher as expert/research funding	Client pays an outside consultant – 'they who pay the piper call the tune'	Outside resources and/or internally generated	Outside resources and/or internally generated
	Differentiated roles	Differentiated roles	Merged roles	Shared roles

Reproduced by permission of the Open University Press from Hart E, Bond M (1995) *Action Research for Health and Social Care: a guide to practice*. Buckingham, Open University Press, pp 40–43.

- new roles are being develop and implemented
- working across traditional conflicting boundaries

More recently, it has been suggested that action research could help nurses better articulate the nature of their practice to address the invisibility of nursing work and to illuminate the significance of their contributions to health care and society (Canam 2008). It has also been suggested that it could have a more significant role in knowledge translation (Kitson 2009).

Action research has much to offer health-care practice. Munn-Giddings *et al.* (2008) found that action research has a strong presence within nursing research but mainly focused on organisational/professional development/education settings. Participation of practitioners within the research process is very strong, though few studies involved service users and/or carers. While many action research studies highlight the difficulties of changing practice (Meyer *et al.* 2000), there have been some more notable successes, for instance, Kilbride (2011).

Exemplar study 1: Local level

Kilbride (2011) looked at the lessons learnt from setting up a new inpatient stroke service in a large NHS London teaching hospital. Key participants included members of the multi-professional stroke team and support staff, the hospital management team and patient/informal carer representatives. Mixed methods were used to generate data. These included focus groups, in-depth interviews, documentary analysis, audits and participant observation. Prior to the study, there was no specialist stroke service, and stroke care was fragmented, uncoordinated and spread over 18 wards. Local and national stroke audits showed there was much room for improvement in care provided with the hospital being placed in the bottom 5% in the country. Over the course of the study and beyond, a culture of sustained service improvement emerged, demonstrated by consistent placement in top 5% in the National Sentinel Stroke Audit (Clinical Effectiveness and Evaluation Unit, 2002, 2004, 2006). This remarkable success of moving from the bottom to the top resulted in the unit receiving a national award for clinical service redesign in 2005.

The success of Kilbride's (2011) action research can be seen in the learning from the systematic monitoring of the emergent processes in the study. Four main themes emerged from the process that had contributed to the local success: building an interprofessional stroke team, developing practice-based knowledge and skills in stroke care, valuing the central role of the nurse in stroke care and creating an organisational climate to support improvement. Whereas the existing body of knowledge had shown stroke units to be linked to better patient outcomes, these findings address a gap in knowledge on how to set up an effective stroke unit. In addition to providing useful practical knowledge, the study also adds to theoretical knowledge by showing how the emergent findings linked to the development of a community of practice. The literature suggests that communities of practice have a key role to play in implementing evidence-based practice (Fitzgerald *et al.* 2006), and this study provides some supporting evidence to this fact and reveals for the first time the practical knowledge and skills required to develop this style of working.

While action research predominately focuses on a local level, as in the aforementioned study, it has also been used to develop national guidance. Interestingly, this also took a community of practice approach.

Exemplar study 2: National level

The principles of appreciative action research (Egan & Lancaster 2005) were used to inform a UK-wide initiative (*My* Home Life (MHL)) to promote quality of life in care homes for older people. Appreciative action research is a positive approach to action research that focuses on what people 'want' and 'what works', rather than the solution of problems. MHL began in 2006 as a small project to synthesise the literature on best practice in care homes (NCHR&D Forum 2007) and is now seen as a social movement for quality improvement in care homes that has crossed national and international borders. Funded by a variety of different sources over time, the MHL team has worked collaboratively with the care homes sector to develop an appreciative, evidence-based and relationship-centred vision for best practice that focuses on making a difference to the lives of those living, dying, visiting and working in care homes. Together, they have co-created and disseminated to 18,000 care homes a range of creative resources (research reports, briefings, bulletins, posters, DVDs, etc.) designed to stimulate dialogue about best practice. The focus is on sharing real stories (from the perspective of residents, relatives and staff) about what works in care homes. A website has been developed to help connect care homes with each other and to share best practice (www.myhomelife.org.uk). In addition, a leadership support and community development programme has been co-produced with care home managers to help facilitate quality improvement (Owen *et al.* 2012). As a bottom-up initiative, MHL has directly influenced the recent White Paper on Care and Support (HM Government 2012). By sticking to the principles of appreciative action research, MHL demonstrates the powerful impact that such research approaches can have both locally and nationally on policy and practice alike.

THE ROLE OF THE RESEARCHER IN ACTION RESEARCH

Critics suggest that action research is no different to what goes on in everyday practice, for example, practice development, medical audit, clinical governance and good management. However, as stated before, the essential difference is the focus on systematically evaluating the process and outcomes of change and reflecting on, and disseminating, findings in relation to what is already known about the topic under study. If, as Stringer (1999) suggests, research is

> 'systematic and rigorous inquiry or investigation that enables people to understand the nature of problematic events or phenomena' (Stringer 1999: 5)

then the role of the researcher in action research is to make this happen. Modifying ideas from Mills (2003) in relation to teaching, we would

Reflection activity

Think about your own area of practice. Identify a research question that could be addressed through an action research study. Why do you think action research would be an appropriate methodology to answer your research question?

argue that it involves a process of working with participants to:

- describe the problem and area of focus
- define the factors involved, for example, the community and agencies involved, the health-care setting within its historical and sociopolitical context, current practice, patient, practitioner and practice outcomes
- develop research questions
- describe the intervention or innovation to be implemented
- develop a timeline for implementation
- describe the membership of the action research group
- develop a list of resources to implement the plan
- describe the data to be collected (qualitative and quantitative)
- develop a data collection and analysis plan
- gain ethical approval and permission to undertake the study
- select appropriate tools of inquiry
- carry out the plan (implementation, data collection, data analysis)
- reflect on and report the results, for example, the final report, professional and academic journals and local newsletters

Not all practitioners have the skills to undertake research, and it is important that they seek adequate levels of support. Action research is often undertaken as part of academic study and supervised by colleagues in higher education. Given its emphasis on learning, action research provides an ideal opportunity for the different agencies involved to personally benefit from the process, for example, submitting work in relation to the study to contribute to academic qualifications. However, academic study is not for all, and other types of support might be more appropriate. There are a number of toolkits for action research (see Hart and Bond (1995) for a good example).

Reflection activity

How is the role of the researcher different in action research to many other forms of research? What specific skills does an action researcher require that are additional to the skills of data collection and analysis needed for other forms of research?

ETHICAL ISSUES

An important role of the researcher in action research is to ensure the well-being of participants. This is normally achieved by going through a process of formal ethical approval. However, the non-predictive nature of action research means that it is additionally important to mutually agree an ethical code of practice at the start of the study. Winter and Munn-Giddings (2001) highlight a number of ethical issues and principles of procedure. First, they emphasise the importance of maintaining a professional relationship, guided by a duty of care and respect for the individual regardless of gender, age, ethnicity, etc., along with a respect for cultural diversity and individual dignity, as well as protection from harm. This last principle is part of any social researcher's role, in addition to the need for informed consent and honesty. However, Winter and Munn-Giddings (2001) suggest that there are other principles of procedure that should be followed in action research (see Box 23.2).

Having an ethical code of practice does not negate the additional need for research governance and formal ethical approval for action research. However, these quality processes are made all the more complex by the action researcher not being able to say in advance what the research will do. Action research proposals need to be written in collaboration with participants, often as co-applicants, with an inbuilt degree of flexibility. The action researcher should indicate the likely course of the study, specify the need for flexibility and enter into open and ongoing dialogue with funders and ethical committees to seek approval for emergent changes in design.

Box 23.2 Ensuring ethical practice: principles of procedure for action research

- Make sure discussions are fully documented.
- Establish procedures for taking joint decisions.
- Ensure the work of the project remains 'visible' to all participants.
- Check back and get any interpretations authorised before wider circulation.
- Enable participants to amend their contribution before its circulation.
- Ensure progress reports and invite suggestions on future developments.
- Differentiate between what is confidential to participants and intended for wider publication.
- Negotiate acceptable rules of confidentiality.
- Give participants the right to withdraw material containing any reference that may identify them.
- Negotiate in advance how disagreements will be resolved.
- Ensure participants seek the group's permission to use material for academic study.
- Draw up clear statement of principles of procedure, early in the work.

Adapted from Winter R, Munn-Giddings C (2001) *A Handbook for Action Research in Health and Social Care*. London, Routledge, pp 220–224.

METHODS OF DATA COLLECTION

While action research is often written up as a case study and tends to draw on qualitative methods (Meyer 2000), an eclectic approach to data collection is taken. Usually, data collection focuses on three stages of the inquiry (exploration, intervention and evaluation) and, where possible, involves participants, as co-researchers, in the design and execution of the study.

Exploration phase

In the exploratory phase of the study, action researchers gather data to explore the nature of the problem and focus of the study. Data are typically generated through questionnaires, interviews and focus groups in order to seek participant opinion as to what needs to change. If the action researcher is an outsider, this phase often includes some participant observation, in order that the researcher can familiarise themselves with the context and establish good working relationships with participants. It helps if the action researcher has some familiarity with the setting, as the clinical credibility of the action researcher can aid entry into the field. Through a process of feeding back findings to participants, the focus of the study (action) is negotiated. The end of the exploration phase usually involves gathering data in relation to the focus of the study in order to establish a baseline from which to measure change over time. Typically, this involves data being generated from audits of practice.

Intervention phase

During this phase, a number of action research cycles usually emerge, as spirals of activity. Each action research cycle comprises a period of planning, acting, observing, reflecting and replanning. Action research should offer the capacity to deal with a number of problems at the same time, and often, spirals of activity lead to other spin-off spirals of further work. It would be wrong to give the impression of order and linearity, although action research is often written up in this way so as not to confuse the reader. During this period of intense activity, it is important to monitor the process of change and reflect on learning being gained.

Data are usually generated through participant observation methods, reflective journals, diaries, field notes and narratives of practice. Throughout the intervention phase, interim findings are fed back to participants to guide their action. Meanwhile, the action researcher should keep self-reflective field notes throughout the study in order to acknowledge their own subjectivity and demonstrate freedom from bias. It is important that they not only represent the views of all participants, including their own, but that they are also clear about whose voice they are representing and when.

Evaluation phase

There is no neat end to an action research project, as often participants wish to continue with the change processes. However, action researchers need to withdraw from the field to analyse and reflect on what has been learnt, in the context of the wider body of knowledge. Before leaving the field, they typically repeat baseline measures to see if change has occurred over time and invite participants to reflect on what has been achieved (or not) and their explanations for this. In the evaluation phase, it is possible to analyse existing documents and protocols to enhance findings and further set the study in context. Most importantly, all findings should be shared with participants to allow them to comment critically on whether they feel their views have been represented adequately and for them to check that they are happy for the material to be shared with a wider audience.

REFLEXIVITY AND ACTION RESEARCH

Reflexivity is a key component of action research practice. Although it is advocated in the research and reflexivity literature that researchers should write themselves into their research accounts, this is often missing from published papers and reports, with those that do include it mainly doing so to enhance the perceived rigour of their studies. Cooper (2013), after undertaking a 3-year action research study with two rehabilitation wards for older people in a healthcare organisation, identified the importance of this aspect of action research in relation to identifying the impact of action research on the researcher and how it can help to inform the study itself.

Feeling that something was missing from her own research account, Cooper (2013) undertook a reflexive analysis of her 3 years of field notes and a review of the action research literature. This process identified difficult, complex and chaotic action researcher journeys riddled with struggles and challenges in relation to working with competing stakeholder agendas, balancing control and participation, managing multiple roles and experiencing uncertainty. These findings were consistent with the writings of other action researchers; however, what Cooper (2013) also identified was the personal impact that experiencing and trying to manage these difficulties and challenges can have on the researcher. The analysis identified a vulnerable and highly emotional experience resulting from a need, at times, to sacrifice personal values and beliefs, the disruption of pre-existing relationships, identity conflicts, intrusion into personal lives, the process of self-reflection and a roller-coaster ride of ups and downs. She highlighted the emotional context of action research and recognised a need for an ethic of care for action researchers, including the provision of support mechanisms that enable emotions to be contained and researchers to feel safe within the research process.

In taking this further, Cooper (2012) identified from her own reflexive analysis that the emotions experienced by researchers can be a reflection of what is going on in the field of study and that support mechanisms are also required that have the ability to contain emotions and help researchers explore their origins so that they can understand them and utilise them to further inform the study itself. She concludes by arguing that the emotional context of action research

> '...needs to be recognised and legitimised as an important aspect of the research process to ensure that those involved in it are supported throughout the process, can capitalise on its potential to gain further understandings, and can prepare themselves adequately for the undertaking of such studies'. (Cooper 2012: 17)

For this to be achieved, she calls for more reflexive accounts of the personal experience of undertaking action research to be written to encourage wider engagement with this critical aspect of action research practice.

ASSESSING QUALITY

What makes action research data trustworthy? Waterman *et al.* (2001) provide 20 questions for assessing action research proposals and projects (see Box 23.3). These criteria were later modified by Greenhalgh *et al.* (2004), but others would question the value of even having such standards or criteria (Lyotard 1979). Reason (2006) argues that quality in action research is not about getting it right, but on stimulating open discussion about the choices being made – for instance, being clear in the first-person sense, being collaborative in the second-person sense and raising the wider debate in a third-person sense. For him, validity includes the practical, the political and the moral, rather than viewing validity as a form of policing research. He suggests the questions that need to be addressed are: 'What are the choices we are making, and are they the best choices?' and 'Can we be transparent about these choices in our reporting of our work?' (Reason 2006: 199).

Reflection activity

Reflexivity is important in the action research process. What strategies can the action researcher use to capture how their own actions, values and perceptions may impact upon the research setting and the research participants?

Box 23.3 Questions for assessing action research proposals and projects

1 Is there a clear statement of the aims and objectives of each stage of the research?
2 Was the action research relevant to practitioners and/or users?
3 Were the phases of the project clearly outlined?
4 Were the participants and stakeholders clearly described and justified?
5 Was consideration given to the local context while implementing change?
6 Was the relationship between researchers and participants adequately considered?
7 Was the project managed appropriately?
8 Were ethical issues encountered, and how were they dealt with?
9 Was the study adequately funded/supported?
10 Was the length and timetable of the project realistic?
11 Were data collected in a way that addressed the research issue?
12 Were steps taken to promote the rigour of the findings?
13 Were data analyses sufficiently rigorous?
14 Was the study design flexible and responsive?
15 Are there clear statements of the findings and outcomes of each phase of the study?
16 Do the researchers link the data that are presented to their own commentary and interpretation?
17 Is the connection with an existing body of knowledge made clear?
18 Is there discussion of the extent to which aims and objectives were achieved at each stage?
19 Are the findings of the study transferable?
20 Have the authors articulated the criteria upon which their own work is to be read/judged?

Reproduced with permission of Department of Health from Waterman H, Tillen D, Dickson R, de Koning K (2001) Action research: a systematic review and guidance for assessment. *Health Technology Assessment Monograph* **5**: 23. London, Department of Health, pp 48–50.

In addition to addressing trustworthiness of data, it is also important to consider their transferability. Action research is often written up as a case study. As such, the findings are reported in their rich contextual detail in order that the reader can judge the relevance to their own practice situation. Sharp (1998) suggests that case studies also lend themselves well to theoretical generalisation, but acknowledges that this is not always attempted. This opens up debates about whether there is any general learning to be gained from specific cases. Bassey (1999) advocates that case study researchers should have more confidence in making fuzzy generalisations about their work. By clearly stating from single cases what researchers consider to be 'possible', 'likely', or 'unlikely' in similar contexts, they protect themselves from the charge of being engaged in trivial pursuit. Meyer *et al.* (2000), drawing on findings that compared a single case of action research with those generated by a systematic review of action research, caution against ignoring the findings from the single case. They argue that the findings from a single case of action research more closely reflect reality and are potentially more valid and meaningful to others. These issues relating to case study research are examined in more detail in Chapter 21.

RESEARCH AS AN AGENT OF CHANGE

It could be argued that the ultimate aim of all research is to improve practice. However, most research relies on practitioners to implement findings. Slowly, the limitations to this segregated approach of research and development are being recognised. A report describing a systematic review of the literature on the spread and sustainability of innovations in health services delivery and organisations (Greenhalgh *et al.* 2004) recommended 'participatory action research' along with 'realistic evaluation' as the way forwards. They saw these approaches as being based on a 'whole-systems' approach, inasmuch as they are:

- theory driven
- process rather than 'package oriented'
- participatory
- collaborative and coordinated
- addressed using common definitions, measures and tools
- multidisciplinary and multimethod
- meticulously detailed
- ecological (relational to people and context)

Whole-systems approaches to change management are now favoured, as they recognise the complexity and inevitability of change.

Clearly, in action research, research is being used as an agent of change. This implies that the action researcher not only needs research skills but also an understanding of change and skills in change management. The literature about change management is large and not easy to access. Sometimes, change is deliberate, a product of conscious reasoning and actions. This type of change is called 'planned change'. In contrast, change sometimes unfolds in an apparently spontaneous and unplanned way. This type of change is known as 'emergent change'.

According to Isles and Sutherland (2001), change can be emergent in two ways: first, managers can make decisions based on unspoken, and sometimes unconscious, assumptions about the organisation, its environment and the future; and, second, external factors (such as the economy, competitors' behaviour and political climate) or internal features (such as the relative power of different interest groups, distribution of knowledge and uncertainty) can influence the change in directions outside the control of managers. This highlights the need to identify, explore and if necessary challenge the assumptions that underlie decisions. Further, it is important to understand that organisational change is a process that can be facilitated. Isles and Sutherland (2001) conclude that it is vital to recognise that organisation-level change is not fixed or linear in nature but contains an important emergent element. Gibbons *et al.* (1994) suggest that there is a need to break away from linear thinking to more flexible and creative systems that allow true expertise to flourish. As can be seen from what has already been written earlier, action researchers take account of these issues in both the design and execution of their studies.

ADVANTAGES AND DISADVANTAGES OF ACTION RESEARCH

Waterman *et al.* (2001) identify eight categories of pivotal factors that can be used to demonstrate the strengths and limitations of action research:

- Participation
- Key persons
- Action researcher–participant relationship
- Real-world focus
- Resources
- Research methods
- Project process and management
- Knowledge

They argue that for each of these factors, there are opposing aspects that help to provide possible avenues for reconceptualising understanding of the process of action research in health care and that offer ideas for its further development. These issues can be summarised into a number of advantages and disadvantages, which are presented in Box 23.4.

Reflection activity

Consider the disadvantages of action research listed in Box 23.4. What can the action researcher do to try to overcome some of these disadvantages?

CONCLUSION

This chapter has explored the nature of action research and demonstrated its value at the 'D' end of the research and development spectrum. It has identified common models of working with action research in nursing and suggests caution in adopting one particular model. It has reflected on the role of the researcher in action research, highlighting the need for a mutually agreed ethical code of practice. In addition, it has described the methods of data collection in relation to three phases of action research (exploration, intervention and evaluation) and given

Box 23.4 Advantages and disadvantages of action research

Advantages	Disadvantages
In situations where: • No evidence exists to support or refute current practice • There is poor knowledge, skills and attitudes to carry out evidence-based practice • Gaps have been identified in service provision • Services are underused or deemed inappropriate • New roles are being developed and implemented • Working across traditional conflicting boundaries	• Not viewed as science • Findings not generalisable • Vulnerability of participants • Depends on collaboration • Difficult to achieve and sustain change • Feedback can be threatening • Change hard to measure • Poor development of theory

some consideration to the idea of research being an agent of change. Finally, consideration has been given to the advantages and disadvantages of action research. In conclusion, it would appear that action research has much to offer health services research, and it is suggested that nurses are making a significant contribution.

References

Bassey M (1999) *Case Study Research in Educational Settings*. Buckingham, Open University Press.

Canam CJ (2008) The link between nursing discourses and nurses' silence: implications for a knowledge-based discourse for nursing practice, *Advances in Nursing Science* **31**(4): 296–307.

Clinical Effectiveness and Evaluation Unit (2002) *National Sentinel Audit of Stroke 2001/2*. Report for site code 175. Prepared on behalf of the Intercollegiate Stroke Group by Clinical Effectiveness and Evaluation Unit, London, Royal College of Physicians.

Clinical Effectiveness and Evaluation Unit (2004) *National Sentinel Audit of Stroke 2004*. Report for site code 230. Prepared on behalf of the Intercollegiate Stroke Group by Clinical Effectiveness and Evaluation Unit, London. Royal College of Physicians.

Clinical Effectiveness and Evaluation Unit (2006) *National Sentinel Audit of Stroke 2006*. Report for site code 230. Prepared on behalf of the Intercollegiate Stroke Group by Clinical Effectiveness and Evaluation Unit, London, Royal College of Physicians.

Cooper J, Meyer J, Holman C (2013) Advancing knowledge on practice change: linking facilitation to the senses framework. *Journal of Clinical Nursing* **22**: 1729–1737.

Dewing J (2005) Admiral nursing competency project: practice development and action research. *Journal of Clinical Nursing* **14**: 695–703.

Egan TM, Lancaster CM (2005) Comparing appreciative inquiry to action research: OD practitioner perspectives. *Organization Development Journal* **23**(2): 29–49.

Fitzgerald L, Dopson S, Ferlie E, Locock L (2006) Knowledge in action. In: Dopson S, Fitzgerald L (eds) *Knowledge to Action? Evidence-based Healthcare in Context*. Oxford, Oxford University Press, pp 155–181.

Gibbons M, Limoges C, Nowotny H, Schwartzman S, Scott P, Trow M (1994) *The New Production of Knowledge: the dynamics of science and research in contemporary societies*. London, Sage.

Greenhalgh T, Robert G, Bate P, Kyriakidou O, Macfarlane F, Peacock R (2004) *How to Spread Good Ideas: a systematic review of the literature on diffusion, dissemination and sustainability of innovations in health service delivery and organization*. Report for the National Co-ordinating Centre for NHS Service Delivery and Organisation R & D (NCCSDO). London, London School of Hygiene and Tropical Medicine.

Hart E, Bond M (1995) *Action Research for Health and Social Care: a guide to practice*. Buckingham, Open University Press.

HM Government (2012) *Caring for Our Future: reforming care and support*. White Paper presented to Parliament by the Secretary of State for Health. London, The Stationery Office.

Isles V, Sutherland K (2001) *Managing Change in the NHS. Organisational Change: a review for health care managers, professionals and researchers*. Report for the National Co-ordinating Centre for NHS Service Delivery and Organisation R & D (NCCSDO). London, London School of Hygiene and Tropical Medicine.

Kilbride C (2011) Developing theory and practice: creation of a community of practice through action research produced excellence in stroke care. *Journal of Interprofessional Care* **25**(2): 91–97.

Kitson A L (2009) The need for systems change: reflections on knowledge translation and organizational change. *Journal of Advanced Nursing* **65**: 217–228.

Koshy E, Koshy V, Waterman H (2011) *Action Research in Healthcare*. London, Sage.

Lyotard JF (1979) *The Postmodern Condition: a report on knowledge*. (trans. Bennington G, Massimi B). Manchester, Manchester University Press.

Meyer J (2000) Using qualitative methods in health related action research. *British Medical Journal* **320**: 178–181.

Meyer J, Spilsbury K, Prieto J (2000) Comparison of findings from a single case in relation to those from a systematic review of action research. *Nurse Researcher* **7**(2): 37–53.

Mills GE (2003) *Action Research: a guide for the teacher researcher*. Upper Saddle River, Merrill/Prentice Hall.

Munn-Giddings C, McVicar A, Smith L (2008). Systematic review of the uptake and design of action research in published nursing research, 2000–2005. *Journal of Research in Nursing* **13**(6): 465–477.

National Care Home Research and Development Forum (NCHR&D) (2007) *My Home Life: quality of life in care homes: literature review*. London, Help the Aged.

Owen T, Meyer J (2012) *My Home Life: promoting quality of life in care homes*. York, Joseph Rowntree Foundation.

Reason P (2006) Choice and quality in action research practice. *Journal of Management Inquiry* **15**(2): 187–203.

Reason P, Bradbury H (2008) 'Introduction' In: Reason P, Bradbury H (eds) *The Sage Handbook of Action Research Participative Inquiry and Practice.* 2nd edition. London, Sage.

Sharp K (1998) The case for case studies in nursing research: the problem of generalisation. *Journal of Advanced Nursing* **27**: 785–789.

Soh KL, Davidson PM, Leslie G, Bin Abdul Rahman A (2011) Action research studies in the intensive care setting: a systematic review. *International Journal of Nursing Studies* **48**(2): 258–68.

Somekh B (1994) Inhabiting each other's castles: towards knowledge and mutual growth though collaboration. *Educational Action Research Journal* **2**(3): 357–81.

Stringer E (1999) *Action Research.* 2nd edition. London, Sage.

Waterman H, Tillen D, Dickson R, de Koning K (2001) Action research: a systematic review and guidance for assessment. *Health Technology Assessment Monograph* **5**: 23.

Whitelaw S, Beattie A, Balogh R, Watson J (2003) *A Review of the Nature of Action Research.* Welsh Assembly Government, Sustainable Health Action Research Programme.

Winter R, Munn-Giddings C (2001) *A Handbook for Action Research in Health and Social Care.* London, Routledge.

Further reading

Reason P, Bradbury H (eds) (2008) *The Sage Handbook of Action Research Participative Inquiry and Practice.* 2nd edition. London, Sage.

Websites

http://www.esri.mmu.ac.uk/carnnew/ – Collaborative Action Research Network, based at Manchester Metropolitan University, provides a network of action researchers linked to the International Journal Educational Action Research.

http://www.aral.com.au/resources/index.html – Site with papers associated with 'areol', action research and evaluation on line, an online course available on the web or by email.

CHAPTER 24

Practitioner Research

Bridie Kent

Key points

- Practitioner research addresses issues and problems that arise in professional practice. It is undertaken by practitioners and generally seeks to bring about change or influence policy in the practice setting.
- Practitioner research follows the same processes as other researches in its quest to generate new knowledge; however, the researchers are different in that their 'insider' role as practitioners in the setting where the research is undertaken provides a closeness to the research setting that 'outsiders' rarely achieve or need.
- Practitioner researchers need to reflect throughout the research process on the impact that their closeness to the research setting has had on the research.
- Practitioner research raises a number of ethical issues that arise from the practitioner researcher's dual roles as researcher and practitioner.

INTRODUCTION

Nurses and other health-care professionals are in a fortunate position in that their places of work are also locations where research can, and should, be conducted. Health care is rapidly changing and dynamic; working in such an environment provides fertile ground for research questions to be identified and for research to be undertaken. Practice settings provide opportunities to identify gaps in evidence that clinicians need to inform their practice and things that really matter to patients and carers.

Whereas many leading nurse researchers are based in university departments, an increasing number of nurses who work in practice settings also undertake research. This may be because engaging in research is a formal aspect of the nurse's role, for example, in the United Kingdom, nurse consultants as advanced practice nurses are expected to undertake their own research. However, many practising nurses and other

The Research Process in Nursing, Seventh Edition. Edited by Kate Gerrish and Judith Lathlean.

Companion Website: www.wiley.com/go/gerrish/research

health-care professionals who undertake research do so as part of an academic course or because they are passionate about answering research questions that arise from their day-to-day practice.

There is a sense in which all registered nurses who undertake research could be considered to be practitioner researchers, irrespective of whether they work in a university or health-care setting. Nurses who undertake research are likely to share a language, values and an outlook that have been shaped by their professional training and subsequent work as a nurse – and this shared understanding of being a nurse will influence the research they undertake. However, in this chapter, the term practitioner researcher is used to refer to those nurses (or other health-care professionals) who work in practice settings and who undertake research in that setting. The research undertaken by these nurses is referred to as practitioner research.

Practitioner research has been defined by McLeod (cited by Shaw 2005) as research by practitioners for the purpose of advancing their own practice. Shaw does, however, consider that additional components should be included in the definition, such as the broader policy or academic rationales for the research as well as the usefulness of this form of research to practice. Gillman and Swain (2006) provide a fuller definition of practitioner research:

> 'Research concerned with issues and problems that arise in professional practice. It is conducted by practitioners, and aims to bring about change, or influence policy in the practice arena. Practitioner research provides a framework for formulating practice knowledge and allows such knowledge to be disseminated to other professionals'. (Gillman & Swain 2006: 233)

Practitioner research follows the same principles and processes as any other research in its quest to generate new knowledge; however, the researchers are different in that their 'insider' role as practitioners in the setting where the research will be undertaken provides a closeness to the research setting that 'outsiders' rarely achieve or need. In this chapter, the issues pertinent to practitioner research will be explored so that these similarities and differences are made clear in order to help enhance the success of this valuable approach to research.

BACKGROUND TO PRACTITIONER RESEARCH

The impetus for practitioner research

Practitioner research is, by its very name, undertaken by practitioners and aims to explore a specific aspect of a service or setting. Campbell (2007) suggests that this practice-based research approach is commonly seen in education, social and health-care settings, and it has an 'improvement' focus, rather than the more traditional one of 'proving'. The impetus for practitioner research often arises from the need for greater understanding of the context in which care is provided and how it might be improved or the need to gain insight into the patient experience in order that their needs might be met more effectively. For example, Clare Warnock, a practice development nurse working in a cancer centre, undertook a qualitative study to explore the experiences of patients with malignant spinal cord compression leading up to diagnosis and during their admission to the cancer centre along with their thoughts about their future. Whereas the findings from this study added to knowledge about an under-researched area of practice, it also provided a clear indication of how services could be improved in the cancer centre to support early discharge planning and family involvement in meeting patients' priorities for care (Warnock & Tod 2014). Thus, new insights gained through practitioner research have the potential to provide genuine practical application of evidence.

Dadds (2014), writing in the field of education, highlights the moral dimensions of practitioner research, which are highly relevant in health care. She sees the orientation towards democracy and social justice as drivers to further inquiry and questioning about our work, which include 'facing up to the values embedded in our thinking'. Nurses are encouraged to develop and foster an enquiring culture in which critical thinking is an essential attribute. Heaslip (2008) argues that this is the ability to think in a systematic and logical manner with openness to question and reflect on the reasoning process used to ensure safe nursing practice and quality care. Practitioner researchers optimise this questioning ethos to try to gain a greater understanding, or clarity, of the everyday world. Generally, the inquiry begins with simple questions being asked such as 'why did this happen?' or 'how will new evidence impact on our current practice?'. Such critical questioning and reflection on practice are a crucial component of practitioner research in order to support professional change and the uptake of research findings into practice.

Practitioner researchers mobilise a number of key attributes as part of the research process, including questioning, expertise in gathering and processing information, passion about the value of nursing (or their own area of practice) to patient care and the ability to put essential insider knowledge to good effect. All these, combined with expertise in research methods, mean that practitioner researchers are well placed to contribute to significant and sustainable changes in practice, policy and education.

Practitioner research approaches

Evidence that can be used to inform practice has grown in amount and in complexity over the past decade (Bucknall *et al.* 2008). Even the traditionally used 'hierarchy of evidence' has changed to reflect this. Whereas in the 1990s, the evidence considered to be most relevant was that generated from quantitative research methods (in particular the randomised controlled trial) and studies focused on determining the effectiveness of interventions, things are now very different. Practising healthcare professionals ask different types of clinical questions that require a broader range of research approaches, such as qualitative methodologies, narrative research, action research and economic analyses. Thus, practitioner researchers are presented with the challenge of choosing the right methodology for the question being asked and require the skills to do this effectively. The perceived separation between quantitative and qualitative approaches is less dominant in the practitioner researcher's world, and the application of methods from critical science, such as action research, or adopting a mixed methodology may be best for this form of 'real-world inquiry'.

Focus of practitioner research

Practitioner research is largely focused on finding real-life solutions to practice-related issues. As Gillman and Swain's (2006) definition quoted earlier in this chapter points out, practitioner research is concerned with bringing about change or influencing policy relevant to practice settings. This focus inevitably raises questions about the relationship between practitioner research and activities such as practice development, quality improvement, audit and service evaluation, each of which generally involve data collection and analysis and often lead to some form of change in practice settings. The boundaries between these different activities are inevitably blurred. However, in referring back to the definition of research given in Chapter 1, research is concerned with the generation of new knowledge that has applicability beyond the immediate setting in which the research was undertaken. Practitioner research is therefore concerned with both investigating local practice with a view to informing or bringing about change and with generating new knowledge that is of relevance beyond the setting in which the research was undertaken. In contrast, practice development, quality improvement, audit and service evaluation are concerned with addressing local issues and gathering evidence to inform local decision-making (Gerrish *et al.* 2009). This differentiation is important not just in terms of the purpose and outcome of the activity but also in terms of ethics and governance. Practitioner researchers will need to seek approval from the appropriate research ethics committee and comply with research governance requirements, whereas practice development, audit and service evaluation projects will need to comply with any local clinical governance requirements in the organisation where the work is to be undertaken (see Chapter 10).

Practitioner researchers are also well placed to undertake research focusing on the implementation of research findings into practice. Research evidence often requires tailoring or modification to suit the local setting, and by working in that setting, practitioner researchers are well placed to lead such work. As discussed in Chapter 38, there is also a need to generate evidence about which strategies may be effective in promoting the use of research evidence in practice. Through examining the knowledge translation process, including the questions being asked and the audiences involved, the practitioner researcher can gain valuable insights into approaches that can be used successfully to bridge the gap between research and practice. Credibility is important, and since the practitioner researcher will be very familiar with the setting and the issues being investigated and will generally be an insider from the perspectives of colleagues and peers, they are well placed to undertake such research.

INSIDER AND OUTSIDER POSITIONS

Reed and Proctor (1995) proposed a 'position continuum' in which a range of positions that a practitioner researcher can adopt is presented (see Box 24.1). *Insiders* are primarily researchers who are engaged with practice or the workplace and conduct research in that setting. *Outsiders* are those who have little or no engagement with practice. Drake and Heath (2011)

Box 24.1 Outsider and insider continuum

Position	'Outsider', primarily a researcher with no or little engagement with practice	'Insider', primarily engaged with practice and carrying out research into this practice
Aims	To explore a social phenomenon (nursing) in order to contribute to the body of social science knowledge	To solve a critical problem, thereby contributing to the body of nursing knowledge
Access	Choice of research setting wide, but contact transient and superficial	Setting limited by practice contacts, but this is sustained and intimate
Role	Researcher is a guest	Researcher is a member
Design and planning	Informed by knowledge of research methods	Informed by knowledge of practice
Analysis	Does not share taken-for granted assumptions and adopts a naïve stance towards the data	Shares taken-for-granted assumptions and needs to reflectively adopt a naïve stance towards the data
Contribution	To academic community and the development of theory	To colleagues and the academic community and the development of practice

Adapted from Reed J and Procter S (1995) *Practitioner Research in Health Care*. London, Chapman and Hall. Reproduced from Reed J (2010) Practitioner research. In: Gerrish K, Lacey A (eds) *The Research Process in Nursing* (p 275) with permission from Wiley Blackwell.

undertook a strengths, weaknesses, opportunities and threats (SWOT) analysis of the benefits of insider research and identified the main challenges to be:

- internal resistance to the process of research
- reliability and validity
- identity as a researcher
- work–research balance, loyalties and values
- relationships with colleagues could become contentious
- power

(Drake & Health 2011: 31)

The primary benefit of practitioner research is the uniqueness of the perspective on the research project that the practitioner researcher develops. However, there are some real challenges that arise when undertaking this form of research within a practice setting. The steps that need to be taken in terms of preparing the ground, choosing the right approach and collecting the data all apply. However, since the practitioner researcher has in essence a dual role, that of practitioner and researcher, it is important that prior to beginning the research, identity and professional issues are clarified.

When embarking on research within your workplace, it is important to reflect upon your status, or position, within the organisation and how others might perceive you, because difficulties do arise directly as a result of this (Drake & Heath 2011). Prior knowledge of the problem or setting, your own insight as a practitioner and the desire to explore an issue that has engaged your attention for some time may conflict with the need as a researcher to maintain a level of distance and rigour. The small-scale nature of the research study, difficulties with maintaining confidentiality and the researcher's closeness to the participants all pose challenges to the practitioner researcher that need to be addressed. Bailey (2007) provides some reflections on her journey as a practitioner researcher undertaking an ethnographic study in the emergency department in which she also worked that might be helpful to novice researchers considering undertaking this approach. At times, she struggled to see where her nursing role ended and her researcher role began. When conducting participant observation, she had to think carefully about the boundaries between her role as observer and participant in the care setting.

Reflection activity

What do you see as the advantages and the disadvantages of undertaking research in your own setting? What steps could you take to address some of the disadvantages?

THE PRACTITIONER RESEARCH PROCESS

Research questions

In practitioner researcher, the close proximity to practice is often the germination point for the research idea or focus. The awareness that there is a gap in the current knowledge or understanding has been the trigger for many small studies that have resulted in practice change. My own doctoral research arose from a desire to understand more fully the reasons for the apparent discrepancies in the recognition of potential organ and tissue donors in the intensive care unit (Kent 2002, 2004). Another example is that of Wen Zeng who, in response to the lack of information about and understanding of older people's needs in his local environment (Macau), undertook a qualitative exploration to document and interpret the lived experiences of older persons with depression in Macau (Zeng *et al.* 2012, 2013). He identified a number of research questions, which were firmly grounded in his experiences from over 15 years practice involving care of the elderly in Macau (see Research Example 24.1).

The questions guiding practitioner research may differ from those of the traditional academic researcher who might have identified the associated gaps in knowledge after significant searching of the existing literature, rather than concentrating on issues affecting the specific context of the practice environment. That is not to say that the practitioner researcher does not need to examine the existing evidence, they do and should since this will help to shape the direction of their research.

RESEARCH EXAMPLE

24.1 Identifying Research Questions

Zeng W, North N, Kent B (2013) Family and social aspects associated with depression among older persons in a Chinese context. *International Journal of Older People Nursing* **8**: 299–308.

Zeng and colleagues undertook a mixed methods study to understand more fully the factors associated with depression among older persons in Macau. The lead researcher (a nurse) had been involved in a study that found that the depression rates among older persons who lived in community settings in Macau were much higher than expected, and yet the reasons for this were unclear. There is stigma associated with depression in this culture, and so Zeng wanted to try to identify what more could be done to help prevent, detect and support those suffering from depression. He identified research questions that included: What are the lived experiences of older people with depression in Macau? What are the principal influences on depression among this population? How can health care be improved to help prevent, detect and support these people? Quantitative (standardised tests) and qualitative (collection of narratives) data were collected from 31 people who were purposively selected community-dwelling older persons affected by depression.

The study revealed the significance of family and social aspects as key determinants of depression. In a society and culture that relies on and values filial support, having poor family support and weak social networks appeared to compound and exacerbate depression. The findings highlight that filial support is seriously strained by the realities of contemporary society in Macau. Since current government policies in Macau rely on and confirm the role of family support, the study identified a clear need for these to be reviewed and modified in light of the realities of family and social support. The findings were used to construct an explanatory framework to inform service development and assist with identification of risk factors for depression.

Sampling

Identifying the research location and accessing participants are the next stages in the research process. Whereas for the traditional researcher identifying settings and participants is largely guided by the need for generalisability of the findings, for the practitioner research, the need to generate locally applicable findings is important. Therefore, the setting and sample are most often determined by workplace access. The sample will reflect the people who need to be studied within that practice setting. As Reed (2010) indicates, if the insider researcher's focus is the environment and people who engage with that practice, then the participants may well be the whole population within that setting, with accessibility being the key determinant for this. This does mean that alternatives to random sampling are clearly acceptable within practitioner research, although the rationale for the choice of sample or setting does need to be stated and the process for sampling made explicit in the research proposal and in subsequent publication of the findings.

Sampling may be just as complex as with other forms of research since there are ethical and professional considerations that must be taken account of. These include dealing with gatekeepers and enthusiastic managers who may want to block access or direct access in particular ways. There is sometimes a vested interest in the research from within the organisation, and it is important that this does not compromise the investigation. A practitioner researcher has to be a skilled negotiator and have a sound awareness of the contextual factors that may be present before, during and after the research has been completed.

RESEARCH EXAMPLE

24.2 Innovative Methods in Practitioner Research

Belman L, Corrigan P (2010) Using action research to develop a thoracic support nurse role to enhance the quality of care. *Nursing Times* **106**(22): 18–21.

This research project, undertaken in a specialist heart centre in the United Kingdom, evolved from clinical nurses' concerns that thoracic patients with complex needs were not receiving optimal care. A senior research nurse and nurse consultant based in the centre led an action research study to develop the role of a thoracic support nurse to enhance the quality of care provided in anticipation that it would lead to a reduction in length of stay. The project aimed to highlight barriers and enablers to developing the role, evaluate the impact of the role and examine the process of change. Several co-researchers who were clinical nurses working in the care setting joined the project team and contributed to data collection as well as being actively involved in the change process. In this article, the authors identify the valuable ongoing learning of participants through first-hand involvement in research in their practice setting. As well as learning about the practicalities of undertaking research in 'the real world', the research team also gained insight into the complexity of implementing and evaluating a new role in practice.

METHODS

Approaches to research vary according to the questions being asked, the paradigm that most closely aligns with these and the contextual issues pertinent to the research setting. So, as with any form of research, the choices are often complex and require careful thought and planning. The methods commonly used in practitioner research are drawn from case study, ethnography, phenomenology, narrative and action research. Research Example 24.2 provides an example of an action research study undertaken in a large hospital to develop a new nursing role to support thoracic patients with complex needs.

Watching, talking or doing both is common data collection activity in practitioner research. Observation, as a participant or non-participant, can generate substantial amounts of data, and when combined with techniques such as 'Think Aloud' (see Chapter 32), it is possible to understand more fully what people are doing and their justifications for the decisions made.

Interestingly, in a review of a sample of 23 practitioner research studies in the field of social care, Mitchell *et al.* (2008) found that the majority adopted qualitative methodologies. Some were descriptive in nature using case study approaches, whilst others focused on individuals such as service users or other practitioners. Most collected data using interviews and no studies using observation were identified in the review. Quantitative and mixed approaches were found in five studies.

In recent years, technological advances have led to developments in data collection within real-world settings. Data collected through novel products such as iBleep™ (www.ibleep.net) have been used to inform service improvement initiatives, such as those aimed at enhancing communication within hospitals at night (see Research Example 24.3) Others have used applications developed for tablet computers, such as Tap Forms™ (http://www.tapforms.com/). These enable rapid collection of data at the bedside in a number of different formats including numeric, audio and photographic. The data collected are easy to download onto spreadsheets for analysis, which is another bonus. As Kimbler *et al.* (2013) indicate, there are existing and emerging technology tools that enable the collection of multimodal data (e.g. textual, visual, aural, spatial and temporal). However, since many of these applications were originally developed for other purposes, there is still much to learn about how they can be used in nursing and health-care research.

RESEARCH EXAMPLE

24.3 Innovative Methods of Data Collection

Pearson R, Madenholt-Titley S, Weatherill F (2008) What the *iBleep* do we know. Presentation at Change Champions Conference, Auckland, New Zealand. Available at http://www.changechampions.com.au/downloads/the-hospital-after-hours_3; http://www.changechampions.com.au/resource/Rosemary_Pearson.pdf (accessed 31 Aug 2014).

At one large urban hospital in New Zealand, a new service was introduced to address several problems that were affecting care in the evenings, nights and at weekend. The 'After-Hours Model of Care' aimed to reduce delays to patient care and improve clinical outcomes by matching clinical skills and competencies to after-hours workload. This initiative involved a single communication system, introduction of an iBleep Coordinator, prioritisation of ward calls and improved response times to ward calls from nursing staff to on-call doctors. iBleep is a system that allows dynamic, two-way, real-time communication with rapid visualisation of essential data such as the reason for the bleep, the ward and bed location, the patient's details and vital observation information such as oxygen level, temperature and respiration rate and the early warning score (EWS). Evidence-based iBleep observation and EWS algorithms were designed and validated by the University of Auckland. Following the implementation of this new model of care, more than 6000 iBleep calls had been made. The hospital saw a reduction in calls to doctors and faster response times by medical staff, and the majority of nursing and medical staff wanted the iBleep to stay. Teamworking was also enhanced, along with more appropriate use of skills.

Using technology may offset, in part, some of the concerns raised about practitioner research being too close to the setting to objectively study practice issues. The use of devices such as tablet computers focuses the researcher on the task required and minimises distractions that can occur. It can also help to ensure that data are being collected consistently and accurately.

Being close to, or familiar with, the research setting and its participants can lead to practitioner researchers anticipating results or actions or behaving in a way that may interfere with the natural course of a study. Participants may feel under an enhanced level of obligation to participate in the study because they know the practitioner researcher. Behaviours may also change as participants strive to support the research. There may also be times when researcher-professional conflict arises during data collection. The practitioner researcher may see something that, as a professional, they recognise as being abnormal and that necessitates some action to be taken; a non-health professional researcher may instead just record the information as part of the data collection process. Bonner and Tolhurst (2002) provide some useful tips for insider researchers when engaged in participant observation to overcome any researcher effect and participant response to the researcher. They advocate reflective examination of assumptions and actions during data collection, as well as several practical strategies:

- Avoiding data collection during scheduled duty times
- Wearing everyday clothes, rather than a uniform when collecting data
- Avoiding inclusion in clinical discussions during data collection periods
- Avoiding, where possible, the provision of nursing care when collecting data
- Maximising the length of time for data collection so that staff adjust to the changed role (researcher, not nurse) for that period

It is important that the practitioner researcher acknowledges the dual position that they hold because they may need to change roles occasionally, for example, when a nursing response is needed to meet a patient's

Reflection activity

What steps can the practitioner researcher take to minimise the possibility that other people's behaviour will change once they know that research is being carried out?

needs. The practitioner researcher should record such occasions in a reflective diary or field notes as they may be incorporated into the research findings. Breen (2007) has written about her experiences as a practitioner researcher undertaking a study to explore experiences following fatal road traffic accidents in Australia. She describes how she adopted neither an insider nor outsider stance, but rather a middle role as a way of helping her to maximise the benefits of the two roles whilst minimising the disadvantages.

Analysis

The phase of analysis is crucial to any research approach. The 'insider as a researcher' has been the focus of some criticism arising from their closeness to the data and difficulties around objectivity. This is not restricted to practitioner research since much of the debate has focused on insider qualitative research (Dwyer & Buckle 2009).

Practitioner researchers should avoid forming assumptions on the basis of their intimate knowledge of the research setting and the participants but should ensure that their analysis is grounded in the data they have collected. It is also important to distinguish between data that have been collected formally as part of the research process and other insights they may have gained through their practitioner role. Only data that have been collected as part of the research, in accordance with ethical and governance principles, can be included in the analysis.

Analysing the data is a complex task, and practitioner researchers have to negotiate 'relational closeness' whilst ensuring 'analytical distance' (Lykkeslet & Gjengedal 2007). Burns *et al.* (2012) comment on this in their study of breastfeeding support by midwives and found that a crucial strategy was to cast a backward critical gaze at their own subjective positioning and engage in ongoing reflexivity, as recommended by Finlay and Gough (2003).

RIGOUR IN PRACTITIONER RESEARCH

Ensuring rigour in the research process is important for all researchers, irrespective of the methodology they have chosen. However, the complexity of practitioner research presents particular challenges. As the earlier sections of this chapter have identified, the insider role occupied by the practitioner researcher raises a number of issues in relation to rigour in the different stages of the research process. These issues should be anticipated when developing the research proposal and strategies put in place to ensure rigour.

Reflexivity is an important way to demonstrate the degree of rigour in practitioner research. It involves the researcher reflecting throughout the research process on how their own actions, values and perceptions impact on the research setting and affect the data collection and analysis. By maintaining a reflective diary, the practitioner researcher can keep a detailed record of how their role as researcher and practitioner undertaking research in their own setting has influenced the research. In Research Example 24.4, Burns *et al.* (2012) provide a detailed account of the reflexivity they engaged in when undertaking a study of postnatal interactions between midwives and women.

There are several actions the researcher can take to enhance rigour in the research process. The criteria for judging the trustworthiness of the research as demonstrated through addressing credibility, transferability, dependability and confirmability (Lincoln & Guba 1985) are particularly pertinent to practitioner research because of its reliance on qualitative approaches. Breen (2007) discusses the actions that she took to maximise research rigour, which included keeping a journal in which she documented daily tasks and memos and member checking, where interview participants were involved in checking the accuracy of her interpretation of the data. She also sent her participants a summary of the results and invited them to comment or provide clarification if needed.

RESEARCH EXAMPLE

24.4 Reflexivity in Practitioner Research

Burns E, Fenwick J, Schmied V, Sheehan A (2012) Reflexivity in midwifery research: the insider/outsider debate. *Midwifery* **28**(1): 52–60.

In this article, the researchers, who were also practising midwives, reflect upon the issues raised regarding the influence of their identity and insider knowledge on a study investigating the provision of breastfeeding support in the first week after birth. Whereas possessing insider knowledge helped them during the 'getting in' and 'fitting in' phases of the research, they experienced unanticipated role ambiguity and encountered moral and ethical challenges due to their insider knowledge and status. Through reflexive analysis of the insider roles, they identified how they occupied a middle ground between being a researcher and a midwife. They conclude that by occupying a middle ground, the midwife researchers can 'draw upon aspects of "self" required to negotiate respectful relationships with colleagues, whilst, also ensuring the maintenance of an analytical degree of distancing'.

Reflection activity

What steps can the practitioner researcher take to ensure the trustworthiness of the research undertaken? How might Lincoln and Guba's notions of credibility, transferability, dependability and confirmability inform the activities that the practitioner researcher might undertake to ensure rigour in the research process? You may find it helpful to refer to Chapter 11.

A further step to enhance the credibility and transferability of the findings is to include details of the participants and the setting in the research report (taking steps to ensure no ethical breaches are made); this allows the reader to make judgements about the similarities between the research setting and their own.

ETHICAL ISSUES

Ethical issues need to be addressed as part of any research project, and therefore, the points raised in Chapter 3 are highly relevant for practitioner research. However, there are added complexities when engaging in practitioner research; the researcher's professional, social, cultural and personal circumstances may all impact, to some degree, on the research (Drake & Heath 2011). When professional roles and research roles become very closely aligned, as they do in practitioner research, various ethical challenges can arise. It is good practice to consider the impact of these two roles early on in the research process and develop a plan that can be activated if the need arises.

One of the primary ethical challenges is that of professional practice. Practitioner researchers remain accountable both legally and professionally whilst conducting their research. At times, unanticipated events or unexpected findings may arise that the practitioner researcher needs to deal with in a professional capacity. So, for example, during observation of clinical activities, if the practitioner researcher notices something that is either unsafe or illegal, then they have a duty to do something about it. As mentioned earlier, a plan developed in advance of the study commencing should guide the practitioner researcher in terms of appropriate actions to take. In my own research, I have had to cease being a researcher and act as a nurse when I noticed an activity that would have severely compromised a patient if I had not stepped in. This is unusual but my plan helped me deal effectively with this as morally and professionally I could not put the research above the needs of the patient.

RESEARCH EXAMPLE

24.5 Ethical Issues in Practitioner Research

Lyford S (2007) The Passage of Rite: the psychosocial impact of liver transplantation on recipient families. Unpublished thesis, University of Auckland.

Solid organ transplantation differs from any other treatment in that a vital organ is transferred from one human being, either living or deceased, to another. The aim of this study was to explore the subjective experiences of family supporting another family member through liver transplantation. This research arose from the personal observations made by Lyford after she received a liver transplant. She found that significant stress was placed on the family whilst they support the recipient, and each other, during the transplant process. For those awaiting a liver transplant, death is often imminent, and this becomes a key stressor for the family. There were a number of ethical issues that needed to be addressed prior to and during this study, not least that the research itself involved a highly stressful and emotive event in the researcher's life. Six participants from two families who had experienced the liver transplant of an adult family member in New Zealand within the preceding 5 years were involved in the study. Semi-structured interviews were conducted, and the analysis revealed key phases of the journey; realisation, readying, reality and renaissance. These interviews inevitably brought to the fore many of the experiences and emotions felt by the practitioner researcher, and so support was provided throughout this process. Although the family journeying was dependent on the recipient's clinical course, all stages were experienced by every family member interviewed. The findings add support for a model of family resilience to be utilised within clinical practice to help in the maintenance of togetherness during the transplant journey.

Another challenge to consider is that of professional power. The practitioner researcher may have an unusual relationship with the research participants if they are also patients or colleagues. This can be seen as having power; commonly, this is explored as part of the ethics review process, and steps must be taken to ensure that this does not create any coercion or pressure on people to participate in a study. Issues of power were highlighted in a study by Lyford (2007) where as a practitioner researcher she had a close, personal interest in the topic being investigated as part of a postgraduate degree (see Research Example 24.5) To ensure that no ethical boundaries were breached, Lyford maintained a research journal to enable self-reflectivity. This was reviewed regularly and used along with professional supervision, particularly during the interview stage of the project. It is quite unusual for a researcher to have such a close connection with the research participants, but in such cases, for example, where the participants are known to the researcher as a result of their illness, it is important that support mechanisms are put in place and frequent checks made during the research to ensure that the researcher's and the participants' well-being is not compromised.

Dissemination of the research findings may present further ethical challenges. There may be some pressure on the practitioner researcher from colleagues or managers to limit reporting of negative findings that may reflect badly on a setting. Furthermore, care must be taken in reporting the findings not to reveal information that may identify an individual or organisation since this will breach ethical principles. When publishing in a journal, author identification is provided, and this can form a link to the potential site of the research, and therefore, steps must be taken to minimise this wherever possible. Betrayal of trust is a real issue, and so the researcher must engage closely with their workplace so that a critical stance can be maintained, without negative outcomes for either party.

Reflection activity

What are the main ethical challenges that arise for a practitioner undertaking research in their own practice setting that involves colleagues with whom they work and patients for whom they provide care? How might the practitioner researcher address these ethical issues?

CONCLUSION

Although much research takes place in practice settings, not all can be classified as practitioner research, since studies are often led by outsiders who are not closely connected with the specific research setting. Practitioner research is a useful and practical way to investigate questions arising from the practice setting.

Despite the often small-scale nature of practitioner research, the findings can have many uses including practice change, service improvements and enhancements to care. They can also provide the fertile ground needed for growing larger projects that have wider generalisability and impact. Therefore, practitioner research has a rightful place in the array of research approaches that can be used to explore nursing issues, and as Fox *et al.* (2007) state, 'it is through practitioners researching their own practice, their own service and their own profession, that positive change will happen in the public services' (page 201).

References

Bailey CJ (2007) Practitioner to researcher: reflections on the journey. *Nurse Researcher* **14**(4): 18–26.

Belman L, Corrigan P (2010) Using action research to develop a thoracic support nurse role to enhance the quality of care. *Nursing Times* **106**(22): 18–21.

Bonner A, Tolhurst G (2002) Insider outsider perspectives of participant observation. *Nurse Researcher* **9**: 7–19.

Breen LJ (2007) The researcher 'in the middle': negotiating the insider/outsider dichotomy. *The Australian Community Psychologist* **19**: 163–174.

Bucknall T, Kent B, Manley K (2008) Evidence use and evidence generation in practice development. In: Manley K, McCormack B, Wilson V (eds) *International Practice Development in Nursing and Healthcare.* Oxford, Blackwell, pp 84–104.

Burns E, Fenwick J, Schmied V, Sheehan A (2012) Reflexivity in midwifery research: the insider/outsider debate. *Midwifery* **28**: 52–60.

Campbell A (2007) *Practitioner Research.* London, Teaching and Learning Research Programme. Available at http://www.tlrp.org/capacity/rm/wt/campbell (accessed 21 Feb 2014).

Dadds M (2014) Perspectives on Practitioner Research. *Development and enquiry programmes: Teacher researchers* Cranfield, National College for School Leadership Network Learning Group.

Drake P, Heath L (2011) *Practitioner Research at Doctoral Level.* London, Routledge.

Dwyer SC, Buckle JL (2009) The space between: on being an insider-outsider in qualitative research. *International Journal of Qualitative Methods* **8**(1): 54–63.

Finlay L, Gough B (2003) *Reflexivity: a practical guide for researchers in health and social sciences,* Malden, Blackwell Science.

Fox M, Martin P, Green G (2007) *Doing Practitioner Research.* London, Sage.

Gerrish K, Mawson S, Hill C, Gerrish P (2009) A pragmatic approach to resolving tensions between the educational validity of masters projects in health care settings and ethical and governance requirements. *Learning in Health and Social Care* **8**(2): 123–134.

Gillman M, Swain J (2006) Practitioner research. In: Jupp V (ed) *The SAGE Dictionary of Social Research Methods.* London, Sage, pp 233–235.

Heaslip P (2008) Critical Thinking and Nursing. Available at http://www.criticalthinking.org/pages/critical-thinking-to-think-like-a-nurse/834 (accessed 22 April 2014).

Kent B (2002) Psychosocial factors influencing nurses' involvement with organ and tissue donation. *International Journal of Nursing Studies* **39**: 429–440.

Kent B (2004) Protection behaviour: a phenomenon affecting organ and tissue donation in the 21st century? *International Journal of Nursing Studies* **41**: 273–284.

Kimbler J, Moore D, Schladen MM, Sowers B, Snyder M (2013) Emerging Technology Tools for Qualitative Data Collection. Available at http://www.nova.edu/ssss/QR/TQR2013/Kimbler_etal.pdf (accessed 22 April 2014).

Lincoln Y, Guba E (1985) *Naturalistic Inquiry.* Thousand Oaks, Sage.

Lyford S (2007) *The Passage of Rite: the psychosocial impact of liver transplantation on recipient families*. Unpublished thesis, University of Auckland.

Lykkeslet E, Gjengedal E (2007) Methodological problems associated with practice-close research. *Qualitative Health Research* **17**: 699–704.

Mitchell F, Shaw IF, Lunt N (2008) Practitioner Research in Social Services: a literature review. Available at http://lx.iriss.org.uk/sites/default/files/resources/practitioner_research_literature_review_report.pdf (accessed 22 April 2014).

Pearson R, Madenholt-Titley S, Weatherill F (2008) What the *iBleep* do we know. Presentation at Change Champions Conference, Auckland, New Zealand. Available at http://www.changechampions.com.au/downloads/the-hospital-after-hours_3; http://www.changechampions.com.au/resource/Rosemary_Pearson.pdf (accessed 31 Aug 2014).

Reed J (2010) Practitioner research. In: Gerrish K, Lacey A (eds) *The Research Process in Nursing*. 6th edition. Oxford, Wiley-Blackwell. pp 271–283.

Reed J, Proctor S (1995) *Practitioner Research in Health Care,* London, Chapman and Hall.

Shaw I (2005) Practitioner research: evidence or critique? *British Journal of Social Work* **35**: 1231–1248.

Warnock C, Tod A (2014) A descriptive exploration of the experiences of patients with significant functional impairment following a recent diagnosis of metastatic spinal cord compression. *Journal of Advanced Nursing* **70**(3): 564–574.

Zeng W, North N, Kent B (2012) A framework to understand depression among older persons. *Journal of Clinical Nursing* **21**: 2399–2409.

Zeng W, North N, Kent B (2013) Family and social aspects associated with depression among older persons in a Chinese context. *International Journal of Older People Nursing* **8**: 299–308.

Further reading

Groundwater-Smith S, Mitchell J, Mockler N, Ponte P, Ronnerman K (2013) *Facilitating Practitioner Research: developing transformational partnerships*. Abingdon, Routledge.

Freshwater D, Lees J (2012) *Practitioner Research in Healthcare: transformational research in action*. London, Sage.

CHAPTER 25

Systematic Reviews and Evidence Syntheses

Andrew Booth, Angie Rees and Claire Beecroft

Key points

- Evidence syntheses, in particular systematic reviews, contribute to evidence-based practice by using explicit methods to identify, select, critically appraise and summarise large quantities of information to aid the decision-making process.
- The three main types of evidence syntheses are systematic reviews, practice guidelines and economic evaluations.
- Regardless of the type of evidence synthesis, several discrete, but interconnected, stages are followed: writing a protocol; systematically searching the literature; selecting relevant studies; assessing the quality of the literature; extracting key information from the selected studies; summarising, interpreting and presenting the findings; and writing up the research in a structured manner.

INTRODUCTION

This chapter builds upon Chapters 7 and 8 to provide a practical introduction to conducting evidence synthesis (i.e. reanalysing and combining existing research), with specific reference to systematic reviews. Readers are advised to refer to these two earlier chapters regarding the skills required to access and appraise research literature. A worked example relating to antibiotics and antiseptics for venous leg ulcers (taken from a completed Cochrane review from the Cochrane Library) is used throughout (see Research Example 25.1).

BACKGROUND TO EVIDENCE SYNTHESIS

The knowledge base for any evidence-based profession is founded on evidence syntheses. By reanalysing previously collected data from original (primary) studies

The Research Process in Nursing, Seventh Edition. Edited by Kate Gerrish and Judith Lathlean.

Companion Website: www.wiley.com/go/gerrish/research

RESEARCH EXAMPLE

25.1 A Cochrane Plain Language Summary and Review Abstract

Summary

Antibiotics and antiseptics to help healing venous leg ulcers

Venous leg ulcers are a type of wound that can take a long time to heal. These ulcers can become infected and this might cause further delay to healing. Two types of treatment are available to treat infection: systemic antibiotics (i.e. antibiotic tablets or injections) and topical preparations (i.e. applied directly to the wound). Whether systemic or topical preparations are used, patients will also usually have a wound dressing to cover the wound and maybe a bandage too. This review was undertaken in order to find out whether using antibiotics and antiseptics works better than usual care for healing venous leg ulcers, and if so, to find out which antibiotic and antiseptic preparations are better than others. In terms of topical preparations, there is some evidence to support the use of cadexomer iodine. Further good quality research is required before definitive conclusions can be made about the effectiveness of systemic antibiotics and topical agents such as povidone iodine, peroxide-based preparations, ethacridine lactate and mupirocin in healing venous leg ulceration.

This record should be cited as: O'Meara S, Al-Kurdi D, Ologun Y, Ovington LG. Antibiotics and antiseptics for venous leg ulcers. *Cochrane Database of Systematic Reviews* 2010, Issue 1. Art. No.: CD003557. DOI: 10.1002/14651858.CD003557.pub3.

Abstract

Background

Venous leg ulcers are a type of chronic wound affecting up to 1% of adults in developed countries at some point during their lives. Many of these wounds are colonised by bacteria or show signs of clinical infection. The presence of infection may delay ulcer healing. There are two main strategies used to prevent and treat clinical infection in venous leg ulcers: systemic antibiotics and topical antibiotics or antiseptics.

Objectives

The objective of the review is to determine the effects of systemic antibiotics, topical antibiotics and antiseptics on the healing of venous ulcers.

Search methods

For the update of this review we searched the Cochrane Wounds Group Specialised Register (searched 24 September 2009); The Cochrane Central Register of Controlled Trials (CENTRAL) – *The Cochrane Library* – 2009 Issue 3; Ovid MEDLINE – 1950 to September Week 3 2009; Ovid EMBASE – 1980 to 2009 Week 38; and EBSCO CINAHL – 1982 to September Week 3 2009. No language or publication date restrictions were applied.

Selection criteria

Randomised controlled trials recruiting people with venous leg ulceration and evaluating at least one systemic antibiotic, topical antibiotic or topical antiseptic that reported an objective assessment of wound healing (e.g. time to complete healing, frequency of complete healing and change in ulcer surface area) were eligible for inclusion. Selection decisions were made by two authors working independently.

Data collection and analysis

Information on the characteristics of participants, interventions and outcomes were recorded on a standardised data extraction form. In addition, aspects of trial methods were extracted, including randomisation, allocation concealment, blinding of participants and outcome assessors, incomplete outcome data and study group comparability at baseline. Data extraction and validity assessment were conducted by one author and checked by a second.

Main results

Twenty-five trials reporting 32 comparisons were identified. Five trials evaluated systemic antibiotics and the remainder evaluated topical preparations – cadexomer iodine (10 trials); povidone iodine (5 trials); peroxide-based preparations (3 trials); ethacridine lactate (1 trial); mupirocin (1 trial) and chlorhexidine (1 trial) (Note: One trial was assigned to two categories). For the systemic antibiotics, the only comparison where a statistically significant between-group difference was detected was that in favour of the antihelminthic levamisole when compared with placebo. This trial, in common with the other evaluations of systemic antibiotics, was small and so the observed effect could have occurred by chance or been due to baseline imbalances in prognostic factors. For topical preparations, there is some evidence to suggest that cadexomer iodine generates higher healing rates than standard care. One study showed a statistically significant result in favour of cadexomer iodine when compared with standard care (not involving compression) in the frequency of complete healing at 6 weeks (RR 2.29, 95% CI 1.10–4.74). The intervention regimen used was intensive, involving daily dressing changes, and so these findings may not be generalisable to most everyday clinical settings. When cadexomer iodine was compared with standard care with all patients receiving compression, the pooled estimate from two trials for frequency of complete healing at 4–6 weeks indicated significantly higher healing rates for cadexomer iodine (RR 6.72, 95% CI 1.56–28.95). Surrogate healing outcomes such as change in ulcer surface area and daily or weekly healing rate showed favourable results for cadexomer iodine, peroxide-based preparations and ethacridine lactate in some studies. These surrogate outcomes may not be valid proxies for complete healing of the wound. Most of the trials were small and many had methodological problems such as poor baseline comparability between groups, failure to use (or report) true randomisation, adequate allocation concealment, blinded outcome assessment and analysis by intention-to-treat.

Authors' conclusions

At present, there is no evidence to support the routine use of systemic antibiotics to promote healing in venous leg ulcers. However, the lack of reliable evidence means that it is not possible to recommend the discontinuation of any of the agents reviewed. In terms of topical preparations, there is some evidence to support the use of cadexomer iodine. Further good quality research is required before definitive conclusions can be made about the effectiveness of systemic antibiotics and topical preparations such as povidone iodine, peroxide-based preparations, ethacridine lactate, mupirocin and chlorhexidine in healing venous leg ulceration. In light of the increasing problem of bacterial resistance to antibiotics, current prescribing guidelines recommend that antibacterial preparations should only be used in cases of clinical infection and not for bacterial colonisation.

within research syntheses, it is possible to summarise large volumes of information in a succinct manner. Instead of basing practice on a single study, and the uncertainty that surrounds such a result, a practitioner can access a more precise result based on multiple studies. The inclusion of multiple studies increases the generalisability of findings and prompts the practitioner to examine conflicting results. Practitioners can also identify gaps in the current knowledge base as a prelude to planning their own research.

Systematic reviews

A *systematic review* (or *overview*) is

> 'a review of the evidence on a clearly formulated question that uses systematic and explicit methods to identify, select and critically appraise relevant primary research, and to extract and analyse data from the studies that are included in the review' (Khan *et al.* 2001: 4)

Whereas 'review' (sometimes referred to as a narrative or traditional review) is a general term used to describe a synthesis of the results and conclusions of two or more publications on a given topic, a systematic review tries to find and then synthesise all relevant studies on a given topic. A systematic review aims to be:

- systematic (e.g. in its identification of literature)
- explicit (e.g. in its statement of objectives, materials and methods)
- reproducible (e.g. in its methodology and conclusions) (Greenhalgh 2010)

The term '*meta-analysis*' is often used interchangeably with 'systematic review'. However, meta-analysis describes a statistical technique used to combine the results of several studies into a single estimate (Akers *et al.* 2009).

Examples of systematic reviews in nursing include reviews on specialist home-based nursing services for children with acute and chronic illnesses (Parab *et al.* 2013), interventions designed to prevent health-care bed-related injuries in patients (Anderson *et al.* 2012) and telephone support for women during pregnancy and the first 6 weeks of postpartum (Lavender *et al.* 2013). All these examples can be found on The Cochrane Library at http://www.thecochranelibrary.com/.

Practice guidelines and economic evaluations

Other examples of evidence syntheses are practice guidelines and economic evaluations. Practice guidelines are

> 'directions or principles presenting current or future rules of policy for the health care practitioner to assist him in patient care decisions regarding diagnosis, therapy or related clinical circumstances.... The guidelines form a basis for the evaluation of all aspects of health care and delivery'. (Clinical Practice Guidelines, National Library of Medicine, MeSH Browser)

Many evidence-based guidelines, such as those produced in the United Kingdom by the National Institute for Health and Care Excellence (NICE), have implications for nursing. Examples of clinical guidelines include 'service user experience in adult mental health (CG136)' (2011), 'feverish illness in children (CG 160)' (2013) and 'varicose veins in the legs (CG 168)' (2013). These guidelines can be accessed on the NICE website: http://guidance.nice.org.uk/.

An '*economic evaluation*' represents a balance sheet of the advantages (benefits) and disadvantages (costs) associated with different health-care options so that a practitioner can make choices (Robinson 1993). Published examples include an economic evaluation of the cost-effectiveness of a multifactorial fall prevention programme in nursing homes (Heinrich *et al.* 2013) and another of the cost-effectiveness of nurse practitioners or community health workers in reducing cardiovascular health disparities (Allen *et al.* 2014).

Advantages of evidence synthesis

Well-conducted evidence syntheses offer several advantages over single primary research studies (Mulrow 1995; Greenhalgh 2010). For example:

- Large amounts of information can be assimilated quickly and efficiently to assist in making timely decisions.

- Explicit review methods help to limit bias in identifying and excluding studies.
- Conflicting or unusual results can be identified and examined to establish generalisable findings and an overall pattern of results.
- Reasons for inconsistency in results across studies can be identified and new hypotheses generated.
- Quantitative techniques, such as meta-analysis, increase the precision of the overall result.
- Conclusions are thus considered to be more reliable and accurate.

Stages in conducting evidence synthesis

Booth and colleagues (Grant & Booth 2009; Booth *et al.* 2011) have identified four discrete, but interconnected, stages to any evidence synthesis, encapsulated in the SAlSA mnemonic:

- **S**earch: systematically searching and selecting the literature
- **A**ppraisa**l**: writing a research protocol and outlining the purpose and methods of the research
- **S**ynthesis: bringing the results together to facilitate the identification of commonalities, differences and patterns
- **A**nalysis: explaining and making sense of the patterns in the data

This chapter focuses on systematic reviews, the most common of research syntheses, but the described methods apply, to varying degrees, to other types of evidence syntheses.

WRITING A SYSTEMATIC REVIEW PROTOCOL

The first step in undertaking a systematic review is to establish whether there is sufficient need for a review. The process starts with a comprehensive search for existing reviews addressing the same (or similar) research question(s) and critical appraisal of the quality of any potentially relevant reviews. Existing and ongoing systematic reviews can be identified by searching the following databases:

- The Cochrane Database of Systematic Reviews (CDSR) – http://www.thecochranelibrary.com/view/0/index.html.
- The Database of Abstracts of Reviews of Effects (DARE) – http://www.crd.york.ac.uk/crdweb/Homepage.asp.
- Major health-related databases, such as MEDLINE, using methodological search filters designed to retrieve systematic reviews (e.g. http://www.nlm.nih.gov/bsd/pubmed_subsets/sysreviews_strategy.html).

Box 25.1 provides an example of such a filter. Local health-care librarians can provide advice and support in identifying and using search filters.

If existing reviews are outdated or of poor quality, it may be necessary to update them or to conduct a new review from scratch. The key to a successful systematic review lies in the reviewer's ability to be precise and specific when stating the problems to be addressed. A structured approach to framing questions should be used. To the four components of PICO (**P**atients (or population), **I**nterventions (or exposures), **C**omparison and **O**utcomes) that apply to all types of question (see Chapter 7), you will find it helpful to add a further component specifically for the purpose of a systematic review, namely, the **S**tudy design(s) that is(are) suitable for addressing the review question (Khan *et al.* 2011). This stage in the systematic review process is perhaps the most difficult, yet most important to get right. A review protocol is drawn up specifying the plan that the review will subsequently follow. It is a key reference document throughout the review process. Modifications should only be made to the protocol if there is a genuine reason (e.g. if an additional outcome measure is identified upon closer examination of the literature).

A review protocol typically includes the following:

- *Background and rationale to the review.* This section includes a justification for the review being undertaken, as well as a preliminary assessment of potentially relevant literature and its size.

Box 25.1 Methodological search filter designed to retrieve systematic reviews in PubMed MEDLINE

This strategy is intended to retrieve citations identified as systematic reviews, meta-analyses, reviews of clinical trials, evidence-based medicine, consensus development conferences, guidelines and citations to articles from journals specializing in review studies of value to clinicians. This subset can be used in a search as systematic [sb].

http://www.nlm.nih.gov/bsd/pubmed_subsets/sysreviews_strategy.html

Example: exercise hypertension AND systematic [sb]

Strategy	Explanation
systematic review [ti] OR meta-analysis [pt] OR meta-analysis [ti] OR systematic literature review [ti] OR (systematic review [tiab] AND review [pt]) OR consensus development conference [pt] OR practice guideline [pt] OR cochrane database syst rev [ta] OR acp journal club [ta] OR health technol assess [ta] OR evid rep technol assess summ [ta] OR drug class reviews [ti]) OR (clinical guideline [tw] AND management [tw])OR (evidence based[ti] OR evidence-based medicine [mh] OR best practice* [ti] OR evidence synthesis [tiab]) AND (review [pt] OR diseases category[mh] OR behaviour and behaviour mechanisms [mh] OR therapeutics [mh] OR evaluation studies[pt] OR validation studies[pt] OR guideline [pt] OR pmcbook))OR	*Includes certain known types of publication more likely to be systematic*
((systematic [tw] OR systematically [tw] OR critical [tiab] OR (study selection [tw]) OR (predetermined [tw] OR inclusion [tw] AND criteri* [tw]) OR exclusion criteri* [tw] OR main outcome measures [tw] OR standard of care [tw] OR standards of care [tw]) AND (survey [tiab] OR surveys [tiab] OR overview* [tw] OR review [tiab] OR reviews [tiab] OR search* [tw] OR handsearch [tw] OR analysis [tiab] OR critique [tiab] OR appraisal [tw] OR (reduction [tw]AND (risk [mh] OR risk [tw]) AND (death OR recurrence))) AND (literature [tiab] OR articles [tiab] OR publications [tiab] OR publication [tiab] OR bibliography [tiab] OR bibliographies [tiab] OR published [tiab] OR unpublished [tw] OR citation [tw] OR citations [tw] OR database [tiab] OR internet [tiab] OR textbooks [tiab] OR references [tw] OR scales [tw] OR papers [tw] OR datasets [tw] OR trials [tiab] OR meta-analy* [tw] OR (clinical [tiab] AND studies [tiab]) OR treatment outcome [mh] OR treatment outcome [tw] OR pmcbook))	*Includes processes more likely to be present in a systematic review (e.g.inclusion criteria and handsearching)*
NOT (letter [pt] OR newspaper article [pt] OR comment [pt])	*Excludes (NOT) publication types [PT] unlikely to be systematic reviews*

- *Review question(s).* The review question(s) should be well focused in terms of the population, intervention and outcome(s).
- *Inclusion criteria.* These should follow on logically from the review question(s) and cover any restrictions regarding study design or publication type, language or year of publication. Any exclusion criteria should be stated explicitly and reasons given. Where feasible, criteria should be applied to the studies by two independent reviewers.
- *Literature search strategy.* This section outlines details of the sources to be searched and a sample search strategy.
- *Quality assessment strategy.* This section provides details of the critical appraisal checklist or scale (preferably validated) used to assess the quality of the included studies.
- *Data extraction strategy.* Where possible, a sample data extraction form should be included, indicating the information to be collected from each study (e.g. details about the participants, methods, interventions, results, etc.).
- *Proposed analysis.* This section documents the type of data most likely to be found (e.g. quantitative or qualitative) and the proposed data synthesis and presentation strategy (e.g. meta-analysis).
- *Plans for reporting and dissemination.* This section describes the strategy for reporting and disseminating the findings to relevant audiences.
- *Members of the review team.* Ideally, a systematic review should be undertaken by a review 'team', although many smaller reviews are written by lone researchers. Members of a review team should include an information specialist to identify, locate and store relevant references; someone to review the literature; a methodologist (such as a statistician) and content experts, possibly an advisory group or academic supervisors.
- *Project timetable.* Include a draft timetable outlining each stage in the systematic review.
- *Proposed costings.* Even small-scale reviews entail costs (e.g. staff time, obtaining articles, etc.). It is important to be aware of these costs at the outset and, if necessary, apply for additional funding.

Reflection activity

Based on your knowledge of protocols in general (e.g. in clinical care and/or in conducting primary research), what good reasons can you think of for writing a protocol before you start undertaking a systematic review? Can you think of any disadvantages from documenting what you are going to do in advance of starting your review?

SYSTEMATICALLY SEARCHING THE LITERATURE

The aim of a systematic literature search is 'to provide a list as comprehensive as possible of primary studies, both published and unpublished' (Khan *et al.* 2001: 21).

Refining the review question

The search starts with refining the review question and translating it into a search strategy that can be used to interrogate electronic bibliographic databases. As well as searching the literature to identify existing systematic reviews, 'scoping' searches ensure that the final strategy reflects all components of the review question(s) and enables reviewers to gain an early indication of the volume of the literature to be reviewed and how research is distributed in terms of study design. Research Example 25.2 applies the PICOS approach to the review of antibiotics and antiseptics for venous leg ulcers.

Selecting relevant sources to search for a systematic review

A review team should search a wide variety of sources for published, as well as unpublished literature including:

- large electronic bibliographic databases, such as MEDLINE, CINAHL, EMBASE and the Web of Knowledge[1]

[1]While some database names originated as meaningful acronyms it is common practice to identify and to refer to common databases by their abbreviated forms.

RESEARCH EXAMPLE

25.2 A Refined Review Question: Antibiotics and Antiseptics for Venous Leg Ulcers (O'Meara *et al.* 2010)

	Components	Keywords	Synonyms(i.e. alternative search terms)
P	Patient/problem/population	Venous leg ulcers	Varicose ulcer (MeSH) Leg ulcer (MeSH) Venous ulcers
I	Intervention	Antibiotics	Exp antibacterial-agents (MeSH) Antibiotics Penicillin Cephalosporin Aminoglycosides Gentamicin Quinolones Ciprofloxacin Clindamycin Metronidazole Trimethoprim
C	Comparison	Antiseptics	Exp anti-infective agents, local (MeSH) Antiseptics Disinfectants
O	Outcomes	Wound healing	Wound healing (MeSH) Ulcer healing Wound size Wound duration
S	Study design	Randomised controlled trials	Randomised controlled trial [publication type] Clinical trial [publication type] Randomized controlled trials (MeSH) Random*control*trial*

- subject-specific electronic bibliographic databases, such as AMED (for allied health literature and complementary and alternative medicine), PsycINFO (for psychological and psychiatric literature), AgeINFO (for literature relating to older people) and so on
- research and trials registers, such as CCTR (formerly the Cochrane Controlled Trials Register), Current Controlled Trials, National Research Register, Index to Theses and Dissertation Abstracts
- grey literature databases, such as the Health Management Information Consortium (HMIC) database, a compilation of data from the library and information services of the Department of Health and the King's Fund
- the Internet, including generic search engines (e.g. Google Scholar) and subject-specific search engines (e.g. Evidence Search (https://www.evidence.nhs.uk/), a free online service from NHS Evidence providing a database of hand-selected web resources for health and social care research)

- reviewing the table of contents of key journals, either on the Web or from the journal issues themselves
- checking the reference lists of selected articles
- contacting experts and key organisations
- conducting citation searches on key articles and authors using the Web of Knowledge or Google Scholar

Developing sensitive search strategies

Systematic literature searches use highly sensitive search strategies to ensure that no relevant studies are overlooked. A reviewer will look through a larger set of references (usually hundreds or even thousands) to minimise the chance of missing relevant items. Using 'specific' search strategies would mean that the search retrieves fewer, highly relevant references, but the reviewer runs the risk of missing relevant studies. The reviewer, therefore, aims to achieve the right balance between 'sensitivity' and 'specificity' when designing search strategies.

The sensitivity of a search strategy can be increased by:

- including more search terms and thesaurus terms (identified from previously retrieved references)
- using truncation ('*' or '$') or wildcards ('?' or '#') in free text searches
- using 'OR' to combine terms within the same concept
- using 'NEAR' or 'ADJ' (to indicate adjacency) to retrieve terms within the same sentence
- utilising a combination of free text and thesaurus search terms
- 'exploding' thesaurus search terms
- selecting 'all subheadings' for thesaurus search terms
- searching only on the 'population' and 'intervention', that is, not introducing 'outcomes' or 'comparisons' into the strategy
- not applying date, language or study design limits to the search strategy
- using 'sensitive' methodological search filters (see 'Methodological search filters' section)

Methodological search filters

Methodological search filters are strategies that are added to the subject search to retrieve different types of evidence from the search. Filters have been developed for the major types of question (i.e. therapy, prognosis, diagnosis and aetiology) and the major types of study (i.e. qualitative research, economic evaluations and clinical guidelines). Sample filters can be found at the InterTASC Information Specialists' Sub-Group Search Filter Resource (https://sites.google.com/a/york.ac.uk/issg-search-filters-resource/home).

Most major databases (e.g. Ovid MEDLINE and PubMed) now include a pre-stored facility to make it easier to use methodological filters. Methodological filters should be used with caution when conducting a *sensitive* search for systematic review purposes. However, they do provide a useful and *specific* way of scoping the quantity and quality of the literature prior to developing a review protocol.

Addressing publication bias

Publication bias means that studies with significant results are more likely to be published (Khan *et al.* 2011). Debate centres on whether systematic reviews should identify and include non-English-language or unpublished research (Egger *et al.* 2003; Song *et al.* 2013). For example, McAuley *et al.* (2000) have shown that if unpublished studies are not included in meta-analyses, the effectiveness of an intervention may be overestimated. However, even the most comprehensive literature search cannot eliminate the possibility of publication bias. For example, some studies are published two or more years after the research was conducted; other studies are never published; there is a tendency towards 'selective reporting', that is, where only studies that show statistically significant results are published and multiple publication of the same results from a single study in several different journals is common. Techniques to address 'publication bias' are suggested under 'SUMMARISING, INTERPRETING AND PRESENTING THE FINDINGS' section.

Reflection activity

Why do you feel that so much effort is spent in a systematic review on identifying the literature? If you were a clinician or a policy-maker what criticisms might you make if a reviewer is unable to demonstrate that they have comprehensively searched the literature? Ultimately, how might such criticisms determine how you, as a clinician or policy-maker, respond to findings from the review?

Managing large sets of references

It is essential to use a reference management system to manage the large numbers of references. Chapter 8 introduced electronic reference management software packages such as Reference Manager and EndNote. Reference management packages allow the reviewer to:

- store and maintain references (journals, books, reports, websites, theses, etc.)
- import references directly from major electronic bibliographic databases, such as MEDLINE
- keep track of references ordered from libraries
- assign keywords to references (e.g. the keyword 'RCT' can be applied to references retrieved from a clinical trials search)
- retrieve sets of references by author, publication year, title, keywords and so on
- insert personal notes and comments relating to individual references
- automatically create reference lists in the reviewer's preferred journal style
- insert references directly into word-processed reports

Documenting a systematic literature search

The review team should keep an accurate record of the search strategy used. Good documentation helps to avoid duplicated effort and provides a basis for updating the review in the future. Information to be recorded includes the date of the search, the sources searched, the search terms used and the number of references retrieved.

Selecting relevant studies

When selecting studies for inclusion, the aim is to identify only those articles that address the question(s) being posed. It is important to screen all the references retrieved and obtain the full text of studies that potentially meet the inclusion criteria. Inclusion criteria should stem directly from the review question(s) and relate to the core components of the question, that is, participants, interventions, outcomes and study design. Research Example 25.3 lists criteria for considering studies for inclusion in the antibiotics and antiseptics for venous leg ulcers review.

Criteria should be set in advance and piloted to check that they can be applied consistently. Final decisions about inclusion and exclusion are made after reading the full text of articles. Reasons for exclusion are recorded. Errors of judgement in study selection can be reduced by using two independent reviewers. However, double review is not always feasible, and it may be acceptable to assess a sample (e.g. 20%) of studies independently and then compare consistency.

Reflection activity

As a student, it is not usually possible (both for practical reasons and concerns of inappropriate collusion, that is, unauthorised cooperation on student assignments) to perform double review of included articles. What alternatives might you suggest? How might you take the fact that you only used a single reviewer into account when writing up your review assignment? Is there anything else you could do if you subsequently decided to try to publish that same review in a peer-reviewed journal?

RESEARCH EXAMPLE

25.3 Criteria for Considering Studies for Review: Antibiotics and Antiseptics for Venous Leg Ulcers (O'Meara *et al.* 2010)

Types of participants

Trials recruiting people described in the primary studies as having venous leg ulcers were eligible for inclusion. Trials recruiting people with different types of wounds (e.g. arterial ulcers, diabetic foot ulcers) were included if the results for patients with venous ulcers were presented separately or if the majority of participants (at least 75%) had leg ulcers of venous aetiology. Selection of trials was not restricted to those with a certain wound status at baseline (i.e. those with colonised or infected wounds); where information was given about these variables, it was recorded (see data extraction).

Types of intervention

The primary intervention is antibiotics (topical or systemic) or antiseptics (topical) prescribed for venous leg ulceration. Systemic preparations could be given orally or parenterally (e.g. by intravenous administration) and administered singly or in combination. Control regimens could include placebo, an alternative antibiotic or antiseptic, any other therapy, standard care or no treatment. Both intervention and control regimens could consist of combinations of antibiotics and antiseptics. Interventions could be delivered in any setting (inpatient, outpatient, nursing home plus any others). Trials evaluating topical silver-based preparations or the use of honey in wound healing were excluded as these interventions have been, or will be, covered in other Cochrane reviews).

Types of outcome measures

Primary outcomes

Trials reporting any of the following outcomes at any endpoint were eligible:

1 Time to complete ulcer healing
2 Proportion of ulcers completely healing during the trial period (frequency of complete healing)
3 Objective measurements of change in ulcer size
4 Healing rate (e.g. mm2 ulcer surface area reduction per week)

Secondary outcomes

Where reported, the following outcomes were also recorded:

1 Changes in signs and/or symptoms of clinical infection
2 Changes in bacterial flora
3 Development of bacterial resistance
4 Ulcer recurrence rates
5 Adverse effects of treatment
6 Patient satisfaction
7 Quality of life
8 Costs

Studies were only eligible for inclusion if they reported a primary outcome since those reporting solely secondary outcomes could introduce reporting bias. Findings from methodological research suggest that failure to report the full range of available outcomes assessed within a trial is associated with statistically non-significant results. This can result in the presentation of a selective and biased subset of study outcomes.

Types of studies

Prospective randomised controlled trials (RCTs) evaluating topical or systemic antibiotics or antiseptics in the treatment of venous ulcers were included.

ASSESSING THE QUALITY OF THE LITERATURE

Study quality refers to the degree to which a study takes steps to minimise bias and error in its design, conduct and analysis (Khan *et al.* 2011). Once studies of a minimum acceptable quality (based on the study design) have been selected, an in-depth critical appraisal is required. It is important to determine whether there is a quality (or study design) threshold, which defines the weakest acceptable study to be included. For example, many Cochrane reviews only include RCTs.

Detailed quality assessment of studies within a systematic review (Khan *et al.* 2011) aims to:

- describe the quality of studies included in the review
- explore whether different effects in different studies can be explained by variations in their quality
- decide whether to pool the effects observed in included studies
- determine the strength of inferences from the data
- recommend how future studies should be conducted

When conducting a systematic review, it is essential to identify suitable checklists for each study design that meets the inclusion criteria. If a checklist does not exist, then adapting existing tools that reflect generic issues relating to validity, reliability and applicability is preferable to developing an unvalidated checklist. Within the Cochrane Collaboration, the Risk of Bias Tool has gained increasing acceptance, partly because graphical indicators allow instant recognition of weaknesses of individual studies as well as those present across a whole group of related studies (Higgins *et al.* 2011).

Reflection activity

Why would you still want to perform quality assessment even if all your included studies found the same overall result (e.g. that treatment X is effective)? Is the fact that studies agree sufficient grounds for trusting that they are of good quality? Hint: Think of a comparable situation where all your friends and family give you consistent advice? Does that automatically make that good advice?

EXTRACTING KEY INFORMATION FROM THE SELECTED STUDIES

'*Data extraction*' involves identifying and recording important items (such as details of the author, the setting, the participants, the interventions, the outcomes and the main results) from each study. Data extraction forms are used to facilitate this process; forms should be piloted so as to reduce

RESEARCH EXAMPLE

25.4 Data Extraction and Management: Antibiotics and Antiseptics for Venous Leg Ulcers (O'Meara *et al.* 2010)

Details of the studies were extracted and summarised using a standardised data extraction sheet. If data were missing from reports, study authors were contacted and asked to provide missing information. Studies that had been published in duplicate were included only once, ensuring that all relevant data from all publications were included. Data extraction was undertaken by one author (DAK) and checked for accuracy by a second author (SO).

Types of data extracted included the following:

1. Study authors
2. Year of publication
3. Country where study performed
4. Study design (RCT)
5. Method of randomisation
6. Unit of randomisation
7. Overall sample size and methods used to estimate statistical power (relates to the target number of participants to be recruited, the clinical difference to be detected and the ability of the trial to detect this difference)
8. Outcomes measured
9. Setting of treatment
10. Duration of treatment
11. Participant selection criteria
12. Details of interventions (including specific antibiotics and antiseptics used) per study group, including concurrent interventions such as compression
13. Numbers per study group
14. Baseline characteristics of participants per treatment group (gender, age, ethnicity, baseline ulcer area, ulcer duration, prevalence of co-morbidities such as diabetes, prevalence of clinically infected wounds with definition as used in the trial, prevalence of colonised wounds with definition as used in the trial, identity of microorganisms isolated)
15. Methods used for identifying microorganisms
16. Statistical methods used for data analysis
17. Results per group for each outcome
18. Withdrawals (per group with numbers and reasons).

errors and minimise bias. For example, the data extraction form must accommodate all eligible study designs and ensure that the researcher consistently collects the same type of data from each study. Sample data extraction forms are provided in the 2nd edition of CRD Report Number 4 (Khan *et al.* 2001). Research Example 25.4 documents the proposed data extraction strategy for the antibiotics and antiseptics for venous leg ulcers example.

SUMMARISING, INTERPRETING AND PRESENTING THE FINDINGS

Once all relevant data have been extracted, they must then be synthesised. In many cases, synthesis entails providing a descriptive summary ('*narrative commentary*'), possibly supported by a tabular presentation ('*summary tables*'). Where possible, quantitative data are combined in a '*meta-analysis*' to quantify the benefits (or harms) of an intervention. Before undertaking such an analysis, it is important to establish whether it is appropriate to do so. For example, there is no value in pooling results if:

- only one study has estimated the effect of an intervention
- significant differences in participants, interventions and/or setting could substantially affect the outcomes (*'clinical heterogeneity'*)
- there is excessive variation in the results of the studies (*'statistical heterogeneity'*)
- outcome(s) have been measured in different ways in each study
- studies do not contain the required information

In simple terms, a meta-analysis involves taking individual results for the same outcome from several studies and calculating a 'single summary statistic' (sometimes referred to as an *'effect measure'*). Standard effect measures include 'odds ratio' (OR), 'relative risk' (RR), 'risk difference', 'number needed to treat', 'standardised mean difference' and 'weighted mean difference'. RR and OR are the most common measures. Both measures relate the proportion of participants who are observed to experience an event in the intervention group to the proportion of participants who experience the same event in the control group. Although the way the statistics are calculated is slightly different, it is easy to remember that for both measures an RR/OR of 1 indicates no difference between the groups being compared (Khan *et al.* 2001).

Where studies examine 'similar' groups, effect sizes across studies should be compared and an overall effect calculated by taking a weighted average of the individual study effects. However, not all readers are comfortable with interpreting the statistical measures involved. Results of a meta-analysis can be presented graphically as a *'forest plot'*, sometimes referred to as a 'blobbogram' or 'OR diagram'. Such a diagram represents the individual study results within the review together with the combined result of the meta-analysis. An example is provided in Figure 25.1.

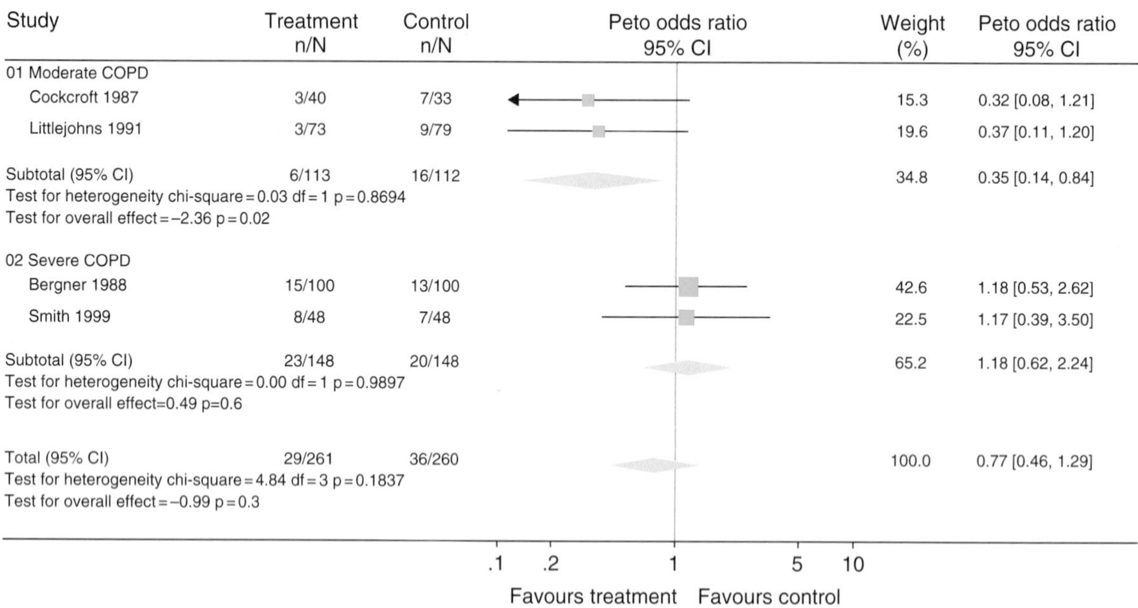

Review: Home care by outreach nursing for chronic obstructive pulmonary disease
Comparison: 01 Respiratory outreach nurse vs control
Outcome: 05 Mortality
Study
Treatment n/N
Control n/N
Peto odds ratio 95% CI
Weight (%)
Peto odds ratio 95% CI
01 Moderate COPD
Cockcroft 1987 3/40 7/33 15.3 0.32 [0.08, 1.21]
Littlejohns 1991 3/73 9/79 19.6 0.37 [0.11, 1.20]
Subtotal (95% CI) 6/113 16/112 34.8 0.35 [0.14, 0.84]
Test for heterogeneity chi-square = 0.03 df = 1 p = 0.8694
Test for overall effect = –2.36 p = 0.02
02 Severe COPD
Bergner 1988 15/100 13/100 42.6 1.18 [0.53, 2.62]
Smith 1999 8/48 7/48 22.5 1.17 [0.39, 3.50]
Subtotal (95% CI) 23/148 20/148 65.2 1.18 [0.62, 2.24]
Test for heterogeneity chi-square = 0.00 df = 1 p = 0.9897
Test for overall effect=0.49 p=0.6
Total (95% CI) 29/261 36/260 100.0 0.77 [0.46, 1.29]
Test for heterogeneity chi-square = 4.84 df = 3 p = 0.1837
Test for overall effect = –0.99 p = 0.3
.1 .2 1 5 10
Favours treatment Favours control

Figure 25.1 An example of a forest plot from the Cochrane review 'Home care by outreach nursing for chronic obstructive pulmonary disease' (Smith *et al.* 2008). Reproduced with permission from John Wiley & Sons

The vertical line represents the line of no effect, that is, where the group receiving the intervention are no better or worse off than the control group or, in other words, where the OR is equal to 1. The small 'blobs' represent the results of individual trials. The area of each 'blob' represents the weight given to each study in the meta-analysis. Larger, higher-quality studies receive more weight than smaller, lower-quality ones. The larger diamond-shaped 'blob' next to the 'total' row represents the overall meta-analysis result when all the studies are pooled together. The horizontal lines associated with each 'blob' represent the confidence interval (in this case, 95%) for each result. The confidence interval tells us how much uncertainty is associated with each result. Narrow confidence intervals indicate that the same result is likely to occur were the study to be repeated many times. Wider confidence intervals mean that different results are more likely to occur. In the example in Figure 25.1, comparing respiratory outreach nurses with a control, the overall pooled result indicated by the diamond lies to the left of the line of no effect. This positioning indicates less of the outcome (mortality) in the treatment (respiratory outreach nurse) group. However, the horizontal points of the diamond, indicating the confidence interval when all the studies are pooled together, cross the line of no effect, which means that the result is not significant. Closer examination of the plot and the text of the review reveals that the authors have pooled studies including people with both moderate and severe chronic obstructive pulmonary disease and the overall effect 'mixes up' people most likely to benefit from the treatment with those who are less likely to benefit.

A meta-analysis is a complex mathematical calculation often requiring input from a statistician. Fortunately, several software packages (such as Review Manager – http://ims.cochrane.org/revman) are available to facilitate meta-analysis.

Even rigorously conducted systematic reviews cannot eliminate the risk of '*publication and related biases*'. Therefore, every review should incorporate a formal assessment of such risks. Statistical and modelling techniques, such as '*funnel plots*', exist to assist in highlighting these biases. Funnel plots map individual effects from studies against some measure of study information (e.g. study size). An asymmetrical inverted funnel may indicate the presence of bias, although the possibility of chance cannot be excluded.

WRITING UP THE REVIEW

A succinct report of the review allows readers to judge its validity and the implications of its findings (University of York *et al.* 2009). All Cochrane reviews are reported in a consistent manner that includes a structured abstract, background, objectives, criteria for considering studies, search strategy, methods of the review, description of studies, methodological quality, results, summary of analyses, discussion, reviewers' conclusions (including implications for practice and research) and references. A similar structure should be adopted when writing up any systematic review. The Preferred Reporting Items for Systematic Reviews and Meta-Analyses (PRISMA, formerly QUOROM) statement outlines a standard for the quality of reporting of systematic reviews of RCTs (Liberati *et al.* 2009).

SYSTEMATIC REVIEWS OF QUALITATIVE RESEARCH

Techniques for identifying and synthesising qualitative research have been at the forefront of recent methodological developments although there remains little consensus as to which methods should be used for searching, appraising and synthesising good quality studies (Hannes & Macaitis 2012). Some of this uncertainty stems from the diversity of qualitative research. Some argue that a particular method of appraisal or analysis may privilege specific types of qualitative research. Evans and Pearson (2001) provide a good overview of the main issues for qualitative systematic reviews for nurses. They characterise such issues under six stages of the review process:

- Defining the focus
- Locating studies

- Selecting studies for inclusion in review
- Critical appraisal
- Data extraction
- Data synthesis

The stages of the systematic review process are thus common to both quantitative and qualitative research (Seers 2012). However, similarities and differences between methods used and their underlying principles exist for quantitative and qualitative syntheses at each stage of the review process.

Approaches to syntheses of qualitative research tend to divide into those that regard syntheses of qualitative research as broadly equivalent to those for quantitative research and those that state that qualitative evidence synthesis is, in fact, conceptually aligned to primary qualitative research (Booth 2013). Both approaches work from the premise that systematic reviews of qualitative research should be systematic, explicit and reproducible but other concepts, strongly associated with quantitative systematic reviews, such as the requirement to be 'comprehensive' mark the battle lines.

Aside from such conceptual differences, the review community is at least starting to identify some broad operating principles. For example, if an established conceptual framework already exists for a topic under exploration, then some type of framework analysis approach may be appropriate; if, however, the topic is still fluid and being defined, then a grounded theory approach may be chosen. Similarly, if the main intent of the review is descriptive, then an aggregative approach, such as that employed by the Joanna Briggs Institute (Hannes & Lockwood 2011a), may be most suitable. If, however, the primary intent is analytical, requiring some degree of conceptual innovation, then an interpretative approach, such as meta-ethnography or critical interpretive synthesis, may be considered. Such principles cannot be prescriptive, however, and those planning a qualitative evidence synthesis may find it helpful to look at compilations of methodological alternatives such as the books by Pope *et al.* (2007) and Hannes and Lockwood (2011b), the open-access article by Barnett-Page and Thomas (2009) or guidance from the Cochrane Collaboration's Qualitative Research and Implementation Methods Group (http://cqim.cochrane.org/). It will also be useful to examine the emerging standards for reporting qualitative systematic reviews, *Enhancing transparency in reporting the synthesis of qualitative research (ENTREQ)* (Tong *et al.* 2012).

Recent methodological developments in qualitative evidence synthesis have challenged the idea that these simply have to follow the lead of the longer-established quantitative systematic review. It is clear that methods from primary qualitative research can not only inform the conduct of qualitative reviews but can also benefit systematic reviews in general. For example, iterative approaches typically used to develop and refine interpretation of qualitative data challenge the rigidly sequential model of reviews perpetuated by the quantitative model. Furthermore, there is increasing acknowledgement that *comprehensiveness of a search strategy* is not in itself a defining characteristic of a systematic review. Instead, the *appropriateness of the sampling strategy* for identifying the literature, be it comprehensive, purposive, theoretical or random (Suri 2011), is a much more tenable principle focusing, as it does, on 'fitness for purpose'. Liberation from the unforgiving principle of the comprehensive search not only benefits qualitative evidence synthesis but also time-limited quantitative approaches such as health technology assessments.

Syntheses of qualitative research include a meta-synthesis of directly observed therapy in tuberculosis (Research Example 25.6) (Noyes & Popay 2007) and a thematic synthesis of group therapy for postnatal depression (Scope *et al.* 2012). Although it is helpful to recognise that the intent of evidence syntheses, whether quantitative or qualitative, may be primarily aggregative (in bringing the evidence together in an additive way) or configurative (in seeking to make sense of a specific phenomenon) (Gough *et al.* 2012), such positions are best pictured on a continuum. Approaches that can integrate both quantitative and qualitative data and that can fulfil aggregative and configurative functions will become increasingly important especially as mixed-method approaches continue to grow in popularity.

RESEARCH EXAMPLE

25.6 A Qualitative Meta-synthesis of Directly Observed Therapy for Tuberculosis (Noyes & Popay 2007)

Background: DOT is part of a World Health Organization (WHO)-branded package of interventions to improve the management of TB and adherence with treatment (Maher 1999). DOT involves asking people with TB to visit a health worker or other appointed person, to receive and be observed taking a dose of medication. To supplement a Cochrane Intervention review of trials of DOT, we conducted a synthesis of qualitative evidence concerning people with, or at risk of, TB, service providers and policy makers, to explore their experience and perceptions of TB and treatment. Findings were used to help explain and interpret the Cochrane Intervention review and to consider implications for research, policy and practice.

Review questions: Two broad research questions were addressed:

1 What are the facilitators and barriers to accessing and complying with tuberculosis treatment?
2 Can exploration of qualitative studies and/or qualitative components of the studies included in the intervention review explain the heterogeneity of findings?

Method:

Search methods: A systematic search of the wider English-language literature was undertaken. The following terms were used: DOT; DOTS; Directly observed therapy; Directly observed treatment; supervised swallowing; self-supervision; in combination with TB and tuberculosis. We experimented with using methodological filters by including terms such as 'qualitative', but found this approach unhelpful as the Medline MeSH heading 'Qualitative Research' was only introduced in 2003, and even after 2003 many papers were not identified appropriately as qualitative. We searched MEDLINE, CINAHL, HMIC, Embase, British Nursing Index, International Bibliography of the Social Sciences, Sociological Abstracts, SIGLE, ASSIA, Psych Info, Econ lit, Ovid, Pubmed, the London School of Hygiene and Tropical Medicine database of TB studies (courtesy of Dr. Simon Lewin) and Google Scholar. Reference lists contained within published papers were also scrutinized. A network of personal contacts was also used to identify papers. All principal researchers involved in the six randomized trials included in the Cochrane Intervention review were contacted and relevant qualitative studies obtained.

Selection and appraisal of studies: The following definition was used to select studies: 'papers whose primary focus was the experiences and/or perceptions of TB and its treatment amongst people with, or at risk of, TB and service providers'. The study had to use qualitative methods of data collection and analysis, as either a stand-alone study or a discrete part of a larger mixed-method study. To appraise methodological and theoretical dimensions of study quality, two contrasting frameworks were used independently by JN and JP (Popay 1998; Critical Appraisal Skills Programme 2006). Studies were not excluded on quality grounds, but lower quality studies were reviewed to see if they altered the outcome of the synthesis – which they did not.

Analysis: Thematic analysis techniques were used to synthesize data from 1990 to 2002, and an update of literature to December 2005. Themes were identified by bringing together components of ideas, experiences and views embedded in the data – themes were constructed to form a comprehensive picture of participants' collective experiences. A narrative summary technique was used to aid interpretation of trial results.

Findings: Fifty-eight papers derived from 53 studies were included. Five themes emerged from 1990 to 2002 synthesis, including: socio-economic circumstances, material resources and individual agency; explanatory models and knowledge systems in relation to tuberculosis and its treatment; the experience of stigma and public discourses around tuberculosis; sanctions, incentives and support, and the social organization and social relationships of care. Two additional themes emerged from the 2005 update: the barriers created by programme implementation, and the challenge to the model that culturally determined factors are the central cause of treatment failure.

Conclusions: The Cochrane Intervention review did not show statistically significant differences between DOT and self-supervision, suggesting that it was not DOT per se that led to an improvement in treatment outcomes. Variants of DOT differed in important ways in terms of who was being observed, where the observation took place and how often observation occurred. The synthesis of qualitative research suggests that these elements of DOT will be crucial in determining how effective a particular type of DOT will be in terms of increased cure rates. The qualitative review also highlighted the key role of social and economic factors and physical side effects of medication in shaping behaviour in relation to seeking diagnosis and adhering to treatment. More specifically, a predominantly inspectorial approach to observation is not likely to increase uptake of service or adherence with medication. Inspectorial elements may be needed in treatment packages, but when the primary focus of direct observation was inspectorial rather than supportive in nature, observation was least effective. Direct observation of an inspectorial nature had the most negative impact on those who had the most to fear from disclosure, such as disadvantaged women who experienced gender-related discrimination. In contrast, treatment packages in which the emphasis is on person-centred support are more likely to increase uptake and adherence. Qualitative evidence also provided insights into the type of support that people with TB find most helpful. Primarily, the ability of the observer to add value depended on the observer and the service being able to adapt to the widely-varying individual circumstances of the person being observed (age, gender, agency, location, income, etc.). Given the heterogeneity amongst those with TB, findings support the need for locally tailored, patient-centred programmes rather than a single world wide intervention.

Reflection activity

To what extent do you consider it appropriate to base methods for systematic review of qualitative research on established methods for systematic review of quantitative research? Imagine that you are a qualitative researcher who has never conducted a systematic review before – are there any concepts from primary qualitative research that you could usefully take with you into this new area of research activity? Hint: instead of thinking literally in terms of papers, picture each study as a key informant in the community who has something to tell you.

CONCLUSION

Evidence syntheses, in the form of systematic reviews, practice guidelines and economic evaluations, provide the opportunity to generate a synthesis of research evidence to inform practice. Explicit methods are used to identify, select, critically appraise and summarise large quantities of information. Irrespective of the type of evidence synthesis, several discrete, but interconnected, stages are followed. Stages include:

- writing a research protocol
- systematically searching the literature
- selecting relevant studies
- assessing the quality of the literature
- extracting key information from the selected studies

- summarising, interpreting and presenting the findings
- writing up the research in a structured manner.

References

Akers J, Aguiar-Ibáñez R, Baba-Akbari Sari A, Beynon S, Booth A, Burch J *et al.* (2009) *Systematic Reviews: CRD's guidance for undertaking reviews in health care.* York, NHS Centre for Reviews and Dissemination, University of York.

Allen JK, Dennison Himmelfarb CR, Szanton SL, Frick KD (2014) Cost-effectiveness of nurse practitioner/community health worker care to reduce cardiovascular health disparities. *Journal of Cardiovascular Nursing* **29**(4): 308–314. DOI: 10.1097/JCN.0b013e3182945243.

Anderson O, Boshier PR, Hanna GB (2012) Interventions designed to prevent healthcare bed-related injuries in patients. *Cochrane Database of Systematic Reviews*, Issue 1. Art. No.: CD008931. DOI: 10.1002/14651858.CD008931.pub3.

Barnett-Page E, Thomas J (2009). Methods for the synthesis of qualitative research: a critical review. *BMC Medical Research Methodology* **9**(1): 59.

Booth A (2013) *Acknowledging a 'Dual Heritage' for Qualitative Evidence Synthesis: harnessing the qualitative research and systematic review research traditions.* PhD by Publications, Sheffield, University of Sheffield.

Booth A, Papaioannou D, Sutton A (2011) *Systematic Approaches to a Successful Literature Review.* London, Sage.

Critical Appraisal Skills Programme (CASP) (2006) Public Health Resource Unit, Oxford. http://www.phru.nhs.uk/casp/critical_appraisal_tools.htm (accessed 13 September 2014).

Egger M, Juni P, Barlett C, Holenstein F, Sterne J (2003). How important are comprehensive literature searches and the assessment of trial quality in systematic reviews? *Health Technology Assessment* **7**(1): 1–76.

Evans D, Pearson A (2001) Systematic reviews of qualitative research. *Clinical Effectiveness for Nursing* **5**: 111–119.

Gough D, Thomas J, Oliver S (2012) Clarifying differences between review designs and methods. *Systematic Reviews* **1**(1): 28.

Grant MJ, Booth A (2009) A typology of reviews: an analysis of 14 review types and associated methodologies. *Health Information and Libraries Journal* **26**(2): 91–108.

Greenhalgh T (2010) *How to Read a Paper: the basics of evidence based practice.* 4th edition. Chichester, John Wiley & Sons, Ltd.

Hannes K, Lockwood C (2011a) Pragmatism as the philosophical underpinning of the Joanna Briggs meta-aggregative approach to qualitative evidence synthesis. *Journal of Advanced Nursing* **67**: 1632–1642.

Hannes K, Lockwood C (2011b) *Synthesizing qualitative research: choosing the right approach.* Chichester, John Wiley & Sons, Ltd.

Hannes K, Macaitis K (2012) A move to more systematic and transparent approaches in qualitative evidence synthesis: update on a review of published papers. *Qualitative Research* **12**(4): 402–442.

Heinrich S, Rapp K, Stuhldreher N, Rissmann U, Becker C, Konig HH (2013) Cost-effectiveness of a multifactorial fall prevention program in nursing homes. *Osteoporosis International* **24**(4): 1215–1223.

Higgins JP, Altman DG, Gøtzsche PC, Jüni P, Moher D, Oxman AD, Savovic J, Schulz KF, Weeks L, Sterne JA, Cochrane Bias Methods Group; Cochrane Statistical Methods Group (2011) The Cochrane Collaboration's tool for assessing risk of bias in randomised trials. *British Medical Journal* **343**: d5928.

Khan K, Kunz R, Kleijnen J, Antes G (2011) *Systematic Reviews to Support Evidence based Medicine: how to review and apply findings of healthcare research,* 2nd edition. London, Royal Society of Medicine.

Khan KS, ter Riet G, Glanville J, Sowden AJ, Kleijnen J (eds) (2001) *Undertaking Systematic Reviews of Research on Effectiveness. CRD's Guidance for Carrying Out or Commissioning Reviews.* 2nd edition. CRD Report No. 4. York: NHS Centre for Reviews and Dissemination, University of York.

Lavender T, Richens Y, Milan SJ, Smyth RMD, Dowswell T (2013) Telephone support for women during pregnancy and the first six weeks postpartum. Cochrane Database of Systematic Reviews, Issue 7. Art. No.: CD009338. DOI: 10.1002/14651858.CD009338.pub2.

Liberati A, Altman DG, Tetzlaff J, Mulrow C, Gøtzsche PC, Ioannidis JP, Clarke M, Devereaux PJ, Kleijnen J, Moher D (2009) The PRISMA statement for reporting systematic reviews and meta-analyses of studies that evaluate healthcare interventions: explanation and elaboration. *British Medical Journal* **339**: b2700.

Maher D, Mikulencak M (1999) *What Is DOTS? A Guide to Understanding the WHO-Recommended TB Control Strategy Known as DOTS.* Geneva: World Health Organization.

McAuley A, Pharm B, Tugwell P, Moher D (2000) Does the inclusion of grey literature influence estimates of intervention effectiveness reported in meta-analyses? *Lancet* **356**: 1228–1231.

Mulrow C (1995) Rationale for systematic reviews. In: Chalmers I, Altman DG (eds) *Systematic Reviews*. London, BMJ Publishing, pp 1–8.

National Library of Medicine, Medical Subject headings (MeSH) from PubMed, MeSH browser. Available at http://www.ncbi.nlm.nih.gov/entrez/query.fcgi?db=mesh (accessed 31 August 2014).

Noyes J, Popay J (2007) Directly observed therapy and tuberculosis: how can a systematic review of qualitative research contribute to improving services? A qualitative meta-synthesis. *Journal of Advanced Nursing* **57**(3): 227–243.

O'Meara S, Al-Kurdi D, Ologun Y, Ovington LG (2010) Antibiotics and antiseptics for venous leg ulcers. *Cochrane Database of Systematic Reviews* 2010, Issue 1. Art. No.: CD003557. DOI: 10.1002/14651858.CD003557.pub3.

Parab CS, Cooper C, Woolfenden S, Piper SM (2013) *Specialist home-based nursing services for children with acute and chronic illnesses*. Cochrane Database of Systematic Reviews, Issue 6. Art. No.: CD004383. DOI: 10.1002/14651858.CD004383.pub3.

Popay J, Rogers A, Williams G (1998) Rationale and standards for the systematic review of qualitative literature in health services research. *Qualitative Health Research* **8**: 314–351.

Pope C, Mays N, Popay J (2007) *Synthesising Qualitative and Quantitative Health Evidence. A guide to methods*. Milton Keynes, Open University Press.

Robinson R (1993) Economic evaluation and health care. What does it mean? *British Medical Journal* **307**: 670–673.

Scope A, Booth A, Sutcliffe P (2012) Women's perceptions and experiences of group cognitive behaviour therapy and other group interventions for postnatal depression: a qualitative synthesis. *Journal of Advanced Nursing* **68**(9): 1909–1919.

Seers K (2012) What is a qualitative synthesis? *Evidence Based Nursing* **15**(4): 101–101.

Smith B, Appleton S, Adams R, Southcott A, Ruffin R (2008) Home care by outreach nursing for chronic obstructive pulmonary disease (Review). *The Cochrane Library. Issue 3*, Chichester, John Wiley & Sons, Ltd.

Song F, Hooper L, Loke YK (2013) Publication bias: what is it? How do we measure it? How do we avoid it? *Open Access Journal of Clinical Trials* **5**: 71–81.

Suri H (2011) Purposeful sampling in qualitative research synthesis. *Qualitative Research Journal* **11**(2): 63–75.

Tong A, Flemming K, McInnes E, Oliver S, Craig J (2012) Enhancing transparency in reporting the synthesis of qualitative research: ENTREQ. *BMC Medical Research Methodology* **12**(1): 181.

University of York Centre for Reviews and Dissemination, Akers J (2009). *Systematic reviews: CRD's guidance for undertaking reviews in health care*. York, Centre for Reviews and Dissemination.

Further reading

Aveyard, H (2010) *Doing a Literature Review in Health and Social Care: a practical guide*. 2nd edition. Milton Keynes, Open University Press.

Booth A, Papaioannou D, Sutton A (2011) *Systematic Approaches to a Successful Literature Review*. London, Sage.

Khan K, Kunz R, Klejnen J, Antes G (2011) *Systematic Reviews to Support Evidence-based Medicine*. 2nd edition. London, Hodder Arnold.

NHS Centre for Reviews and Dissemination (2009). *Systematic Reviews: CRD's guidance for undertaking reviews in health care*. York, University of York.

Pope C, Mays N, Popay J, (2007) *Synthesising Qualitative and Quantitative Health Evidence. A guide to methods*. Milton Keynes, Open University Press.

Torgerson C (2003) *Systematic Reviews*. London, Continuum International Publishing Group.

Websites

http://www.campbellcollaboration.org – The Campbell Collaboration

http://www.cochrane.org – The Cochrane Collaboration

http://www.thecochranelibrary.com – The Cochrane Library

https://sites.google.com/a/york.ac.uk/issg-search-filters-resource/home – The InterTASC Information Specialists' Sub-Group Search Filter Resource

CHAPTER 26

Realist Synthesis

Jo Rycroft-Malone, Brendan McCormack, Kara DeCorby and Alison M. Hutchinson

Key points

- Realist synthesis is growing in popularity as a review approach. It is particularly appropriate for unpacking the impact of complex interventions because it works on the premise that one needs to understand how interventions work in different contexts and why.
- Realist synthesis is premised on a set of principles rather than a formula. Stages of review include theory formulation, bespoke data extraction form development, finding and appraising evidence, data synthesis and narrative construction. Fundamentally, realist synthesis is concerned with developing and refining theory through this process.
- The demands on a realist synthesiser are different to those expected in a Cochrane-type review. Quality assurance within realist synthesis is dependent on the reviewers' explicitness and reflexivity. In turn, this requires a high level of expertise in reasoning and research methods.

INTRODUCTION

The research evidence base for health-care policy and practice is huge, and most of us would not have the time to search, appraise and interpret this volume of available information. Evidence reviews have become a popular mechanism for the identification, appraisal and synthesis of research-based evidence about the effectiveness of a particular intervention. Traditional systematic reviews, which tend to include research evidence according to specific eligibility criteria that favour the hierarchy of evidence and which answer focused questions, have been criticised for being too specific (Pawson *et al.* 2004, 2005; McCormack *et al.* 2007a). This critique becomes particularly relevant when considering the complexity of implementing health-care interventions. The context of health care is complex, multifaceted and dynamic, which means that rarely, if ever, would the same intervention work in the same way in different contexts. As such, conventional systematic review approaches to evaluating the evidence of whether they work tend to result in limited answers

The Research Process in Nursing, Seventh Edition. Edited by Kate Gerrish and Judith Lathlean.

Companion Website: www.wiley.com/go/gerrish/research

such as 'to some extent' and 'sometimes' (Pawson *et al.* 2004; Pawson 2006). Realist synthesis has emerged as an ever increasingly popular strategy for evidence review that focuses on providing explanations for why interventions may or may not work, in what contexts, how and why.

REALIST REVIEW: PHILOSOPHY AND PRINCIPLES

A realist synthesis has its roots in realism, which as a philosophy of science is situated between the extremes of positivism and relativism (Delanty 1997). Realism involves identifying underlying causal mechanisms and how they work under what conditions (Pawson & Tilley 1997; Pawson 2002, 2013; McEvoy & Richards 2003). Because causal mechanisms always occur in a particular social context, there is a need to understand the complex relationship between these mechanisms and the effect that context has on their effectiveness. Complex interventions according to Pawson *et al.* (2004) and Pawson (2013) are comprised of theories, involve the actions of people, consist of a chain of steps or processes that interact and are rarely linear, are embedded in social systems, are prone to modification and exist in open systems that change through learning. Pawson and Tilley (1997) sum this up as follows: context + mechanism → outcome (CMO), which is a testable proposition.

For Pawson (2006), any synthesis of evidence needs to investigate why and how interventions might work, in what contexts. The aim is

> … to articulate underlying programme theories and then to interrogate the existing evidence to find out whether and where these theories are pertinent and productive. (Pawson 2006: 74)

In this case, 'theory' is construed and defined differently from positivistic interpretations. For realist synthesis, a theory is framed in terms of a proposition, expressed as a CMO, about how interventions work; for example, if you implement an intervention in this way, in this context, you may get x result (Pawson *et al.* 2004, 2005; Pawson 2006).

REALIST SYNTHESIS: EXAMPLES

There are a growing number of published examples of realist synthesis, but few related specifically to nursing. Examples from the health-related literature more broadly include a review by Greenhalgh *et al.* (2007) that sought to understand the efficacy of school feeding programmes and what it is about them that made them work (or not). Wong *et al.* (2010) reviewed Internet-based medical education, developing a preliminary set of questions to aid course developers and learners to consider issues around engagement, interactivity and course–context interaction. McCormack *et al.* (2013) conducted a realist review on change agency, which found that issues such as accessibility, cultural compatibility and attitude influence their overall impact. Other good examples include Best *et al.* (2012) who reviewed large-system transformation and Jagosh *et al.* (2012) who reviewed community-based participatory research approaches.

Key features of realist syntheses have been distilled in publication standards: Realist And Meta-narrative Evidence Syntheses: Evolving Standards (RAMESES) (Wong *et al.* 2013). These standards reinforce the need to focus on the nature of the theory offered, theory building and testing, data to support interpretations and a detailed description of the analysis and synthesis process, among other criteria within the review process. Although it is not advisable to be prescriptive about the process and set of decisions related to realist synthesis, a level of detail that offers transparency is recommended (Wong *et al.* 2013). The RAMESES guidelines include a list of items to be incorporated in published accounts of realist syntheses and are a useful 'checklist' for a realist reviewer.

Reflection activity

In the context of evidence-informed health care (E-IHC), what are the overall benefits of working with the question 'what works, for whom does it work, in what circumstances and why?'

STAGES IN CONDUCTING A REALIST SYNTHESIS

We draw on two examples within this chapter to illustrate the stages in conducting a realist synthesis: first a published example (McCormack *et al.* 2006, 2007a, 2007b, 2007c, 2007d) and second a realist synthesis undertaken by an international team (the Realist Synthesis of Implementation Strategies (ReS-IS) project) (Rycroft-Malone *et al.* 2012; McCormack *et al.* 2013) that answered the question, 'what are the interventions and strategies that are effective in enabling evidence-informed health care?'

A realist synthesis follows similar stages to a traditional systematic review with some notable differences (see Box 26.1). The realist synthesis approach is framed around a number of key principles:

- The review focus is derived from a negotiation between commissioners (of the review) and the researchers. Therefore, the extent of stakeholder involvement throughout the process is high.
- The search and appraisal of evidence is purposive and theoretically driven with the aim of refining theory.
- Multiple types of information and evidence are included.
- The process is iterative.
- The outcome is always 'explanatory', that is, the findings focus on explaining to the reader why (or not) the intervention works and in what ways, to enable informed choices about further use and/or research.

Pawson *et al.* (2004) set out the following steps for a realist synthesis approach.

Phase 1: Concept mining and theory formulation

Developing the focus of the study and the theories to be examined is an important aspect of a realist synthesis study as it provides the structure for examining a diverse body of evidence (Pawson *et al.* 2004). Phase 1 is therefore concerned with concept mining and theory formulation, digging through the literature for key terms, ideas, middle-range theories and hypotheses that begin to provide some explanations to your subject of interest (Pawson *et al.* 2005). The challenge of developing the framework for a realist synthesis is to find the level of abstraction that allows the reviewers to both stand back from the mass of detail and variation in the data set and also meet the purpose of the review. Additionally, as a realist synthesis focuses on determining 'what works' within differing contextual configurations, a theoretical model must be outcome focused.

McCormack *et al.* (2006) developed a theoretical model derived from the project steering group's ideas and questions, the project team's constructions and conceptualisations of practice development found in the literature. These ideas and conceptual connections were referred to by McCormack *et al.* as *theoretical fragments* as they are the basis for constructing the model. Following discussion of these theoretical fragments among the project team and the project steering group, a theoretical model was developed around the 'who, what/why, how and by whom' of practice development (Figure 26.1).

The model has 4 theoretical areas containing 13 areas of focus with themes for exploration as follows:

Theory area 1: Properties of the people and context in practice development

- What impact does the extent of involvement of different stakeholders have on the outcomes of practice development?
- What impact does the scale of a study have on the outcomes of practice development?
- How do contextual factors in the study setting have an impact on the outcomes of practice development?
- How do cultural factors in the study setting have an impact on the outcomes of practice development?
- How do styles of leadership in the study setting have an impact on the outcomes of practice development?

Box 26.1 Approach to realist synthesis (adapted from Pawson *et al.* 2004)

Define the scope of the review	Identify the question	What is the nature and content of the intervention?
		What are the circumstances or context of its use?
		What are the policy intentions or objectives?
		What are the nature and form of its outcomes or impacts?
		Undertake exploratory searches to inform discussion with review commissioners/decision-makers
	Clarify the purpose(s) of the review	Theory integrity – does the intervention work as predicted?
		Theory adjudication – which theories around the intervention seem to fit best?
		Comparison – how does the intervention work in different settings, for different groups?
		Reality testing – how does the policy intent of the intervention translate into practice?
	Find and articulate the programme theories	Search for relevant 'theories' in the literature
		Draw up list of programme theories
		Group, categorise or synthesise theories
		Design a theoretically based evaluative framework to be 'populated' with evidence
Search for and appraise the evidence	Search for the evidence	Decide and define purposive sampling strategy
		Define search sources, terms and methods to be used (including cited reference searching)
		Set the thresholds for stopping searching at saturation
	Appraise the evidence	Test relevance – does the research address the theory under test?
		Test rigour – does the research support the conclusions drawn from it by the researchers or the reviewers?
Extract and synthesise findings	Extract the results	Develop data extraction forms or templates
		Extract data to populate the evaluative framework with evidence
	Synthesise findings	Compare and contrast findings from different studies
		Use findings from studies to address purposes(s) of review
		Seek both confirmatory and contradictory findings
		Refine programme theories in the light of evidence including findings from analysis of study data
Draw conclusions and make recommendations		Involve commissioners/decision-makers in review of findings
		Draft and test out recommendations and conclusions based on findings with key stakeholders
		Disseminate review with findings, conclusions and recommendations

Reproduced from McCormack B, Wright J, Dewer B, Harvey G, Ballintine K (2007a) A realist synthesis of evidence relating to practice development: methodology and methods. *Practice Development in Health Care* **6**(1): 5–24 (pp 9–11) with permission from John Wiley and Sons.

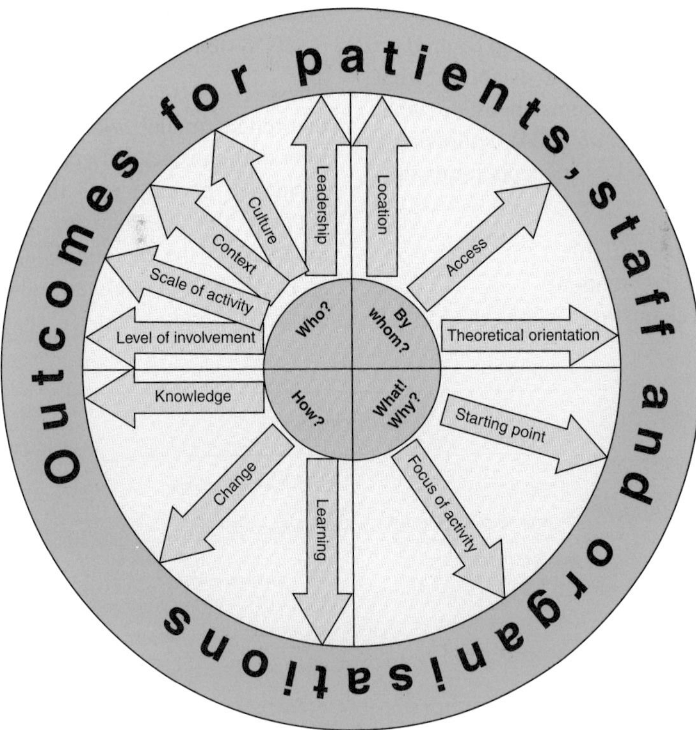

Figure 26.1 Explanatory model for practice development. Reproduced from McCormack B, Wright J, Dewer B, Harvey G, Ballintine K (2007a) A realist synthesis of evidence relating to practice development: methodology and methods. *Practice Development in Health Care* **6**(1): 5–24 (p 15) with permission from John Wiley and Sons.

Theory area 2: Properties of the people involved in developing practice

- How does the location of a practice developer have an impact on the outcomes of practice development?
- How do the means by which the practice developer gains access to the practice environment have an impact on the outcomes of practice development?
- How do the methodological positions taken by practice developers have an impact on the outcomes of practice development?

Theory area 3: Issues surrounding the initiation and carrying out of practice development

- How do factors involved in the initiation of practice development have an impact on its outcomes?
- What are the foci of practice development activity and how do they have an impact on its outcomes?

Theory area 4: Approaches to the use of knowledge, bringing about change and supporting learning in practice development

- How do approaches taken to support learning within practice development have an impact on outcomes?
- How do approaches taken to bring about change within practice development have an impact on outcomes?
- What forms of knowledge use and knowledge generation are used in practice development, and what are the consequences for the outcomes?

In the ReS-IS project, 'theory formulation' occurred through an iterative process of workshops, telephone conferences and 'blog discussions'. All project team members were immersed in knowledge utilisation research. Discussion at the first workshop centred on the purpose of the synthesis being to establish 'what works for whom, in what circumstances, in what respects, and how' (Pawson *et al.* 2004). Following a brainstorming exercise, five key concepts for examination emerged:

- Change agency (person, roles)
- Levels (target of intervention)
- Technology (mechanisms)
- Education and learning strategies
- Systems change (group or social processes)

These concepts were then framed to construct a theoretical model with *dose* (what quantity of an intervention is needed), *theory* and *contextual factors* (evidence of particular theory and context issues shaping the mechanism) as central factors and *outcomes* as the encompassing factor (Figure 26.2).

The ReS-IS model had 4 theoretical areas and 13 theoretical foci:

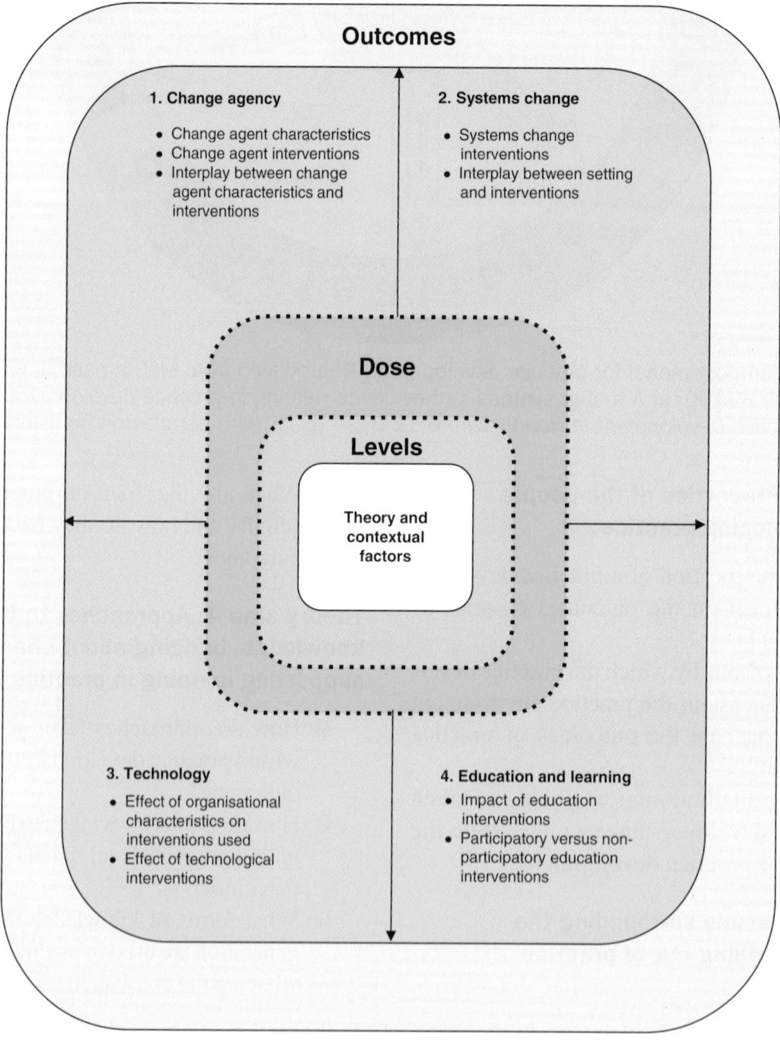

Figure 26.2 A theoretical model to explain knowledge utilisation in the context of evidence-informed health care (the ReS-IS model)

Theory area 1: Properties of change agency in E-IHC

- What impact do the characteristics of the change agent have on E-IHC?
- What is the overall impact of the change agent intervention on E-IHC?
- What impact does the interaction between the change agent and the setting have on E-IHC?

Theory area 2: System change in E-IHC

- What impact do characteristics of the system change intervention(s) have on E-IHC?
- What is the overall impact of the system change intervention(s) used?
- What impact does the interaction between the system change and the setting have on E-IHC?
- What impact do senior leadership roles have in creating practice environments that integrate daily use of evidence at the point of care delivery?

Theory area 3: Properties of technologies (paper and electronic) used in E-IHC

- What impact do the characteristics of the technological intervention(s) have on E-IHC?
- What is the overall impact of the technological intervention(s) used?
- What impact does the interaction between the technological intervention and the setting have on E-IHC?

Theory area 4: Education interventions in E-IHC

- What impact do the characteristics of the education intervention(s) have in enabling E-IHC?
- What is the overall impact of the education intervention(s) used?
- What impact does the interaction between the education intervention and the setting have on E-IHC?

The breadth of the theoretical areas outlined in both these examples clearly suggests a considerable scope and degree of work. Pawson *et al.* (2004) caution that totally comprehensive reviews are impossible and that the task is to prioritise and agree on which theories are to be inspected. For example, McCormack and colleagues used the concerns of the project steering group to focus the work. In addition, the steering group identified their desired use of the review outcomes (e.g. information to inform commissioning, funding and dissemination of practice development approaches) that helped provide a direction for key areas of work to target.

The ReS-IS team engaged in discussion with the wider knowledge utilisation community through workshops, presentations and discussions and as a result adopted a pragmatic approach that resulted in the prioritisation of one theory area for a first review.

Data extraction forms

The theoretical model is made visible in a realist synthesis through the 'data extraction forms'. This is a unique feature of realist synthesis in that unlike traditional systematic reviews, a *bespoke* set of data extraction forms are developed. Box 26.2 provides examples of data extraction forms developed by McCormack *et al.* (2007a).

Phase 2: Evidence synthesis

Finding and appraising the evidence

In a realist synthesis, a systematic approach is adopted to the finding, analysis and synthesis of evidence. The approach needs to reflect the concerns of the research methodology being used; in realist synthesis, the literature needs to be scrutinised to identify 'programme theories' (Pawson *et al.* 2004). It is worth reiterating that from a realist perspective a 'theory' is an intervention *and* it is a theory because it is always based on a hypothesis (evidence of y requires x intervention) and if the intervention is used in a particular context it will bring about a particular outcome (if I do x then y will/might happen).

The search for evidence is guided by the theoretical model developed in Phase 1. A number of

Box 26.2 Example of data extraction form

Full reference

Theory area 1: Properties of the people and context in practice development

What impact does the extent of involvement of different stakeholders have on the outcomes of practice development?

What impact does the scale of a study have on the outcomes of practice development?

How do contextual factors in the study setting have an impact on the outcomes of practice development?

How do cultural factors in the study setting have an impact on the outcomes of practice development?

How do styles of leadership in the study setting have an impact on the outcomes of practice development?

Theory area 2: Properties of the people involved in developing practice

How does the location of a practice developer have an impact on the outcomes of practice development?

How do the means by which the practice developer gains access to the practice environment have an impact on the outcomes of practice development?

How do the methodological positions taken by practice developers have an impact on the outcomes of practice development?

Theory area 3: Issues surrounding the initiation and carrying out of practice development

How do factors involved in the initiation of practice development have an impact on its outcomes?

What are the foci of practice development activity and how do they have an impact on its outcomes?

Theory area 4: Approaches used to the use of knowledge, bringing about change and supporting learning in practice development

How do approaches taken to support learning within practice development have an impact on outcomes?

How do approaches taken to bringing about change within practice development have an impact on outcomes?

What forms of knowledge use and knowledge generation are used in practice development, and what are the consequences for the outcomes?

Critique (from Critical Appraisal Skills Programme 2002)

Was there a clear statement of the aims of the research?

Was the research design appropriate to address the aims of the research?

Was the recruitment strategy appropriate to the aims of the research?

Were the data collected in a way that addressed the research issue?

Has the relationship between researcher and participants been adequately considered?

Was the data analysis sufficiently rigorous?

Is there a clear statement of findings?

Additional comments

Would it be useful to get hold of the full report for this study:

Yes: No:

References to follow up:

Reproduced from McCormack B, Wright J, Dewer B, Harvey G, Ballintine K (2007a) A realist synthesis of evidence relating to practice development: methodology and methods. *Practice Development in Health Care* **6**(1): 5–24 (p 22) with permission from John Wiley and Sons.

approaches can be applied to literature searching, including:

- searching using keywords
- mapping of commonly used subject headings onto concepts (theoretical fragments) of the theoretical model
- mapping keywords onto concepts of the theoretical model

McCormack and colleagues (2006, 2007a) experimented with all three approaches and found that the approach of mapping keywords onto concepts of the theoretical model was the most efficient and yielded the best results. They believe this was the case because the term 'practice development' is not a search term available on most databases and thus does not stand alone as a keyword or as a subject heading. McCormack *et al.* used the concepts from the theoretical model as a checklist to guide the selection of papers found using the terms 'practice' and 'development' across a range of databases. While use of these terms was not specific, it had the advantage of at least identifying those papers that used the terms in the specific way that distinguishes practice development from other forms of managed change. Using the concepts helped to increase the rigour and specificity of the selection of papers for in-depth scrutiny. The possible drawback of this approach is that it assumed the quality of the previous studies and ran the risk of 'closing down' the possible range of programme theories that would be identified. The search included the databases listed in Table 26.1.

A list of 376 references was developed, to which were added 14 papers that the researchers were aware of but were not found in the searches. However, examination of the list showed that entries in different databases may use different conventions resulting in duplication. In this case, 38 papers were entered twice, and a further 183 papers were excluded because they were descriptive papers, editorials and news stories or despite previous searches did not meet criteria as practice development papers. The remaining 169 papers formed the basis of the first phase review. The 169 papers remaining after removing the duplicates were classified as shown in Table 26.2.

Table 26.1 Databases searched

Databases	References identified
British Nursing Index	63
CINAHL	203
First Search	52
MEDLINE	33
National Electronic Library for Health (NeLH)	0
PsycINFO	10
Social Sciences Citation Index	11
AMED	0
HMIC	0
Bandolier (http://www.medicine.ox.ac.uk/bandolier)	4

Reproduced from McCormack B, Wright J, Dewer B, Harvey G, Ballintine K (2007a) A realist synthesis of evidence relating to practice development: methodology and methods. *Practice Development in Health Care* **6**(1): 5–24 (p 19) with permission from John Wiley and Sons.

To ensure reliability, papers were read in parallel by two members of the research team who used the bespoke data extraction form. In addition, the papers were critiqued by the whole research team to ensure congruity with the conceptual framework.

In the ReS-IS study (Rycroft-Malone *et al.* 2012; McCormack *et al.* 2013), two members of the research team developed a directory of terms to accompany and provide context for the theoretical model. They circulated an initial list of terms and invited the whole group to add to the list. The final list of terms, in conjunction with relevant indexing terms, was used to guide the searches. The first search focused on literature relevant to the change agency theory area. Two team members conducted the searches of six online databases: MEDLINE, CINAHL, Embase, PsycINFO, Sociological Abstracts and Web of Science. Health sciences librarians were consulted in the process of constructing the search. Consistent with the purpose of the review to examine the effectiveness

Table 26.2 Classification of papers

Category	Number of papers
1. Explicitly use practice development as a study methodology or study the experience of involvement in practice development	71
2. Scholarly reviews of practice development literature	30
3. Concept analyses	6
4. Studies in which practice development approaches are implicit (e.g. using facilitative approaches to change)	29
5. Papers based on empirical research, but did not contain evidence about practice development processes or outcomes	33

Reproduced from McCormack B, Wright J, Dewer B, Harvey G, Ballintine K (2007a) A realist synthesis of evidence relating to practice development: methodology and methods. *Practice Development in Health Care* **6**(1): 5–24 (p 19) with permission from John Wiley and Sons.

of interventions and strategies to enable evidence-informed E-IHC (in general), the search strategies were deliberately broad and did not include discipline-related terms, with one exception. In CINAHL, the indexing term 'nursing knowledge' was combined, using the Boolean operator 'OR', with the term 'knowledge', in order to capture all papers indexed using either 'knowledge' or 'nursing knowledge'.

A 10-year publication period was searched. As a quality measure, one group member reviewed the indexes of 14 journals that published articles about knowledge utilisation issues. A second group member determined that relevant papers from these journals were adequately indexed in the databases selected. Additionally, using their knowledge of the literature, all team members reviewed the final reference list to ensure that potential relevant papers were not missed by the search strategy.

Over 15,000 electronic references were returned from the *change agency* search strategies. Preliminary screening of the article titles retrieved in the search reduced the list of potentially relevant papers to 196. The preliminary screen was intentionally inclusive to capture all articles potentially relevant to the review's purpose of addressing what change agency interventions worked, for whom, in what circumstances, in what respects and how. At this stage, all seemingly relevant papers were retrieved in full text for a more detailed relevance test. Second-level screening resulted in the exclusion of further papers, bringing the final tally of papers relevant to the theory area to 52.

The group is divided into five subgroups, and the references were divided evenly across the subgroups. Within each subgroup, articles were initially screened for relevance to the theory area and study purpose. If a reviewer considered that an article did not meet the relevancy requirement, a second subgroup member reviewed it. Discrepancies in opinions about relevancy of articles were resolved through discussion. The rationale for exclusion for any articles was documented. If considered relevant, data were extracted from the article, and this extraction was then peer reviewed/validated by a second member of the subgroup.

Once all subgroups had completed data extraction for the articles they deemed relevant to the project, the respective data extraction tables were amalgamated to form a single data extraction table for all articles addressing *change agency*. Data pertaining to the target population and discipline for each study were then extracted within the subgroups.

Pawson *et al.* (2004) argue that a thorough realist synthesis should not rely on published papers alone, but that all forms of evidence should be taken into account. In addition, the non-linear nature of realist synthesis methodology and its focus on meeting the needs of key stakeholders means that an iterative approach needs to be adopted in the appraising of evidence.

DATA SYNTHESIS

In the published works of Pawson and colleagues, little, if any, guidance on data synthesis is offered. They suggest that synthesis should focus on four dimensions:

- Questioning the integrity of a theory
- Adjudicating between competing theories
- Considering the same theory in comparative settings
- Comparing the 'official' theory with actual practice

However, detail about how to undertake the actual synthesis of evidence is not provided.

McCormack *et al.* (2006, 2007a) adopted an eight-step process to data synthesis, drawing on classical approaches to thematic analysis in qualitative research. The data from the individual data extraction forms for the published literature were extracted and copied onto 'theory synthesis forms' for each of the four theory areas. The data consisted of direct quotes, researchers' commentaries and impressions. These data were grouped according to the particular emphasis in the data and researchers' impressions of the specific meanings. Each theory synthesis form was read and reread in order to gain an overall impression of the data. Data from each theory synthesis form were then themed. In some cases, the original papers were revisited in order to clarify meanings and finalise themes. A draft report was formulated and presented to the project steering group for discussion, clarification and challenge.

The grey literature data were then fed into the 'theory synthesis forms' for each of the theory areas in order to form a complete data set. The data were reread and the initial themes reconsidered based on the evidence from the grey literature. Few themes changed significantly, but instead, the grey literature either strengthened or weakened initial themes. The themes were constructed into a narrative, and these narratives formed the structure of the findings section of the report.

The final stage consisted of an analysis of the telephone interviews, which were themed under the questions on the interview schedule. Key quotes and comments were highlighted, and these were fed into the discussion of the data in order to highlight particular issues, confirm themes from the literature, verify or contradict the strength of claims made in the literature analysis and identify novel issues and themes. This final stage resulted in the identification of four overarching themes and nine sub-themes, and these formed the structure for the data synthesis (Box 26.3).

Figure 26.3 shows the iterative approach adopted by McCormack *et al.* (2006, 2007a).

The ReS-IS research team adopted an alternative approach to data synthesis, derived from the principles underpinning realist evaluation. Thematic analysis was first conducted by three subgroups who themed the extracted data according to one of the following three questions:

1. What impact do the characteristics of the change agent have on knowledge use?
2. What is the overall impact of the change agent intervention on knowledge use?
3. What impact does the interaction between the change agent and the setting have on knowledge use?

Subgroup members independently themed the data extracted from each article using the question assigned to their subgroup. The subgroup then collated the themes identified by each of the members. From here, the subgroup members identified overarching themes or 'chains of inference'. A chain of inference is a connection that can be made across articles based on the themes identified. The connection may not be explicit, but a possible relationship between the theme and the outcome under consideration may have been highlighted. Subgroup members each shared the chains of inference they had identified. Figure 26.4 shows the chains of inference identified by the group.

Discussion, amendment and/or confirmation of the chains of inference that had been proposed happened via teleconference. For each chain of inference, articles linking themes and chains of inference were recorded to create an audit trail. Table 26.3 shows an example of some chains of inference linked to themes and original articles.

Box 26.3 Data analysis themes and sub-themes

Theme	Sub-theme
1. Unidisciplinary versus multidisciplinary approaches	• None
2. Stakeholders	• Managers • Service users • Practice development roles and relationships • HEI relationships • Learning
3. Methodologies and methods	• Methodological perspectives • Methodologies in use • Methods • The cost/funding of practice development
4. Outcomes arising from practice development	• None

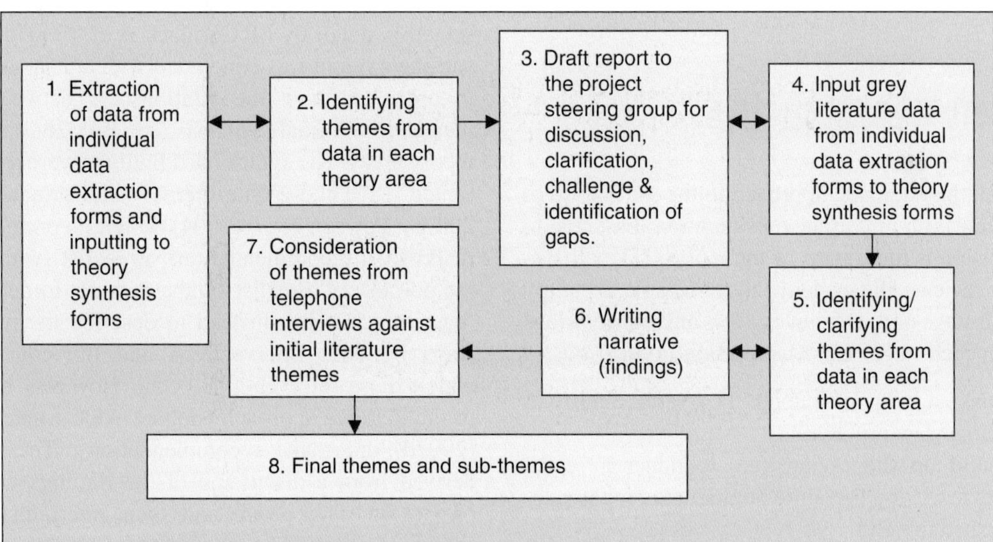

Figure 26.3 Data extraction, analysis and synthesis

In a face-to-face meeting, the team identified connections between the chains of inference and their impact on evidence-informed practice. Having articulated the connections, the group formulated hypotheses regarding the chains of inference. A chain of inference is, therefore, linked to each hypothesis, and for each chain of inference, themes from the literature are also linked. Further, all papers

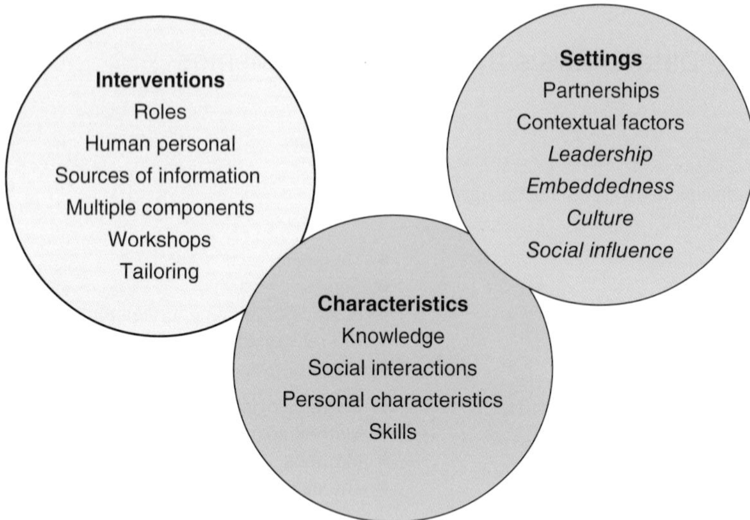

Figure 26.4 Chains of inference

from which the themes related to the respective chains of inference were drawn are clearly identified. Box 26.4 provides an illustration of this process.

NARRATIVE CONSTRUCTION

Adopting a systematic approach to the writing up of the review is an important consideration. Essential to the decision is the format of the report. Like all systematic reviews, the reader needs to be able to clearly see each stage of the review process and the decisions made in each stage. This is important in order to:

- make a judgement about the overall quality of the review processes
- build on the review (e.g. conduct a repeat review using literature not included in the published review)
- make a judgement about the conclusions made by the authors and the implications of the conclusions for practice
- undertake further research drawing on the review conclusions

Typically, the writing of the review follows the theoretical model developed. McCormack and colleagues adopted a two-stage approach to the reporting of findings. Firstly, the literature analysis relating to each of the sub-theory areas (13) was presented in detail by McCormack *et al.* (2007b). Each sub-theory area was concluded with a data summary in order to show the relationships between data themes in the final synthesis (see Box 26.3) and the theory areas. The synthesised findings were then presented using these data themes (McCormack *et al.* 2007c). Pawson *et al.* (2004) do not recommend the making of 'recommendations' in realist synthesis as the purpose of a realist synthesis is not to determine 'best' practice but instead to describe the relationships between interventions and the contexts in which those interventions occur. However, because of the iterative approach adopted, McCormack *et al.* (2007d) did make recommendations. These were derived from a discussion of the findings with the project steering group and their interpretation of actions that should be recommended arising from the synthesised findings. However, recommendations were made concerning the development of a practice development (theoretical) model rather than a list of recommendations for 'doing practice development'.

In the ReS-IS project, the narrative was constructed around the identified hypotheses for the theory area. Four members (the authors of this

Table 26.3 Chains of inference linked to themes and original articles

Chains of inference	Derived from the following themes	Articles
Knowledge	Professional qualifications Expert knowledge Knowledgeable Local knowledge Research knowledge Practice knowledge	1, 3, 6, 7, 10, 11, 13, 14, 15, 16, 18, 19, 20, 21, 22, 23, 25, 29, 35, 36, 37, 39
Skills	Communication skills Leadership skills Thinking skills Clinical skills Cognitive skills Evaluation skills Political skills Facilitation skills Reflective skills	2, 4, 5, 6, 7, 8, 9, 10, 11, 12, 13, 14, 15, 16, 17, 18, 19, 20, 21, 22, 24, 25, 27, 28, 32, 33, 34, 36, 38, 39, 40
Personal characteristics	Role model Positive attitude Responsibility/accountability Respected Information seeking Positive attitude Accessible Age Teacher Culturally compatible Objectivity Years of experience	1, 2, 4, 6, 7, 8, 13, 14, 15, 16, 17, 18, 22, 28, 29, 30, 31, 32, 33, 35, 36, 37, 38, 39
Social interaction	Social influence Networking Shared ownership	5, 8, 12, 15, 18, 31, 39, 40

chapter) worked together to write the narrative. Unlike McCormack *et al.*, the analysis and synthesis was written as one account. This was possible because of the use of hypotheses, which acted as synthesised statements of findings against which the previous stages of analysis could be presented.

STRENGTHS AND LIMITATIONS OF REALIST SYNTHESIS

As Pawson and colleagues (2004, 2005) have noted, unlike some other review processes, one of the strengths of a realist approach to review is that it has firm roots in philosophy and social sciences. Rather than being a method or formula, it is a 'logic of enquiry' (Pawson *et al.* 2004: 37), which enables a flexible, all-embracing approach to explanation (what works for whom, in what circumstances and in what respects) rather than judgement. Rather than controlling for real-life events, realist synthesis has the capacity to work with and untangle complexities. This allows for an equal focus on what works, as much as what does not work in an attempt to learn from failures and maximise learning across policy, disciplinary and organisational boundaries. Furthermore, realist synthesis is inherently stakeholder driven, which facilitates engagement and the inclusion of multiple perspectives.

Box 26.4 Hypotheses linked to chains of inference

Hypotheses	Chain of inference (theory level)	Chain of inference (sub-theory level)	Themes from the literature	Papers addressing the theme
An opinion leader and his/her personal characteristics are dependent on contextual factors in order to have an impact on E-IHC	The nature of the relationship between the change agent's personal characteristics, the role adopted and contextual influences and the impact of E-IHC	Roles	Opinion leader (OL)	*Papers with mixed and positive effects only:*
		Personal characteristics	`Facilitator (FAC) Change agent (CA)	6 OL (Wright, Chaillet, Curran, Moore, Davies, Majumdar)
A facilitator and his/her personal characteristics are dependent on contextual factors in order to have an impact on E-IHC		Contextual factors		6 FAC (internal/ external and external facilitators included) (Stetler, Cranney, Gerrish, Milner, Thomas, Hutt)
				Total 18 CA papers, 12 OL and FAC

Reflection activity

Consider a particular practice topic, for example, rehabilitation of older people following stroke, effectiveness of approaches to incontinence management, teamworking in the emergency department or any other topic that you wish to consider as a focus for service improvement. What would be the advantages of using a realist approach to synthesising the evidence underpinning this topic? What would be the challenges associated with using a realist approach?

The strengths of realist synthesis underpin its limitations. Realist synthesis is premised on a set of principles rather than a formula, and while this allows for flexibility and inclusivity, it means that the review is not reproducible. The two examples used in this chapter are good examples of how taking a set of principles and developing a particularised approach result in similar, but not identical, processes. For example, it follows that if the appraisal and data extraction needs to be bespoke to the particular review questions that arise from the theoretical framework, these will be different for each review. Furthermore, given that the fundamental interest in realist synthesis is about finding out what works in what contexts, the recommendations one can make will not be generalisable. However, findings are theoretically transferable: ideas ('theories') that can be

> ### Reflection activity
>
> Having read the two examples of realist syntheses offered in this chapter, consider how you could adapt the processes described to your particular project.

tested in different contexts, with different stakeholders. Pawson *et al.* (2004) suggest that realist syntheses are not for novices. Unlike a Cochrane review, for example, which relies on standardised protocols and tools, the demands on a realist synthesiser are different. For example, quality assurance within realist synthesis is dependent on the reviewers' explicitness and reflexivity. In turn, this requires a high level of expertise in reasoning, research methods and quality appraisal.

CONCLUSION

Realist synthesis is particularly appropriate for unpacking the impact of complex interventions because it works on the premise that one needs to understand how interventions work in different contexts and why. It is not an easy option to evidence review. As the two examples used in this chapter show, there is no one prescribed approach to doing a realist synthesis; there is a set of principles that the reviewer must particularise to the issue being explored while being sympathetic to the philosophy of realism. This presents unique challenges but with it is the opportunity to develop more pragmatic conclusions than some other approaches to systematic reviewing.

References

Best A, Greenhalgh T, Lewis S, Saul JE, Caroll S, Bitz J (2012) Large system transformation in health care: a realist review. *Milbank Quarterly* **90**(3): 421–456.

Critical Appraisal Skills Programme (2002) *Evidence-Based Health Care: an open learning resource for health care practitioners.* Oxford, CASP.

Delanty G (1997) *Social Science: beyond constructivism and realism*. Buckingham, Open University Press.

Greenhalgh T, Kristjansson E, Robinson V (2007) Realist review to understand the efficacy of school feeding programmes. *British Medical Journal* **335**: 858–861.

Jagosh J, Macaulay A, Pluye P, Salsberg J, Bush PL, Henderson J, Sirett E, Wong G, Cargo M, Herbert CP, Seifer SD, Green LW, Greenhalgh T (2012) Uncovering the benefits of participatory research: implications of a realist review for health research and practice. *Milbank Quarterly* **90**(2): 311–346.

McCormack B, Dewar B, Wright J, Garbett R, Harvey G, Ballantine K (2006) A Realist Synthesis of Evidence Relating to Practice Development. Final Report To NHS Education For Scotland and NHS Quality Improvement Scotland. http://www.healthcareimprovementscotland.org/previous_resources/policy_and_strategy/a_realist_synthesis_of_evidenc.aspx (accessed 9 September 2014).

McCormack B, Wright J, Dewer B, Harvey G, Ballintine K (2007a) A realist synthesis of evidence relating to practice development: methodology and methods. *Practice Development in Health Care* **6**(1): 5–24.

McCormack B, Wright J, Dewer B, Harvey G, Ballintine K (2007b) A realist synthesis of evidence relating to practice development: findings from the literature review. *Practice Development in Health Care* **6**(1): 25–55.

McCormack B, Wright J, Dewer B, Harvey G, Ballintine K (2007c) A realist synthesis of evidence relating to practice development: interviews and synthesis of data. *Practice Development in Health Care* **6**(1): 56–75.

McCormack B, Wright J, Dewer B, Harvey G, Ballintine K (2007d) A realist synthesis of evidence relating to practice development: recommendations. *Practice Development in Health Care* **6**(1): 76–80.

McCormack B, Rycroft-Malone J, DeCorby K, Hutchinson AM, Bucknall TK, Kent B, Schultz A, Snelgrove-Clarke E, Stetler C, Titler M, Wallin L, Wilson V (2013) A realist review of interventions and strategies to promote evidence-informed health care: a focus on change agency. *Implementation Science* **8**: 107. DOI: 10.1186/1748-5908-8-107.

McEvoy P, Richards D (2003) Critical realism: a way forward for evaluation research in nursing? *Journal of Advanced Nursing* **43**: 411–420.

Pawson R (2002) Evidence-based policy: the promise of realist synthesis. *Evaluation* **8**: 340–358.

Pawson R (2006) *Evidence-Based Policy: a realist perspective*. London, Sage.

Pawson R (2013) *The Science of Evaluation. A realist manifesto*. London, Sage.

Pawson R, Tilley N (1997) *Realistic Evaluation*. London, Sage.

Pawson R, Greenhalgh T, Harvey G, Walshe K (2004) *Realist Synthesis: an introduction: RMP methods paper 2/2004*. Manchester, Centre for Census and Survey Research, University of Manchester. Available at http://www.ccsr.ac.uk/methods/publications/documents/RMPmethods2.pdf (accessed 31 August 2014).

Pawson R, Greenhalgh T, Harvey G, Walshe K (2005) Realist review – a new method of systematic review designed for complex policy interventions. *Journal of Health Service Research and Policy* **10**(3): 21–34.

Rycroft-Malone J, McCormack B, Hutchinson AM, DeCorby K, Bucknall TK, Kent B, Schultz A, Snelgrove-Clarke E, Stetler C, Titler M, Wallin L, Wilson V (2012) Realist synthesis: illustrating the method for implementation research. *Implementation Science* **7**: 33. DOI: 10.1186/1748-5908-7-33.

Wong G, Greenhalgh R, Pawson R (2010) Internet-based medical education: a realist review of what works for whom in what circumstances. *BMC Medical Education* **10**: 12. DOI: 10.1186/1472-6920-10-12.

Wong G, Greenhalgh T, Westhorp G, Buckingham J, Pawson R (2013) RAMESES publication standards: realist syntheses. *BMC Medicine* **11**: 21. DOI: 10.1186/1741-7015-11-21.

Websites

http://www.leeds.ac.uk/sociology/realistsynthesis/ – A website companion to the book *Evidence-Based Policy: A Realist Perspective* by Ray Pawson in 2006 that which provides a range of supporting materials for realist synthesis.

http://www.cfhi-fcass.ca/PublicationsAndResources/ResearchReports/articleview/07-09-01/071c5f66-506c-40d5-aba0-d573ae4ad674.aspx – The Canadian Foundation for Healthcare Improvement website provides an overview of realist review for complex healthcare interventions.

https://www.jiscmail.ac.uk/cgi-bin/webadmin?A0=RAMESES – An online discussion forum anyone interested in realist or meta-narrative review.

http://www.ramesesproject.org/index.php?pr=Resources – A website with sources of support and downloadable resources for realist research methods.

http://www.screencast.com/t/rLTVzmGHBX – A webcast that covers some of the underpinning assumptions and philosophy of realist synthesis and evaluation.

CHAPTER 27

Mixed Methods Research

Joanne Turnbull and Judith Lathlean

Key points

- Mixed methods research is a type of research where quantitative and qualitative approaches are integrated within one project.
- Integrating approaches in mixed methods designs should have the potential to generate knowledge or understanding that could not be gained from a qualitative or quantitative study alone.
- Mixed methods are used to investigate complex and multi-faceted healthcare problems and processes.
- Pragmatism is often proposed as the most common or most appropriate epistemology for mixed methods.

WHAT IS MIXED METHODS RESEARCH?

Mixed methods research is that which combines quantitative and qualitative data collection and analysis in the same study. However, this type of research involves more than simply using qualitative or quantitative methods; it is the process of bringing together or *integrating* approaches within a single study that is important. There are many different mixed methods research designs, but examples include a qualitative study undertaken alongside a randomised controlled trial (RCT) (e.g. White *et al.* 2012), the use of a survey to supplement ethnographic work (e.g. Turnbull *et al.* 2012) or an evaluation where quantitative intervention measures were used alongside semi-structured interviews (e.g. Latter *et al.* 2010).

Other terms used to describe this approach include 'combined methods research', 'multi-method', 'multiple methods' or 'blended research' (see Bryman (2008) for a discussion of the different languages used). However, the term 'mixed methods' has become increasingly accepted as standard for this type of research particularly in health and social sciences (O'Cathain *et al.* 2007a). Some researchers may also

The Research Process in Nursing, Seventh Edition. Edited by Kate Gerrish and Judith Lathlean.

Companion Website: www.wiley.com/go/gerrish/research

use such terms to refer to research in which two or more *quantitative* methods are used (e.g. routinely collected statistics on health outcomes and a survey conducted on the relevant population) or combining different *qualitative* methods (e.g. interviews with non-participant observation). In this chapter, the term 'mixed methods' is used to mean the planned mixing of quantitative and qualitative components within a single study. For it to truly count as mixed methods, the data derived from the two methods should be integrated (O'Cathain *et al.* 2007b), and it should offer the possibility of generating knowledge or understanding that could not be gained from a qualitative or quantitative study alone. Mixed methods studies may be viewed as placing together methods like 'pieces of a jigsaw' to create a more complete picture (Bryman *et al.* 2008) or as having a multiplicative effect where mixed methods can generate a whole that is greater than the sum of its parts (Creswell 2010).

CAN – AND SHOULD – METHODS BE MIXED?

Qualitative and quantitative perspectives are often presented as dichotomous (sometimes placed in opposition to each other) in their methods (observations or experiments), reasoning (inductive or deductive) and methods of analysis (interpretive or statistical). In reality, research practice may commonly be on a continuum between the two. The two main perspectives are the constructivist/interpretivist (qualitative) paradigm and the positivist (quantitative) paradigm. There are long-standing arguments in some research fields that methods associated with different theoretical philosophies or paradigms cannot – and should not – be mixed because the two paradigms are incommensurate; that is, the underpinning view on the nature of reality and truth is different in each paradigm. The qualitative paradigm sees reality as constructed by the complex set of meanings people attribute to their experiences and there can be multiple truths. In contrast, the quantitative paradigm holds that reality is a single, known fixed point that can be objectively measured (see Chapter 12 for more discussion of these issues). 'Purist' researchers consider paradigm,

Reflection activity

What are the two main research paradigms and how do they differ? Why is an understanding important to mixed methods research? In what ways could different paradigms influence researchers in how they conduct mixed methods research? In reflecting upon these questions, you may find it helpful to refer Chapter 12.

methodology and methods to be inextricably linked and suggest that mixing qualitative and qualitative methods is not possible. Some researchers believe that while mixing methods across the paradigms is feasible and can broaden the dimensions of the research, in each study, one approach should always be dominant, meaning the philosophical underpinnings or 'theoretical drive' is drawn from this paradigm (Morse & Niehus 2009). In this way, the second method is viewed as supplementary to the main or primary method (see section 'MIXED METHODS DESIGNS' later in this chapter).

Some researchers have adopted paradigms that are appropriate to mixed methods research, such as pragmatism and realism. Here, a different stance is taken, so that one method is not prioritised over another and there is the belief that mixing methods, to some extent, overcomes the paradigm arguments. First, there are those who consider methods as 'techniques', emphasising the sampling, collection and analysis of data (Bryman 2012). These are not necessarily tied to a particular philosophical position, and so can be fused, thus *transcending* the paradigm wars. Second, by taking a pragmatic approach, it is argued mixed methods can *supersede* the paradigm wars. Pragmatism emphasises choosing a research design and thus methods that are most appropriate to the research question (Creswell 2010). It recognises that all research methods have their limitations and the use of more than one method may allow the researcher to understand a phenomenon that cannot be understood by the use of another method. Pragmatism has an appeal in its 'right tools for the job' approach, but there may be difficulties in

Reflection activity

Why do you think pragmatism has gained popularity amongst mixed methods researchers?

integrating methods where researchers uncritically accept a pragmatic approach, without giving due consideration to the assumptions that underlie qualitative and quantitative paradigms (Biesta 2010).

WHY ARE MIXED METHODS USED IN NURSING AND HEALTH SCIENCES RESEARCH?

Researchers have increasingly recognised that different research approaches are equally good at answering different types of research questions. Interest in the use of mixed methods has partly stemmed from the view that research methods need to account for, and reflect, the complexity of health and healthcare processes and problems (Östlund *et al.* 2011). Added to this is the recognition by many that this complexity is best explored by tapping a multiplicity of sources of knowledge, and this is where mixed methods research can excel (Wisdom *et al.* 2012). For example, a researcher might be interested in both how many people attend primary care outside usual surgery hours ('out of hours') (Turnbull *et al.* 2008) and their experiences of, and views about, the use of these services (see Research Example 27.1). Generating the knowledge to answer these questions will require more than one research approach.

Mixed methods designs are increasingly used in the health sciences although reports suggest that mixed methods research designs account for less than 3% of studies published in top-ranking journals in nursing (Mantzoukas 2009) and health services research (Wisdom *et al.* 2012). However, many research funding bodies are increasingly receptive to, and sometimes demand, mixed methods designs (Curry *et al.* 2013). In the United Kingdom, the proportion of mixed methods studies commissioned by the English Department

RESEARCH EXAMPLE

27.1 Complementarity of Mixed Methods

Turnbull J, Pope C, Martin D, Latimer V (2010) Do telephones overcome geographical barriers to general practice out-of-hours services? Mixed-methods study of parents with young children. *Journal of Health Services Research and Policy* **15**: 21–27.

This study focused on the role of place (geographical distance and rurality) on access to general practitioner services outside normal surgery hours ('out of hours'). The mixed methods design included a quantitative geographical analysis of the rates of telephone calls to an out-of-hours service, followed by a qualitative study to understand the experience of access from the point of view of service users. The quantitative analysis revealed that patients from rural areas and those who lived at greater distances from primary care centres made fewer contacts with out-of-hours services. Those at greater distances were also more likely to receive GP telephone advice. The greatest variation in call rates was seen for children aged 0–4 years, and therefore, the qualitative study focused on the parents of young children. Qualitative analysis suggested that this geographical variation was linked to familiarity with the system (notably previous contact with health services) and the availability of services, legitimacy of demand (particularly for children) and negotiation about mode of care. The integration of findings demonstrated how place may affect parents' help-seeking behaviour in relation to out-of-hours services (see also Turnbull *et al.* 2008).

of Health Research and Development programmes increased from 17% in the early 1990s to 30% by 2004 (O'Cathain *et al.* 2007a).

With any given research question, it is important to be clear about what a mixed methods design will add or achieve. A number of typologies have been developed to summarise the reasons for mixing methods. Some of these run into many items, creating an exhaustive catalogue of reasons and attempting to list every possible combination of methods that could occur. However, most of these reasons can be organised under key concepts in relation to mixed methods – convergence (sometimes described as 'triangulation'), facilitation (or development) and complementarity.

KEY CONCEPTS IN MIXED METHODS RESEARCH

Convergence and divergence

Convergence is used to describe the notion of adopting two or more methods to study the same phenomenon to *corroborate* the findings from one method with the other. With this process of cross-checking, it is intended that the confidence in the entire study will be enhanced. Some authors refer to this as triangulation, which is proposed as a way of enhancing the validity of findings, based on the idea that convergent validity may be inferred where the viewpoints agree. The term triangulation derives from a loose analogy with navigation and surveying in which different bearings are taken in order to arrive at a precise physical location – the point where the bearing lines *converge*.

However, there are some problems with the notion of triangulation as a test of validity, particularly if the findings from different methods within a mixed methods study do not converge on the same point. From this perspective, if the two sources contradict, it may be assumed that differences occur because of weakness of one of the methods. However, it may also be the case that different methods simply reveal a more complex picture where one set of methods uncovers further data that may *diverge* from the findings of the other method. For this reason, triangulation may be better viewed as examining both convergence and divergence of findings. The use of mixed methods may be better viewed as a way of gaining deeper or greater understandings of a phenomenon by investigating it from different perspectives. Indeed, Morse (2003: 190) has defined triangulation as 'the combination of the results of two or more rigorous studies conducted to provide a more *comprehensive* picture of the results than either study could do alone'.

While this purpose of combining methods to achieve a broader, more comprehensive picture is not disputed, the use of the term triangulation in this context is. The etymology of the term suggests very clearly the idea of *convergence* and coming together at a particular point, whereas the idea of more comprehensive picture suggests a widening out, a *divergence* away from the initial ideas. When this happens, the researcher must carefully consider these divergences and reflect on the complexity revealed by mixed methods. Using the term triangulation to signify both processes serves to confuse. However, this dual meaning of the term may stem from the issue that it is almost impossible to know at the outset of a mixed methods study whether the findings will converge or diverge. The term *complementarity* better describes the process in which mixed methods result in a more comprehensive understanding of the phenomena under study, so that one method can be used to elaborate, clarify, explain or illustrate the results of another.

Although the term triangulation is sometimes used to describe the process of corroborating findings by converging on a *single point*, there is a further issue in that this suggests alignment with the quantitative paradigm, where there is belief in a single fixed reality (i.e. one truth) that can be objectively known through the use of multiple methods. However, as suggested earlier, many researchers operate from an ontological assumption of *multiple realities* (i.e. many truths). Indeed, many of the arguments used earlier in the chapter to justify the use of mixed methods recognise the multiple ways of knowing and the need for a range of ways of understanding the world to advance knowledge.

A further caution needed with triangulation is that while the corroboration process might suggest a greater air of validity or confidence in the findings, it is important to examine the way in which the methods have been applied in every study. Flawed methods might lead to a single point, but this does not mean that additional confidence should be taken from the resultant findings. For these reasons, we suggest that, in the context of mixed methods research at least, the notion of convergence (and divergence) better describes the use of different methods to provide a more *comprehensive* picture of the results.

An example of convergence featured in a study that explored a new type of health call-centre work (Turnbull *et al.* 2012). Ethnographic (non-participant observation and semi-structured interviews) and survey methods were used to examine the everyday work of non-clinical call handlers using a computer decision support system (CDSS) to triage urgent and emergency calls (see Research Example 27.2). Ethnographic data suggested that these workers demonstrated high levels of skills and expertise, drawing on their experience, experiential knowledge and teamwork in their everyday use of the CDSS. The survey was designed to provide further data on the skills that call handlers perceived to be important as well as on some aspects not fully captured by the ethnography (e.g. call handlers' qualifications, previous work experience). Some of the findings from each method were found to corroborate and explain each other, most notably confirming the range of skills and expertise that call handlers used and identifying the skills that call handlers believed were important to do their job.

Facilitation

The acceptance that there are alternative modes of knowing or understanding about a health problem can substantiate the use of mixed methods for the *development* or *facilitation* of research. Here, one method is used to facilitate the next stage of the research, for example, in relation to the sampling strategy, for instrument development, as a process evaluation within an RCT, or to develop or improve health interventions. Research Example 27.3 provides

RESEARCH EXAMPLE

27.2 Convergence in Mixed Methods Research

Turnbull J, Prichard J, Halford S, Pope C, Salisbury C (2012) Reconfiguring the emergency and urgent care workforce: mixed methods study of skills and the everyday work of non-clinical call-handlers in the NHS. *Journal of Health Services Policy* **17**: 233–240.

This study examined a new type of health call-centre work in urgent and emergency care. A comparative mixed methods case study approach was used to describe in detail the design, development, management and use of a computer decision support system (CDSS) in three healthcare settings. This article specifically focuses on the everyday work of non-clinical call handlers, as well as their skills and expertise in providing telephone triage and assessment, supported by a CDSS. The study combined ethnographic (non-participant observation and semi-structured interviews) and survey methods. These methods were ordered sequentially (ethnographic followed by a survey) so that the qualitative work informed the design of the survey. The survey included aspects identified as important in the ethnography (e.g. skills and views about the CDSS) and also covered aspects that were not fully captured by the ethnography (e.g. qualifications and previous work experience). Data analysis was an iterative process, moving backwards and forwards between the ethnographic and survey datasets so that the data were checked against each other and the research team was able to critically question emergent findings. The survey data were used to substantiate themes derived from the qualitative data, as well as highlighting some divergent findings. The use of mixed methods revealed and corroborated the key finding that while these workers are often portrayed simply as 'trained users' of technology, they demonstrate high levels of experience, skills and expertise in using the CDSS.

RESEARCH EXAMPLE

27.3 Using Mixed Methods to Facilitate Sampling

Hanna L, May C, Fairhurst K (2011) Non-face-to-face consultations and communications in primary care: the role and perspective of general practice managers in Scotland. *Informatics in Primary Care* **19**: 17–24.

This study explored attitudes of general practice managers to non-face-to-face consultation and communication technologies in the routine delivery of primary care. This mixed methods study included a postal survey followed by in-depth qualitative interviews. The survey was sent to all practice managers in Scotland. The survey results then informed the sampling process. Qualitative interviews were based on the survey results to achieve a maximum variation sample of 20 survey respondents incorporating a range of characteristics including gender, age, practice list size, geographical location and practice area deprivation indices. The findings of this study suggested that practice managers supported the use of new technologies for routine tasks to manage workload and increase convenience for patients. However, contextual factors (such as practice list size, practice deprivation area and geographical location) affected whether managers would pursue the introduction of these technologies.

an example of a facilitative mix of methods in relation to sampling. Here, the researchers adopted the *sequential* use of quantitative and then qualitative phases. A survey was implemented, the results of which were used to purposively sample participants who held a range of views about the topic under investigation.

Another important way in which methods are combined to facilitate the research is to design, develop and test a research instrument. Most often, this would take the form of qualitative methods, for example, individual interviews or group discussions being used to understand the context, detail and language associated with an issue to enable the design of a survey instrument or questionnaire. In this way, the questionnaire should be more relevant to the issue being investigated and appropriate for the population under study than if the preliminary work had not been undertaken. This might be most useful for researching populations that have different characteristics from the research team, for example, young people or populations from different cultural backgrounds. By undertaking preliminary work to better understand their perspectives and importantly their preferred way of talking about the issues being investigated, a research instrument, such as a questionnaire, is more likely to be relevant to those being asked to complete it.

Complementarity

The notion of complementarity in mixed methods research is grounded in the argument that the weaknesses of one method can be offset by combining them with an alternative method that offers different strengths – that is, methods are combined to complement one another. This broad concept covers a whole range of different rationales for why two or more methods can offer advantages over a single method approach. First, there is the issue of *completeness* or *comprehensiveness*. As discussed previously, not everything can be known or discovered through one way of looking at the social world; therefore, by combining methods, knowledge that is not accessible through one route can be included in a study by the employment of alternative methods. A questionnaire can collect data on what people report they do or intend to do in a certain situation, for example, how a clinician provides information to a patient during a consultation. However, by observing the clinic setting, data can be collected on how they actually do communicate with the patient.

Second, another way in which different methods complement each other is where qualitative methods are used to provide a detailed examination of the *context* for understanding the information gleaned with broad-brush quantitative methods. In the presentation of findings from the research, qualitative data can then be used to *illustrate* some of the themes arising from the quantitative data. Alternatively, as in the example in Research Example 27.2, quantitative data can be used to *substantiate* the findings emerging from the interpretative analysis of qualitative data.

Third, qualitative methods might be combined with quantitative methods in order to help *explain* any association found between the factors (or variables) being studied. For example, quantitative methods can provide a snapshot of a particular issue and explore whether associations between various factors (or variables) are apparent. However, these methods would not shed light on why these associations have been found. Complementing the quantitative work with qualitative work can enable explanatory factors to be explored with the population under study. This was the rationale for using mixed methods in the study presented in Research Example 27.1, where the study was designed to explore the role of place (i.e. urban or rural locations and geographical distance) in people's use and experiences of access to out-of-hours general practitioner services. By using a *sequential* design, the associations and patterns identified in the quantitative phase were further explored in the follow-on qualitative phase. In this way, the qualitative work was able to develop further the insights gained from the initial results and at the same time offer some explanations as to why the associations between place and access to out-of-hours services had been found in the quantitative analysis.

Another example of where qualitative work can help explain quantitative work is within RCTs (Lewin *et al.* 2009). This is most useful when complex interventions are being evaluated, such as psychological therapy or the organisation of specialist services (Medical Research Council 2000). Here, the quantitative method will be able to answer the question of whether one approach is more effective than another. Complementing an RCT study with qualitative methods will help to explain why this effect has been observed. In other words, the trial methodology focuses on the *outcome* of the intervention, and the qualitative methods will focus on the *process* of the intervention, which, as suggested earlier in the chapter, can have a significant effect on health outcomes. An example of combining qualitative methods with an RCT is given in Research Example 27.4.

RESEARCH EXAMPLE

27.4 Mixed Methods in the Design of a Randomised Controlled Trial

Bruton A, Kirby S, Arden-Close E, Taylor L, Webley F, George S, Yardley L, Price D, Moore M, Little P, Holgate S, Djukanovic R, Lee AJ, Raftery J, Chorozoglou M, Versnel J, Pavord I, Stafford-Watson M, Thomas M (2013) The BREATHE study: breathing retraining for asthma. Trial of home exercises. A protocol summary of a randomised controlled trial. *Primary Care Respiratory Journal* **22**(2): PS1–PS7.

The BREATHE study is a three-arm parallel randomised controlled trial of people with asthma to assess the effect of home exercises (incorporating a breathing exercise training programme delivered by DVD format with supporting booklet) in comparison with 'usual care' and with that of face-to-face physiotherapist-led training of similar content. As part of the trial, qualitative methods are used to pilot the educational materials with a panel of 20–30 members using face-to-face and telephone interviews. Qualitative methods are also designed to evaluate patient experiences of the trial and identify factors that may have influenced trial outcomes and include telephone interviews with patients in each arm of the trial, purposively sampled for diversity and seeking to ensure representation of participants with poor adherence or outcomes.

MIXED METHODS DESIGNS

There are different strategies for combining qualitative and quantitative research methods and a number of typologies of mixed methods designs exist (e.g. see Creswell & Plano Clark 2010; Morgan 2013), but they commonly include the timing (sequence), weighting (dominance) and the mixing (integration) of quantitative and qualitative methods (Creswell 2010).

Sequence

Methods may be used *concurrently* or *sequentially* (Creswell 2010). A concurrent design is one in which quantitative and qualitative data are collected at the same time and analysed together. In a sequential design, the researcher conducts a qualitative phase of the study followed by a quantitative phase, or vice versa. The different quantitative and qualitative components are kept separate, which does allow each component to stay true to its own paradigm and methodology requirements.

Weighting (dominance)

As we outlined earlier in the chapter, Morgan (2013) suggested that researchers should consider if one method is *dominant* over another so that one method is the principal method used to collect data and the other is complementary or supplementary (e.g. in terms of resources devoted to them, the depth of analysis and how study components are reported and disseminated). For example, a qualitative component may be added to a quantitative survey, but both methods would still be driven by the deductive assumptions of the quantitative paradigm. Morgan (2013) took this approach in his 'Priority-Sequence Model', which consists of four basic research designs depending firstly whether a qualitative or a quantitative approach is the principal method (priority) and secondly if the complementary method serves as a preliminary or a follow-up method to the principal method (sequencing). However, other researchers may design their study so that equal status is given to the quantitative and qualitative components, as is the case with the study presented in Research Example 27.1. It is also possible that the relative importance of different study components may not emerge until the later phases of a research study.

INTEGRATION IN MIXED METHODS RESEARCH

Increasingly, an indicator of quality in mixed methods studies is the way in which the methods interact with each other (O'Cathain *et al.* 2007b; Östlund *et al.* 2011). As argued earlier, it is precisely the fact that mixed methods can bring something extra to the research process that distinguishes this approach from single method research or two methods used in tandem. It is this *integration* that ensures the added value. Integration may occur at one or many stages of the research process, from devising the research questions through to writing up, including the stages of research design, sampling, analysis and interpretation of the results (O'Cathain *et al.* 2007b).

Research question

This is a key stage in the integration of mixed methods in any study, because it is the research question that is the driver for the choice of research design. In the study presented in Research Example 27.1, it was the interest in both how *often* patients used out-of-hours services and their *experiences* of those services that set the direction of the mixed methods study. The quantitative part was designed to provide information about the use of out-of-hours services and the qualitative part to consider peoples' experiences of out-of-hours services.

Research design

Integration in the design stage has been highlighted previously where mixed methods are used for facilitation and complementarity. An often-cited good example of integrated research design is summarised in Research Example 27.4, where qualitative data collection is embedded in an RCT. This study allows the researchers both to evaluate patient experiences of the trial *and* identify factors that may influence the outcomes of the trial.

Sampling

Methods are integrated where the sampling for one phase of a mixed methods study is informed by the analysis of an earlier phase. It might be appropriate to sample case studies from the results of a survey as in the study described in Research Example 27.3. In this example, the whole population of interest was surveyed about their experience and attitudes towards service user involvement in mental health service development. Following this, a purposive sample of respondents holding a range of views towards involvement was invited to take part in an in-depth interview.

In a study that explored community mental health nurses' experiences of delivering brief interventions for anxiety and depression in the context of an RCT (Simons *et al.* 2008), nurses were sampled on the basis of the different interventions they had delivered. In the analysis of the interviews, the commonalities and differences between the nurses' experiences were sought, depending upon the type of intervention they had provided. It would not have been appropriate, in this instance, to only look for themes that were common across the whole dataset, because the participants had been sampled for this part of the study specifically because they had experience of the different interventions in the trial.

Analysis

In many cases, it may be better to analyse qualitative and quantitative datasets separately, using techniques suited to each form of data. In this situation, integration should take place at the interpretation stage (see following text). However, at the analysis stage, in some studies, there are ways in which datasets can be combined or transformed into a single dataset. The process of transforming qualitative data into quantitative data has been referred to as *quantitising*, while the process of converting quantitative data into qualitative data has been referred to as *qualitising* (Bazeley 2012).

One way of quantitising qualitative data is transforming responses from a qualitative interview into variables for numerical analysis. This was the approach taken in a study in which 173 people were interviewed after discharge from an acute psychiatric hospital admission (Simons *et al.* 2002).Semi-structured interviews were used to ask people about their experience of the discharge procedure. After the interview, the researcher completed a pro forma in which the person's experience was converted into a number of broad categorical variables, for example, the length of notice the person received about discharge from hospital and whether or not the person was involved in the decision to discharge. These data were then analysed statistically, while the full interview data were analysed using qualitative analysis techniques. This type of transformation should be approached cautiously because the sample size for many qualitative components would not yield sufficient data for a meaningful statistical analysis.

Interpretation

A key stage in mixed methods research is bringing together the insights gained from both methods. This often takes place in the latter stages of the study once the main analysis has been completed. This further stage is referred to by some as 'crystallisation' (O'Cathain *et al.* 2007b), where there is a purposeful search for convergence, divergence and discrepancy between the findings from the different methods. It is important to ensure that this additional process in mixed methods research is deliberately planned into the time and resources for the study at the outset. It is disappointing when reading a mixed methods study to find that in the presentation of the results and subsequent discussion, both parts of the study are presented separately with no attempt made to bring the insights from the parts together.

Specific examples have been used to illustrate integration at different stages of the research, but integration is often not restricted to one stage of the research in any one project. High-quality mixed methods studies may have integrated elements throughout. To ensure that integration is apparent to readers of mixed methods studies, it may be appropriate when presenting such

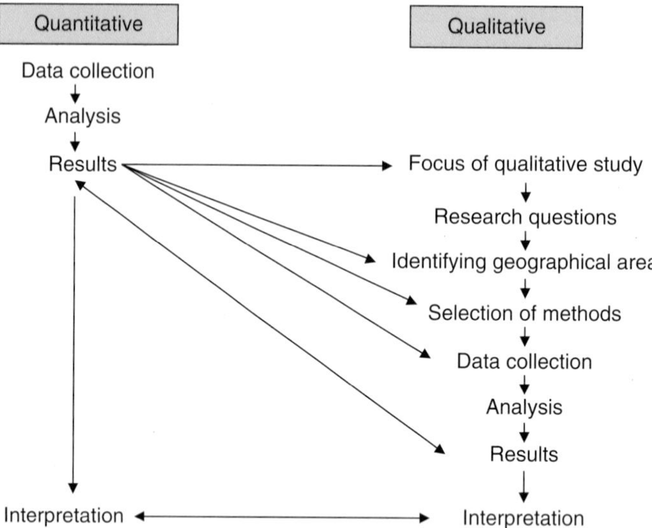

Figure 27.1 An example of how to represent mixed methods integration in a diagram. Reproduced from Turnbull J (2008) *Out-of-Hours General Practice: an investigation of patients' use and experiences of access to services.* Unpublished PhD thesis. Southampton, University of Southampton with permission from Joanne Turnbull.

Reflection activity

Why is it so important to consider how different methods are integrated within a single study?

studies to devise a diagram to demonstrate where it takes place. For the study described in Research Example 27.1, a diagram was used in the written presentation of the research to clearly demonstrate the way in which the two components of the study were integrated (Figure 27.1).

CHALLENGES WITH MIXED METHODS STUDIES

Although mixed methods research can bring many advantages to the research endeavour, careful consideration is needed before embarking on such a study. It should not be undertaken simply because it is assumed to be inherently better than a single method study. As with all research, the design should be driven by the research question and good rationale is required for any design adopted. Some of the challenges with mixed methods research are summarised in the following.

The strategic use of mixed methods

Researchers might propose a mixed methods design as they believe it is favoured by funding bodies and that using this design will increase their chance of gaining funding. This is not sufficient justification to attempt a mixed methods study, since the research topic and question may not warrant such a design.

Mixed methods requires a range of expertise and skill

There are limited training programmes that specifically focus on how to conduct good quality mixed methods studies. It is therefore unlikely that one researcher will have the range of necessary skills to ensure the quality of both methods within a mixed methods study. This means mixed methods studies are usually conducted by teams of researchers with complementary skills.

Multidisciplinary or interdisciplinary team working

Diversity and complementary expertise within mixed methods teams are an integral part of multidisciplinary working, and while this can often be a rich and rewarding experience, the nature of such teams also has the potential to give rise to tensions and challenges. This might include dealing with differences between quantitative and qualitative approaches, trusting the 'other', handling conflicts and tensions and establishing effective leadership roles (Curry *et al.* 2012). It is important to adopt respectful and collaborative practice to guard against 'silos' developing where a series of separate mini-projects are conducted rather than integrated mixed methods. This is particularly pertinent where one method has been the dominant approach in a particular discipline and there may be limited understanding of the other approach.

Maintaining quality in mixed methods research

If both qualitative and quantitative methods are being applied, there is a danger that neither approach will be conducted well. The overall quality of a mixed methods study will always be constrained by the individual components. While there are as yet no established criteria or checklists for assessing the quality of mixed methods studies, this issue is being debated. For example, researchers in the field are asking whether it is appropriate to apply both sets of criteria to a mixed methods study. However, as the discussion about integration indicated, it may be the aspects of the research that are *distinctive* to mixed methods that should be assessed, rather than applying criteria developed for a different purpose.

> **Reflection activity**
>
> How might researchers ensure quality and rigour when undertaking a mixed methods study?

CONCLUSION

Mixed methods research has gained greatly in popularity in recent years, but therein lies a danger. While it has the potential to provide positive and enriching experiences for researchers, as well as answers to complex healthcare questions, the term has been used as a 'catch-all' to lend credence to research that is not truly adopting the underpinning philosophy and principles. To ensure that the value, robustness and integrity of mixed methods approaches are maintained, attention must be paid to the integration of qualitative and quantitative data in a way that produces outcomes that are greater than the sum of the parts.

References

Bazeley P (2012) Integrative analysis strategies for mixed data sources. *American Behavioral Scientist* **56**: 814–828.

Biesta G (2010) Pragmatism and the philosophical foundations of mixed methods research. In: Tashakkori A, Teddlie C (eds) *Sage Handbook of Mixed Methods in Social and Behavioral Research*, 2nd edition. London, Sage, pp 95–117.

Bruton A, Kirby S, Arden-Close E, Taylor L, Webley F, George S, Yardley L, Price D, Moore M, Little P, Holgate S, Djukanovic R, Lee AJ, Raftery J, Chorozoglou M, Versnel J, Pavord I, Stafford-Watson M, Thomas M (2013) The BREATHE study: breathing retraining for asthma. Trial of home exercises. A protocol summary of a randomised controlled trial. *Primary Care Respiratory Journal* **22**(2): PS1–PS7.

Bryman A (2008) Why do researchers integrate/combine/mesh/blend/mix/merge/ fuse quantitative and qualitative research? In: Bergman M (ed) *Advances in Mixed Methods Research*. London, Sage, pp 87–100.

Bryman A (2012) Mixed methods research: combining quantitative and qualitative research. In: Bryman A (ed), *Social Research Methods,* 4th edition. Oxford, Oxford University Press, pp 628–652.

Bryman A, Becker S, Sempik J (2008) Quality criteria for quantitative, qualitative and mixed methods research: a view from social policy. *International Journal of Social Research Methodology* **11**: 261–276.

Creswell JW (2010) Mapping the developing landscape of mixed methods research. In: Tashakkori A, Teddlie C (eds) *Sage Handbook of Mixed Methods in Social and Behavioral Research*, 2nd edition. London, Sage, pp 45–68.

Creswell JW, Plano Clark VL (2010) *Designing and Conducting Mixed Methods Research*, 2nd edition. London, Sage.

Curry LA, O'Cathain A, Plano Clark VL, Aroni R, Fetters M, Berg D (2012) The role of group dynamics in mixed methods health sciences research teams. *Journal of Mixed Methods Research* **6**: 5–20.

Curry LA, Krumholz HM, O'Cathain A, Plano Clark VL, Cherlin E, Bradley EH (2013) Mixed methods in biomedical and health services research. *Circulation: Cardiovascular Quality and Outcomes* **6**: 119–123.

Hanna L, May C, Fairhurst K (2011) Non-face-to-face consultations and communications in primary care: the role and perspective of general practice managers in Scotland. *Informatics in Primary Care* **19**: 17–24.

Latter S, Sibley A, Skinner TC, Craddock S, Zinken KM, Lussier MT, Richard C, Roberge D (2010) The impact of an intervention for nurse prescribers on consultations to promote patient medicine-taking in diabetes: a mixed methods study. *International Journal of Nursing Studies* **47**: 1126–1138.

Lewin S, Glenton C, Oxman AD (2009) Use of qualitative methods alongside randomised controlled trials of complex healthcare interventions: methodological study. *British Medical Journal* **339**: b3496.

Mantzoukas S (2009) The research evidence published in high impact journals between 2000–2006: a quantitative content analysis. *International Journal of Nursing Studies* **46**: 479–489.

Medical Research Council (2000) *A Framework for Development and Evaluation of RCTs for Complex Interventions to Improve Health*. London, Medical Research Council.

Morgan DL (2013) *Integrating Qualitative and Quantitative Methods: a pragmatic approach*. London, Sage.

Morse JM (2003) Principles of mixed methods and multimethod research design. In: Tashakkori A, Teddlie C (eds) *Handbook of Mixed Methods in Social and Behavioral Research*. Thousand Oaks, Sage, pp 189–208.

Morse JM, Niehus L (2009) *Mixed Method Design: principles and procedures*. Walnut Creek, CA, Left Coast Press.

O'Cathain A, Murphy E, Nicholl J (2007a) Why, and how, mixed methods research is undertaken in health services research in England: a mixed methods study. *BMC Health Services Research* **7**: 85. DOI: 10.1186/1472-6963-7-85.

O'Cathain A, Murphy E, Nicholl J (2007b) Integration and publications as indicators of 'yield' from mixed method studies. *Journal of Mixed Methods Research* **1**: 147–163.

Östlund U, Kidd L, Wengström Y, Rowa-Dewar N (2011) Combining qualitative and quantitative research within mixed method research designs: a methodological review. *International Journal of Nursing Studies* **48**: 369–383.

Simons L, Petch A, Caplan R (2002) *'Don't They Call It Seamless Care?': a study of acute psychiatric discharge*. Edinburgh, Scottish Executive Social Research.

Simons L, Lathlean J, Squire C (2008) Shifting the focus: sequential methods of analysis with qualitative data. *Qualitative Health Research* **18**: 120–132.

Turnbull J (2008) *Out-of-Hours General Practice: an investigation of patients' use and experiences of access to services*. Unpublished PhD thesis. Southampton, University of Southampton.

Turnbull J, Martin D, Lattimer V, Pope C, Culliford D (2008) Does distance matter? Geographical variation in GP out-of-hours service use: an observational study. *British Journal of General Practice* **58**: 471–477.

Turnbull J, Pope C, Martin D, Latimer V (2010) Do telephones overcome geographical barriers to general practice out-of-hours services? Mixed-methods study of parents with young children. *Journal of Health Services Research and Policy* **15**: 21–27.

Turnbull J, Prichard J, Halford S, Pope C, Salisbury C (2012) Reconfiguring the emergency and urgent care workforce: mixed methods study of skills and the everyday work of non-clinical call-handlers in the NHS. *Journal of Health Services Policy* **17**: 233–240.

White P, Bishop FL, Prescott P, Scott C, Little P, Lewith G (2012) Practice, practitioner, or placebo? A multifactorial mixed-methods randomized controlled trial of acupuncture. *Pain* **153**: 455–62.

Wisdom JP, Cavaleri MA, Onwuegbuzie AJ, Green CA (2012) Methodological reporting in qualitative, quantitative, and mixed methods health services research articles. *Health Services Research* **47**: 721–745.

Further reading

Andrew S, Halcomb E (2009) *Mixed Methods Research for Nursing and the Health Sciences*. Oxford, Wiley-Blackwell.

Bergman MM (ed) (2008) *Advances in Mixed Methods Research: theories and applications*. Thousand Oaks, Sage.

Tashakkori A, Teddlie C (eds) (2010) *Sage Handbook of Mixed Methods in Social and Behavioral Research*, 2nd edition. London, Sage.

Websites

http://mmr.sagepub.com/ – *Journal of Mixed Methods Research*. Information about the journal and table of contents for each edition and requesting free sample copy.

http://www.ncrm.ac.uk/ – The ESRC National Centre for Research Methods training centre for innovations in methods. Hosted workshops on mixed methods that are detailed on the site plus a discussion paper about mixed methods written by Julia Brannen. Also, seminars within the individual research programmes relevant to mixed methods.

SECTION 4

Collecting Data

This section contains six practical chapters dealing with the common methods used in nursing research to collect data. A generic approach has been maintained, with several of the methods such as interviewing and observation being used in both qualitative and quantitative research.

Chapter 28 begins by tackling interviews, a versatile data collection method widely used in nursing research. This is followed by Chapter 29 that describes focus groups, which are increasingly popular as an adjunct to individual interviews, or as a stand-alone tool. Both these chapters deal with the purposes to which the methods are best suited, the essential preparation for, and conduct of, the interview or focus group, and the practical and ethical issues raised.

Chapter 30 then deals with questionnaires, perhaps being the most widely used method of data collection in health care research. This chapter discusses in detail some of the ways of testing validity and reliability of existing questionnaires, as well as giving advice to the nurse researcher who is developing her own measure.

Observation, structured or unstructured, participant or not, forms the focus of Chapter 31. It is a powerful tool for data collection that is used less often than it might be, perhaps because of the demands made upon the researcher. Observation is used differently in qualitative than in quantitative research, and this chapter discusses each approach carefully. Ethical issues raised are considered, as are the problems of ensuring validity, reliability and trustworthiness of the data collected.

The final two chapters in this section, Chapters 32 and 33, consider less commonly used methods of data collection but which are important to nursing research. Think aloud is a technique for data collection that has unique ability to increase our understanding of clinical decision making in nursing. It can be combined with other data collection tools to increase the richness and validity of data gathered. Finally, Chapter 33 deals with outcome measures. Evaluation of clinical treatments is increasingly measured by patient-based outcomes, as well as scientifically observable physiological measures, although the latter are still, of course, important. This chapter therefore considers the range of measures that can be used to assess the effects of nursing care and which are also vitally important in many research studies.

The Research Process in Nursing, Seventh Edition. Edited by Kate Gerrish and Judith Lathlean.

Companion Website: www.wiley.com/go/gerrish/research

CHAPTER 28

Interviewing

Angela Tod

Key points

- Interviews can be used to collect qualitative and quantitative data and can vary in their degree of structure. The degree of structure is dictated by the research design and purpose.
- Key skills in conducting rigorous interviews include developing a well-designed data collection tool, selecting a suitable environment, establishing rapport and balancing the direction and flexibility of questioning.
- Interviews can generate rich data reflecting the perspective of participants. Interviews can be of particular value when the research focus is a sensitive area.
- Interviews are labour intensive and expensive and can introduce bias.
- Interviews provide a unique opportunity to gain insight into a range of subjects and experiences related to nursing and health services.

INTRODUCTION

This chapter considers some of the key issues confronting the researcher in conducting a research interview. Brief attention is paid to the purpose and nature of the research interview. This is followed by an overview of different types of interview and some of the advantages and disadvantages of the different forms. The main issues to reflect on when undertaking research interviews are reviewed followed by an outline of some factors relating to validity, reliability and ethics.

THE PURPOSE OF THE RESEARCH INTERVIEW

Conducting a research interview is one of the most exciting and fascinating methods of data collection in nursing and healthcare research. This may explain why it is one of the most commonly used data collection methods. Interviews are used in both qualitative and quantitative research as the primary data collection method or as a supplementary method in mixed-method studies.

The Research Process in Nursing, Seventh Edition. Edited by Kate Gerrish and Judith Lathlean.

Companion Website: www.wiley.com/go/gerrish/research

Reasons for undertaking interviews

The purpose of undertaking a research interview varies widely. The research aim will dictate the exact nature and form of the interview in terms of structure, direction and depth. Generally, the more that is known about a topic beforehand, the more structured and less in-depth the exploration.

A structured interview approximates to a standardised interviewer-administered questionnaire in that the wording and order of questions is the same for all participants. Structured interviews normally generate quantitative data. Some include limited open questions and have some capacity to produce qualitative data. Structured interviews could be used for a survey in order to measure variables in a specific population. They are useful when a certain amount is already known about the subject under examination and are used to explore differences between people with varying characteristics or experiences (Murphy *et al.* 1998: 112–123). The inclusion of open questions facilitates the collection of data to illuminate survey responses.

The majority of interview-based studies in nursing are qualitative in nature and so adopt a less structured, more 'in-depth' and flexible approach. Such methods are recommended when the research purpose is to:

- explore a phenomenon about which little is known
- understand context
- generate a hypothesis or theory to explain social processes and relationships
- verify the results from other forms of data collection, for example, observation
- illuminate responses from a questionnaire survey
- conduct initial exploration to generate items for questionnaires

Interviews, therefore, have the capacity to describe, explain and explore issues from the perspective of participants.

RESEARCH EXAMPLE

28.1 Using Interviews as a Single Method of Data Collection in a Qualitative Study

Warnock C, Tod A (2014) A descriptive exploration of the experiences of patients with significant functional impairment following a recent diagnosis of metastatic spinal cord compression. *Journal of Advanced Nursing* **70**: 564–574.

In this study, 10 patients with a diagnosis of metastatic spinal cord compression (MSCC) were interviewed (3 women and 7 men with an age range of 59–81). Time from cancer diagnosis to MSCC diagnosis varied from 1 month to 17 years. The aim of the study was to explore the experiences, concerns and priorities of patients who were newly diagnosed with advanced MSCC and had significant problems with mobility at presentation. The semi-structured interviews were conducted and audio-recorded. The recordings were transcribed verbatim and analysed using Framework Analysis (Ritchie & Lewis 2003). Two main interconnected themes were identified: thinking through the implications of MSCC and meeting the challenges of MSCC. Participants emphasised the importance of being able to cope and described the actions they were taking to improve their situation. Participants balanced talking about their problems while emphasising ways in which they could cope and remain hopeful. The study revealed patients' main concerns were reduced mobility, losing their independence, the impact of the diagnosis on their family and getting home.

Using interviews, the researchers were able to explore patients' experiences and priorities in a sensitive and challenging clinical context. Responses to the diagnosis of MSCC were revealed along with implications for nursing and multi-disciplinary care, for example, the importance of support regarding increasing mobility and returning home where possible.

Research Examples 28.1, 28.2 and 28.3 illustrate different uses of the research interview. Warnock and Tod (2014) used semi-structured interviews to explore the experience of patients with a new diagnosis of metastatic spinal cord compression (see Research Example 28.1). This study demonstrates how interviews can generate qualitative data to explore patient experience in a sensitive and challenging clinical context. McDonnell *et al.* (2013) used interviews in the qualitative component of a mixed-method study

RESEARCH EXAMPLE

28.2 Using Interviews in a Mixed-Method Study

McDonnell A, Tod A, Bray K Bainbridge D, Adsetts D, Walters S (2013) A before and after study assessing the impact of a new model for recognizing and responding to early signs of deterioration in an acute hospital. *Journal of Advanced Nursing* **69**(1): 41–52.

This before- and- after, mixed-method study evaluated the impact of a new intervention for detection and management of deteriorating patients on the knowledge and confidence of nurses working in an acute hospital. The intervention included a training session, new observation charts and a new track and trigger system. Fifteen nurses were interviewed before the training, and 6 weeks after, the intervention was introduced on their ward. Interviews occurred alongside a survey of 213 nurses. A topic guide was used in the interview. It was developed in the light of existing literature, the content of the questionnaire and emerging findings from the survey.

The survey demonstrated an increased knowledge and confidence in detecting and managing patient deterioration following the intervention. The findings from the interviews reinforced those from the survey, but they also offered insights into the reasons for the observed changes and increase the confidence. This allowed conclusions to be drawn from the data about why the intervention had prompted a positive impact. The interview data also allowed some insight into what aspect of the intervention had helped and in what ways. The implications for practice generated by the study are more likely to be rooted in the reality of practice when enhanced by the experience shared in interviews.

RESEARCH EXAMPLE

28.3 Using Interviews to Collect Data in a Quantitative Study

Laws R (2004) Current approaches to obesity management in UK primary care: the counterweight programme. *Journal of Human Nutrition and Dietetics* **17**: 183–190.

This study aimed to examine obesity management in 40 primary care practices in the United Kingdom. A total of 141 general practitioners and 66 practice nurses were interviewed using a structured approach. A researcher-administered questionnaire was used to establish which of five obesity management approaches participants used. The approaches were based on time spent with patients and the nature of advice given. Referral practice and attitudes to obesity management were also recorded. Reported practice in the interviews was compared to recorded practice in the clinical notes.

The approach revealed that obesity was under-reported and under-recognised in primary care. However, it demonstrated the challenge of collecting data from busy clinical staff as one third of the participants did not complete the questionnaire/interview.

to explore the impact of a new model to detect and manage patient deterioration (see Research Example 28.2). It demonstrates how interview data can be used alongside a questionnaire to illuminate nurses' experiences of a new intervention to improve practice. In this study, the interview data reinforced the findings of the survey and provided greater insight into the reality of the clinical context within which the intervention was implemented. Laws (2004) uses structured interviews to collect quantitative data from doctors and nurses on obesity management (see Research Example 28.3).

The difference between a clinical and research interview

Nurses are trained to use interviews to obtain information from patients in clinical settings. While this clinical experience may be a good preparation for undertaking research interviews, the research context and purpose is different and requires different skills. In research interviews, the focus of data collection is broad, as it is necessary to understand meanings regarding the area of study from the participants' viewpoint.

In the clinical context, data collection is focused on identifying a problem; fitting it into a predetermined category, for example, diagnosis; and deciding a management or intervention strategy (Britten 1995). This means that clinical situation lends itself to being more controlled by the clinician. In addition, a nurse would freely respond to patients' questions related to the clinical situation. In a research interview, this is not appropriate. To respond to questions may deviate away from the interview focus and may bias responses by changing the participant's knowledge base. Judgements made by researchers therefore differ from those of the nurse.

TYPES OF INTERVIEW

Structure

Robson (2011) states that the most common distinction made between different types of interview is the degree of structure and standardisation. A continuum exists from completely structured to unstructured interviews (Figure 28.1). In general, the less structured an interview, the more in-depth and flexible the questioning. An unstructured interview is likely to be led more by the informant's agenda rather than the interviewer. It will generate qualitative data.

In structured or standardised interviews, the balance of control lies with the interviewer. Such an approach would be adopted for survey purposes or when less in-depth data are required. Structured interviews are also used if it is not possible for the participant to self-administer a questionnaire, for example, if the participant does not have the ability or concentration to read. In nursing research, a structured interview may be used to gain some insight where competing work or home demands would make a more in-depth interview impossible. Interviewing nurses on a busy ward might be an example of this.

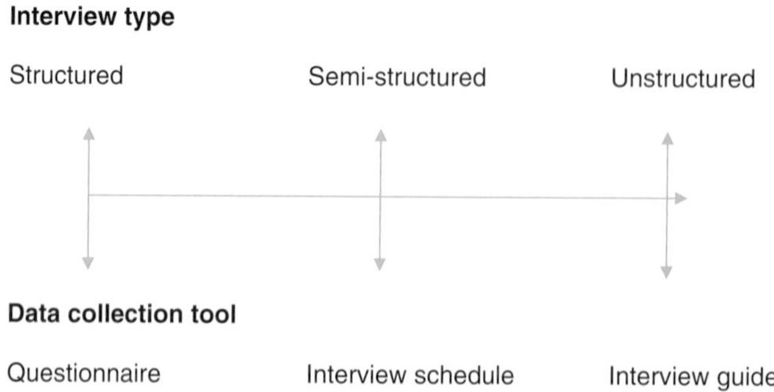

Figure 28.1 The continuum of interview structure and data collection tool required

In many qualitative studies, semi-structured and unstructured interviews are used. Semi-structured interviews will have predetermined topics and open-ended questions laid down in an interview schedule. They retain the flexibility necessary to follow issues raised by participants that had not been anticipated. Control and direction of interviews of this nature still lies with the researcher, but there will be capacity to be responsive to the interviewee's agenda and views. Semi-structured interviews are widely used in qualitative studies adopting a number of methodological approaches in nursing research.

Unstructured interviews are the most in-depth and least directive. The aim here is often to explore in great detail a general area of interest or a phenomenon from the participant's perspective. A few themes may guide the interview, but it will be led by the participant's perspective and viewpoint. Interviews of this nature are very informal and can appear more like a conversation than an interview. The interview guide will comprise a list of topics rather than predefined questions. This approach is more commonly adopted in qualitative research methodologies where little previous knowledge exists regarding the area of study.

The degree of structure employed in an interview will depend on the purpose of the study and the depth of inquiry required. It will also vary according to the resources available. With structured interviews, questioning techniques are standardised to ensure the reliability of the data. Unstructured interviews can be labour intensive and expensive. Their informal and unguided structure means they can take a long time to conduct and also to transcribe and analyse. As is always the case with research, it is important to choose the right tool for the job and to make sure the approach adopted is achievable within the time and cost restraints of a study.

Reflection activity

Identify a research question that you are interested in answering where interviews would be a good method to use to collect data. What are the advantages of taking a more structured or an unstructured approach to conducting the interviews?

Face-to-face versus telephone interviews

The vast majority of individual interviews are conducted face-to-face. The researcher is able to probe and investigate hidden and suppressed views and experiences. The ability to observe body language and eye contact helps to interpret what is being said. It also helps to interpret emotion, distress, anxiety and silence and to respond accordingly. For example, if a respondent displays emotion, it may provide an appropriate opportunity to collect data on a sensitive and upsetting experience of great value to the study. On the other hand, it may be appropriate to appraise the situation with regard to stopping the interview. Making this judgement is difficult if the interview is not face-to-face.

Telephone interviews are increasingly being used to conduct structured and semi-structured interviews. In some circumstances, it may be a cheaper, more convenient mode of inquiry. Telephone interviews are limited in their ability to detect detailed information, misinformation and the emotional implications and subtext relating to the interview topic. However, there are situations where telephone interviews have clear advantages, particularly for structured interviews. Midanik and Greenfield (2003) compared the use of telephone and in-person interviews to collect data for a national survey on alcohol use. They found no differences in the number and quality of responses and so advocate the use of telephone interviews for national surveys. Telephone interviews are cheaper, requiring less travel and the equipment needed is minimal (a simple connecting cable between phone and recorder).

In a qualitative research project, Garbett and McCormack (2001) were able to capture the views of 26 nurses working in different roles and settings across the United Kingdom by using telephone interviews. To undertake face-to-face interviews would have been expensive and required long distances to travel. Using the telephone also helped to ensure participants were not under any pressure to participate as they found it easier to refuse.

> **Reflection activity**
>
> In relation to the research question you have identified in the earlier activity for which interviews would be appropriate, list the advantages and disadvantages of using telephone interviews. Which do you think will be most appropriate to use and why?

Telephone interviews can offer a more sensitive and less threatening approach when the nature of the research topic may create a risk of participants thinking they would be judged. It also provides a more convenient option if people are busy and have conflicting commitments. Smith (2005) engages in a wider discussion on contexts where telephone interviews may be appropriate or preferable.

One-off or longitudinal interviews

Numerous studies use interviews as a one-off strategy of data collection where interviews are collected at one point in time. Longitudinal or sequential interviews provide the opportunity to collect data at different time points, for example, during the course of a patient's illness. This captures the evolving experience of the participant and tracks changes and gaps, for example expectations and experiences or health status.

Sequential interviews can generate richer data. Field and Morse (1985) claim that it is often impossible to collect good quality data at the first interview. The increased trust that develops over time between researcher and interviewee will also facilitate more in-depth and better quality data. For example, Henning *et al.* (2013) used sequential interviews for a study involving caregivers of people with dementia.

UNDERTAKING AN INTERVIEW

On the surface, an interview may appear to be a process of asking a few questions. In reality, conducting a sound and rigorous interview can be a testing and complex enterprise (Robson 2011). The researcher has a responsibility to master certain techniques in order to produce results that are meaningful, useful and ensure the interviewee's generous contribution is not in vain.

Developing the data collection tool

It is important to develop the right tools to address the research purpose and answer the research question. Key to this is developing a data collection tool with the right level of structure. Examples are provided in Box 28.1. A structured interview will require a structured, inflexible schedule akin to a questionnaire. It has to be administered in the same way and the same order, with the same wording for each participant. An unstructured interview will have maximum flexibility and often requires a guide comprising only a few core items. With a semi-structured interview, a suitable schedule is essential to achieving the right balance of direction and flexibility. This means the central research question will be addressed, it will also allow new and interesting responses to be explored further. An unstructured interview has no set of questions and may be more discursive. It may just consist of an opening question or an invitation for the participant to share their experience of the issue being explored.

A number of factors should be considered in constructing an interview schedule. How important these are may depend upon the purpose of the study (i.e. to generate quantitative or qualitative data) and the nature of the questioning (i.e. level of structure and sensitivity of the subject).

First, it is necessary to be clear about the types of questions to be asked. Six main types of questions (Patton 1987; Britten 1995) have been identified:

- Behaviour or experience
- Opinion or belief
- Feeling
- Knowledge
- Sensory experience
- Background information such as demographics

Some are easier to ask about and answer than others. Questions related to behaviour and knowledge may

Box 28.1 Examples of interview structure, purpose and questions

Interview structure	Research purpose	Example of a question(s)
Structured or standardised interview	To identify (i) the nature, range and frequency of angina symptoms experienced by the population of a geographical area and (ii) variation in symptom experience between and within the population according to characteristic for example, age, gender and ethnicity	a) Which of the following angina symptoms do you experience? (Provide a list of symptoms with boxes to tick) b) How often do you experience them? (Provide a scale for participants to indicate frequency of experience)
Semi-structured interview	To explore and identify barriers to angina symptom reporting and diagnosis	Can you tell me a bit about yourself? How old are you? Are you married? Do you have any children? When did you first notice that there was something wrong with your heart? What symptoms or discomfort did you experience? What did you think was causing these feelings at first?
Unstructured interview	To understand an individual's experience of living with angina and the meaning it has for them in their life	Can you tell me about your experience of living with angina?

elicit short and specific responses. In comparison, questions about beliefs and feelings are more challenging, complex and potentially sensitive. They may need to be approached gradually and only after non-threatening questions have been asked.

It is common for the sequence of the schedule to be divided into sections, for example, introduction, 'warm-up' or opening questions, the main interview questions, 'wind-down' questions and closing the interview (see Box 28.2).

Inappropriate timing of questions can sabotage the interview. If rapport and trust have been established, it is possible to ask questions of an extremely sensitive nature. It is necessary continually to judge the appropriateness of an interview question in terms of the timing and how it will be interpreted and received by the interviewee.

Prompts can be built into the interview. These are particularly important in semi-structured interview schedules. Prompts have been described as questions that derive from the researcher (Robson 2011). They are intended to test an a priori assumption of the researcher or facilitate the interviewee to reflect on or expand upon a certain theme issue (Legard *et al.* 2003). They can also be used if participants lose their thread as a way of encouraging them to re-engage with the interview. Box 28.3 provides examples of broad questions, followed by more focused questions

Box 28.2 Sequence of questions in an interview

Interview sequence	Type of questions
Introduction	• Introducing the study • Explain the purpose of the interview • Check the participant understands the purpose and nature of the study • Obtain or verify consent • Promote a relaxed atmosphere by making conversation
Warm-up	• Ask neutral, unthreatening questions • Ask for factual background information, for example, age, children and job • Seek clarification or expansion if necessary
Main interview questions	• Ask questions relating to the main research aim • Ensure sequence follows some logic and sense • Start with broad questions followed by more focused ones • Leave the most sensitive and difficult questions until last • Use prompts and probes to generate deeper and richer data
Wind-down	• Round off with a few simple questions especially if the interview has been tense, emotional or sensitive • Let the interviewee know the interview is winding up, e.g. say 'to finish with ...' • Ask if there is anything else they would like to add
Close of interview	• Check again that there is nothing else they want to add • Check if people know and remember what will happen to the data • Thank the participant

(Compiled with reference to Legard *et al.* 2003; Robson 2011.)

Box 28.3 Example of questions used in a semi-structured interview

Broad question *(asked at the beginning of the interview to gain an overview of the patient's experience, develop rapport and influence subsequent questioning)*
Can you tell me something about your general health?

Focused question *(asked afterwards to elicit information about diagnosis of angina and any other chronic condition)*
Do you have any longstanding illness or disability?

Structured questionnaire *(administered as a way of verifying the patient has angina)*
Administer the 'Rose Angina Questionnaire' (Rose *et al.* 1977). This is a short questionnaire eliciting information on the patients' chest pain and is an objective measure of angina symptoms.

Prompt *(if not mentioned investigate further whether they have angina)*
Has your doctor told you what is wrong with you, that is, what causes the chest pain?
(The results of this study are found in Tod *et al.* (2001).)

with predetermined prompts. These were used in a study where people with angina were interviewed (Tod *et al.* 2001).

CONDUCTING THE INTERVIEW

Selecting a suitable environment

Maintaining a suitable interview environment will often require a trade-off between accessibility, comfort and level of distraction. If a venue is considered inappropriate or inaccessible, people will be reluctant to take part. Common choices are the interviewee's home or workplace. A more neutral location may be required if people are likely to be distracted by or protective of their personal or professional setting. Interviewing people in their own home may be preferable in some situations, for example, where it is helpful to understand the impact of the home environment on the person's experience of a health condition.

The comfort of the environment is essential if interviewees are to feel relaxed, at ease and able to concentrate. On occasions, however, it may be necessary to sacrifice some comfort in order to involve participants from certain groups, for example, interviewing patients on bed rest or nurses on or near their ward. Choosing an environment with minimum risk of disruption is also a concern. There are certain things that a researcher can do to facilitate this, such as turning off telephones and other equipment and putting up a 'do not disturb' sign.

Even the best-laid plans can go astray, and sometimes, the unexpected occurs, for example, a participant having unexpected childcare commitments resulting in a child being present at the interview. The researcher then needs to make a judgement about whether to proceed with the interview with the knowledge that the quality may be affected or whether to cancel the interview and risk offending the participant.

Establishing rapport

A successful interview will be reliant upon developing a sense of trust and rapport. The attitude and demeanour of the interviewer is a key, and it is essential that they appear genuine and interested in the participant's views. Legard *et al.* (2003) suggest that the researcher displaying confidence, tranquillity and credibility facilitates this. Humour and adaptability are also tools. Being organised, efficient and focused; having a well-planned and paced schedule of questions; and being responsive to the mood, body language and priorities of the interviewee all help to develop a good interview relationship. The posture and bearing of the researcher should convey attention and interest.

Questioning technique

Techniques used to facilitate questioning need to maintain a balance between direction and flexibility. Where the balance lies will reflect the research aim, method and level of structure. Techniques include active listening, being clear and unambiguous, not leading respondents towards particular views or beliefs and keeping interested. The tradition is to advise researchers to say as little as possible because of the risk the interviewer may contaminate, influence or confuse the interviewee. Some researchers argue for more interaction in qualitative interviews on the grounds that it allows the researcher to test out emerging ideas and discussion helps to explore more complex issues (Melia 2000). One approach to being more interactive is what Melia refers to as 'verbal memo-ing' where the interviewer investigates initial arguments emerging from analysis. Another option that can be used in both qualitative and quantitative research would be to construct vignettes or scenarios from earlier accounts to draw out opinion in subsequent interviews.

The appropriate use of prompts and probes can help to achieve the right balance of breadth and depth in the questioning (Legard *et al.* 2003). In structured interviews, they may be used to clarify a question if it is misunderstood. In unstructured and semi-structured interviews, some questions lead the respondent to broad statements that may set the stage or reveal a range of issues and dimensions. Probes may then be used to uncover layers of meaning. Probing questions have the capacity to amplify, explore, explain or clarify (Legard *et al.* 2003). The astute use of silence to help participants reflect and respond, is a valuable interview technique. An interested look, maintaining eye contact or summarising can all help to prompt a response.

Managing the interview

An interview is a sensitive interaction and needs careful handling. This should start from the outset by considering how the researcher is perceived by the participant. Difference or similarity in age, ethnicity, gender or social status can all make a difference to how people respond. The interviewer's demeanour and appearance may vary depending on whether they are interviewing a chief executive of a hospital or a teenager. Clarity in introducing the researcher and the project can help. This will also minimise any risk of role conflict for a nurse conducting a research interview.

Setting the scene for the respondent is essential. Points to explain include the following:

- There are no right or wrong answers.
- They have the right to withdraw or stop at any time.
- They can interrupt or ask for explanations whenever they want.
- The interview will be recorded (usually on digital recorder) with their permission.

COMMON PITFALLS IN CONDUCTING INTERVIEWS

A common concern in interviewing patients is the risk of losing the research role and slipping into that of a teacher, preacher or counsellor (Allmark *et al.* 2009). This risk is particularly dangerous in less structured interviews where the discussion is more in-depth. On occasions, it is difficult to avoid role conflict, especially for nurses and others with a clinical training. The interviewer must avoid putting their own view and perspective forward. This is a particular hazard when the respondent has said something the researcher disagreed with or finds offensive. To explore such views gently will be more productive than challenging them (Legard *et al.* 2003).

Handling a situation that is emotionally charged can be testing if a participant becomes upset, anxious or angry. Sensitive questioning can help, as will communicating empathy and interest with body language and eye contact. However, it is important not to be frightened of such emotional situations. Not only do they often produce the most valuable and insightful data, the participant may find it a positive experience to discuss the issue in this way.

Selecting the most appropriate way of recording an interview is a key factor in its success. The most common form of recording is a digital audio recording, supplemented by field notes. Other media include video recording, video conferencing or Internet chat rooms. The use of photographs taken by participants to guide interviews is becoming more popular in studies, especially with more marginalised groups (Catalani & Minkler 2010). In making a decision, it is important to consider how intrusive the technology will appear to the participant, ease of use of the technology, reliability and ethical aspects regarding confidentiality and privacy. It is always important to check that recording equipment is working before the interview. Following the interview the recording is normally transcribed verbatim and ready for analysis.

When taking field notes, researchers need to be aware of how this may be interpreted by the respondent. If the researcher appears more absorbed in scribbling notes than in participating in the interview, it is easy for the participant to think that the researcher is not listening or interested.

Additional challenges in managing an interview can occur if the researcher and participant do not speak the same language and an interpreter is used. Developing rapport and trust can be more difficult if

> **Reflection activity**
>
> Think about the ways in which you can improve the environment when interviewing someone outside of their home? What can you do to make the interview environment conducive to a comfortable conversation?

Reflection activity

How can you plan ahead to make sure an interview runs smoothly? Draw up an action plan for undertaking an interview.

conducting an interview through a third person. It is therefore necessary to ensure that the interpreter is acceptable to the participant and culturally appropriate, in addition to having good language skills. Maintaining accuracy in collecting data is also difficult. The interpreter should be skilled and practised in research interview work and be able to demonstrate accuracy of translation between interviewee and interviewer.

Managing an interview well is a difficult task and needs practice. Piloting is recommended, especially when the researcher is new to the interview process. Piloting allows questions to be tested and refined and practice gained in using recording equipment. A novice interviewer is advised to secure good supervision, not just to support the research design and data analysis, but also to aid reflection of the interview experience. Mistakes are inevitable, but it is always worth reflecting back on these and discussing ways to avoid the same pitfalls in the future.

ADVANTAGES AND DISADVANTAGES OF INTERVIEWS

Interviewing is a flexible and adaptable method of data collection and can be an efficient way of collecting data on a myriad of subjects, including participants' views, attitudes, behaviours and experiences. The flexibility of the interview format and structure is one of its greatest advantages. The interview is malleable and can be adapted to fit the needs and purpose of different studies from quantitative surveys to detailed phenomenological explorations of individuals' experiences.

Structured interviews have the capacity to generate a large volume of data from a large sample. They are an excellent means of collecting data that are predominantly quantitative but can incorporate qualitative questioning. It is possible to use structured interviews to test the findings of smaller, in-depth interview studies with a larger population.

Semi- and unstructured interviews have an unrivalled ability to generate data of depth and complexity. The forum of the interview provides the opportunity to explore the intricacy of an issue from the perspective of individual participants.

Interviews may provide the only method of eliciting the views of people who are often 'hard to reach' in terms of research and who would be reluctant or unable to participate in research using other methods. There is some indication that, while not intentionally having a direct therapeutic effect, people do find the experience of being interviewed a positive one.

Many of the disadvantages are reflected in the challenges referred to earlier, for example, the risk of introducing bias by inadequate sampling or questioning. Following the advice and techniques outlined earlier can avoid this. However, one danger to be considered is that the involvement in the interview itself may change the views or perceptions of the participants. The researcher should be continually vigilant of this risk of a 'Hawthorne effect' throughout data collection and analysis.

Finally, interviewing can be expensive in terms of time and funding. Resources may be required to support the researchers' or participants' involvement, for example, travel, care of participants' dependants, reimbursement for loss of earnings and refreshments. The cost of reliable technical recording equipment and transcription are not insignificant and need to be considered when making the decision to use interviews as a data collection method.

ISSUES OF VALIDITY AND RELIABILITY

The degree of reliability (the accuracy and consistency of data collection) required from an interview will vary. In a structured interview, high levels of reliability will be sought. Training and a robust schedule will ensure standardised practice between different researchers. With a more in-depth, semi- or unstructured interview, reliability is less achievable. Such an interview will be flexible and interactive in order to understand the participant's social construction and representation of the research phenomenon. However, a competent researcher with a consistent approach and well-designed schedule will be able to maximise the rigour of the results (Lincoln & Guba1985).

The validity of a study considers how 'true' the data are. The challenge is to demonstrate that the findings are an accurate account of the participant's representation of the topic, and not due to bias or inappropriate interpretation.

Data collection bias may arise in interviews because of the way the sample has been selected, how the interview is conducted or because of the researcher's influence. In order to protect against these risks, it is necessary to monitor and reflect on the following questions:

- Does the sample have any inbuilt bias, for example are some groups excluded or under-represented?
- Are the questions addressing the participant's concerns, views and experiences?
- Have the interviewees been given the opportunity to adequately present their views?
- Has the researcher led or influenced the participant's responses in any way?

Having clear and well-prepared documentation will help to address these questions, for example interview schedules and field notes.

ETHICAL ISSUES WITH INTERVIEWING

Some of the major ethical issues relating to interview-based studies are outlined here. For a more detailed discussion, see Allmark *et al.* (2009).

Consent

Chapter 11 gives details of the procedures that need to be followed to obtain informed consent. Potential interviewees should be approached with sufficient time to reflect on the implications of participation, and not feel pressurised into taking part. A signature is required to indicate informed consent has been given. When this is obtained some time prior to the interview taking place, consent should be verified immediately before the actual interview.

Anonymity and confidentiality

The names and identity of participants should not be revealed as a result of the collection, analysis and reporting of the study in order to preserve their anonymity and confidentiality. It is important to ensure that first contact with participants about the study is via someone with a legitimate role and right to identify them, for example, the medical consultant or senior nurse involved in the patient's care.

There are circumstances when complete anonymity is not possible to guarantee, for example, when reporting the age, gender and medical condition/role that would identify a person. This is a real risk in smaller interview-based studies recruiting from a limited sampling frame. Where this threat occurs, it should be pre-empted and included in the informed consent procedure. Sometimes, people are prepared to be involved despite the risk of being identified, but they should be given the chance to agree any direct references and quotes from them used in any reports or publications.

In order to protect anonymity, interviewees are sometimes referred to by number or pseudonym. Asking a person to choose their own pseudonym can help them understand the confidentiality implications of participation.

Once an interview has been transcribed, all identifiable references need to be removed from the transcript. These ought then to be stored in locked, secure storage and on password-protected computers.

Protecting participants' and researchers' rights and protecting them from harm

Ensuring interviewees' understanding of the study and its requirements is a key concern when protecting them from harm. It is important to make certain participants know what subjects will be covered, especially where these are sensitive or distressing in nature. Where necessary, support for the participant may be required and, where available, stated in the information sheet.

When explaining the study, it is important not to raise participants' expectations regarding its impact on their own care, other people's care or the development of services. People often participate in interviews where they share their views and experiences for altruistic reasons. Researchers should endeavour to be realistic in any claims that the study has the capacity to make change.

One major risk in conducting interviews is where a risk to the participant or someone else is revealed. Examples include:

- a patient revealing suicidal thoughts
- a patient or staff member describing an incident of negligence or abuse
- a patient revealing that their medical condition has deteriorated.

These challenging dilemmas should be considered on a case-by-case basis. The risk–benefit balance of reporting what the participant has disclosed or remaining silent may vary tremendously. Where possible, the risk of this should be pre-empted, and a reporting process put in place and made clear in the information sheet. For example, the situation might be discussed with a patient's doctor or nurse.

Finally, the researcher has a requirement to protect themselves. If an interview has been particularly emotional, tense or challenging, the availability of experienced, trusted supervision to facilitate reflection is invaluable. The other main risk for a researcher relates to issues of personal safety. It is standard practice for interviewers to inform an identified person of the time and location of an interview and inform them when it is over and they have left the venue. This is a particular requirement when interviewing in people's own home or unknown environments. A mobile phone and panic alarm are sometimes carried as additional means of communication if the researcher feels exceptionally threatened.

CONCLUSION

Conducting an interview involves sharing an aspect of someone's life. As such, the decision to employ interviews as a data collection method should not be taken lightly. The practical, procedural, ethical and cost implications all have to be considered. However, if these are addressed and a researcher has the required expertise and support, conducting an interview can be a vehicle to gaining a unique insight into the area of study and a privilege and pleasure to undertake.

References

Allmark P, Boote J, Chambers E, Clarke A, McDonnell A, Thompson A, Tod AM (2009) Ethical issues in the use of in-depth interviews: literature review and discussion. *Research Ethics Review* **5**(2): 43–88.

Britten N (1995) Qualitative research: qualitative interviews in research. *British Medical Journal* **311**: 251–253.

Catalani C, Minkler M (2010) Photovoice: a review of the literature in health and public health. *Health Education and Behaviour* **37**(3): 424–451.

Field PA, Morse JM (1985) *Nursing Research: the application of qualitative approaches*. London, Chapman & Hall.

Garbett R, McCormack B (2001) The experience of practice development: an exploratory telephone interview study. *Journal of Clinical Nursing* **10**: 94–102.

Henning J, Froggatt K, Payne S (2013) Spouse caregivers of people with advanced dementia in nursing homes: a longitudinal narrative study *Palliative Medicine* **27**(7): 683–691.

Laws R (2004) Current approaches to obesity management in UK primary care. *Journal of Human Nutrition and Dietetics* **17**: 183–190.

Legard R, Keegan J, Ward K (2003) In-depth interviews. In: Ritchie J, Lewis J (eds) *Qualitative Research Practice*. London, Sage, pp. 138–169.

Lincoln Y, Guba E (1985) *Naturalistic Inquiry*. London, Sage.

McDonnell A, Tod A, Bray K, Bainbridge D, Adsetts D, Walters S (2013) A before and after study assessing the impact of a new model for recognizing and responding to early signs of deterioration in an acute hospital. *Journal of Advanced Nursing* **69**(1): 41–52.

Melia KB (2000) Conducting an interview. *Nurse Researcher* **7**(4): 75–89.

Midanik LT, Greenfield TK (2003) Telephone versus in-person interviews for alcohol use: results of a 2000 National Alcohol Survey. *Drug and Alcohol Dependence* **72**: 209–214.

Murphy E, Dingwall R, Greatbatch D, Parker S, Watson P (1998) Qualitative research methods in health technology assessments: a review of the literature. *Health Technology Assessment* **2**(16): 1–274.

Patton MQ (1987) *How to Use Qualitative Methods in Evaluation*. London, Sage.

Ritchie J, Lewis J (2003) *Qualitative Research Practice: a guide for social science students and researchers.* London, Sage.

Robson C (2011) *Real World Research.* 3rd edition. Chichester, John Wiley & Sons, Ltd.

Rose GA, McCartney P, Reid DD (1977) Self-administration of a questionnaire on chest pain and intermittent claudication. *British Journal of Preventive and Social Medicine* **31**: 42–48.

Smith E (2005) Telephone interviews in healthcare research: a summary of the evidence. *Nursing Research* **12**(3): 32–42.

Tod A, Read C, Lacey A, Abbott J (2001) Overcoming barriers to uptake of services for coronary heart disease: a qualitative study. *British Medical Journal* **323**: 214–217.

Warnock C, Tod A (2014) A descriptive exploration of the experiences of patients with significant functional impairment following a recent diagnosis of metastatic spinal cord compression. *Journal of Advanced Nursing* **70**: 564–574.

Further reading

King N, Horrocks C (2010) *Interviews in Qualitative Research*. London, Sage.

CHAPTER 29

Focus Groups

Claire Goodman and Catherine Evans

Key points

- Focus groups are a useful data collection method when the aim is to clarify, explore or confirm ideas with a range of participants on a predefined set of issues.
- Group interactions are an important feature of focus groups and an integral part of the data collection process.
- It requires considerable preparation and skill to run a successful focus group; ideally, one person should act as the moderator of the group, whilst a second researcher acts as observer.
- Analysis of focus group data should ask specific questions about the group process and interaction as well as the content of the discussion.

PURPOSE OF FOCUS GROUPS

A focus group is an in-depth, open-ended group discussion that explores a specific set of issues on a predefined topic. Focus groups are used extensively as a research method in nursing research in two ways:

- To obtain the views and experiences of a selected group on an issue (see Research Examples 29.1 and 29.2)
- To use the forum of a group discussion to increase understanding about a given topic (see Research Example 29.3)

Focus groups seldom aim to produce consensus between participants and are unlikely to be the method of choice if this is the study's aim. The key premise of focus groups is that individuals in groups do not respond to questions in the same way that they do in other settings and it is the group interaction that enables participants to explore and clarify their experience and insights on a specific issue. Participants can share and discuss their knowledge and even revise their original ideas and understanding. This data collection method allows the researcher to expose inconsistency within a group as well as providing examples of conformity

The Research Process in Nursing, Seventh Edition. Edited by Kate Gerrish and Judith Lathlean.

Companion Website: www.wiley.com/go/gerrish/research

RESEARCH EXAMPLE

29.1 The Use of Focus Groups with Marginalised Groups and to Address Sensitive Topics

Culley L, Hudson N, Rapport F (2007) Using focus groups with minority ethnic communities: researching infertility in British South Asian communities. *Qualitative Health Research* **17**: 102–112.

This study set out to explore community understandings of infertility and involuntary childlessness in British South Asian communities. The study had two phases: the first explored a cross section of public attributes and perceptions surrounding infertility and provided the context and insight for the second phase that involved in-depth interviews with individuals who had experienced infertility problems. By not involving people with infertility problems in the focus groups, the researchers were able to explore the social context and stigma and ask direct questions about their views of childless couples. Groups were single sex (important for the Muslim groups and older South Asians) and involved people of similar age. There were 14 focus groups that ranged in size from 3 to 10 with a mode of 6. The involvement of focus group facilitators from the different South Asian ethnic groups represented to work as translators, group facilitators and advisors on what was said in the discussions was costly. Recruitment to the groups was labour intensive. When leading the group discussions, attempts to 'depersonalise' what was a very sensitive topic by asking about community constructions of infertility were not always successful. Participants often 'repersonalised' the issue and gave examples of personal and family experience. There was concern that this may have led to over disclosure because there were so few opportunities in these communities to discuss these issues. They also had experience of people attending the groups to seek help for their own fertility problems. This posed ethical dilemmas for the researchers on how they should respond. The researchers concluded that focus groups were a powerful and versatile tool in accessing community attitudes and allowed them to understand cultural norms and meanings. However, it was time consuming and costly, produced complex and messy data, and was further complicated because multiple languages were involved.

and agreement. Focus groups, therefore, have the potential to provide a rich source of data.

Focus groups were first developed for market research at Columbia University in the United States and used to gauge audience responses to propaganda and radio broadcasts during World War II. Twohig and Putnam (2002), in a review of studies that have used focus groups in health-care research, did not identify any studies cited by MEDLINE before 1985 but noted that it has been a widely used method in sociology, education and political science.

Focus groups are not aligned with a particular tradition of qualitative research. It is therefore important that researchers who use this method are sure that it fits with the overall research approach. As the discussion is organised *outside* the everyday experience and there is a preset focus to the interaction, there are inevitable tensions in employing focus group methods in studies that have a strong emphasis on naturalistic inquiry and immersion in the participants' lived experience. For example, the researcher would need to justify how the use of focus groups would fit with a study that is based on grounded theory or phenomenology (see Chapters 14 and 15 for more detailed consideration of this issue).

There is considerable variation in how focus groups are reported in nursing research literature and little agreement about optimum group size and numbers of groups to include within a study. There is also criticism that focus groups encourage a superficial approach to enquiry and therefore have limited value as a stand-alone data collection method.

RESEARCH EXAMPLE

29.2 The Use of Focus Groups as Part of a Mixed Method Study

Seymour JE, Almack K, Kennedy S, Froggatt K (2013) Peer education for advance care planning: volunteers' perspectives on training and community engagement activities. *Health Expectations*, **16**: 43–55.

This paper reports on an evaluation of a 3-day training programme to prepare volunteers to undertake community-based peer education for advance care planning and associated end-of-life care issues. The training programme was developed as a part of a larger community-based study exploring end-of-life concerns and educational needs among older adults and their care providers. The paper describes the 32 volunteers' perspectives on the peer education training programme, their feelings about assuming the role of volunteer peer educators and the community engagement activities with which they engaged during the year after training. The methodological framework for the study was participatory action research, and focus groups were used at the follow-up workshop, and complementary data were obtained through immediate evaluative activities during and at the end of each training day, individual interviews and a postal survey. The results from the survey were used to inform the development of an aide-memoire for four focus groups held 6 months after the end of the training. Quantitative data were analysed to provide descriptive statistics about the participants, evaluative activities and survey data were subject to content analysis, and interview and focus group data were transcribed and analysed qualitatively with the support of NVivo. Findings were presented in relation to the different stages of the evaluation process. The focus groups demonstrated how participants had developed over time and gained confidence in talking with others about advance care planning. Findings also suggested that those people who were already part of a community group or who had completed the training as a staff volunteer were more likely to report success as a peer educator. They concluded that the ability to sustain being a peer educator (as demonstrated by participation in the focus groups 6 months after training) is closely related to a social identity nurtured by group connections and membership.

CONDUCTING A FOCUS GROUP

It is a misconception to regard focus group interviews as a simple way of gathering data from multiple participants. A focus group requires the researcher to give time to preparation and have skills in facilitating group discussion. It is labour intensive and often involves two researchers, one as moderator of the group discussion and the other as observer. Consideration is given here to sampling strategy and group size, developing a topic guide and how to conduct a focus group, including managing the discussion and recording information.

Sampling strategy and group size

Major challenges in using focus groups include identifying, sampling and recruiting participants, group size and composition, and decisions on how many focus groups should be held. How individuals are recruited to groups can affect what is talked about and the dynamics of the group (Farnsworth & Boon 2011).

The identification and sampling of members of the target population are guided by the aims or research questions for the study. It can be useful to develop a topic-specific sampling strategy to encompass the diversity of people involved in the subject area (Kitzinger & Barbour 1999). For example, in order to obtain a spread of views of how minority ethnic groups understood infertility and involuntary childlessness, Culley *et al.* (2007) used a sampling strategy that included participants from four main South Asian communities and involved group facilitators fluent in their different languages (Research Example 29.1).

Focus groups undertaken with young people and children require a different approach to sampling and group composition. Gibson (2007) suggests that age

RESEARCH EXAMPLE

29.3 The Use of Focus Groups to Increase Understanding of a Given Topic

Dickinson A, Machen I, Horton K, Jain D, Maddex T, Cove J (2011) Fall prevention in the community: what older people say they need. *British Journal of Community Nursing* **16**(4): 174–180.

Little is known about the barriers and facilitators to the uptake by older people of fall prevention services. The aim of this research was to explore the views, preferences and experiences of older people in relation to fall prevention interventions. The research involved a diverse sample of older people, including those from two specific ethnic minority groups (South Asian and Chinese).

A total of 17 focus groups were conducted, facilitated by two researchers. Each focus group lasted about an hour and comprised older people ($n=122$) who were attending (or who had previously attended) a fall prevention intervention. Where possible, focus groups were held directly following group-based interventions. Participants were purposively sampled from a broad range of interventions (including falls clinics, postural stability classes, T'ai Chi classes and exercise classes). Topic guides were developed in consultation with the study steering group and incorporated issues raised by a systematic review undertaken as part of the study. Recordings of the focus groups were fully transcribed and analysed drawing on a constant comparative approach. Overall, adherence to interventions was greatly facilitated by participants experiencing a multiplicity of benefits. These included improvements in physical strength and balance, receiving advice and having a thorough assessment, as well as social and emotional benefits such as making new friends, enjoyment, improved confidence and less social isolation. Attendance was adversely affected if there were no perceived benefits or if there was an expectation that benefits would quickly be apparent. Other influences on uptake were accessibility of services, how groups were facilitated, the level of activity, language ability, lack of time and poor health. The authors concluded that a detailed understanding of what enabled older people's uptake and participation in fall prevention activities was key to the design and review of community-based programmes.

should inform how large the group is and recommends only a 1–2 year age difference in members of the group and that limited language ability and skills may mean that a focus group is not a suitable method for children under 6 years.

To gain access to the possible participants from the target population, it is often helpful to approach a stakeholder or group representative. For example, a director of nursing in a health-care organisation is a useful stakeholder to gain access to clinical nurses. Identifying participants from populations not necessarily associated with an organisation, for example, 'healthy' older people, can be assisted by approaching places they visit, such as a drop in centre and advertising the project or recruiting a pre-existing group (Seymour *et al.* 2002).

Non-random sampling techniques such as purposive and convenience sampling are normally used because the intention of the focus group is usually to increase understanding of a phenomenon, not providing evidence directly generalisable to a wider population. Moreover, a randomly selected group may not hold a shared perspective on the research topic, prohibiting meaningful group discussion (Smithson 2008). Purposive sampling is preferable when sampling participants with specific characteristics, experience or knowledge, such as older people that have experienced falls (see Research Example 29.3). If the target population is small and difficult to identify or access, convenience sampling can be helpful. When all participants within the target population would be eligible to participate, selection can be based upon interest in participating in the study and availability.

Group composition and size are both contentious issues within the focus group literature. Again, decisions are based upon the nature of the enquiry, the study design and the amount of time and funding available. Debates on group composition focus on homogeneity (similar participants) versus heterogeneity (diverse participants) and the use (or not) of pre-existing groups. Homogeneous groups segmented by, for example, a shared experience (see Research Example 29.3), language group or role (Research Examples 29.1 and 29.2) are generally preferable to ensure free discussion and enable cross-group comparisons. Differences, however, between participants in a heterogeneous group are often illuminating, and the use of pre-existing groups can enable the context to be captured within which ideas are formed and decisions made (Smithson 2008). Using pre-existing groups can also be useful in recruiting people unlikely to come forwards to participate in a focus group if they feel marginalised by society or are unwilling to participate with people they do not know. However, in groups where participants are very familiar with each other, existing group norms and hierarchies may inhibit the contributions of members (Kitzinger & Barbour 1999).

The size of a focus group varies typically from between 5 members to no more than 12. The group must be large enough to ensure diversity of perspectives and be small enough to ensure everybody has a chance to participate. Decisions on group size are informed by:

- the nature of the subject area (the more sensitive the area, the smaller the group)
- the level of group structure (the more structure, the larger the group)
- the resources available (funding for more than one group, size of room space)
- moderator expertise (the less experienced the moderator, the smaller the group)

Generally, it is advisable to invite more than the required number of group members to counter the inevitable problems of no-shows. Telephoning people who have agreed to participate a few days beforehand can reduce this problem. The focus group needs to be conducted at a convenient time in an accessible venue, possibly apart from their place of work. In practice, it is often the financial resources and time available for the study that influence venue choices.

Focus groups need more preparation and anticipation than individual interviews. On the day of the focus group, the moderator should arrive sufficiently early to signpost the location, arrange the room and have refreshments for participants. An ideal room is one that is private, large enough to accommodate the group, quiet and comfortable. If working with an observer, it is important to talk through the anticipated process and the topic guide and agree seating arrangements.

Reflection activity

Identify a research question that you are interested in answering where focus groups would be a good method to use to collection data. Identify your target population and consider how you will sample and recruit participants. What size group do you consider appropriate and why?

Structuring group discussion and developing a topic guide

The level of group structure depends upon the intention of the focus group. A structured group using a topic guide is preferable when the research questions are clear, for example, using focus groups to inform further research (see Research Example 29.1). A less structured group framed around one or two topic areas is useful in exploratory research when little is known about the area of study (see Research Example 29.3). Both approaches have advantages and disadvantages. The structured approach ensures consistency across groups enabling comparisons to be made between groups, but a narrow set of questions may limit the discussion and inhibit contributions on related issues. Less structure often creates a livelier group discussion. A compromise between the two approaches may also be used. Morgan (1997) describes this as a 'funnel-based' approach in which

> 'each group begins with a less structured approach that emphasizes free discussion and then moves toward a more structured discussion of specific questions' (Morgan 1997: 41)

The research aims and the literature should inform the development of the topic guide. The intention of the guide is to create a natural progression through the topic areas and stimulate group discussion without influencing the responses. A structured guide uses at most five to six questions. A less structured approach is to organise the guide around two or three broad discussion topics, loosely phrased as questions, like 'We are interested in ….?', 'What can you tell us about this area?' (Morgan 1997). In both instances, the questions are ordered to move from general to specific and non-sensitive to more sensitive, the aim being to enable all group members to participate. The topic area should be familiar to all, not be intimidating or require personal exposure. More sensitive or probing questions come nearer the middle of the interview. This provides participants with time to feel safe to speak within the group. Open-ended questions prefixed by either how, what, where or why allow participants freedom to respond. Direct questions such as 'why?' can be experienced as confrontational and provoke defensive responses in the group.

Managing the discussion

Sufficient time should be allowed to greet and seat participants. Begin the session by welcoming participants, introducing yourself and the observer and clarifying the purpose of the session and the anticipated finish time. Ensure participants understand how the discussion will be recorded, who has access to these recordings and how confidentiality will be maintained. Ask if participants have any questions about the group format and agree ground rules. Ground rules are intended to facilitate group discussion, not confine it. The agreed rules should be concise, few in number and displayed for participants (e.g. on flip chart). They may state:

- that issues discussed in the group are confidential to the participants and the researchers
- that everyone can expect to be listened to and that their views should be respected
- that only one person can speak at a time.

Introductions to the topic should be brief and clear, and instructions kept to a minimum. This helps participants to understand the focus of the session, without directing their thinking and emphasises that the ownership of the group discussion belongs to both the participants and the moderator. Participant introductions create an opportunity for all to speak and provide identification markers to differentiate participants for the observer and when transcribing the audio recording. Plan for latecomers and ensure that participants are informed prior to the interview whether or not they will be able to take part if they arrive after the indicated start time.

Moderators should promote debate by asking open questions and probing for more detail on points of interest, reflecting a comment made to confirm understanding and summarising points to check that all areas have been covered, particularly before changing a topic. Comments such as 'that's interesting, can you say more?' or 'does anyone else have a comment?' can encourage reflection and interaction. These techniques reinforce for participants that the points they make are valued and encourage participation in the discussion. The discussion should include all areas in the topic guide, particularly if conducting several focus groups. Incomplete data sets restrict comparative analysis between groups and may compromise the aims of the study.

Moderators need to encourage participation by inviting group members to comment on an individual's views, especially if someone is dominating the discussion. Avoid expressing personal opinions or correcting participants' knowledge. If there is something that requires challenging or correcting, for example, if someone states something that is untrue, then this can be tactfully addressed at the end as part of the summing up.

Group exercises may be used within the session to explore understanding about a particular issue or to indicate preferences. Such exercises encourage participants to focus on each other rather than the

Reflection activity

Careful planning of a focus group will help ensure its success. What factors do you need to consider when planning a focus group?

moderator. For young people and children, Gibson (2007) suggests that the inclusion of activities and exercises to maintain interest and concentration as well as facilitate a sense of working together can help stimulate discussion and responses to research questions.

Timekeeping is essential and shows respect for participants' time. Leave 5–10 min to round up the group discussion. This provides an opportunity for participants to offer further comments and reflect on their experience of participating in the group.

Recording information

Group interactions are the crucial feature of focus groups and mark them as different from individual interviews. Digital recording, video camera and an observer can be used alone or in combination to record the group interaction. Ideally, transcribed recording is preferable, with an observer and/or videotaping. Videotapings can be poor at recording speech and are normally used in combination with audio recording. An observer is useful for recording, for example, the group's seating arrangement and non-verbal cues of supportive or aggressive behaviour. An observation sheet with headings for particular areas of interest can help to structure the observations.

Recording equipment should be reliable and have a high-quality microphone for recording groups, rather than individuals. The quality of the digital recording directly influences the precision of the transcribing and the consequent validity of the transcript analysis. Ensure sound files are labelled with an identification number, date and time, to prevent recording over data and as a reference point for transcribing.

ONLINE FOCUS GROUPS

Internet-based data collection is receiving increasing attention in health science research. It can be a good way of accessing seldom heard (often referred to as hard to reach) groups, and for tackling subjects that are sensitive. It also facilitates dialogue between participants who may not otherwise have encountered each other and for the ill, disabled, housebound respondents, and it has obvious advantages for people who are socially or geographically isolated. The visual anonymity provided by online focus groups may mean that participants feel more comfortable expressing their views and thus achieve a greater equality of participation.

When running an online focus group, there are two choices: to do it in real time (synchronous) when the moderator and participants are all logged in at the same time, or when messages are posted in response to the moderator and participants respond at different times (asynchronous) (Smithson 2008). A particular feature in asynchronous group discussions is that it enables participants to take time in answering questions, allowing more time to reflect. As well as cost benefits, responses can be transferred directly in a database where they are immediately accessible for analysis, without the need for transcription (Tates *et al.* 2009).

It can be difficult for the moderator to follow conversation threads and responses if they are happening simultaneously, and also, participants may be less inclined to give full responses, only indicating agreement or disagreement to statements made.

DATA ANALYSIS

The principles and process of analysis for focus group data are very similar to those applied to qualitative data obtained from individual interviews. When undertaking analysis of a focus group discussion, it is important to be clear about the purpose of the analysis and whether it is the group discussion as a whole or the range of contributions to that discussion that is of interest. The research question and the rationale for using focus groups guide the analysis and inform how the data are organised and read.

It is seldom practical to ask focus group participants to check the validity of transcripts or preliminary analysis. It is therefore useful to summarise at the end of the group what the moderator believes to be the main issues to emerge from the discussion for confirmation or clarification by the group. This not only helps understanding but also represents the first stage in analysis where tentative themes can be identified and subsequently tested within the detailed analysis of the group transcripts. At the end of the focus group, it is also good practice for the group's moderator to debrief with the observer to record initial impressions of how the group went and to identify issues that may directly affect the analysis. Factors such as dominance of the discussion by particular individuals, impressions of how engaged participants were with the issues raised and whether non-participation in the group indicated disagreement or affirmation with what was being said should be noted. These first impressions are useful as memoranda that can subsequently inform analysis.

In contrast to analysis of individual interviews, an important part of the analytic process is identifying areas of agreement and controversy and how views are modified or reinforced during the group discussion. When coding data, it is helpful to think about the data as a group process. It is therefore sensible to organise the data to reflect how the discussion progressed. Most groups will take some time to establish a rapport, and there will be some issues and questions that generate more interest and contributions than others. Coding the data into narrative units can be helpful as there will be some major issues identified within the group discussion that either generate the most contributions or the strongest responses. This means that individual responses to a particular issue or question, the asides, challenges and elaborations that occur within the group are coded together and in relation to each other. Software that supports qualitative analysis is invaluable as it can track individual contributions as well as interactions and responses and allows interrogation of the data in different ways. Furthermore, by tracing the development and sequence of statements of the discussion on an issue, it is possible to judge which ideas participants offered as tentative thoughts at the beginning of a focus group became, by the end of the group, established views.

The approach to analysis of focus group data is often descriptive with little attention given to the interaction that occurred within groups. Analysis should consider if certain statements provoked the most emotion, reaction or conflict, if there were discernible alliances that emerged within the group or particular interests that were emphasised over others. Redwood *et al.* (2012) in a study that based data collection within a group art activity with South Asian women noted that women rarely spoke more than a sentence or two in one turn, but what emerged from these interactive data sequences were 'small stories'. Often, it is these personal narratives nested within the discussion that can provide valuable insights about individuals' experiences that would otherwise not have been heard. However, if analysis of a focus group discussion reveals that the priority of participants is to *only* tell their life accounts and not engage in interactive discussion, then it is worth considering if the focus group format was the most appropriate approach.

The use of descriptive statistics to summarise the frequency with which issues were raised and the amount of time spent discussing an issue can be helpful, particularly when comparing responses between different focus groups. When marked differences are identified between groups, this should prompt another look at what it was about these groups, their membership or setting, that could explain the variation. However, there should be considerable caution in suggesting that a particular subject or issue was more important or significant because it was raised more frequently than something else. Counting statements made on particular topics will generate a list of what participants said, but attributing meaning to this can be problematic unless the analysis also accounts for how people interacted within the group.

ISSUES OF VALIDITY AND RELIABILITY

Validity is the extent to which a procedure actually measures what it proposes to measure. Typically, focus groups have high face validity as a credible method that can directly capture the views of participants in response to the study focus. Threats to face validity are those that threaten the accuracy of the participants' views on the topic areas of interest. These can include research questions that are unsuitable for a focus group because they are concerned with the narrative on individual experience. Idiosyncratic and opportunistic recruitment from the population of interest can make it difficult to interpret findings. A lack of transparency in how the group discussion was organised, the prompts used, the amount of direction given to the group by the moderator and approaches to analysis can also threaten the confidence with which the results from focus group research can be interpreted.

Reliability concerns the degree of consistency in observing the area of interest over time. For focus groups, reliability is most relevant as it relates to the consistency in the data gathered within each respective group. Threats to consistency across groups include:

- the structure and delivery of the topic guide
- the impact of moderator bias
- differences between the groups' membership, for example, regarding gender
- the interview environment
- accuracy in transcription and analysis

However, in groups where the emphasis is on discovery, the diversity of the participants may enhance the breadth of understanding.

ADVANTAGES OF FOCUS GROUPS

Whereas focus groups can appear to be a quick and flexible method of data collection, they are not an inexpensive or time-saving method (see Research Example 29.1). Considerable time is required to recruit participants, set up the groups, transcribe and analyse the data generated. There are, however, some clear advantages that focus group methods have over other data collection methods. In the early stages of a study, the discussion and data generated by a focus group can identify complex problems and areas that need further exploration and clarification. A group discussion held at the end of the study provides the opportunity for participants to respond to the findings and offer explanations or alternative interpretations. The exploratory and illuminatory function of focus groups can thus extend and challenge how researchers define their research questions and report their findings. Used in conjunction with other methods such as interviews and observation, focus group data can confirm, extend and enrich understanding and provide alternative narratives of events and beliefs.

Focus groups are frequently used when the opinions of laypeople are sought. The method does not require participants to be able to read and write, and people can feel safe within a group. If facilitated well, participants can express their views in relation to the opinions and experiences of others without feeling pressure to respond all the time. It is participant driven and enables the language, priorities and attitudes of a group to be expressed. It is one of the few data collection methods that allow people to modify their initial thoughts and ideas as part of the data gathering process. Paradoxically, focus groups can be a good way of researching topics that are taboo or controversial when participants who hold an experience in common can give each other permission to discuss. For example, focus groups may be used to enable people who are HIV positive to discuss freely their attitudes to sexual health and the issues they encounter as a result of their health status.

The synergy generated from a group discussion often enables participants to consider the topic with more enthusiasm than an individual interview can achieve. However, questions examining feelings or requiring personal reflection may only be suited to a focus group approach when participants have self-selected or they know each other and are comfortable with that level of public self-disclosure such questions require. It is the level of engagement expressed within a group, the range of participation and the ability to develop the discussion around certain issues that are often a good measure of how successful a focus group has been.

LIMITATIONS OF FOCUS GROUPS

Focus groups can have high credibility and face validity, but equally they can be susceptible to researcher manipulation and bias. The limitations of the method are the reliance on the skill of the group moderator, the risk of individual participants dominating discussion and excluding the contributions of others, and the possibility that the structure and format of focus groups excludes certain groups from participation.

Focus group facilitation is difficult. The novice researcher should take the opportunity to observe some focus groups before taking on the moderator role, consider training on group dynamics and talk through with an experienced colleague how they will lead the group. The moderator has to maintain a balance between encouraging discussion and participation and being careful not to bias responses by giving preference to speakers whose views are perceived as the most 'interesting'. The moderator also needs the confidence to be able to refocus the group if participants break into two or three separate discussions at the same time and intervene if the discussion threatens to become destructive or lead to conflict.

Most authors writing on the subject of focus groups raise the spectre of the dominant group member as a major limitation of the method. Participants who are very assertive in their views can discourage participation from those who disagree or who are less certain in their opinions. Where participants have different levels or authority or education, this too can affect willingness to participate. Nevertheless, if the focus group is seen as an opportunity to capture how a group expresses their opinions and if certain people can make statements that are unchallenged and allowed to dominate, then the analysis must capture this. Reed and Payton (1997) argue that if one considers focus groups as 'displays of group perspectives', then *how* groups negotiate and develop their views can be as revealing as what is said.

Focus groups can discriminate against an individual's ability to participate. People who have different communication disabilities such as deafness, partial paralysis affecting speech and dementia may be able to participate in interviews but struggle in a focus group,. although a review of the evidence of people with dementia's participation in research (van Baalen *et al.* 2011) suggested that individuals with early-stage dementia are able to participate in focus groups. The authors provided practical guidelines for focus groups with this population based on the studies reviewed. Most focus groups also require people to be able to communicate in the language of the researcher that may exclude some people from minority ethnic groups who do not share a common language. It is possible to involve translators, although this can make the discussion more stilted and meanings harder to interpret. Halcomb *et al.* (2007), in a review of studies that had used focus groups with linguistically diverse groups, found that focus groups are particularly useful for studies on service provision and community needs for minority and multicultural groups.

The location of focus groups may also affect the ability to participate and exclude some potential participants. For example, where a focus group is held may favour participation by people who have easy access to transport or live close to the proposed venue.

Reflection activity

Refer back to the earlier reflection activity where you identified a research question. What are the advantages and disadvantages of using focus groups in your proposed study?

ETHICAL ISSUES

The particular ethical issues that arise within focus group research are the maintenance of confidentiality, consent, the management of disclosure and maintaining the respect and feelings of self-worth of each participant. It is important that participants agree that the discussions held within the group are confidential and not shared outside the group. The moderator needs to ensure that each participant agrees to this, especially in situations where the group members know each other.

The discussion format of a focus group can mean that people forget that the reason they are meeting is to participate in a research project. Frequently, discussion will prompt disclosures that may not have been made within the context of an interview. Although this can interrupt the flow of the conversation, it is the moderator's responsibility to remind group members how the discussion will be used and why.

Consent is more problematic; apart from staying silent, it is very difficult for an individual within a group to withdraw their consent to participate. The right to withdraw consent should be discussed prior to the focus group, and although silence can be a useful option, it may be wrongly interpreted as a form of assent to what others are saying. Researchers should consider offering participants the opportunity to withdraw consent after the group has met if they believe that the discussion did not reflect their views or it was a process they no longer wanted to be associated with. This would mean their contributions could not be reported.

The process of group participation can lead to unanticipated consequences. It can raise consciousness, expose underlying conflicts and falsely create an expectation that something will be done about the issues raised. Sometimes distinctions between focus groups and therapy groups can become blurred especially if participants share painful personal experiences. It requires skilled facilitation to recognise if someone is becoming distressed and either change the subject or recognise that a break is needed to allow people to leave the group or recover.

Although these kind of data are very rich, it is exploitative if people expose their feelings and reveal their needs, but there is then no means of offering further support. It is therefore important to have mechanisms in place for individuals to revisit the issues raised and if necessary to discuss them further. As part of this process, the moderator also needs to consider their role within the group discussion, ensuring that it is understood by participants, and consider the extent to which they are prepared to disclose their own views.

Finally, the moderator has a responsibility to ensure that participants do not feel devalued by their experience in the group. This can happen when opinions that are expressed are ridiculed or strongly opposed by other group members. In these situations, the moderator should reinforce the right of each person to have an opinion and for it to be listened to, even if people are not in agreement. If this is not possible, then the moderator should change the focus of the group's discussion or bring it to a close.

Reflection activity

Identify the ethical issues associated with using focus groups to answer the research question you have identified earlier. What steps could you take to address these ethical issues?

CONCLUSION

This chapter has provided an overview of the purpose and usefulness of focus groups for nursing research. It has emphasised that this method of data collection requires careful preparation and skill in leading and managing group discussion. The method is particularly useful when researchers wish to understand and clarify thinking on a topic from a group perspective. The need to be transparent about the purpose and process of the focus group, and sensitive to the particular ethical challenges this method poses, has been emphasised throughout. In conclusion, focus groups are a useful and versatile data collection method that can be used within a wide range of study settings and with diverse groups to great effect.

References

Culley L, Hudson N, Rapport F (2007) Using focus groups with minority ethnic communities: researching infertility in British South Asian Communities. *Qualitative Health Research* **17**: 102–112.

Dickinson A, Machen I, Horton K, Jain D, Maddex T, Cove J (2011) Fall prevention in the community: what older people say they need. *British Journal of Community Nursing* **16**(4): 174–180.

Farnsworth J, Boon B (2011) Analysing group dynamics within the focus group. *Qualitative Research* **10**(5): 605–624.

Gibson F (2007) Conducting focus groups with children and young people: strategies for success. *Journal of Research in Nursing* **12**: 473–483.

Halcomb EJ, Gholizadeh L, DiGiacomo M, Phillips J, Davidson P (2007) Considerations in undertaking focus group research with culturally and linguistically diverse groups. *Journal of Clinical Nursing* **16**: 1000–1011.

Kitzinger J, Barbour RS (1999) Introduction: the challenge and promise of focus groups. In: Barbour RS, Kitzinger J (eds) *Developing Focus Group Research: politics, theory and practice* London, Sage, pp 1–20.

Morgan DL (1997) *Focus Groups as Qualitative Research.* 2nd edition, London, Sage.

Redwood S, Gale NK, Greenfield S (2012) 'You give us rangoli, we give you talk': using an art-based activity to elicit data from a seldom heard group. *BMC Medical Research Methodology* **12**: 7. DOI: 10.1186/1471-2288-12-7.

Reed J, Payton V (1997) Focus groups: issues of analysis and interpretation. *Journal of Advanced Nursing* **26**: 765–771.

Seymour J, Bellamy G, Gott M, Ahmedzai SH, Clark D (2002) Using focus groups to explore older people's attitudes to end of life care. *Ageing and Society* **22**(4): 517–526.

Seymour JE, Almack K, Kennedy S, Froggatt K (2013) Peer education for advance care planning: volunteers' perspectives on training and community engagement activities. *Health Expectations*, **16**: 43–55.

Smithson J (2008) Focus Groups. In: Alasuutari P, Bickman L, Brannen J (eds) *The Sage Handbook of Social Research Methods.* London, Sage, pp 357–370.

Tates K, Zwaanswijk M, Otten R, van Dulmen S, Hoogerbrugge PM, Kamps WA, Bensing JM (2009) Online focus groups as a tool to collect data in hard-to-include populations: examples from paediatric oncology. *BMC Medical Research Methodology* **9**: 15. DOI: 10.1186/1471-2288-9-15.

Twohig PL, Putnam W (2002) Group interviews in primary care research: advancing the state of the art of ritualised research. *Family Practice* **19**: 278–284.

van Baalen A, Vingerhoets AJJM, Sixma HJ, de Lange J (2011) How to evaluate quality of care from the perspective of people with dementia: an overview of the literature. *Dementia* **10**(1): 112–137.

Further reading

Barbour R (2008) *Doing Focus Groups* (qualitative research kit). 3rd edition. London, Sage.

Gibbs A (1997) Focus Groups, *Social Research Update*, Issue 19, University of Surrey, Guilford. Available at http://sru.soc.surrey.ac.uk/SRU19.html (accessed 31 August 2014).

Smithson J (2008) Focus Groups. In: Alasuutari P, Bickman L, Brannen J (eds) *The Sage Handbook of Social Research Methods.* London, Sage, pp 357–370.

CHAPTER 30

Questionnaire Design

Martyn Jones and Janice Rattray

Key points

- Questionnaires are a quick, relatively inexpensive method of gathering standardised information that is convenient for both participant and researcher.
- It is important to understand the process of questionnaire design, both for the design of own questionnaires and the appropriate use of existing measures.
- Establishing the reliability and validity of a measure is important in using and adapting previously validated questionnaires, particularly when constructing shortened scales.
- Developing a new measure is a lengthy process, with key theoretical and psychometric considerations for item generation, scale construction and response format.
- Pilot testing of a new questionnaire is likely to influence the quality of data returned and response rates.

INTRODUCTION

This chapter considers methodological issues involved in the design and administration of questionnaires. It will:

- examine the strengths and limitations of questionnaires to gather self-report data
- introduce and critique basic psychometric evaluation methods for evaluating the worth of established questionnaires
- identify methods for developing a new questionnaire

Establishing the worth of an existing questionnaire or developing new measures of sufficient methodological rigour is of great importance. Understanding the process of questionnaire design is essential in allowing the researcher to evaluate whether a questionnaire is of sufficient quality for use in a study. It is important that nurses understand the theoretical issues associated with questionnaire design, so that they can interpret study findings and generate and validate their own questionnaires.

Questionnaires enable us to collect data in a standardised manner and to make inferences to a wider population when those data are obtained from

The Research Process in Nursing, Seventh Edition. Edited by Kate Gerrish and Judith Lathlean.

Companion Website: www.wiley.com/go/gerrish/research

an appropriate sample of that population. Standardised questionnaires have undergone rigorous psychometric analysis to demonstrate their reliability and validity, and wherever possible, these should be used. Where this is not possible, the researcher may have to design their own measure.

Questionnaires allow for the collection of self-report data that would be difficult to gather in any other manner (Polit & Beck 2014) and have led to an increase in understanding of health and well-being, including patient experiences and outcomes.

PURPOSE OF QUESTIONNAIRES

Nurse researchers use questionnaires to measure knowledge (Furze *et al.* 2003), attitudes (Ruzafa-Martinez *et al.* 2011), emotion (Zigmond & Snaith 1983), cognition (Moss-Morris *et al.* 2002) and health behaviour (Conner & Sparks 2005). This approach captures the self-reported observations of the individual and is commonly used to measure patient perceptions of their health and well-being (see Box 30.1 for examples). The main benefits are that questionnaires are usually relatively quick to complete, inexpensive to produce and easy to analyse (Bowling 2009). Standardised questionnaires allow data to be gathered at different levels of specificity. For example, data on quality of life might be gathered using a generic measure such as the Short-Form 36 (Ware & Sherbourne 1992) or using a health-specific measure such as the Cardiovascular Limitations and Symptoms Profile (Devlen *et al.* 1989). Questionnaires may also inform a sampling strategy to recruit participants for individual interviews or focus groups (Barbour 2008).

Reflection activity

Consider the research question: In general medical and surgical wards in one hospital, does monthly clinical supervision improve staff well-being?

In order to demonstrate whether or not clinical supervision improves staff well-being, you will need to compare nurses who receive monthly supervision with those who do not. How could you design a questionnaire-based study to answer this question? How would you plan to measure staff well-being?

Box 30.1 Examples of what questionnaires can measure

Area	Questionnaire
Knowledge	The York Angina Beliefs Questionnaire (Furze *et al.* 2003)
Attitude/beliefs/ intention	Operationalising the Theory of Planned Behaviour (Conner & Sparks 2005) Developing a questionnaire to measure nurses' attitudes towards older people (Ruzafa-Martinez *et al.* 2011)
Cognition	The Revised Illness Perception Questionnaire (Moss-Morris *et al.* 2002)
Emotion/mood	Hospital Anxiety and Depression Scale (Zigmond & Snaith 1983)
Health status	Short-Form 36 (Ware & Sherbourne 1992)
Quality of life	EQ-5D (EuroQoL Group 1990)
Behaviour	Functional Limitations Profile (FLP) (Patrick & Peach 1989)

USING AND ADAPTING VALIDATED QUESTIONNAIRES

There are several challenges associated with the use of existing questionnaires. It is important to appraise questionnaires to determine their suitability. The researcher must consider a number of questions to inform their choice (see Box 30.2). The process of demonstrating the reliability and validity of a questionnaire is not easily accomplished. Wherever possible, researchers should use existing questionnaires with established reliability and validity.

Box 30.2 Key questions in choosing a questionnaire

Key questions	
Will the questionnaire provide data to answer the research questions?	When evaluating findings from a questionnaire study or when deciding whether a questionnaire should be used, the research questions should be revisited to ensure that this is an appropriate approach.
Is there a standardised questionnaire with demonstrated reliability and validity that can be used?	Using an established standardised questionnaire is preferable to developing one from scratch. Findings can be benchmarked with other respondent groups that may allow comparisons with population norms for example, Short-Form 36 (Ware & Sherbourne 1992).
If so, how were reliability and validity established?	Reliability and validity of a standardised questionnaire must be established by the developers. It is advisable to access original papers to review this. If the questionnaire has been used by other researchers, they too should present reliability and validity data.
How widely used is the questionnaire?	If a questionnaire has been widely used, it is likely to have good psychometric properties. For example, the Hospital Anxiety and Depression Scale (Zigmond & Snaith 1983) has been used in different patient populations internationally and continues to be valid and reliable. However, this is not always the case, and evidence of good psychometric properties should always be established.
Is the questionnaire responsive to change over time, and are there ceiling and floor effects?	In a longitudinal study that seeks to identify change over time, responsiveness of a questionnaire is important so that small changes can be detected. Ceiling effects mean that continued improvement can not be detected and floor effects that continued deterioration cannot be detected. Such effects limit the usefulness of many measures.
Is the questionnaire appropriate for the proposed participants?	It may be tempting to use a standardised questionnaire on a different group other than the one the questionnaire was designed for. This may be possible but further psychometric evaluation of its performance will be required.
If not, can I adapt an existing questionnaire or do I need to develop my own?	In the absence of a suitable standardised measure, this may be the only option. Developing a questionnaire is a rigorous process and needs to be planned in a well-considered, systematic manner.

RELIABILITY

Reliability refers to the repeatability of a questionnaire, that is, that it will measure what it is supposed to measure in a consistent manner. This can be demonstrated statistically in a number of ways: test–retest, inter-rater and internal consistency (Polit & Beck 2014).

Test–retest reliability refers to consistency over time, that is, will a questionnaire yield the same results in the same situation when administered twice over a short period of time such as days or a week (Polgar & Thomas 2011)? Statistical tests that can demonstrate this include Cohen's kappa coefficient and Pearson's correlation (Bowling & Ebrahim 2005). A correlation coefficient exceeding 0.8 indicates good test–retest reliability (Polgar & Thomas 2011). Test–retest reliability is particularly important if the questionnaire is to be used to assess change over time.

Inter-rater reliability is used to establish the degree of agreement between two or more raters or interviewers. The kappa statistic or correlational analysis quantifies this (Bowling & Ebrahim 2005).

Internal consistency reflects how well items are related to each other, that is, do scale items measure the same concept or construct? Cronbach's alpha (α) statistic calculates average inter-item correlations (Bowling & Ebrahim 2005). A questionnaire is judged to have good internal consistency when α exceeds 0.70 (Macnee & McCabe 2008). Cronbach's alpha statistic can be reported for the whole questionnaire or separately for each domain or subscale.

As an alternative to Cronbach's alpha statistic, item–total correlations can be used. This provides additional information about how each item is related to the total score from the questionnaire or domain and can be used to identify items that either do not relate to the construct the questionnaire is measuring or those that are too similar. However, this score can be biased if sample sizes are small. Calculating corrected item–total correlation is recommended where the item score is removed from the total score prior to the correlation. Kline (1993) recommends removing any questionnaire item with a corrected item–total correlation of <0.3. High inter-item correlations (>0.8) suggest that these are repetitions and the removal of the duplicate is indicated (Kline 1993).

VALIDITY

Validity refers to whether the questionnaire measures what it is supposed to measure and if it measures it correctly and accurately. There are different types of validity.

Face validity is a subjective assessment that the items in a scale appear to be relevant, clear and unambiguous.

Content validity is assessed by asking experts to judge whether questionnaire items fully represent the concept or construct to be measured. This relatively weak form of validity is a useful starting point.

Criterion validity establishes the relationship of a questionnaire with an established 'gold standard' measure. Concurrent and predictive validity are two types of criterion validity.

Concurrent validity examines the relationship of a variable that respondents are known to differ on (Bryman & Cramer 2011). For example, students vary in their levels of course attendance and may be absent for reasons other than illness. Does a measure of course satisfaction relate to such absence, or not? If not, the measure of course satisfaction may be suspect.

Predictive validity examines the utility of a questionnaire in predicting cross-sectional associations or a criterion variable measured at a point in the future (Bowling 2005).

Construct validity relates to how well the items in the questionnaire represent the underlying conceptual structure. For example, does a measure of disease-specific quality of life capture the domains theorised to exist? Factor analysis is a statistical technique that can be used to determine the constructs or domains within the questionnaire and can contribute to establishing construct validity. Related to this, ***convergent validity*** is demonstrated when the questionnaire correlates with a related measure and does not correlate with a dissimilar measure *(**discriminant validity**)* (Bowling 2005).

The cultural and temporal relevance of the measure must also be considered when deciding whether to use an existing questionnaire. Making use of measures derived in other cultures and developed in the past is not without difficulty. For example, the Hospital Anxiety and Depression Scale (HADS) (Zigmond & Snaith 1983) was developed in United

States in the early 1980s for use in non-psychiatric patients. Is this measure appropriate for use in UK research settings? Several studies have suggested that this is the case. The reliability of the HADS has been established in the United Kingdom (Crawford *et al.* 2001). Other studies have established its use in long term conditions (Zetta *et al.* 2011). However, there may be some caveats in its use in particular patient groups. For example, the HADS contains items that may relate to physical abilities of the person as well as depression, for example, 'I feel as if I am slowing down' (Martin & Thompson 2000). This makes it important to assess psychometric properties when a questionnaire is used in settings other than those where validity has already been demonstrated. The adaptation of measures for use in other language groups is also likely to require translation and back translation strategies and re-establishment of the measures' psychometric qualities (Al-lela *et al.* 2011).

As a general rule of thumb, if a questionnaire requires amendment for use in a particular sample, the researcher should demonstrate the reliability and validity of the revised questionnaire (Rattray & Jones 2007). Furthermore, it is good practice to present results from an established standardised questionnaire by detailing the reliability, for example, Cronbach's alpha, or validity of the measure.

DEVELOPING A QUESTIONNAIRE

From deciding to develop a questionnaire to producing the final standardised measure can be a lengthy process. Research Examples 30.1, 30.2 and 30.3 provide examples of researchers who have undertaken a rigorous process of developing and testing new questionnaires in different fields of enquiry. There are several pitfalls to avoid including how to

RESEARCH EXAMPLE

30.1 A Questionnaire Examining Evidence-Based Practice in Nurses

Arvidsson S, Bergman S, Arvidsson B, Fridlund B, Tingstrom P (2012) Psychometric properties of the Swedish Rheumatic Disease Empowerment Scale. *Musculoskeletal Care* **10**: 101–109.

This paper reports on the development and psychometric evaluation of a Swedish Rheumatic Disease Empowerment Scale and examines the construct validity, internal consistency reliability, inter-item correlations and discriminant validity. The 23-item measure was adapted from an existing Swedish Diabetes Empowerment Scale and used a 5-point Likert scale (strongly disagree (1) to strongly agree (5)). The measure was developed in two stages, with the item development consisting of a replacement of diabetes-related terms by those with a more rheumatic disease focus. A test of the face validity of the measures with 58 patients with rheumatic disease reviewed the relevance, clarity and readability of the items. Exploratory factor analysis, using principal component analysis with varimax rotation, tested the construct validity of the measure. In total, 260 patients were surveyed and 5 factors were established. Floor and ceiling effects were examined. Cronbach's alphas ranged from 0.59 to 0.91 for the five factors including 'goal achievement', 'self-knowledge', 'managing stress', 'assessing dissatisfaction and readiness to change' and 'support for caring'. Discriminant validity was established with those patients reporting better self-rated health (a single item, perceived health, from the SF-36) also scoring significantly more highly on three empowerment scales. A similar but non-significant trend was found for the two further factors. The authors concluded that this measure showed acceptable psychometric qualities but recognised the need to establish the test–retest reliability of the newly developed questionnaire. This robust, well-developed measure has the potential to evaluate the effects of a patient education programme.

RESEARCH EXAMPLE

30.2 A Questionnaire Examining Children's Views of the Quality of Hospital Care

Frank C, Asp M, Fridlund B, Baigi A (2010) Questionnaire for patient participation in emergency departments. *Journal of Advanced Nursing* **67**(3): 643–651.

This paper reports the three phases of development of the questionnaire for patient participation in emergency departments (PPED). In phase 1 (item generation), previous qualitative work led to the development of items in three areas of practice by three nurses and two patients. A 4-point Likert scale was used (1 strongly disagree to 4 strongly agree). In phase 2 (content validity), the PPED was examined for face validity (assessed by three nurses and three patients). Cognitive testing using think-aloud techniques led to adjustment of 42 items. Exploratory factor analysis with varimax rotation was used in phase 3; testing reported from 356 patients recently cared for in the emergency department to examine construct validity, criterion-related validity and reliability (Cronbach and test–retest) of the PPED. This resulted in a 17-item four-factor solution: 'fight for participation', 'requirement for participation', 'mutual participation' and 'participation in getting basic needs satisfied'. Cronbach's alpha (0.63–0.84) and test–retest reliability (0.59–0.93) were acceptable. Criterion-related validity was also acceptable, revealing moderate correlations between factor scores on the PPED with five items from a well-established, validated QPP instrument (Wilde & Larsson 2002). This measure was judged to have acceptable reliability and validity to enable its use in the routine evaluation of PPED, producing data for use by a wide range of healthcare professionals.

RESEARCH EXAMPLE

30.3 A Questionnaire Regarding Patient Involvement in Myocardial Infarction Care

Brunt D, Rask M (2012) A suggested revision of the Community Oriented Program Environmental Scale (COPES) for measuring the psychosocial environment of supported housing facilities for person with psychiatric difficulties. *Issues in Mental Health Nursing* **33**: 24–31.

This paper reports on the development of a revised 36-item short version of the COPES, examining the construct validity and reliability of the emergent structure using item analysis and factor analysis (using principal component analysis and varimax rotation). The study examines the relevance and usability of the instrument in people with psychiatric disabilities and tested the hypothesised factor structure of the original scale. A short-scale version was required to reduce the burden of the original questionnaire, which comprised 3 higher-order domains and 10 subscales. Sixty-seven residents and 154 caregivers completed the short-scale version (the first 4 items from each of the 10 subscales, i.e. those with the highest corrected item total correlation scores). A Likert scale was used with four options, 'not at all' (1) to 'a very high degree' (4). Results from both the resident and staff datasets are presented. In the resident reports, a 6-factor solution was revealed, accounting for 66.8% of the variance, but only two of the subscales reached acceptable levels of reliability (Cronbach's alpha). In the staff data set, 6 factors explained 53% of the total variance; however, only a single subscale was reliable. The authors suggest an amended simplified factor structure, but conclude that the established subscale structure of the shortened COPES was not sufficiently reliable for use in this setting. This study revealed the difficulties of amending measures for use in mental health settings, and showed that resident accounts were more reliable than staff perceptions.

avoid bias and error, including non-responder, acquiescent response bias and measurement error.

Non-responder bias occurs when those who do not consent to take part in the study differ from those who do. For example, the non-responder group might be younger than those who consent, or there may be gender differences. This may present difficulties in making generalisations from findings. Optimising recruitment is one way to avoid this.

Acquiescent response bias is the tendency for respondents to agree with a statement or respond in the same way to all items. This may be avoided by including both positively and negatively worded items.

Measurement error may be reduced by establishing reliability and validity of the measure.

Developing items

When developing a questionnaire, items or questions are generated that require responses to a series of questions or statements. The responses are generally converted into numerical form, summed and statistically analysed. Care must be taken in developing and piloting the items to ensure they reflect the key concepts identified in the research questions. The researcher can use different sources to develop items and ensure face and content validity. Reviewing the literature will be helpful, and consulting with experts may generate relevant items (Bowling & Ebrahim 2005). There are compelling reasons for engaging potential respondents in developing items. They can prevent the inclusion of unnecessary items or identify items that may be sensitive or controversial.

It is at this stage that the proposed domain or factor structured should be proposed (Ferguson & Cox 1993). It is not common to develop a questionnaire that relies upon a response to a single item, and multi-item scales are generally used in preference to avoid bias and misinterpretation and to reduce measurement error (Bowling 2005). For example, the Student Nurse Stress Index (Jones & Johnston 1999) comprises 22 items representing 4 subscales. However, single items may have some advantage and are used on occasion to assess general perceptions of health status (Bowling 2005). Single items are usually simple to complete and reduce respondent burden.

The developer must also consider relevance and acceptability of the questionnaire to the target group. The items need to be written in language that respondents find easy to understand. For example, it is important to avoid the use of technical terms when recruiting lay persons, for example, 'breathing machine' rather than 'ventilatory support'and 'water pill' rather than 'diuretic'. However, care needs to be taken not to oversimplify language, which may offend.

Items or questions should be clearly written to avoid misinterpretation and leading questions avoided. Age can be collected as a continuous or categorised variable. If the latter is the case, the categories must be clearly identified and be mutually exclusive. For example, in question 1a, a respondent who is 30 years old would identify with the first and second category, whereas in question 1b, they would identify with just the first category:

1a What age are you? 18–30 30–50 50–70 over 70
1b What age are you? 18–30 31–50 51–70 71+

As another example, if a researcher is interested in how social support receipt influences patient adjustment to a long-term condition, they might ask the following questions:

2a Did you receive practical and emotional support? Yes/No
2b Was this support helpful? Yes/No

On the face of it, question 2a might be reasonable, but if the patient had received practical rather than emotional support, or vice versa, the item would be ambiguous. A better way would be to ask four questions:

3a Did you receive practical support? Yes/No
3b If yes, was this practical support helpful? Yes/No
4a Did you receive emotional support? Yes/No
4b If yes, was this emotional support helpful? Yes/No

Level of data

The type of question, language used, order of items and how the questionnaire is presented may all bias responses and influence response rates. Participants need to be clear about the purpose of the questionnaire and understand what they are being asked to do. It is important to engage the participant's interest early on to encourage completion. It is best to avoid presenting controversial or emotive items at the beginning of the questionnaire. To prevent boredom, demographic and/or clinical data may be presented at the end.

Closed questions, which offer a restricted range of responses, can be viewed as too restrictive by some respondents. There may not be an appropriate response option, and therefore, consideration should be given to including the option for free text responses or open questions. This is a particularly useful when developing a questionnaire.

There are a range of scales and response styles that may be chosen that produce different types or levels of data. Probably, the lowest level of measurement is *categorical* or *nominal* data, which can be grouped into distinct categories. The most common questionnaire item that provides data at a categorical or nominal level is gender. Respondents may be categorised according to clinical condition or demographic data such as diagnosis or gender.

Ordinal data imply an order to responses, but there is no equal distance between each option. For example, the assumption is often made that the same distances exist between strongly agree and agree as between strongly disagree and disagree. However, this is not the case. A measurable or quantifiable difference between each item on the scale can only exist at the next level of data, which is *interval* or *ratio*. In this instance, the difference in temperature of 37 and 38 °C is the same as between 36 and 37 °C, that is, of 1° of temperature. The level of data collected by a questionnaire will influence the nature of subsequent analysis. Therefore, when developing a new questionnaire, the developer must be clear which scale and response format should be used in light of this. Chapter 35 discusses types of data and their analysis in more detail.

Range of scales

A range of response format scales are available. The *Likert-type* or *frequency* scale is commonly used. This provides ordinal-level data, and Likert-type scales generally measure level of agreement. Respondents may be given a range of 5, 7 or even 9 pre-coded options ranging from strongly agree to strongly disagree. This scale makes the assumption that attitudes can be measured, although there is no assumption that the differences between strongly agree and agree are equivalent to those between strongly disagree and disagree. There is controversy about whether to offer a neutral point, that is, 'undecided' or 'no opinion' in such scales of agreement. If the respondent has no opinion about an item, it may cause confusion not to offer that choice and therefore increase the possibility of non-response bias (Burns & Grove 1997).

Less commonly used in nursing research are Thurstone and Guttman scales. Thurstone scales are constructed following analysis of empirical data provided often by expert panels, such that attitudes and behaviours measured by the items are equally spaced along a continuum from favourable to unfavourable, and each item is given a weighting. Items included in the final questionnaire usually have a dichotomous response format and are chosen to represent the range of assigned weights. An example is the Nottingham Health Profile (Hunt *et al.* 1985). Guttman scaling uses methods that establish a hierarchy of items such that when participants agree with an item, they will also agree with items of a lower ranking, for example, Katz Index of Activities of Daily Living (Katz *et al.* 1963) and the Rivermead Mobility Index (Collen *et al.* 1991). Further details of the questionnaire development process for Thurstone and Guttman is provided by Oppenheim (1992).

Response formats

A range of response formats are possible. Participants may be asked to indicate an appropriate response from a choice of five boxes. For example:

	All of the time	*Most of the time*	*Some of the time*	*Rarely*	*Never*
I feel anxious					

Alternatively, a horizontal or vertical linear scale may be used, and the respondent asked to mark where they would position themselves on the line.

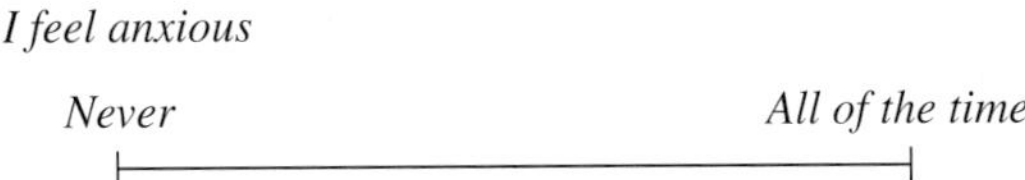

Before deciding on the response format, it is important to be clear about how the data will be analysed.

Certain questions should be avoided, for example those that lead or include double negatives or double-barrelled questions (Bowling 2005). A mixture of both positively and negatively worded items may minimise the danger of acquiescent response bias, that is, the tendency for respondents to agree with a statement or respond in the same way to items.

If it is appropriate for respondents to expand upon answers and provide more in-depth responses, free text response or open questions may be included. While this approach may be welcomed by respondents and provide rich data, such material can be difficult to analyse and interpret (Polgar & Thomas 2011). Such problems may be outweighed by the benefits of including this option, particularly in the early development of a questionnaire. Free text comments can inform future questionnaire development by identifying poorly constructed items or new items for future inclusion.

ADMINISTERING QUESTIONNAIRES

Questionnaires can be administered via a variety of routes, that is, either postal, face-to-face or increasingly online. They may be self-completed by participants or be presented by interviewer either face-to-face or via the telephone.

Presentation and layout of the questionnaire is important as this can affect response rates. Always try to make it easy for the participant to complete. A covering letter and/or a participant information sheet is used to introduce the study to the participant. This is to establish the credibility of the study and to convince the participant of its worth (Czaja & Blair 2005). The covering letter should explain what the study is about, why it is important, how findings will be used and how the respondent was selected. It must clarify issues surrounding confidentiality and anonymity and provide a contact number for respondents to contact if they have questions (Czaja & Blair 2005). Participant information sheets fulfil a similar purpose and are required by ethics committees (Barrett & Coleman 2005).

There are some simple principles to follow to encourage responses and reduce the number of missed items:

- Simple instructions before each section of the questionnaire are helpful. This may include a worked example.
- The font size should be large enough to be read easily.
- Items or questions should be clearly numbered.
- Avoid the overuse of capital letters, and use lower case wherever possible, which is easier to read.
- If the questionnaire is to be administered by post, it is best to have questions on one side of the paper only.
- Consider the length of your questionnaire and keep it as brief as possible.
- Reminders may be sent to participants. This can increase the response rate but must be detailed as part of an ethics application.
- The respondent should be thanked for participating in the study.

The use of coding systems ensures the confidentiality and anonymity of participants, with the researcher maintaining and storing securely a codebook linking the code on a questionnaire to the participant's name. This protects the identity of participants but allows the linking of questionnaire data with other forms of data, which may include data in existing secondary data sets or data held in other health-related records. Questionnaire packs must be adequately prepared and coded and include the covering letter, consent form, return and contact details. If presumed consent was part of the ethical approval, return of the questionnaire may be taken to indicate consent (Czaja & Blair 2005).

Online administration will have to consider many of the aforementioned issues and the computer interface and navigational issues (Norman *et al.* 2001). If some participants do not have computer access, there is a danger of sample bias. However, the increased use of computers, tablets and smartphones makes this less problematic.

Reflection activity

Refer back to the research question posed earlier to examine the effect of monthly clinical supervision on staff well-being. Think through the advantages and disadvantages of delivering the questionnaire by hand, by post or electronically for the respondents to self-complete, or presenting it via an interviewer either face-to-face or by telephone. Decide which approach is best suited for the proposed study. What factors have influenced your decision?

Research governance procedures must be adhered to and ethical approval obtained for questionnaire-based studies. Less experienced researchers will benefit from the support of more senior researchers and appropriate training. Polit and Beck (2012) provide an example of a training manual that includes the research protocol, detailing study procedures and the role of the researcher in gaining consent and/or administering the questionnaire pack by the chosen administration route. They also include a data collection protocol, which identifies the conditions necessary for collecting data, the time and setting data can be collected and replies to frequently asked questions (identified during piloting the questionnaire).

PILOTING

Piloting is a key stage in the development of the questionnaire. This allows the pretesting of the measure ahead of the main study. Piloting enables evaluation of the performance of the measure in meeting the study objectives. This is an essential stage, particularly if the study is using a newly constructed questionnaire. It allows the researcher to establish whether questions are intelligible or unambiguous. It establishes whether the items are acceptable and inoffensive and how long the measure takes to complete (Polit & Beck 2012). Such pilots can be relatively informal with small numbers of participants. It is also appropriate at this stage to develop a plan for validation of the measure (Czaja & Blair 2005; Rattray & Jones 2007). The opinion of experts may be sought to establish the face or content validity of the measure.

The measure may be piloted more formally with up to 50 participants to test the acceptability of questionnaire items and should include an initial examination of reliability and validity (Bowling 2002). As part of this evaluation, item analysis provides a strategy to decide on whether all items in the measure should remain. An item–total correlation cut-off of <0.3 can be used to identify items that do not add to the explanatory power of the measure and that should be discarded (Kline 1993). Questionnaire items that have high endorsement of particular response options add little to the discriminatory power of the measure and should be deleted (Priest *et al.* 1995). A more detailed discussion of these issues can be found in Rattray and Jones (2007).

RESPONSE RATES

Response rate has been defined as 'the number of eligible sample members to complete, divided by the total number of eligible sample members' (Czaja & Blair 2005: 37). Response rates of 75% and above are considered good (Bowling 2002), although response rates far less than this are common. Lower response rates are problematic in that those sample

Reflection activity

Think about the proposed study to examine the effective of monthly clinical supervision on staff well-being. How might the design of the questionnaire influence the response rate? What strategies could you use when administering a questionnaire to maximise the response rate?

members who have not completed may differ from responders. Strategies to establish the nature of any response bias are recommended.

The return route also has an impact on response rates. Response rates for questionnaires presented by interviewer may be increased. This may be because the interviewer can clarify items and motivate the respondent (Polit & Beck 2012).

COMPARISON BETWEEN FACE-TO-FACE STRUCTURED INTERVIEW AND POSTAL QUESTIONNAIRES

Each method of administration has strengths and limitations, and different methods may be combined. For example, in a face-to-face study, the researcher may make an initial approach to gain consent and, having given the person time to consider (usually at least 24 hours), may then administer the questionnaire to the participant for self-completion and return in the setting or for return by post. Alternatively, the researcher may administer the questionnaire as a structured interview that may be delivered face-to-face or by telephone. Response rates for structured interviews tend to be higher than for postal surveys, fewer missing items are found, and the researcher can ensure that the participant completed the questionnaire in the required sequence (Bowling 2002). Having the interviewer present to clarify any questions the participant has may promote a good response. However, the interviewer must avoid influencing the response given by respondents (Polit & Beck 2012).

STRENGTHS AND LIMITATIONS OF QUESTIONNAIRES

The standardised questionnaire has many advantages. It allows the collection of considerable data quickly and relatively cheaply. It is generally convenient and can be administered in a range of settings. It allows for a count of issues and occurrences in a systematic and standardised manner and can be supplemented with routinely gathered information or objective data from case notes (Bowling 2002).

Social desirability is a potential limitation of questionnaire data, with participants attempting to influence the impression they provide through their answers (Bowling 2005). Self-completed questionnaires are less prone to such bias than those administered by interviewers (Bowling 2002). The researcher may consider using a measure of social desirability to evaluate this form of self-presentation bias (Stober 2001).

Questionnaire data is almost exclusively retrospective based and is gathered by asking a respondent to report on a construct of interest and rate their response considering the recent past. Such accounts normally rely on memory, which can be affected by the participant's current affective state. Recall effects can bias data, for example, current depression may bias reports of previous symptoms (Shiffman & Stone 1998). Such introspection effects create systematic bias, with the attitudes of the person influencing their retrospective account. Gathering information retrospectively about thoughts or decisions in a particular situation may also be compromised by the person's knowledge of the outcome.

Administering a questionnaire may actually change participant behaviour. For example, asking a participant about their alcohol consumption may influence subsequent reports. Repeated use of a measure may also lead to familiarity with the questionnaire, which may make it difficult to discriminate such practice effects from actual change over time.

ETHICAL ISSUES

Ensuring that informed consent is obtained is vital in questionnaire studies. Participants must be given sufficient time to consider the request before being asked to provide information. Questionnaire studies should ensure confidentiality, that is, the respondents' identity will not be linked to the information they provide, and their identity will not be revealed in any dissemination of findings (Polit & Beck 2014). Anonymous responses may allow the respondent to feel more ready to provide information. However, true anonymity is difficult to achieve, particularly in small surveys, and does not allow linkage of data or sending of reminder letters. Where anonymity cannot be assured, data must be treated as confidential, and the respondent reassured that only the researchers will access the data (Oppenheim 1992). Some postal surveys assume implied consent, with the return of the questionnaire indicating informed consent, but this may not be justified in situations involving vulnerable participants (Polit & Beck 2014).

The researcher must have strategies to deal with situations where the subject area might cause distress to the respondent or where there is an indication of a worsening of clinical condition. For example, if a participant's score on a screening measure of depression suggests a potential depressive disorder, then it may be appropriate to refer that patient to their general practitioner. Furthermore, questionnaires that include intrusive or offensive items, items that are not needed, or that do not have established reliability and validity may be ethically suspect. Ethics committees will offer guidance in this area.

CONCLUSION

This chapter has considered issues associated with the design and use of questionnaires, including the decision process involved in either choosing an established measure or developing a questionnaire. Questionnaires are increasingly used in research, and researchers should have a good understanding of design and administration issues. A systematic approach should be adopted when designing and appraising a questionnaire. This involves consideration of items, demonstrating the reliability, validity and acceptability of a questionnaire appropriate to a particular research setting and participants. Presentation, wording, order and layout are important factors in influencing validity and response rates. There are several strategies to improve this, but good representative responses are important to minimise bias and measurement error.

Reflection activity

Identify the ethical issues associated with using questionnaires to answer the research question posed earlier. What steps could you take to address these ethical issues?

References

Al-lela O, Bahari M, Al-abbassi M, Basher A (2011) Development of a questionnaire on knowledge, attitude and practice about immunization among Iraqi parents. *Journal of Public Health* **19**: 497–503.

Arvidsson S, Bergman S, Arvidsson B, Fridlund B, Tingstrom P (2012) Psychometric properties of the Swedish Rheumatic Disease Empowerment Scale. *Musculoskeletal Care* **10**: 101–109.

Barbour R (2008) *Introducing Qualitative Research: a student guide to the craft of doing qualitative research.* London, Sage.

Barrett G, Coleman M (2005) Ethical and political issues in the conduct of research. In Bowling A, Ebrahim E (eds) *Handbook of Health Research Methods: investigation, measurement and analysis.* Maidenhead, Open University Press, pp 555–583.

Bowling A (2002) *Research Methods in Health.* Buckingham, Open University Press.

Bowling A (2005). *Measuring Health: a review of quality of life measurement scales*, 3rd edition. Maidenhead, Open University Press.

Bowling A (2009) *Research Methods in Health: investigating health and health services*, 3rd edition. Maidenhead, Open University Press.

Bowling A, Ebrahim E (2005) *Handbook of Health Research Methods: investigation, measurement and analysis.* Maidenhead, Open University Press.

Brunt D, Rask M (2012) A suggested revision of the Community Oriented Program Environmental Scale (COPES) for measuring the psychosocial environment of supported housing facilities for person with psychiatric difficulties. *Issues in Mental Health Nursing* **33**: 24–31.

Bryman A, Cramer D (2011) *Quantitative Data Analysis with IBM SPSS 17, 18 & 19.* London, Routledge.

Burns N, Grove SK (1997) *The Practice of Nursing Research Conduct, Critique, and Utilization*, 3rd edition. Philadelphia, WB Saunders.

Collen FM, Wade DT, Robb GF, Bradshaw CM (1991) The Rivermead Mobility Index: a further development of the Rivermead Motor Assessment. *International Disabilities Studies* **13**: 50–54.

Conner M, Sparks P (2005) The theory of planned behaviour and health behaviours. In: Conner M, Norman P (eds) *Predicting Health Behaviour*, 2nd edition. Buckingham, Open University Press, pp 170–222.

Crawford JR, Henry J, Crombie C, Taylor E (2001) Normative data for the HADS from a large non-clinical sample. *British Journal of Clinical Psychology* **40**(4): 429–434.

Czaja R, Blair J (2005) *Designing Surveys: a guide to decisions and procedures*. Thousand Oaks, Pine Forge Press.

Devlen J, Michaelson S, Maguire P (1989). *Cardiovascular Limitations and Symptoms Profile*. Manchester, Manchester Center for Primary Care Research.

EuroQol Group (1990) A new facility for the measurement of health-related quality of life. *Health Policy* **16**: 199–208.

Ferguson E, Cox T (1993) Exploratory factor analysis: a user's guide. *International Journal of Selection and Assessment* **1**(2): 84–94.

Frank C, Asp M, Fridlund B, Baigi A (2010) Questionnaire for patient participation in emergency departments. *Journal of Advanced Nursing* **67**(3): 643–651.

Furze G, Bull P, Lewin RJP, Thompson DR (2003) Development of the York Angina Beliefs Questionnaire. *Journal of Health Psychology* **8**(3): 307–315.

Hunt S, McEwen J, McKenna SP (1985) Measuring health status: a new tool for clinicians and epidemiologists. *Journal of the Royal College of General Practitioners* **35**: 185–188.

Jones MC, Johnston DW (1999) The derivation of a brief student nurse stress index. *Work and Stress* **13**(2): 162–181.

Katz S, Ford A, Moskowitz R (1963) Studies of illness in the aged: the index of ADL. A standardised measure of biological and psychosocial function. *Journal of American Medical Association* **185**: 914–919.

Kline P (1993) *The Handbook of Psychological Testing*. London, Routledge.

Macnee CL, McCabe S (2008) *Understanding Nursing Research: reading and using research in evidence-based practice*, 2nd edition. Philadelphia, Wolters Kluwer Health/Lippincott Williams and Wilkins.

Martin CR, Thompson DR (2000) A psychometric evaluation of the Hospital Anxiety and Depression Scale in coronary care patients following acute myocardial infarction. *Psychology, Health and Medicine* **5**(2): 193–201.

Moss-Morris R, Weinman J, Petrie K, Horne R, Cameron LD, Buick D (2002) The Revised Illness Perception Questionnaire (IPQ-R). *Psychology and Health* **17**(1): 1–6.

Norman KL, Friedman Z, Norman K, Stevenson R (2001) Navigational issues in the design of online self-administered questionnaires. *Behaviour and Information Technology* **20**(1): 37–45.

Oppenheim AN (1992) *Questionnaire Design, Interviewing and Attitude Measurement*. London, Pinter.

Patrick D, Peach H (1989) *Disablement in the Community*. London, Continuum.

Polgar S, Thomas SA (2011) *Introduction to Research in the Health Sciences*. Edinburgh, Churchill Livingstone.

Polit D, Beck C (2012) *Nursing Research: generating and assessing evidence for nursing practice*, 9th edition. Philadelphia, Wolters Kluwer/Lippincott Williams and Wilkins.

Polit D, Beck C (2014) *Essentials of Nursing Research: appraising evidence for nursing practice*, 8th edition. Philadelphia, Wolters Kluwer/Lippincott Williams and Wilkins.

Priest J, McColl BA, Thomas L, Bond S (1995) Developing and refining a new measurement tool. *Nurse Researcher* **2**(4): 69–81.

Rattray J, Jones MC (2007) Essential elements in questionnaire design and development. *Journal of Clinical Nursing* **16**: 234–243.

Ruzafa-Martinez M, Lopez-Iborra L, Madrigal-Torres M (2011) Attitude towards Evidence-Based Nursing Questionnaire: development and psychometric testing in Spanish community nurses. *Journal of Evaluation in Clinical Practice* **17**: 664–670.

Shiffman S, Stone A (1998) Introduction to the special section: ecological momentary assessment in health psychology. *Health Psychology* **17**(1): 3–5.

Stober J (2001) The Social Desirability Scale-17 (SDS-17): convergent validity, discriminant validity, and relationship with age. *European Journal of Psychological Assessment* **17**: 222–232.

Ware J, Sherbourne C (1992) The MOS 36-item short-form health survey (SF-36) I: conceptual framework and item selection. *Medical Care* **30**: 473–483.

Wilde B, Larsson G (2002) Development of a short form of the Quality from the Patient's Perspective (QPP) questionnaire. *Journal of Clinical Nursing* **11**: 681–687.

Zetta S, Smith K, Jones M, Allcoat P, Sullivan F (2011) Evaluating the angina plan in patients admitted to hospital with angina: a randomized controlled trial. *Cardiovascular Therapeutics* **29**(2): 112–124.

Zigmond AS, Snaith RP (1983) The Hospital Anxiety and Depression Scale. *Acta Psychiatrica Scandinavica* **67**: 361–370.

CHAPTER 31

Observation

Jo Booth

Key points

- The use of observation in research provides a first-hand account of behaviours or events, collected systematically for analysis and theory development.
- Depending on the theoretical approach of the research, observation may range from completely unstructured to highly structured; observer roles may vary from complete observer to full participant.
- Participant observation is more commonly used within the qualitative paradigm, and requires immersion of the researcher in the field.
- Structured observation is more common in quantitative research and requires the rigorous use of checklists and categories to record the observed data.

THE PURPOSE OF OBSERVATION

Observation involves using our senses to gather information and develop an understanding of the world around us. It can entail using all of the senses, judging and interpreting what we perceive to enable us to make sense of the information. When providing clinical care for patients, nurses observe patients' physical and mental condition while also observing for signs of pain or emotional and psychological distress.

In nursing research, observation is an active process by which data are collected about people, behaviours, interactions or events. The aim of data collection through observation is to gain detailed information that can contribute to understanding the phenomena being studied. Observational data provide a first-hand account of behaviours or events witnessed by the observer and collected systematically to facilitate the development or testing of theories.

Observation can be used as the principal data collection method in both quantitative and qualitative studies. Whyte *et al.* (2006) used observation in two ways, firstly by directly observing the ward setting where nurse–patient contact and interaction took place (see Research Example 31.1) and secondly by observing the verbal exchanges between nurses and

The Research Process in Nursing, Seventh Edition. Edited by Kate Gerrish and Judith Lathlean.

Companion Website: www.wiley.com/go/gerrish/research

RESEARCH EXAMPLE

31.1 Using Observation in Qualitative Research

Whyte R, Watson HR, McIntosh J (2006) Nurses' opportunistic interventions with patients in relation to smoking. *Journal of Advanced Nursing* **55**(5): 568–577.

This study aimed to identify the extent to which nurses recognise and utilise opportunities to provide health education on smoking to patients in hospital. A qualitative case study, using facets of ethnography, evaluated the smoking-related health education role of 12 diplomate nurses. Data were collected through lifestyle questionnaires, tape-recorded nurse–patient interactions and interviews, observation, field notes and examination of patients' nursing documentation. Triangulation of data enabled in-depth exploration of the nurses' health education interactions in acute wards and contributed to rigour in the study.

The findings indicated that smoking was part of nurses' health agenda, as evidenced by their recognition of opportunities to introduce the topic, although the content of their interactions was variable.

RESEARCH EXAMPLE

31.2 Non-participant Structured Observation in Quantitative Research

Doherty-King B, Yoon JY, Pecanac K, Brown R, Mahoney J (2014) Frequency and duration of nursing care related to older patient mobility. *Journal of Nursing Scholarship* **46**(1): 20–27.

This observation study evaluated the frequency and duration of nursing care activities related to mobilising 47 older patients in acute care settings. It also identified who initiated the mobility event (patient or nurse). Observers shadowed 15 registered nurses (RNs) each for two to three 8-hour periods. Data on frequency and duration of mobility events were recorded on handheld computer tablets. Six mobility events were observed: standing, transferring, walking to and from the patient bathroom, walking in the patient room and walking in the hallway. Results showed one third of older patients were not engaged in any mobility event during an 8-hour period. Mean duration for ambulation was less than 2 minutes per observation period and patients who were dependent had fewer mobility events. The majority of mobility events were initiated by patients.

patients. These exchanges were captured through audio-recorded indirect observation where the researcher was not a direct witness, but the tape recorder served this purpose. Whyte's study provides an example of how observation can be used with a range of data collection methods in a qualitative study. The studies conducted by Doherty-King *et al.* (2014) and Ampt *et al.* (2007) illustrate the use of observation within the context of quantitative research (Research Examples 31.2 and 31.3).

As a preliminary phase in research, observations can be used to identify routines, activities and happenings that occur in settings to provide the basis for more focused observations during the main study. As the exploratory phase of a study of nurse–patient interactions, Booth *et al.* (2005) conducted non-participant observation to determine the structure and content of morning care activities in stroke rehabilitation units. The aim was to collect data about nursing activities and interactions to

RESEARCH EXAMPLE

31.3 Non-participant Observation in Experimental Design

Ampt A, Westbrook J, Creswick N, Mallock N (2007) A comparison of self-reported and observational work sampling techniques for measuring time in nursing tasks. *Journal of Health Services Research and Policy* **12**(1): 18–24.

In this study, self-reported and observational work sampling techniques were compared when applied to ward-based nurses. Nine nurses self-reported on their work over an 8-week period, followed by an observational work sampling study over 4 weeks. Field notes were also recorded. In total, 3910 data points were collected, 667 during the self-report study and 3243 in the observational study. The two techniques indicated significant differences in registered nurses' work patterns. The observational study showed that compared with the self-reported study, patient care (40% vs. 33%, $P<0.000$) and ward-related activities (7% vs. 3%, $P<0.001$) were recorded significantly more frequently and documentation less frequently (8% vs. 19%;,$P<0.000$). Both techniques generated similar proportions of time spent in breaks (12%), medication tasks (13%) and clinical discussion (15%). The study concluded that the self-report work sampling technique is not a reliable method for obtaining an accurate reflection of the work tasks of ward-based nurses.

Reflection activity

Consider the types of phenomena (activities and interactions) in your work area that would be suitable to investigate using observational methods. Identify which phenomena would be most suited to qualitative observation and which would be suited to quantitative observation.

inform the development of data collection methods for the pilot and main studies.

Observation can also be used to confirm, support or refute data that have been collected through other methods, such as questionnaire survey or interview. Providing a record of behaviours or events as they occur can help to overcome sources of bias such as the effect of time on memory, or of participants giving socially acceptable answers. Instead, they provide a means of recording what people actually do as opposed to what they say that they do. When used in longitudinal studies, observation methods can uncover processes that evolve over time.

Observer roles

Depending on the theoretical approach of a study, the researcher may be a participant or a non-participant observer. In participant observation, the researcher participates in the activities of those who are being observed, while in non-participant observation, the researcher remains detached from those being observed. In a seminal paper, Gold (1969) identified four observational roles that researchers might adopt:

- Complete participant – the researcher participates fully in the activities of those being observed and attempts to act as one of the group. Observation may be conducted overtly or covertly.
- Participant-as-observer – the researcher participates in the activities of those being observed, but the role is made explicit and observation is conducted overtly.
- Observer-as-participant – the researcher participates briefly with those being observed but spends most of the time observing behaviours/events.
- Complete observer – the researcher is chiefly concerned with observing behaviours and has no interaction with those being observed.

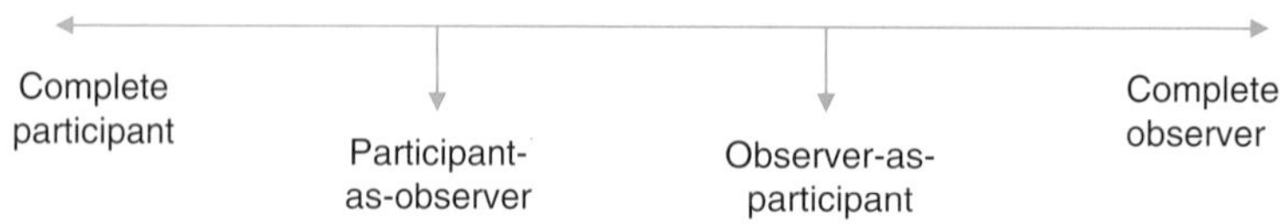

Figure 31.1 Observations roles (from Gold 1969)

This may be seen as a continuum ranging from the researcher's complete participation with the work and activities of those being observed to complete detachment from them (Figure 31.1).

Where the researcher is a participant, irrespective of the extent of the participation, the research approach is generally qualitative, whereas in quantitative research, the researcher usually assumes a non-participant role, that is, that of a complete observer.

The observer role may not be as rigid as Gold's typology would suggest and researchers may find their role changing as a study progresses. For example, during the course of a study, the researcher's role of participant-as-observer may change to that of observer-as-participant, depending on the needs of the study (Melnyck & Fineout-Overholt 2005). Similarly, in a practice environment, it is challenging to maintain a complete observer role as presence alone will have an impact.

There is also the possibility of observer role confusion, especially when nurse researchers conduct research in their specialist area. Millard *et al.* (2006), in a study on community nursing, adopted the role of observer-as-participant. As a practising community nurse, Millard reported a tendency for nurse participants to involve her in discussions or to seek her advice.

Collecting observational data

Researchers who use observational methods may choose one of two forms of sampling, namely, *event sampling* or *time sampling*. Event sampling involves identifying specific events, such as used by Doherty-King *et al.* (2014). The 'events' in their study were standing, transferring, walking to and from the patient bathroom, walking in the patient room and walking in the hallway (Research Example 31.2). In time sampling, the researcher records on an activity sheet behaviours, which have previously been identified within a category system, at regular intervals throughout a specified period of time. Booth *et al.* (2005), for example, observed each participating patient every 20 seconds over a period of 1.5 hours.

Observation data can be collected directly by the researcher 'on the spot' in the research setting, in which case observations are coded using an observation schedule. Alternatively, various forms of recording equipment may be used. The activities to be observed can be video recorded, with the advantages that the researcher does not need to be present and that a permanent record of the observed phenomena is obtained that can be repeatedly viewed. In this way, multiple layers of analysis can be undertaken, such as an exploration of patients' activities and exploration of nursing activities during the same encounter. Thus, a diverse range of activities and interactions can be explored and analysed from different perspectives (Francis 2004; Pan *et al.* 2013). In addition, both verbal and non-verbal interactions may be captured simultaneously.

When a range of behaviours are being observed, such as physical activity and non-verbal and verbal interactions, an activity checklist can be used simultaneously with audio or video recording, allowing the observer to concentrate on a limited range of phenomena at the time. There is a limit to the number of activities that can be recorded in a given time period, and observer fatigue must be acknowledged and avoided.

Reflection activity

What do you think the issues and practical choices might be in deciding whether to video or audio-record observations in your workplace?

PARTICIPANT OBSERVATION

This form of observation, associated with the qualitative paradigm, is used in order to explore, understand and interpret a culture or group from an insider's or *emic* perspective. Participant observation has its origins in social anthropology where data are collected in the normal surroundings of the people or events being studied. For example, the anthropologists Mead (1935) and Malinowski (1922) studied the lives and traditions of groups of people in their social surroundings by immersing themselves in the cultures of the groups, sometimes for several years (see Chapter 15 for a more detailed account of the use of participant observation in ethnography).

Characteristics and purpose of participant observation

According to Gold's (1969) typology, there are three roles the researcher might adopt as a participant observer, namely, the complete participant, participant-as-observer and observer-as-participant (see Figure 31.1).

As a complete participant, observation may be conducted covertly to ensure that those being observed are not aware of the researcher's purpose and do not change their behaviour. Covert observation has been used in sociological and anthropological studies often with the purpose of investigating sensitive topics, thereby promoting an understanding of events and behaviours (Petticrew *et al.* 2007); however, there are ethical implications to consider when using this approach in health care. In a study by Rosenhan (1973), eight participants were admitted to different psychiatric hospitals in America in order to observe the way in which psychiatric wards operated and the behaviour of staff towards psychiatric patients. The participants gained entry to the hospitals by claiming to 'hear voices'. Seven of the participants were diagnosed with schizophrenia and one with manic-depressive psychosis. Once admitted, the pseudo-patients stopped pretending to exhibit symptoms and reverted to 'normal' behaviour although the diagnoses of schizophrenia remained. Through covert participant observation, the pseudo-patients recorded their experiences and those of other patients and demonstrated the powerlessness and depersonalisation that was the reality for psychiatric patients at that time. The data collected in the study could not have been obtained had the research been conducted overtly. However, the ethical issues associated with covert observation, such as deception and observing participants without their knowledge and consent, make this a problematic role for nurse researchers.

In participant-as-observer and observer-as-participant, the researcher's role is known and consent is obtained from the study participants. The openness of the role allows the researcher to ask group members to explain activities or events that have been observed. The amount of time the researcher spends in participation in each of these roles will depend on the data to be collected, and the researcher may, in fact, switch between roles, spending more time on participation or more time on observation as required (Melnyck & Fineout-Overholt 2005).

Negotiating access and building rapport

As discussed in Chapter 11, those who wish to conduct research must obtain permission to access the study site. The process will require approval of the ethics committee and local research and development departments and negotiation with local nursing and medical personnel/gatekeepers before potential participants can be approached. Familiarity with aspects of nursing culture and the language and traditions of hospitals and/or primary care will assist nurse researchers when entering a setting for the first time. The researcher may be considered an 'insider', which can facilitate the exploration of practice processes and the understanding of the phenomenon being studied (Carnevale *et al.* 2008). Nonetheless, this is only the first step and the researcher must spend time learning to integrate with people in the setting to gain trust and acceptance.

Negotiating access and building rapport with participants should be considered, not as a one-off event, but as a continuing process that requires patience and diplomacy to ensure that essential data are collected (Hammersley & Atkinson 1995; Robson 2011).

Without the trust of participants, researchers may find they are not accepted and are unable to access the data they seek.

Working in the field and minimising disruption

Researchers conducting participant observation first enter the setting with a broad idea of what they want to observe. The researcher's intention is to gain a 'feel' for the setting, the participants, how activities are conducted and the context in which they occur. Participation in the work and activities of a group and a developing rapport with participants enable the researcher to refine the areas of observation, a process that Spradley (1980) referred to as 'forming a funnel'. This allows the observation to become more focused.

Researchers may spend long periods of time working alongside study participants to familiarise themselves with the environment and the culture. This enables them to join in day-to-day activities and share experiences with participants. Polit and Hungler (2006) call this 'getting backstage' to discover the reality of a group's experiences and behaviour, free from 'protective facades'. How well this is achieved is dependent on the trust and rapport that is developed between researcher and participants.

Spending time in a site prior to data collection also enables participants to become familiar with the presence of the researcher and any recording equipment that might be used. It is essential that the researcher's presence during data collection causes minimal disruption so that observed behaviours or events accurately reflect normality. While it is not possible to remove the impact of the researcher completely, it is important that researchers try to minimise observer effects – the extent to which their presence is felt.

Recording observations: field notes

Field notes are a record of the observations the researcher has made and should be recorded as soon as possible after observing an event to ensure accuracy. They may be written in a notebook used specifically for the purpose or may be audio recorded. Whichever method is used, the security and confidentiality of the material is essential.

As a participant and an observer, it may be difficult to record field notes when and where they occur. The researcher may have to move out of an area to do so. It may also be useful to record field notes in a place that is conducive to thinking about and interpreting observed data, away from an area that is busy or noisy.

The way in which field notes are organised may be revised or refocused as observation progresses, or they may reflect themes that have been identified in the course of observation. The material constitutes collected data and, as the researcher attempts to make sense of observations and their contexts, the analytical process begins. An example of recorded field notes is presented in Box 31.1.

Most qualitative researchers keep a diary/journal record of their personal reflections during the periods of participant observation. In it, they record their feelings, experiences and thoughts and acknowledge their position as a research instrument through which data pass.

Researchers as participant observers must recognise their potential effect on the study participants and the setting and hence the data they collect. This process, called reflexivity, is the process of a continual internal dialogue and critical self-evaluation of researcher's positionality as well as active acknowledgement and explicit recognition that this position may affect the research process and outcome (Berger 2013). In qualitative research, reflexivity contributes to the trustworthiness of the data. It is an inherent consideration in addressing the rigour of all forms of observational research.

NON-PARTICIPANT OBSERVATION

In non-participant observation, the researcher assumes the role of a complete observer and endeavours to have no influence on the phenomena under observation. In quantitative research, a validated structured schedule is used for data collection, whereas in qualitative research, less structured forms

Box 31.1 Fieldnotes

Readiness to learn

Assessing readiness to learn is important for any strategy for health education. Field notes made during observation demonstrate a patient's lack of readiness not only to stop smoking but for information about smoking (Whyte 2004).

Case study 7

11.15 am – Nurse B (nurse participant) is working in the ward with a patient who is not in the study. I am in the ward dayroom with Sheila (patient participant).

Sheila is talking with three patients, all of whom are smoking. The talk is about smoking - ways of giving up, feeling like outcasts and problems caused by smoking. Sheila says she has spent a lot of money trying to give up and she wishes she hadn't bothered and just spent it on cigarettes instead. Doctors have been telling her for years that smoking is the cause of her heart trouble but she doesn't believe it as all of her family has had heart, trouble and none of them smokes. She thinks it's in her genes and has nothing to do with smoking, although she admits that she might be kidding herself (observation and field notes).

I don't think Sheila is ready to stop smoking.

2 pm – Nurse B and Sheila are sitting talking beside Sheila's bed. They appear quite relaxed.

Nurse B uses the opportunity to introduce the subject of smoking. Sheila's tone of voice becomes defensive when she is asked if she is a heavy smoker and she tries to change the subject. Nurse B talks about the harmful effects of smoking, but Sheila eventually stops the conversation by saying: '... nobody nags me to do anything about my smoking because they know what I've been through' (observation, field notes and tape-recorded data).

Sheila is not ready to stop smoking – assessment of readiness would have identified that.

of data collection are used. However, a systematic process to both the collection and analysis of data is equally important for both forms of research.

Recording unstructured observations

As outlined in Research Example 31.1, Whyte *et al.* (2006) assumed a non-participant observer role in a qualitative study of the provision of smoking-related information and used an unstructured approach to observation by audio recording nurse–patient interactions. The audio recordings were transcribed verbatim, and the data were analysed qualitatively using a framework developed specifically for the study, based on the literature on verbal communication and health education.

Observation methods using a structured method of data collection are appropriate for quantitative studies, collecting data about actions and behavioural interactions (see Research Examples 31.2 and 31.3).

Recording structured observations

In studies that use structured observation, the researcher is a non-participant observer who records the phenomena under examination using a framework for data collection. Such a framework is developed prior to commencement of the study. The researcher's aim is to devise a tool to facilitate the systematic collection of data in a way that will, as far as possible, limit subjectivity and observer bias, thereby enhancing validity and reliability. This involves a process that is similar to that followed when developing a questionnaire or structured interview schedule.

Category system

The first stage is to draw up a category system from which activity checklists and/or rating scales are developed for completion by the observer. A category system comprises a comprehensive list of the behaviours likely to arise within the situation under observation.

In developing the category system, the researcher needs to be clear about the phenomena to be observed. Expressing these as concise written statements is an important discipline in helping to ensure clarity. This also enables the researcher to identify subcategories for each category.

In observation research, the categories often comprise the following:

- Location
- Time
- Activity
- Facial expression
- Verbal interaction
- Personnel

Each category has within it a range of attributes or sub-categories that are amenable to observation.

In designing observation schedules, it is important that the categories are mutually exclusive so that the observed phenomena can only be coded within one category (e.g. see the example of 'weeping' in Box 31.2).

Box 31.2 Category system for structured observation

Location
Bed, bedside, day room, treatment room, bathroom

Time
Starting time, finishing time

Activity
Sleeping, eating, walking, reading, watching television

Facial expression
Natural repose, smiling, laughing, grimacing, weeping[a]

Verbal interaction
The nature of the interaction – for example, question, explanation, reassurance, humorous exchange

The tone of voice – for example, soft, harsh

Personnel
Patient, nurse, doctor, occupational therapist, family member

[a]Note that the word 'weeping' is used rather than 'crying', which could be interpreted as 'crying out' as, for example, in pain or anger. The careful use of descriptive words is crucial in avoiding ambiguity and subsequent errors in coding.

Patient	Sleeping	Eating	Walking	Reading	Watching TV
1		✓			
2	✓				
3	✓				
4			✓		
5					✓

Figure 31.2 A simple activity checklist

Box 31.3 An activity checklist used in structured observation

Walking

1 Unable to walk, even with maximum assistance.
2 Constant assistance of one or two persons is required during ambulation.
3 Assistance is required with reaching aids and/or their manipulation. One person is required to offer assistance/support.
4 The patient is independent in walking up to 50 yards/m, or may require supervision for confidence or safety.
5 The patient must be able to assume the standing position, sit down and use necessary walking aids correctly. The patient must be able to walk 50 yards/m without help or supervision.

When the category system has been developed, the next stage is to assess its face and content validity. This can be achieved by seeking the views of a panel of individuals who have expertise in the topic of the investigation. When testing for face validity, the individuals are asked to comment on the appropriateness of the categories and the clarity of the wording. Assessing the content validity involves asking for views of the appropriateness of each item of the category system and whether, in their view, it is sufficiently complete or whether additional behaviours should be recorded.

Activity checklist

Activity checklists are developed from the subcategory systems. These can be simple lists that require to be coded, as shown in Figure 31.2. Alternatively, they can be more complex. Using a numerical coding scheme to rate the activity can provide a more qualitative level of observation, as indicated in Box 31.3 where 'walking' is rated using the criteria given for ambulation in the Modified Barthel Index (Shah *et al.* 1989).

The next stage in the process is to establish the reliability of the schedule. Reliability in observational methods refers to the consistency with which categories of observation are identified and recorded when the same behaviours are observed and recorded, either by different observers or by the same observer on different occasions. There are therefore two aspects of reliability that ought to be tested during the development of the schedule. These are the *inter-observer* reliability, that is, the level of reliability of the schedule when used by more than one observer, and its *intra-observer* reliability, also described as test–retest reliability, that is, the level of reliability of the schedule when used by the same observer on more than one occasion.

If more than one observer is used to collect data on the same phenomena, it is important that they are trained in using the observation schedule and that the *inter-observer* reliability is evaluated. This involves each observer collecting and recording data on the same situation at the same time and using statistical procedures to analyse the results. The kappa statistic is a measure of agreement based on the proportion of subjects who give the same responses (Armitage & Berry 1994). The value of kappa can range from zero, which indicates no agreement, to 1.0 which indicates perfect agreement. A value that exceeds 0.75 represents excellent agreement; values less than 0.4 indicate poor agreement. *Intra-observer* reliability can be assessed using the same statistical procedure, but in this case, the data are collected and recorded on the same behaviours on different occasions by only one observer. It may be difficult to ensure that the same behaviours can be observed on separate occasions. This can be overcome by using a video recording of the activity and making recordings during a series of showings.

The observation schedule can be used in conjunction with a diagram of the physical environment, and field notes can be made to provide a verbal description to place the quantitative recordings in context.

Reflection activity

Which of the two major observational approaches, participant and non-participant, would you be most likely to use and why?

ADVANTAGES AND DISADVANTAGES OF OBSERVATION

Observational methods have the advantage that they can uncover and describe practice and behaviours as they actually happen, rather than what people think or say they do. This is a fundamental advantage in fast-moving, rapidly changing health-care environments where accurate self-rating of activities is poor (Ampt *et al.* 2007). Observation also allows researchers to access the context in which study participants are operating and so can help to explain the phenomena that are observed. Unlike studies that rely on self-report data, real-time observational data is not subject to the effects of recall or to misinterpretation by the participant. They are therefore inherently more reliable. Observation can offer verification of self-report data and contribute to the reliability, validity, trustworthiness and rigour of a study.

Using a structured observation schedule helps to minimise observer bias in that the data that are collected are predetermined, as is the coding scheme (Schnelle *et al.* 2005). An advantage of using a previously validated observation schedule is that it allows researchers to replicate the work of others in different settings or with different populations. Since structured observation offers a means of collecting quantitative data, this method of data collection can be incorporated into descriptive or cross-sectional surveys or experiments (Curtis *et al.* 2003; Booth et al 2005; Pan *et al.* 2013). Designing a schedule provides other researchers with a tool with which to conduct replication studies.

While structured observation schedules undoubtedly have advantages in terms of reliability and validity, highly structured systems for coding and recording behaviour may prevent the capture of complex activities that occur spontaneously. Use of a rating scheme can have the effect of 'pigeonholing' observed behaviours such that inappropriate judgements are made about events under examination. In addition, any form of interruption during a period of observation is likely to result in incomplete data collection with the consequent need to abandon the unit of observation.

While useful in helping us to understand *what* people do, structured observation offers little insight into *why* they do it. Underlying meanings that are ascribed to behaviours remain inaccessible when structured observation is used as the primary and sole source of data. Participant observation, on the other hand, is intrinsically more flexible, but this is traded against issues of rigour.

Participant observation allows the researcher to reflect the reality of events as they occur and can be used to provide in-depth descriptions of behaviours, events and activities (Carnevale *et al.* 2008), thereby contributing to explaining them in their natural contexts (Oeye *et al.* 2007). The opportunity for the researcher to assume a participant role facilitates the development of trust between researcher and those being observed. This may help to break down barriers and lead to enhanced understanding of the subtleties of complex behaviour and dynamic interpersonal interaction. Participant observation offers a means of studying the art of nursing, whereas structured observation can be used to investigate its science. For any form of observation study, however, it has to be remembered that events that are observed represent only a 'snapshot' of the overall activity.

Throughout participant observation the researcher has two roles – as both nurse and researcher. This dual role has the potential to be a source of conflict. There is a risk that researchers may become immersed in the culture and fail to maintain sufficient distance between themselves, the culture and the participants, thereby losing their research perspective and threatening the credibility of the data.

One of the strongest criticisms that can be levelled at observation methods is that the presence of the observer, be that a person or a camera, may influence the very behaviours that are the focus of the study. Schnelle *et al.* (2005) have argued that prolonged exposure to observation reduces the likelihood of behaviour resulting from the 'observer effect'. However, this contention is problematic since one cannot know what the behaviour would have been had the subjects not been observed.

Observational methods of data collection are relatively time-consuming as the researcher needs to be present during the period of direct observation or when conducting or viewing video recordings and hence are considered costly to undertake.

VALIDITY AND RELIABILITY

As has been seen, observation can be used in both qualitative and quantitative studies. In qualitative studies, the terms used to encompass the concepts of validity and reliability have been described as 'trustworthiness' or 'rigour' (see Chapter 12).

In structured observation, the terms 'reliability' and 'validity' are pertinent. The use of a carefully designed tool for recording the observations is important. Using a structured observation schedule helps to minimise observer bias in that the data collected are predetermined, as is the coding scheme. All personnel who are involved as observers need to undergo training in using the schedule and in coding and recording the data to ensure consistency and inter-observer reliability of the study. Careful piloting can help identify problems such as observer bias so that corrective action can be taken before the main study is conducted.

The trustworthiness or validity of an observation study can be affected if the observer misconstrues certain phenomena, misinterprets their importance or is temporarily distracted or tired. Some behaviours may be outside the range of the observer's field of vision or specified observation period. Actions may be misinterpreted because the observer is not sufficiently knowledgeable about the topic of the study, or the observer may be influenced by a preconception of the situation that is observed.

The presence of the observer can also influence the behaviour of those being observed and hence the trustworthiness and validity of the data. The likelihood of this increases when a researcher conducts an observation study in his or her own workplace (Mulhall 2003). It also occurs when the observation is overt and the observed are aware of the process (Pan *et al.* 2013).

ETHICAL ISSUES

There are key principles that govern the ethics of nursing research. Adherence to these principles ensures that practitioners involved in undertaking research respect the autonomy and personhood of all participants.

Covert observation

In studies where covert observation is used, researchers should ensure that disclosure is made and debriefing provided for each participant when their participation in the study is completed. However, as a general principle, covert observation is not considered ethical because the autonomy of the individuals being observed, their right to information about the study and their right to consent are breached. In cases where covert observation is considered, alternative, more open ways of addressing the problem should be sought.

Overt observation

The researcher should plan the study such that all individuals who may be present during any period of observation are given full information about the study in advance so they can decide whether or not to take part. This may, however, prove difficult if, during the observation, an unanticipated event occurs that necessitates the presence of another individual or group of people. In this instance, the researcher may be required to seek consent retrospectively.

A further dilemma concerns what constitutes 'full information'. It could be argued that failure to provide full information diminishes the autonomy of the individual to make an informed decision regarding consent to participate. On the other hand, by providing full details of the phenomena to be observed, the researcher may risk influencing the participant's behaviour, thereby diminishing the validity of the study findings. As it is unethical to undertake research that is rendered less valid by the information that is given, it may be necessary to reach a compromise.

The principle of non-maleficence requires that the research does not cause harm. The researcher may come across an incident where they feel the need to intervene in clinical care, perhaps because of a sense of the need to 'help out' when clinical colleagues are overstretched, or where they observe inappropriate practice. This poses problems on at least two fronts. Firstly, such a distraction will prevent the continuous observation of the focus of the study. Secondly, it raises ethical issues concerning the professional clinical role of the nurse researcher. The Code of Professional Conduct for Nurses and Midwives (Nursing and Midwifery Council 2008) is clear in stating the necessity for intervention if patient care or safety is compromised. In situations that do not involve patients, researchers may need to discuss what has been observed with members of staff or colleagues. In such cases, the researcher's role as a participant observer may be changed to such an extent that the study can no longer continue.

CONCLUSION

Recording and analysing observed events and activities as they actually occur in naturalistic settings can enhance a study's scope to provide reliable and valid findings. This method of data collection is appropriate for qualitative and quantitative studies, and depending on the nature of the study, the researcher's role may involve participation to varying degrees. Importantly, when using observation, the researcher must consider the ethical issues associated with this method of data collection.

References

Ampt A, Westbrook J, Creswick N, Mallock N (2007) A comparison of self-reported and observational work sampling techniques for measuring time in nursing tasks. *Journal of Health Services Research and Policy* **12**(1): 18–24.

Armitage P, Berry G (1994) *Statistical Methods in Medical Research*. Oxford, Blackwell Science.

Berger R (2013) Now I see it, now I don't: researcher's position and reflexivity in qualitative research. *Qualitative Research* E-publication ahead of print. 1–16. DOI: 10.1177/1468794112468475.

Booth J, Hillier VF, Waters KR, Davidson I (2005) Effects of a stroke rehabilitation education programme for nurses. *Journal of Advanced Nursing* **49**(5): 465–473.

Carnevale FA, Macdonald ME, Bluebond-Langer M, McKeever P (2008) Using participant observation in pediatric health care settings: ethical challenges and solutions. *Journal of Child Health Care* **12**(1): 18–32.

Curtis V, Biran A, Deverell K, Hughes C, Bellamy K, Drasar B (2003) Hygiene in the home: relating bugs and behaviour. *Social Science and Medicine* **57**: 657–672.

Doherty-King B, Yoon JY, Pecanac K, Brown R, Mahoney J (2014) Frequency and duration of nursing care related to older patient mobility. *Journal of Nursing Scholarship* **46**(1): 20–27.

Francis D (2004) Learning from participants in field based research. *Journal of Education* **34**: 265–277.

Gold R (1969) Roles in sociological field observation. In: McCall G, Simmons J (eds) *Issues in Participant Observation: a text and reader*. London, Addison Wesley.

Hammersley M, Atkinson P (1995) *Ethnography: principles and practice*, 2nd edition. London, Routledge.

Malinowski B (1922) *Argonauts of the Western Pacific*. London, Routledge, Keegan and Paul.

Mead M (1935) *Sex and Temperament in Three Primitive Societies*. New York, Morrow.

Melnyck BM, Fineout-Overholt E (2005) *Evidence-Based Practice in Nursing and Healthcare. A guide to best practice*. Philadelphia, Lippincott Williams and Wilkins.

Millard L, Hallet C, Luker K (2006) Nurse-patient interaction and decision-making in care: patient involvement in community nursing. *Journal of Advanced Nursing* **55**(2): 142–150.

Mulhall A (2003) In the field: notes on observation in qualitative research. *Journal of Advanced Nursing* **41**: 306–313.

Nursing and Midwifery Council (2008) *Code of Professional Conduct*. London, NMC.

Oeye C, Bjelland AK, Skorpen A (2007) Doing participant observation in a psychiatric hospital – research ethics resumed. *Social Science and Medicine* **65**: 2296–2306.

Pan S, Tien K, Hung I, Lin Y, Sheng W, Wang M, Chang S, Kunin C, Chen Y (2013) Compliance of health care workers with hand hygiene practices: independent advantages of overt and covert observers. *PLoS ONE* **8**(1): e53746.

Petticrew M, Semple S, Hilton S, Creely KS, Eadie D, Ritchie D, Ferrell C, Christopher Y, Hurley F (2007) Covert observation in practice: lessons from the evaluation of the prohibition of smoking in public places in Scotland. *BMC Public Health* **7**: 204. DOI: 10.1186/1471-2458-7-204.

Polit D, Hungler B (2006) *Essentials of Nursing Research: methods, appraisal and utilisation*, 6th edition. Philadelphia, Lippincott.

Robson C (2011) *Real World Research*, 3rd edition. Chichester, John Wiley & Sons, Ltd.

Rosenhan D (1973) On being sane in insane places. *Science* **179**: 250–258.

Schnelle JF, Osterweil D, Simmons SF (2005) Improving the quality of nursing home care and medical-record accuracy with direct observational technologies. *The Gerontologist* **45**(5): 576–582.

Shah S, Vanclay F, Cooper B (1989) Improving the sensitivity of the Barthel Index for stroke rehabilitation. *Journal of Clinical Epidemiology* **42**: 703–709.

Spradley JP (1980) *Participant Observation*. New York, Holt, Rinehart & Winston.

Whyte RE (2004) *The Provision of Health Education on Smoking to Patients in Hospital: a critical evaluation of the role of diplomate nurses*, Unpublished PhD Thesis. Glasgow, Glasgow Caledonian University.

Whyte R, Watson HR, McIntosh J (2006) Nurses' opportunistic interventions with patients in relation to smoking. *Journal of Advanced Nursing* **55**(5): 568–577.

CHAPTER 32

Think Aloud Technique

Tracey Bucknall and Leanne M Aitken

Key points

- Think aloud is a technique that allows for the examination of an individual's thinking processes and decisions that are being considered at that point in time. Participants are asked to think aloud while carrying out specific tasks such as problem solving, diagnosis or patient management.
- Think aloud can be used in both simulated and natural settings, as well as conducted concurrently during the task and/or retrospectively during follow-up interviews.
- When planning to conduct a study using think aloud, it is necessary to consider the study setting, recruitment plans, data collection and data analysis processes and strategies to optimise validity and reliability of the data.
- Think aloud technique can be used as a single method or in a combination of methods.

INTRODUCTION

The process of comparing and evaluating information to form an opinion or decision about future actions is fundamental to human behaviour. Not surprisingly, making sound clinical decisions is a key attribute required of clinicians. Clinical decisions are usually made in a climate of uncertainty and with incomplete information. They frequently consist of a combination of factual information and value judgements, and as a result, practices may vary amongst clinicians even when similar information is available to them. The variation in clinical practice has been the subject of much debate, particularly with the growing interest in evidence-based practice. Patient, clinician and organisational characteristics have been shown to alter the context of a situation, thus changing the availability of information and subsequent patient outcomes (Bucknall *et al.* 2008). Yet in spite of a growing knowledge on the influence of context on clinical decision making, there remains limited understanding of the decision-making processes

The Research Process in Nursing, Seventh Edition. Edited by Kate Gerrish and Judith Lathlean.

Companion Website: www.wiley.com/go/gerrish/research

underlying clinical practice decisions. The think aloud technique, also referred to as verbal protocols, has been widely used in research to elicit information underlying thinking processes and actions.

WHAT IS THINKING ALOUD?

Thinking aloud is a technique that allows for the examination of an individual's thinking processes and decisions that are being considered at that point in time. Participants are asked to think aloud while carrying out specific tasks such as problem solving, diagnosis or patient management. Participants may be unaware of the topic of interest and are required to report only the information being considered and their intentions as they actually occur (Payne 1994).

Think aloud reports provide a sequential record of the participant's thinking and behaviour while completing the specific task. They supply the cues, context, processes, goals and strategies that comprise the affective and behavioural responses mediated by thinking (Schragen *et al.* 2000). In particular, it measures alternative information choices accessed and their sequence of selection, identifying the decision rules that guide an individual's search patterns (Johnson 1993).

BACKGROUND TO THINK ALOUD

As early as 1890, William James noted the importance of introspection as a method of scientific inquiry (James 1890). Verbal protocols were collected by behavioural psychologists to gather detailed descriptions of subjects' thinking. However, the validity of this approach was highly criticised as the subjects required prior training in introspective techniques in order to specify and interpret their own thinking as they proceeded. Then about 40 years ago, Newell and Simon (1972) used the think aloud part of introspection to pioneer verbal protocol analysis. Think aloud research has since been guided by the highly regarded work of Ericsson and Simon (1984, 1993) who assumed that verbal reports could be analysed like other behaviours.

Based on the principles of information theory, think aloud was used to concurrently report on subjects' thinking during problem-solving tasks (Newell & Simon 1972). Describing an interaction between the problem solver and the specified task, information processing assumes that decisions are based on information that has been processed and transformed by the human brain. This information may be stored in short- or long-term memory. Although short-term memory is readily accessible, it holds limited information for a short duration. In contrast, long-term memory is less accessible but has an unlimited capacity for storing information and is a combination of factual information and personal experiences. Using a complex system of integrated nodes, information is retrieved from long-term memory and transferred to short-term memory for quick response. A clinician's performance is then dependent on the acquisition, storage and retrieval of basic and updated knowledge and the integration of experience into long-term memory (Schmidt *et al.* 1990).

In clinical practice, health professionals are constantly confronted with large volumes of information that can only be partially processed at any one time. Clinical research based on information-processing theory has attempted to describe the process clinicians use to adapt to differing task complexities. Many believe clinicians adapt to task complexity and storage limitations by reducing information into workable chunks in order to quickly process information and focus on priorities (Newell & Simon 1972).

APPLYING THINK ALOUD IN NURSING RESEARCH

Close analysis of verbal protocols obtained from problem solvers as they worked out diagnostic or treatment decisions has provided valuable evidence of information use in clinical settings. In nursing, much of the research originally focused on the approaches that nurses used to decide on a diagnosis, with little emphasis on the management of patient problems. More recently, researchers have applied think aloud to study nurses' decision making during patient assessment and patient care as a means of improving patient outcomes (Aitken & Mardegan 2000). Think aloud research assists us to understand how nurses use information on which to base their practice decisions. As well as understanding the cognitive processes and inferences being drawn at the time, it can also be used to identify faulty reasoning (Offredy & Meerabeau 2006). Payne (1994) also suggests that think aloud may be useful:

- in providing early insight into behaviours
- for pretesting questionnaires to improve clarity
- to compare it with data collected by other methods
- to test hypothesis about behaviour
- to build and test models of behaviour such as expert systems

Think aloud can be used in both simulated and natural settings, as well as conducted concurrently during the task and/or retrospectively during interviews following observation.

Think aloud has also been used in combination with other methods to offer greater insight into a phenomenon than a single method alone. Given that all research methods have strengths and weaknesses, think aloud may be used to reinforce or offer alternative viewpoints from the findings from other approaches. For example, a recent study by Bucknall and colleagues used participant think aloud following observation of clinical nurse handover, observations from a non-participant observer and a ward environment assessment that included staffing resources and patient profiles. From these data, we could analyse the type of information given in handover, the type of data sought following handover, the influencing contextual characteristics and the use of the information in planning nursing care.

Research Example 32.1 provides an overview of six studies that illustrate the different uses of the think aloud methodology in gaining an understanding of the decision-making processes and products of nursing across different clinical settings.

Reflection activity

Identify a research question that you are interested to answer where think aloud would be a good method to use to collect data. What thinking and decision-making processes are you keen to learn more about?

HOW TO USE THINK ALOUD

When planning to conduct a study using think aloud, it is necessary to consider a variety of questions regarding the aims of the study that will influence the specific method that is used. These questions concern the study setting, recruitment plans, data collection and analysis processes and strategies to optimise validity and reliability of the data.

Possibly, the most fundamental question regarding method is whether the work can be conducted in the natural setting or whether a simulated setting provides an environment that will adequately answer the questions being considered. Natural settings enable you to study your research question in the usual practice environment, thereby enhancing external validity of your findings; however, it is limited by needing to conform to the restrictions of usual practice and does not allow you to control the research setting (Aitken & Mardegan 2000).

In contrast, simulated settings allow easy control and reproducibility of the decision scenario and the ability to preselect the task that you wish to study in order to optimise the relevance to the research question and to compress the elements of the decision task, thereby reducing the time and resources required (Fonteyn *et al.* 1993; Aitken & Mardegan

RESEARCH EXAMPLE

32.1 Different Approaches to Using Think Aloud

Study 1 Using think aloud in simulations

Fossum M, Alexander GL, Goransson KE, Ehnfors M, Ehrenberg A (2011) Registered nurses' thinking strategies on malnutrition and pressure ulcers in nursing homes: a scenario-based think-aloud study. *Journal of Clinical Nursing* **20**: 2425–2435.

The aim of this study was to explore the thinking strategies and clinical reasoning processes registered nurses use during simulated care planning for malnutrition and pressure ulcers in nursing home care. Thirty registered nurse participants were asked to work through four written scenarios using a concurrent think aloud approach. A variety of thinking strategies were identified after qualitative deductive content analysis; the most common of these included 'making choices', 'forming relationships' and 'drawing conclusions'. Structured risk assessments related to malnutrition or development of pressure ulcers were not performed by any of the study participants who moved very rapidly from assessment into the planning phase of their thinking. The think aloud method of data collection was effective in highlighting the lack of systematic risk assessment and the focus on planning within the clinical reasoning cycle.

Study 2 Using think aloud in natural settings

Tower M, Chaboyer W, Green Q, Dyer K, Wallis M (2012) Registered nurses' decision-making regarding documentation in patients' progress notes. *Journal of Clinical Nursing* **21**: 2917–2929.

Situated in clinical practice, this study examined 17 registered nurses' decision making when documenting care in patients' progress notes. Participants were supplied with a digital recorder after training in think aloud. They were asked to record their think aloud strategies as they were documenting their end of shift reports. Results from data collected during think aloud research in the natural setting are considered more reliable than data collected in simulated situations of practice. In this study, follow-up interviews were also used to confirm interpretations and expand on data collected. In documenting progress notes, three scenarios were evident: the new patient, as expected patient progress and the discharging patient. Nurses used mental models for decision making with cues directing their assessments. In addition, situation awareness was demonstrated at different levels in decision making highlighting both the present situation and anticipation of future events.

Study 3 Using think aloud concurrently and retrospectively in natural settings

Aitken LM, Marshall AP, Elliott R, McKinley S (2009) Critical care nurses' decision making: sedation assessment and management in intensive care. *Journal of Clinical Nursing* **18**: 36–45.

The purpose of this study was to investigate the decision making of Australian critical care nurses as they assessed and managed the sedation needs of critically ill patients. Using the think aloud approach, the researchers studied the nurses while they cared for critically ill patients over a 2 hour period. Nurses were asked to describe the data they were collecting and their responses to those data. They were advised not to try and explain their thinking as that information would be followed up during the interviews. Data analysis used the transcripts from both concurrent and retrospective think aloud sessions. Attributes and concepts used in the assessment and management of sedation were identified, with an average of approximately 50 relevant attributes raised during 2 hours of care. The complexity of decision making in this environment is demonstrated through the results of this study. In addition, the detail of the types of attributes, including assessment, physiology and treatment, provides important detail to inform education and skills development in the field.

Study 4 Using think aloud to compare nurses' decision-making accuracy

Goransson KE, Ehnfors M, Fonteyn ME, Ehrenberg A (2008) Thinking strategies used by registered nurses during emergency department triage. *Journal of Advanced Nursing* **61**: 163–172.

This study of 16 RNs was set in an emergency department triage area in Sweden. The aim of this study was to describe and compare nurses' thinking processes, strategies and triage accuracy. Nurses were preselected from the results of a previous study examining triage accuracy. Five scenarios based on real patient situations were developed. Participants read the scenario aloud and verbalised their thinking as if they were actually reviewing a triage patient. Content analysis was used to analyse verbatim transcripts. The research demonstrated a wide variety of thinking strategies being used by nurses with surprisingly little difference between nurses based on the previous study of accuracy.

Study 5 Using think aloud to compare nurse practitioners and general practitioners

Lundgren-Laine H, Kontio E, Perttila J, Korvenranta H, Forsstrom J, Salantera S (2011) Managing daily intensive care activities: an observational study concerning *ad hoc* decision making of charge nurses and intensivists. *Critical Care* **15**(4): R188.

The purpose of this study was to describe the ad hoc decision making of ICU shift leaders including both nursing and medical shift leaders. Twelve charge nurses and eight intensivists used think aloud in the clinical setting while coordinating the activities within an ICU. Concurrent observation and recording of situation-related notes by one of the researchers also occurred. Qualitative content analysis was used to identify each decision, with protocol analysis applied to identify the level of verbalisation that occurred and the nature of ad hoc decisions made by participants. Data were collected on morning, evening and night shifts with between 2 and 6 hours of data collection occurring for each participant. This data collection and analysis process was effective in identifying that on average 10 ad hoc decisions were made by each participant every hour, with these decisions forming eight categories including (i) adverse events, (ii) diagnostics, (iii) human resources and know-how, (iv) material resources, (v) patient admission, (vi) patient discharge, (vii) patient information and vital signs and (viii) special treatments.

Study 6 Using think aloud to validate patient management tools

Hagen N, Stiles C, Nekolaichuk C, Biondo P, Carlson L, Fisher K, Fainsinger R (2008) The Alberta breakthrough pain assessment tool for cancer patients: a validation study using a Delphi process and patient think-aloud interviews. *Journal of Pain and Symptom Management* **35**(2): 136–152.

Breakthrough pain in cancer patients is difficult for clinicians to manage. To measure the effectiveness of interventions requires a standardised validated tool that can be appropriately used by patients. This study used think aloud by patients as an additional measure of validating a questionnaire on pain assessment. Nine patients completed the survey. They were told to talk about what they were thinking as much as possible while completing the form. The information provided specific feedback on areas of improvement with revisions being made when multiple patients reported similar difficulty. The think aloud method was reported to be useful in providing both clarity and feasibility of tool completion.

Reflection activity

What are the advantages and disadvantages of undertaking think aloud in natural or in simulation settings? Which approach would you select to examine the research question you identified earlier and why?

2000). However, depending on the research question being investigated and the level of complexity of the simulated environment, it may not truly replicate the characteristics that influence practice or allow for interaction between the participant and either patients or colleagues, thereby limiting the external validity of findings (Lutfey *et al.* 2008). Where simulations are used, it is essential that they are developed through thorough review of real practice, with extensive review by experts in the field to ensure content validity (Fonteyn *et al.* 1993; Goransson *et al.* 2007; Fossum *et al.* 2011).

RECRUITMENT

Elements to determine when developing a plan for recruitment of participants into a study using think aloud include the number of participants, any particular levels or types of experience or expertise of the participants and the process to be used to recruit participants.

Participant numbers in think aloud studies are generally relatively low due to the depth and richness of data that are usually gained from each participant, with some reports suggesting that as few as five or six participants produce reasonably stable results (Van Den Haak *et al.* 2003). As participant numbers increase, there is the ability to synthesise findings from individual participants and make some comparisons across the participants, as well as to draw some inferences about the overall reasoning process (Fonteyn *et al.* 1993). Large participant numbers are more likely to be found in short decision scenarios studied in the simulated setting (Lutfey *et al.* 2008).

Consideration of whether participants' prior experience or expertise might influence the study question is essential. A number of studies using think aloud have limited investigation to participants with specific expertise, for example, novices or experts, or specific experience, for example, extensive triage experience. Alternatively, groups of participants at opposing ends of the spectrum have been included to allow comparison of findings to determine common and unique cognitive processes (Hoffman *et al.* 2009).

DATA COLLECTION

The process used for data collection in think aloud studies will vary depending on the research question being answered, the setting for the study and the time frame needed to collect sufficient data to answer the question. Despite these differences, the common principles of audio recording, training of participants, provision of instructions and interaction with the participant will need to be considered for all think aloud studies.

Data collected from the participant will be recorded on an audio recorder (in some instances video recording will also be used). It is essential that the audio recorder is an appropriate size and placed to avoid interruption to the participant's usual processes. A small lapel-mounted microphone attached to a pocket-size recorder is often ideal. Pilot work using the study equipment within the study environment is essential to determine the quality of the audio recording and the amount of background noise so as to ensure the think aloud is able to be adequately heard for transcription purposes.

Training participants in the technique of think aloud is an important component of data collection and provides an opportunity for the researcher to explain to participants that they should only be attempting to verbalise, not rationalise, their thought processes. Training also allows participants to practice the process and ask any questions they might have, particularly those regarding what elements of information should be verbalised (Li 2004). One of the most common exercises given to participants to train them in the method of think aloud is to ask them to 'count the number of windows in their home' as it requires sequential progression through various rooms in their home while being a simple exercise that most participants are able to complete rapidly, thereby giving confidence in the technique. Other exercises include counting the number of dots on a page or performing an arithmetic exercise. Some investigators consider that it is important to select practice tasks where the researcher can verify the accuracy of the verbalisations (Nicholls & Polman 2008).

Other information provided to participants prior to beginning data collection include the need to keep talking as long as the participant is thinking, as well as the lack of need to provide an explanation or rationale for thoughts or actions, or to make thoughts rational (Aitken & Mardegan 2000; Nicholls & Polman 2008). If a follow-up interview is being used, it is useful to emphasise that this interview is able to be used for clarification of decision processes. The clarity and simplicity of instructions to participants are particularly important in limiting the bias to participants' cognitive processing. Wherever possible, participants should not be told the explicit hypotheses being investigated in the study but instead be given general information. For example, in a series of studies investigating critical care nursing practice, participants have been advised that the investigator was interested in how they cared for critically ill patients rather than advice that indicated a specific interest in haemodynamic monitoring (Aitken 2000) or sedation assessment and management (Aitken *et al.* 2009). Such strategies help to reduce the likelihood that participants will be tempted to concentrate on a specific area of practice in a way that does not reflect usual processes.

Interaction with the participant should be minimal during data collection, preferably limited to prompts to 'keep talking' or 'keep thinking aloud' when the participant stops verbalising (Ericsson & Simon 1993; Van Den Haak *et al.* 2003). This guidance is intended to reduce any influence or change to the usual cognitive processes. Throughout the data collection session, it is helpful if the researcher takes notes regarding the activities that are being undertaken. These notes will help to inform a follow-up interview if one is being used and also to provide clarity and context during data analysis.

DATA ANALYSIS

Analysis of think aloud data generally consists of three steps including transcribing, segmenting and coding.

Transcribing

The first stage of data analysis requires converting the verbal data from an audio recording to a verbatim transcription. Depending on whether the think aloud process was conducted within the natural or simulated setting, this transcription may be time-consuming and problematic if there is significant background noise, poor quality recording or lack of clarity of the participant's speech. Transcription may be more accurate if it is carried out by someone who is familiar with the content area (Fonteyn *et al.* 1993); however, care must be taken that they transcribe only the words that were actually verbalised rather than what the transcriber might be expecting.

Segmenting

This phase of data analysis involves dividing the transcription into meaningful components so that each segment deals with a single, but complete, decision process (Yang 2003). At this point, most investigators remove data that are not relevant to the decision task, for example, social interaction with colleagues.

Coding

Coding involves assigning categories or concepts to each of the identified segments. These codes may consist of a single level or alternatively incorporate multiple levels of categories and subcategories. Within the coding component of analysis, there is a requirement to develop the coding schemes and protocols – this may be undertaken prior to data collection with categories determined a priori based on current literature or practice (Ericsson & Simon 1993) or may be developed inductively throughout data analysis with the data informing development of categories (Fonteyn *et al.* 1993; Yang 2003; Bloem *et al.* 2008; Nicholls & Polman 2008).

Box 32.1 An example of think aloud analysis

Think aloud transcript

Hi, just woken him up a little bit, just assessed him neurological, so he's just opened his eyes a tiny bit. .... It's alright; your daughters are here with you; you're doing really well. Just woken up, that's good. You want to put your hand out for a while? I'm just putting your arm down, so your elbow's not touching the rail there... there you go. .... It's alright. That's fine.

I'm just going to do his fluids, his noradrenaline; he's had 18mls this last hour. The milrinone is still on 5 and his insulin is on 15, which is 3 units of heparin an hour, and I've put his morphine down to one because his respiratory rate was dropping, dropped down to 8, and since we've woken him up, etc., his respiratory rates come up to 10, which is good. Just doing his urinary output, he's got good urine output of 260 ml, and I'm going to turn this [noradrenaline] down a little because he's awake and his blood pressure is good at the moment.

.... Yeah, that's fine because like with the sedation tonight, he had quite a bit, and his respiratory rate dropped down a little, so we thought we'd just lighten him a little bit. See how he goes, but if he gets restless, agitated or indicates that he has pain or anything, we'll give him a bit more analgesia. The other thing is I've just come on duty so I've just neurologically assessed him, so I've spoken to him and got him to move his arms and things.

We just like to know that he's awake and doing all the right things, which he is. He's restoring from painful stimuli, which is good, and he's, um, you know he's got a lot of analgesia on board because pupils are quite pinpoint. But they're reactive, yeah, but they're very tiny.

Phrase	Category	Cues used
Hi, just woken him up a little bit, just assessed him neurological, so his just opened his eyes a tiny bit	Assessment	Responsiveness
It's alright; your daughters are here with you; you're doing really well	Management	
Just woken up, that's good	Assessment	Responsiveness
I've put his morphine down to one because his respiratory rate was dropping, dropped down to 8, and since we've woken him up, etc., his respiratory rates come up to 10, which is good	Diagnosis	Respiratory rate Morphine dose
I'm going to turn this [noradrenaline] down a little because he's awake and his blood pressure is good at the moment	Planning	Wakefulness Blood pressure Noradrenaline dose
Yeah, that's fine because like with the sedation tonight, he had quite a bit, and his respiratory rate dropped down a little, so we thought we'd just lighten him a little bit	Planning	Sedation dose Respiratory rate Responsiveness
But if he gets restless, agitated or indicates that he has pain or anything, we'll give him a bit more analgesia	Planning	Agitation Pain

Continued

Phrase	Category	Cues used
We just like to know that he's awake and doing all the right things, which he is	Evaluation	Wakefulness
He's withdrawing from painful stimuli, which is good	Assessment	Response to painful stimuli
He's, um, you know he's got a lot of analgesia on board because pupils are quite pinpoint. But they're reactive, yeah, but they're very tiny	Evaluation	Pupil size Dose of analgesia

There are two perspectives regarding how to approach coding, with Ericsson and Simon (1993) recommending that segments are coded in random order, thereby reducing the possibility of introducing bias as a result of the contextual information provided prior to and following the segment. Using this process is believed to increase the likelihood that the analysis is an accurate reflection of what was actually said, rather than what the analyst believed the participant was thinking or how the analyst would have thought in a similar situation.

The alternative, and most common, perspective is to code the data in sequential order, thereby allowing the contextual information to inform the interpretation of the data. Throughout this process, the analyst builds up an overall understanding of the data including different patterns between individual participants. To reduce the chance of bias, strategies such as dual coding by two analysts and limited knowledge of the study hypotheses and participants' background should be used (strategies are discussed under 'Issues of validity and reliability').

Detailed steps within the coding phase have been described, with one of the most clear processes put forward by Fonteyn and colleagues (Fonteyn *et al.* 1993). These authors propose a three-step coding process involving:

- referring phrase analysis – identification of all nouns and noun phrases to allow identification of the concepts used by the participant
- assertional analysis – identification of the assertions made by participants to determine the relationships between concepts
- script analysis – identification of the operators used by participants and how they structured the problems, made choices and progressed through the decision process

Box 32.1 demonstrates an example of think aloud analysis.

VALIDITY AND RELIABILITY

There has been limited investigation of the reliability and validity of think aloud as a data collection technique within various settings including health care. Considerations to optimise validity and reliability include specifying what level of verbalisation is being sought from participants, the timing of data collection and processes to optimise each phase of data analysis.

Ericsson and Simon (1993) describe three levels of verbalisation identified below:

1. Vocalisation of covert articulation that requires no intermediate processes and the subject is not required to expend special effort to achieve this.
2. Description and explication of the thought content that does not require bringing new information, but simply explicating or labelling information that is held in a compressed internal format.
3. Explanation and discussion of thought processes that involves linking information from both short- and long-term memories.

Ericsson and Simon (1993) argue that level 1 and 2 verbalisations do not change the sequence of information; however, level 3 verbalisation requires an additional process of information retrieval that changes the sequence of heeded information and therefore no longer reliably reflects the usual cognitive processes. This view is supported by a number of other researchers in the field (Yang 2003; Nicholls & Polman 2008) but argued against by others (Davison *et al.* 1995; Nielsen & Yssing 2004; Guan *et al.* 2006). The opposing view, although in the minority in the literature, does suggest that practitioners think faster than they speak, have difficulty verbalising the complexity of their thought processes and consider that think aloud interferes with their usual problem-solving process (Nielsen & Yssing 2004).

The reliability of data collection through think aloud may be affected by the timing of the data collection. Concurrent think aloud is often considered to accurately and completely reflect the usual cognitive processes used in performing the task (Fonteyn *et al.* 1993), while retrospective think aloud is more likely to be open to error through either inaccurate memory of the decision task or the requirement to explain a procedure and therefore access long-term memory (Yang 2003). Despite this, a benefit of retrospective think aloud is that it does not require the participant to verbalise until after the task is complete, therefore reducing the interference with usual task processes (Guan *et al.* 2006). A combination of concurrent and retrospective think aloud is considered as a potential strategy to provide the most accurate and full description of the reasoning used during a particular problem-solving task (Fonteyn *et al.* 1993; Whyte *et al.* 2009). Whyte and colleagues (2009) demonstrated that concurrent think aloud provided a more complete representation of decision processes, but that retrospective think aloud added additional unique data not captured in the concurrent verbal reports. This combination of concurrent and retrospective data collection has been used in a number of studies into nursing practice (Aitken 2000; Goransson *et al.* 2008; Aitken *et al.* 2009) as well as other fields (Bloem *et al.* 2008).

Each phase of the data analysis should be checked by a second person to ensure inter-coder reliability. In the transcribing phase, this is relatively easy and involves someone other than the transcriber listening to the audio tapes as they check the content against the transcription and should be carried out on all the data from each participant. Within the segmenting phase, reliability testing can be achieved by having a second coder segment a component of the transcriptions, with segments compared between the coders (Ericsson & Simon 1993). If significant differences are present between the two versions of analysis, further discussion and clarification of the rules guiding this phase of the analysis are required, before repeating the process. Reliability testing of the coding phase of data analysis should also be undertaken, using a similar process to that outlined for the segmenting phase. Assessment of inter-coder reliability for the segmenting and encoding phases is usually carried out on 10–20% of the study data (Goransson *et al.* 2008).

Bias in data analysis may also occur, generally as a result of the data coders having prior knowledge of the research question or hypotheses under investigation and therefore subconsciously wanting to support or disprove the hypotheses. Alternatively, data coders may expect participants to think in the same way that they do and therefore add meaning to the analysis that is not explicit in the data. In regard to the first source of bias, if possible, data coders should be limited in their knowledge of the explicit hypotheses under investigation, as well as group membership, for example, if there are both novice and expert participants in the study (Goransson *et al.* 2008). The second source of bias can be limited by coders randomly coding segments of information rather than coding them in sequential order, by having coders without domain-specific knowledge (Li 2004) or alternatively by computerising as much of the analysis as possible (Li 2004; Goransson *et al.* 2007).

One technique that has been suggested to improve the trustworthiness of think aloud data is to return the analysis to each participant to verify whether the protocols compiled for them truly reflect their cognitive processes (Li 2004; Nicholls & Polman 2008). The value of this process may be limited as it is unlikely that participants can accurately recall their cognitive

Reflection activity

What steps could you take to enhance the rigour of your proposed study using the think aloud technique?

processes (Fonteyn *et al.* 1993) or alternatively participants may actually proceed through a decision scenario in a different manner to how they believe, although it is reasonable to expect they may be able to confirm broad concepts.

ETHICAL ISSUES

Earlier studies by nursing researchers were mostly conducted in simulated settings due to ethical concerns about disruption to the participant's thinking that may potentially lead to patient care errors in real clinical settings. However, there is evidence to suggest that the talking that occurs is similar to discussions that routinely take place between students and educators or doctors and nurses and therefore should not compromise patient care (Greenwood & King 1995; Aitken 2000; Aitken & Mardegan 2000).

Two processes can be followed to reduce the risk of harm to patients. First, an explanation of the process to the patients and families should be provided prior to commencing data collection. In this situation, explanations are usually given to them about the process and a reassurance that the data collection will be stopped if they find it upsetting. Second, the participants are encouraged not to verbalise any information which they believe would be upsetting for the patient to hear. Information can be discussed either away from the bedside or at a later point in time during the interview process (Greenwood & King 1995; Aitken & Mardegan 2000).

Other ethical considerations regarding privacy and anonymity of patient information can be addressed by deleting any identifying information that is audio recorded inadvertently from the written transcripts.

Reflection activity

Identify the ethical issues associated with using think aloud to answer the research question you identified earlier. What steps could you take to address these ethical issues?

Given the focus of the study is on the individual nurse's thinking and the low level of risk for patients, then patient consent may not always be required.

Other ethical issues concerning recruitment and data collection are not unique to think aloud. Similar concerns were documented in an observational study by Bucknall (2000, 2003) where audio recordings of an observer following a nurse were collected. However, in think aloud, it is particularly important that participation is voluntary in order to minimise the chance that participants strive to provide data that they believe is being sought and to be truthful in their responses (Li 2004). Ensuring that the conduct, particularly the recruitment and data analysis, is not undertaken by anyone in a management role within the study setting will also help to increase the truthfulness of the data provided.

STRENGTHS AND LIMITATIONS

Think aloud provides a unique opportunity to study decision making in the natural clinical setting in that it offers a greater understanding of observed behaviour compared with the same subject working under silent conditions (Ericsson & Simon 1993). In particular, it makes available detailed information concurrently being processed by the decision maker. Although it is relatively inexpensive to collect the information, data analysis is detailed and very time-consuming.

Importantly, participants do not need to be trained in the process of introspection in order to carry out the task, as interpretation is not required. Subjects need to be instructed only to verbalise their thoughts as they arise, not to try and explain them (Ericsson & Simon 1993). Retrospective recall during interviews and field observations can later be used for this purpose. However, retrospective reports are subject to recall bias, where reconstruction of the decision process may occur rather than the actual processing, and as a result are less valued than concurrent reports. Nevertheless, Ericsson and Simon (1998) have recognised that when subjects are asked to retrospectively explain their thinking, their performance is changed and, indeed, mostly improved. Such cases offer an educational opportunity to improve student reasoning and have been likened to researchers expressing their analysis in writing.

However, three main concerns have been raised about think aloud reports. These are:

- the validity of reports equating to thinking
- the reactivity of subjects when reporting their thinking
- the objectivity of the reports compared with other behavioural research (Crutcher 1994)

Critics of think aloud argue that verbalisations may reflect the norms for behaviour rather than verification of the underlying processes because people are unable to report on higher-order mental processes. It is also recognised that heavy cognitive loads may limit verbalisations, although their completeness may depend on conscious processing of information (Ericsson & Simon 1993).

In addition, think aloud has been criticised for increasing reaction times for task performance and changing the outcomes of decisions. In using cognitive resources to verbalise thinking, think aloud may alter the process or at the very least focus the person on information that is more readily available to report. However, Barber and Roehling (1993) found that think aloud reports using two different mediums (written or verbal reports) did not affect task performance of information requested or decision outcomes. They also investigated the effect of prompts on task performance and found no discernable differences between the control and experimental groups. Similarly, Williamson and colleagues (2000) argued that prompts do not lead to reactivity but rather encouraged the subject to articulate their thoughts in more detail. Sudden insight from the subject may be in fact the retrieval of prior knowledge from long-term memory, reorganised into new schemata (Smagorinsky 1998).

Similar to all research, the quality and objectivity of the research is dependent on the process. Apart from deciding if think aloud is the most appropriate method for studying the decision task, the objectivity of reports depends on the preparation of the subject in the think aloud process and quality of the data collection process. Evidence to support the validity of think aloud was demonstrated by Biggs *et al.* (1993) study comparing data from concurrent verbal protocols with a computer search. Although think aloud increased the time to process, it did not affect the type of information, the amount selected or the accuracy of the decision.

More generally, a criticism of the approach is one levelled at most qualitative research methods, that is, a consequence of using small numbers means the results are not generalisable outside the study population. Although think aloud generally uses small numbers, the analysis of many decision-making instances is similar to repeating an experiment multiple times over – this is also known as replication logic. This process does allow for theoretical generalisation to existing theory rather than generalisation to other populations.

CONCLUSION

The think aloud approach provides a unique way of eliciting information about the cues, context, processes, goals and strategies that comprise an individual nurse's response to information in clinical or simulated settings. Identifying alternatives and their sequence of selection offers researchers an opportunity to view and understand the decision rules that guide clinicians during patient care. Think aloud can be used concurrently or retrospectively, as a single method or in a combination of methods. Data analysis can comprise both qualitative and quantitative techniques depending on the focus of the study. Notably, the think aloud technique is a low-risk, economical way of increasing our understanding of clinical decision making and offers greater insight into problem solving than methods where behaviour is viewed in silence.

References

Aitken LM (2000) Expert critical care nurses' use of pulmonary artery pressure monitoring. *Intensive and Critical Care Nursing* **16**: 209–220.

Aitken LM, Mardegan KJ (2000) 'Thinking aloud': data collection in the natural setting. *Western Journal of Nursing Research* **22**: 841–853.

Aitken LM, Marshall A, Elliott R, McKinley S (2009) Critical care nurses' decision making: sedation assessment and management in intensive care. *Journal of Clinical Nursing* **18**: 36–45.

Barber AE, Roehling MV (1993) Job postings and the decision to interview: a verbal protocol analysis. *Journal of Applied Psychology* **78**: 845–856.

Biggs SF, Rosman AJ, Sergenian GK (1993) Methodological issues in judgment and decision-making research: concurrent verbal protocol validity and simultaneous traces of process. *Journal of Behavioral Decision Making* **6**: 187–206.

Bloem EF, van Zuuren FJ, Koeneman MA, Rapkin BD, Visser MR, Koning CC, Sprangers MA (2008) Clarifying quality of life assessment: do theoretical models capture the underlying cognitive processes? *Quality of Life Research* **17**: 1093–1102.

Bucknall TK (2000) Critical care nurses' decision-making activities in the natural clinical setting. *Journal of Clinical Nursing* **9**: 25–36.

Bucknall TK (2003) The clinical landscape of critical care: nurses' decision-making. *Journal of Advanced Nursing* **43**: 310–319.

Bucknall TK, Kent B, Manley K (2008) Evidence use and evidence generation in practice development. In: Manley K, McCormack B, Wilson V (eds) *International Practice Development in Nursing and Healthcare*. Oxford, Wiley-Blackwell, pp 84–104.

Crutcher R (1994) Telling what we know: the use of verbal report methodologies in psychological research. *Psychological Science* **5**: 241–243.

Davison GC, Navarre SG, Vogel RS (1995) The articulated thoughts in simulated situations paradigm: a think-aloud approach to cognitive assessment. *Current Directions in Psychological Science* **4**: 29–33.

Ericsson KA, Simon HA (1984) *Protocol Analysis: verbal reports as data*. Cambridge, MA, MIT Press.

Ericsson KA, Simon HA (1993) *Protocol Analysis: verbal reports as data*. Cambridge, MA, MIT Press.

Ericsson KA, Simon HA (1998) How to study thinking in everyday life: contrasting think-aloud protocols with descriptions and explanations of thinking. *Mind, Culture, and Activity* **5**: 178–186.

Fonteyn ME, Kuipers B, Grobe SJ (1993) A description of think aloud method and protocol analysis. *Qualitative Health Research* **3**: 430–441.

Fossum M, Alexander GL, Goransson KE, Ehnfors M, Ehrenberg A (2011) Registered nurses' thinking strategies on malnutrition and pressure ulcers in nursing homes: a scenario-based think-aloud study. *Journal of Clinical Nursing* **20**: 2425–2435.

Goransson KE, Ehrenberg A, Ehnfors M, Fonteyn M (2007) An effort to use qualitative data analysis software for analysing think aloud data. *International Journal of Medical Informatics* **76**(Suppl 2): S270–S273.

Goransson KE, Ehnfors M, Fonteyn ME, Ehrenberg A (2008) Thinking strategies used by registered nurses during emergency department triage. *Journal of Advanced Nursing* **61**: 163–172.

Greenwood J, King M (1995) Some surprising similarities in the clinical reasoning of 'expert' and 'novice' orthopaedic nurses: report of a study using verbal protocols and protocol analyses. *Journal of Advanced Nursing* **22**: 907–913.

Guan Z, Lee S, Cuddihy E, Ramey J (2006) The validity of the stimulated retrospective think-aloud method as measured by eye tracking. Paper presented at the Proceedings of ACM CHI 2006 Conference on Human Factors in Computing Systems, Montreal, Canada.

Hoffman KA, Aitken LM, Duffield C (2009) A comparison of novice and expert nurses' cue collection during clinical decision-making: verbal protocol analysis. *International Journal of Nursing Studies* **46**: 1335–1344.

James W (1890) *The Principles of Psychology*. New York, Holt.

Johnson M (1993) Thinking about strategies during, before, and after making a decision. *Psychology and Aging* **8**: 231–241.

Li D (2004) Trustworthiness of think-aloud protocols in the study of translation processes. *International Journal of Applied Linguistics* **14**: 301–313.

Lundgren-Laine H, Kontio E, Perttila J, Korvenranta H, Forsstrom J, Salantera S (2011) Managing daily intensive care activities: an observational study concerning *ad hoc* decision making of charge nurses and intensivists. *Critical Care* **15**(4): R188.

Lutfey KE, Campbell SM, Renfrew MR, Marceau LD, Roland M, McKinlay JB (2008) How are patient characteristics relevant for physicians' clinical decision making in diabetes? An analysis of qualitative results from a cross-national factorial experiment. *Social Science and Medicine* **67**: 1391–1399.

Newell A, Simon HA (1972) *Human Problem Solving*. Englewood Cliffs, Prentice-Hall.

Nicholls AR, Polman RC (2008) Think aloud: acute stress and coping strategies during golf performances. *Anxiety Stress Coping* **21**: 283–294.

Nielsen J, Yssing C (2004) *Working paper: the disruptive effect of think aloud.* Copenhagen, Department of Informatics, Copenhagen Business School.

Offredy M, Meerabeau E (2006) The use of 'think aloud' technique, information processing theory and schema theory to explain decision-making processes of general practitioners and nurse practitioners using patient scenarios. *Primary Health Care Research and Development* **6**: 46–59.

Payne JW (1994) Thinking aloud: insights into information processing. *Psychological Science* **5**: 241–248.

Schmidt HG, Norman GR, Boshuizen HP (1990) A cognitive perspective on medical expertise: theory and implications. *Academic Medicine* **65**: 611–621.

Schragen J, Chipman S, Shalin V (eds) (2000) *Cognitive Task Analysis.* Mahwah, NJ, Lawrence Erlbaum Associates.

Smagorinsky P (1998) Thinking and speech and protocol analysis. *Mind, Culture, and Activity* **5**: 157–177.

Tower M, Chaboyer W, Green Q, Dyer K, Wallis M (2012) Registered nurses' decision-making regarding documentation in patients' progress notes. *Journal of Clinical Nursing* **21**: 2917–2929.

Van Den Haak MJ, De Jong M, Schellens PJ (2003) Retrospective vs concurrent think-aloud protocols: testing the usability of an online library catalogue. *Behaviour and Information Technology* **22**: 339–351.

Whyte J, Ward P, Eccles DW (2009) The relationship between knowledge and clinical performance in novice and experienced critical care nurses. *Heart and Lung* **38**: 517–525.

Williamson J, Ranyard R, Cuthbert L (2000) A conversation-based process tracing method for use with naturalistic decisions: an evaluation study. *British Journal of Psychology* **9**: 203–221.

Yang SC (2003) Reconceptualizing think-aloud methodology: refining the encoding and categorizing techniques via contextualized perspectives. *Computers in Human Behavior* **19**: 95–115.

CHAPTER 33

Outcome Measures

Peter Griffiths and Anne Marie Rafferty

Key points

- Selecting outcome measures is a vital part of designing a study.
- Researchers need to be clear about the intended outcomes of care before identifying outcomes.
- Having identified the intended outcomes, appropriate measures with evidence of reliability and validity must be selected or developed.
- Researchers need to carefully assess the properties of research instruments and not simply accept the claims of others that a measure is valid.
- Researchers need to consider the sensitivity of the outcome to change and the timing of outcome measurement.

INTRODUCTION

Nursing care is complex and has many facets. However, at its core is the attempt to make a difference in some way to the lives of the people who receive care. Consequently, research exploring the 'outcomes' of care has a central role in the history of the discipline. Florence Nightingale is often credited with developing the modern profession of nursing. What is less often recognised is her contribution to research through her use of outcome data to demonstrate variations in the quality of care in field hospitals in the Crimea and, on her return, hospitals in England. Working with a statistician, John Farr, Nightingale identified the extremely high mortality rates that existed in hospitals and demonstrated the impact of reforms to the system of care, including basic hygiene measures and provision of space, which dramatically improved the situation.

Nightingale's work showed that more soldiers died from neglect than their battle wounds. The relatively simple nursing interventions that she implemented could do much to improve the situation, and this was demonstrated by improving mortality. Where the benefit of change is so dramatic and the outcome as clear-cut as death, there is little more

The Research Process in Nursing, Seventh Edition. Edited by Kate Gerrish and Judith Lathlean.

Companion Website: www.wiley.com/go/gerrish/research

required than to measure the outcome of interest over a period of time and watch it change.

Fortunately, in modern health-care systems, while death rates may still be a key measure of success, we can turn our attention to other aspects of care and aim to promote health and better or faster recovery, alleviate suffering and generate positive experiences for patients. But modern health care is far more complex and fast moving than it was in Nightingale's day. Variation in mortality will have far more to do with the underlying prognosis of the patient with only a few being at significant risk of death. Most people will recover, but variations in recovery after surgery will be affected by many factors including nutrition, speed of remobilisation, infection prevention measures, early identification and correct treatment of complications and a patient's sense of well-being. These factors are in themselves important since infections, for example, are costly to treat and distressing to patients in their own right irrespective of their overall contribution to the speed of recovery.

Nurses might play a significant part in all these areas, but they will not do so alone. Furthermore, these outcomes are less clear-cut and present more challenges than the observation and recording of death. Issues include how we might measure the speed and extent of recovery and at what point it would be best to do so? How could experiences such as 'distress' and 'well-being' be measured? How can we be sure if relatively small differences in a patient's condition are due to nursing when so many other professions contribute and the underlying condition of patients matters so much?

We have simplified our description of the situation in the Crimea in order to emphasise that it is not so easy to identify the outcomes of care. In this chapter, we examine the key principles in identifying, selecting and using outcome measures to research the impact of nursing care: these are principles only, since the potential 'outcomes' of nursing care are too vast too be enumerated.

Reflection activity

What kind of study design would you use to identify the effect of nursing and control for the effects of other potentially influential variables?

NURSE-SENSITIVE OUTCOMES

Many factors contribute to the outcome of care for a particular patient, including care given by other professionals, organisational, environmental and demographic variables as well as those of the individual patient. To this, we must add changes in patient well-being (positive or negative) that may occur irrespective of external intervention. For a researcher, the challenge is to identify outcomes that are sensitive to the inputs of nursing. This can be defined as

> '...a variable patient or family caregiver state, behaviour, or perception responsive to nursing intervention...'. Maas *et al.* 1996: 296)

There are two key aspects to identifying a nurse-sensitive outcome for a particular study. Firstly, if a researcher intends to examine the impact of a specific nursing intervention, they need to be clear about what the intended consequence of that intervention is. While this might sound self-evident, it is not always a straightforward endeavour. Sometimes, there can be a lack of clarity about what the intended outcome is. In these cases, the remedy is clear. The researcher needs to examine critically what might be realistically achieved by a given intervention. Such theory must be strong in the sense that there should be a clear and plausible hypothesis about the mechanism that links an intervention to a particular outcome. It is not sufficient to simply suppose that doing 'X' will 'make someone better'. For example, a programme of meditation and relaxation during the post-operative recovery period might be introduced because it is thought that it might reduce pain and hence reduce the use of analgesics and promote earlier mobilisation. The link between these outcomes and the intervention is clear. If we added 'quality of life' to the list of possible outcomes, the link becomes general and somewhat tenuous and speculative. Equally, if the only outcome measured was 'relaxation', then the purpose of implementing such an intervention would be missed.

However, in many cases, the relevant outcomes are quite general. For example, there is a growing literature that links aspects of good quality nursing organisation and leadership to quality of care as measured by mortality (Kazanjian *et al.* 2005). However, mortality is not the only outcome that could be measured and may not be the best measure to use for a variety of reasons, not least that it might not be as sensitive to nursing as other outcomes. In these cases, researchers wishing to study the results of variation and change need to consider a wide range of outcomes that might result.

There are many possible outcomes and not all will apply in all circumstances. Recent reviews of possible outcome measures for nursing quality (Griffiths *et al.* 2008, 2012) reveal the huge diversity of phenomena that have been considered as nurse sensitive. Box 33.1 shows those most frequently identified, but many other phenomena have been considered and

Box 33.1 Frequently identified nurse-sensitive outcomes (based on Griffiths *et al.* 2008)

Indicator	**Type**
Cardiac arrest/shock	Safety
Communication and successful giving of information	Effectiveness/experience
Complaints	Patient experience
Confidence and trust	Patient experience
Continence	Effectiveness
Failure to rescue	Safety
Falls	Safety
Infection	Safety
Instrumental activities of daily living and self-care	Effectiveness
Knowledge of condition and treatment	Effectiveness/experience
Length of stay	Effectiveness/safety
Medication administration errors	Safety
Mortality	Safety/effectiveness
Nutrition	Effectiveness/safety
Pain	Effectiveness
Pulmonary embolus/deep vein thrombosis	Safety
Pressure ulcer	Safety
Respiratory failure	Safety
Satisfaction with care	Patient experience
Symptom control	Effectiveness

supported as nurse sensitive. This list is by no means exhaustive but does give an indication of the diverse and diffuse impacts of nursing.

Degrees of sensitivity

A researcher will need to consider just how sensitive to nursing a particular outcome is. This will vary across different settings and according to the precise focus of a study. A study examining the effectiveness of a programme of pressure ulcer prevention would clearly be designed in the expectation that this outcome is sensitive to it. A well-designed controlled trial would ensure that the nursing intervention was the only *difference* in professional input that patients received. However, other factors would still be important in determining whether or not a patient actually acquired a pressure ulcer. An examination of previous literature and local data is necessary to give some indication of baseline rates of the problem. Problems that are more frequent or severe may have more potential for improvement and are thus potentially more sensitive. Existing literature may also give an indication of how much change might be expected. For example, if other programmes of pressure ulcer prevention have shown only small benefits, a researcher might be alerted to the likelihood that changes will be relatively small.

This issue is even more significant where a study is focussed on something that is intended to alter quality of care more generally. Clearly, a study of pressure ulcer prevention *must* consider pressure ulcers. But what if the study is exploring something more general such as the impact of levels of nurse staffing on patient outcomes? A systematic review of the association between nurse staffing and patient outcomes in acute hospitals illustrates this (Kane *et al.* 2007). Several outcomes were identified as consistently associated with staffing levels, but the degree of sensitivity to nursing varied considerably across outcomes and care settings (see Table 33.1).

Reflection activity

Given the variation in sensitivity of different outcomes to staffing, which would you select for inclusion in a study and why? What factors would influence your choice?

OUTCOMES VERSUS PROCESS

A focus on outcomes appears to be an obvious one. If nursing is intended to deliver benefit to patients, then the best way of studying interventions and care delivery is to demonstrate improvement in those patient outcomes that are influenced by nursing. However, there are many circumstances where this is not possible or is not the highest priority. Outcomes of care can be distinguished from the processes of care: the activities undertaken to deliver care and treatments (Donabedian 1978). The aim of many interventions is to change the *process* of care on the assumption that the process will lead to better outcomes. If an intervention is designed to improve care processes, it is important to examine if the changes did in fact occur.

However, it should not be assumed that changes in process lead to improvements in outcomes. Because of the complexity of nursing, it is often unclear which (if any) particular aspects of care processes are important in delivering outcomes. For example, despite their widespread use, there is no clear evidence that using pressure ulcer risk assessment tools has an impact upon ulcer incidence (Pancorbo-Hidalgo *et al.* 2006). Researchers designing studies need to assure themselves of the relative importance and priority of assessing outcomes and should certainly not assume that many cherished nursing processes are validated by a link with outcomes. Assessment of process alone is only sufficient when the evidence base for the link to outcomes is clear.

CHARACTERISTICS OF MEASURES

Outcomes can be broadly classified as relating to effectiveness (positive impacts), safety (prevention of harm) and patients' experience of care (Griffiths

Table 33.1 Percentage reduction in the odds of adverse outcomes associated with an increase of one registered nurse per patient day (based on Kane *et al.* 2007)

All patients	
Cardiopulmonary resuscitation	28%
Hospital-acquired pneumonia	9%
Mortality	4%
Pulmonary failure	6%
Intensive care patients	
Cardiopulmonary resuscitation	28%
Hospital-acquired pneumonia	30%
Mortality	9%
Pulmonary failure	60%
Relative change in length of stay	24%
Unplanned extubation	51%
Surgical patients	
Cardiopulmonary resuscitation	28%
Failure to rescue	16%
Hospital-acquired bloodstream infection	36%
Mortality, surgical patients	16%
Relative change in length of stay	31%
Surgical wound infection	85%

et al. 2008). Box 33.1 gives examples of these types of outcome. In this section, we will explore characteristics of measures in more depth.

Measuring subjective states

Subjective measures are generally areas where there is self-report of individual interpretations and assessments. Many such outcomes are of great importance, and the role of subjective measurement extends to areas beyond what is typically considered 'experience' into evaluations of the effectiveness of care. Increasingly, 'Patient-Reported Outcome Measures' (PROMs) are recognised as having a central role in researching and evaluating health-care services. For example, pain is a subjective state that must largely rely on patient report. To examine changes and to research interventions, researchers must attempt to turn such subjective assessments into measures so that comparison can be made.

There is a variety of approaches to measuring such subjective states. A single concept (e.g. pain, happiness, satisfaction) can be assessed using a single item with various approaches taken to quantifying it. One frequently used approach, particularly in pain assessment, is the use of a visual analogue scale. Typically, a visual analogue scale is a 100 mm line with anchors at either end describing extremes of the state. The patient is asked to mark a position on the line to indicate their current state. The researcher can then measure this line to get a numerical estimate (see Figure 33.1). Some versions will have additional descriptors at intermediate points. Such approaches generally work well for pain assessment and have been widely used in

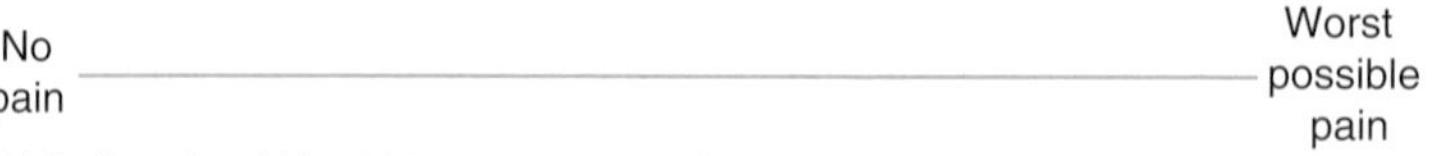
No
pain
Worst
possible
pain
N.B. line should be 100 mm – not produced to scale here

Figure 33.1 Visual analogue pain scale

research, but they may not be suited to everyone or in all circumstances. For example, visual analogue scales cannot be used over the telephone, and there is some question over their use with children and those with cognitive impairment. A frequently used alternative is the numerical rating scale where patients are asked to give a number (generally from 0 to 10) with similar anchors given. Alternatively, descriptions of pain intensity can be used to form a verbal rating scale (e.g. no pain, mild pain, moderate pain, severe pain, excruciating pain) or a series of faces indicating increasing distress can be used.

A commonly used alternative to this approach is the Likert scale where respondents are asked to rate the extent to which they agree or disagree with a statement (e.g. 'my pain is well controlled'). Typically, there are five response categories offered ranging from 'strongly agree' to 'agree' through to 'agree' and 'strongly disagree'. There is some controversy about the most appropriate middle response category, but 'undecided' or 'neither agree nor disagree' is typical. The most positive response is conventionally assigned a score of 5, running down to 1 for the most negative response.

Measurement scales and batteries

For other outcomes, there may not be a simple, single item that can be measured directly, even where there might be directly observable elements. Outcomes such as independence (or dependence) in activities of daily living or stress are complex. For example, while stress could be measured by a single question (are you feeling stressed?), the subjective response to this question would not properly capture the more complex theoretical underpinning of what psychologists understand and define as stress. In these cases, a series of items are needed to assess the underlying concept. These items form a scale that aims to give an overall measure. In order to do this, there needs to be a clear conceptual basis for the underlying variable and a clear basis on which the items on a scale can be summed to give an overall score. See Box 33.2 for examples of measurement scales commonly used in health-care research.

Developing scales requires rigorous testing to ensure that the items selected genuinely reflect and relate to the underlying construct. Procedures used include assessing the extent to which each item correlates with the overall score and the statistical procedure of factor analysis to determine whether meaningful groupings of items emerge that are clearly related to the construct and underlying theory.

It is important that researchers distinguish such scales, where individual items have little significance on their own, from batteries, where a series of questions each represent an outcome or item of interest. Since there are likely to be numerous 'outcomes' of nursing care, it is important to be clear if a series of questions (e.g. Was your pain well controlled? Were you given explanations about your medications you could understand?) are seen as part of a scale or not. If these items are seen as a scale measuring a single outcome, then it is the summary score from the group of questions that is of interest. If each is a question in its own right, then issues of the relationship of one question to a 'score' is not relevant. Each item must be considered in its own right.

Objective measurement

Measures of a person's own psychological state and perceptions are of necessity subjective, and this in itself is not a problem for researchers. However, in other cases, subjective judgement may be incorporated into an attempt to rate what might be regarded as an objective characteristic. An objective characteristic or measure is one that can be directly measured or assessed. While absolute 'objectivity' is never attainable, there is considerable difference between

Box 33.2 Examples of measurement scales

Outcome	Scale	Source
Anxiety	State-Trait Anxiety Inventory (STAI)	Spielberger *et al.* (1970)
Anxiety and depression	The Hospital Anxiety and Depression Scale (HADS)	Zigmond and Snaith (1983)
Functional dependence	The Barthel Index	Mahoney and Barthel (1965)
Functional independence	Functional Independence Measure (FIM)	Linacre *et al.* (1994)
Health status	Short Form Medical Outcomes Survey 36 (SF36)	Ware and Sherbourne (1992)
Pressure sore risk	The Braden Scale	Bergstrom *et al.* (1987)
Quality of life	EuroQol	The EuroQol Group (1990)
Self-esteem	Rosenberg Self-Esteem Scale	Rosenberg (1979)
Stress	The Perceived Stress Scale	Cohen *et al.* (1983)

Inclusion on this list does not imply that the scale is conceptually clear, reliable or valid.

assessing (say) whether or not someone has been discharged from hospital compared to grading a pressure sore.

In the former case, any judgements made can be clearly verified, and there is little room for inconsistency. In the latter case, there are fine judgements to be made. There must be precise and clear definitions of the parameters to be assessed and the characteristics that define whether a pressure sore is to be graded at one given level or another. These need to be specified in such a way as to ensure that the definitions are interpreted in the same way by different observers (see Research Example 33.1). Other examples may be where patients or clinicians report on a patient's performance in activities of daily living. Interpretations of whether or not a task can be performed can be confused with how difficult it is. Furthermore, if rating is not based on direct observation, there may be inexact recall or other sources of error.

Some subjective states such as pain or stress may have objective correlates, such as physiological measurements that are associated with these states. For example, both pain and stress are associated with elevated serum cortisol and elevated blood pressure. Pain is associated with a raised pulse. Although it might seem appealing to avoid 'subjective' measures and use these measures instead, such physiological measures are not themselves measures of pain or anxiety (or any other psychological state) and should not be given precedence because of their seeming objectivity. Such objective measures are of most significance when they are of interest in their own right (e.g. blood pressure).

VALIDITY AND RELIABILITY

No measurement of outcomes can ever be perfect. In many cases, measurement is direct and fairly precise, but even then, there can be a small margin of error. For example, the length of hospital stay, while reasonably clear-cut, is based upon an assessment of

RESEARCH EXAMPLE

33.1 Comparison of Pressure sore Grading Systems

Pedley GE (2004) Comparison of pressure ulcer grading scales: a study of clinical utility and inter-rater reliability. *International Journal of Nursing Studies* **41**(2): 129–140.

This study measured inter-observer agreement of three different grading systems for pressure sores. All three classified pressure sores into four stages and were apparently very similar. Thirty-five observations were made by 2 registered nurses on 35 recorded ulcers on 30 adult inpatients using all 3 systems. The 2 nurses agreed on presence of an ulcer in 29/35 cases. One or other nurse identified a pressure ulcer in 34 cases, and both agreed that there was no ulcer in 1 case. However, when it came to grading the ulcer, they agreed in only 54% of cases for the best system and 49% for the worst. Qualitative data identified problems with scale construction relating to visualisation of the base of the wound, discolouration of the skin, abrasions and shallow ulcers. The authors concluded that while refinements in scale construction may improve agreement between raters, there is a need to develop objective measures of pressure-induced tissue damage.

when a stay begins (arrival in A&E? admission to the ward?) and is recorded with a degree of precision (hours or minutes) that is never absolutely precise. In general, the level of precision in these measurements is sufficient for the likely purposes of research although the potential of different definitions means that care needs to be taken to ensure that like is being compared to like and all outcomes are assessed using a consistent approach. Similarly, if studies are conducted across different sites, it is important that definitions and approaches to assessment are standardised. However, in many cases, outcome assessment is considerably more problematic.

In selecting outcomes, it is important to determine both the reliability and validity of the assessment. For clinical outcomes, there are several issues to be considered. We will consider validity first. In essence, validity refers to the extent to which we are measuring what we desire to measure.

Often, consideration of validity focuses on the extensive procedures for validating scales where a subjective state (latent construct), for example, anxiety, is assessed by a series of items. Some similar issues apply to single-item rating scales, for example, a global rating of satisfaction. There needs to be a careful assessment that the answer (or score) 'means' exactly what we think it means. The process of validation begins with an assessment of face and content validity. Face validity is a subjective assessment that items are relevant and clear. Content validity is a more formal judgement that the content of an instrument logically and comprehensively covers the domain of interest. While both these procedures may increase the chances that a measure that has been developed is indeed valid, neither can be used to directly demonstrate that validity has been achieved (Beckstead 2009). Factor analysis is often used to select an initial set of items from a wider pool and to assess the extent to which a final set of items reflects theoretically meaningful underlying variables. However, of far more significance is evidence of 'criterion validity', which demonstrates that theoretically expected relationships do in fact exist. This can take the form of showing a strong correlation with another, similar outcome or scale (concurrent validity) or that the scale predicts future events in the way that would be expected (predictive validity). For example, a functional status measure, examining people's abilities in activities of daily living, would be expected to predict ability to live independently at home.

Ideally, to validate a measure, there should be an objective 'gold standard' for the outcome, and while this is not always available, the issue needs to be considered. Where an outcome measure is the presence or absence of disease or disorder, it is often necessary to use a less than perfect measure because a full diagnostic procedure is complex or unfeasible for another reason. This is often the case with psychological states or condition. For example, the Edinburgh Postnatal Depression Scale (EPDS) is often used to assess the outcomes of supportive and preventative interventions by midwives and health visitors in the antenatal and postnatal period rather than undertaking a full diagnostic interview to determine whether postnatal depression is actually present. Such interviews are time consuming, expensive and potentially burdensome for research participants. The EPDS is a short questionnaire that can be quickly completed and is easily assessed. Validating such a scale is problematic and often researchers simply compare the results of the EPDS to another, similar scale. However, the criterion used to validate the outcome measure should be the 'gold standard' approach to making the diagnosis or assessment. This will vary, but in the case of postnatal depression, it is a full standardised psychiatric assessment. The validity of the EPDS can only assessed by its ability to predict an actual diagnosis of postnatal depression.

Where the criterion is a category, generally presence or absence of disease or a problem as opposed to some measure of 'amount' of a problem, the researcher needs to seek evidence of *sensitivity* and *specificity*. These relate to the extent to which the instrument misclassifies people using the gold standard as a reference. Sensitivity is the percentage of people who have the diagnosis (according to the gold standard) who are correctly identified by the instrument. Specificity is the percentage of people who do not have the diagnosis (according to the gold standard) who are correctly classified. Researchers must seek evidence that these figures are sufficiently high in a population similar to that currently being investigated. To do this, researchers must look at the description of the population in previously published research and consider if the frequency and severity of the disorder are likely to be similar in the population at hand.

Reliability refers to the extent to which the same measure of the same outcome can vary irrespective of changes in the underlying outcome. Any measure is subject to some degree of imprecision, and many human characteristics vary naturally over time without any underlying changes. Variation can occur because of imprecision in the measure, either because of the measurement equipment or procedure itself (e.g. a device to measure blood pressure) or because of variation in the way the measure is applied (e.g. variation in the way the operator uses the device). Often, in research, different people conduct measurements and they may vary in their approach. In such cases, the same measurement applied at the same time would give different results. The outcome itself may also vary somewhat over time, irrespective of change in a person's underlying state. For example, blood pressure varies from moment to moment, but these changes do not necessarily reflect alterations in an underlying condition leading to hypertension.

Typically, two forms of evidence are sought for reliability. One is inter-rater reliability, where two measures are taken at approximately the same time by two people. The assumption is made that the underlying characteristic (say blood pressure) has not changed during any brief interval between assessments. Over a series of ratings (covering the full range of possible values), the extent to which the two ratings agree is assessed. The other approach is test–retest reliability when the measurement is repeated over time. Again, the assumption is made that the underlying 'outcome' has not varied over the interval between measures. This approach to reliability assessment is primarily designed to assess unreliability due to 'natural' variation although it would also be influenced by unreliability in the measurement procedure itself.

The approach taken to assessing reliability will depend upon the outcome to be measured. Test–retest reliability is unlikely to be particularly relevant if measuring a fixed or slow-changing characteristic such as height, but inter-rater reliability is important in that there is scope for variation in the measurement procedure. In other cases, both assessments are important. There is natural variation in blood pressure over the course of the day. If the outcome 'hypertension' is to be assessed by a single measure, it is important to explore how reliable this single measure is by assessing agreement between measures over a period of weeks when the underlying condition will not change but blood pressure will. The individual measurement is also subject to unreliability due to the measurement procedure itself and so in this case both forms need to be assessed. For most patient-completed scales (e.g. psychological measurement based on questionnaires), test–retest reliability is the key since asking the same person to complete the same questionnaire twice at the same time is logically impossible, but it is important to establish that the measure is constant over periods when it is thought that the outcome is also constant.

BIAS IN MEASUREMENT

In addition to error, which is random, there is also the potential for *systematic* differences in measurement, also referred to as bias (although this is not intended to reflect deliberate or motivated misreporting). For example, where two observers are making measurements (or where two devices are used to assess the same measurement), there is potential for *systematic* differences arising from different approaches and interpretations. One observer might consistently (perhaps subconsciously) round a pulse measurement up to the nearest 5. There is certainly ample evidence that some 'terminal digits' are preferred to others with numbers ending in 5 or 0 being recorded far more frequently than others (Wen *et al.* 1993). Such an observer would give a rating that was consistently higher than one who rounded down. Assessment of agreement between raters or two approaches to measurement on interval measures needs to consider more than just correlation. It needs to explore the extent to which the assessment of two raters or repeated measures using the same instrument might differ consistently (Bland & Altman 2010; Griffiths & Murrells 2010). Correlation coefficients do not give any indication of such systematic difference (Brennan & Silman 1992).

Because of the linked issues of error and bias, the oft-quoted solution of using a single observer to undertake outcome assessment creates a false sense of security. A single observer will be less prone to random 'error' because they are likely to be consistent with themselves. However, they are still subject to observer drift, where criteria or procedures are applied differently over time as fatigue or carelessness sets in, leading to systematic differences in recordings at the beginning compared to the end of observation periods. More significantly, having a single observer does nothing to protect against systematic 'bias' where that one rater uses the measures in a way that consistently over- or under-represents the true value. The key solution is to pick instruments with known reliability, train observers properly and consistently and check their levels of agreement. If there is considerable disagreement, further training and standardisation of administration must be sought.

SELECTING OUTCOME MEASURES

In selecting outcomes and measures to assess them, researchers should never simply rely on the previous use of a measure as evidence of validity or reliability. Furthermore, they should be wary of taking other researchers' claims of validity at face value. Selecting an outcome measure requires a full assessment of the current evidence of validity. The complexity of validation and reliability testing means that the process is a significant undertaking in itself; the development of a new instrument should not be undertaken lightly without considerable resource. However imperfect it may be, researchers with limited resources are generally advised to use an existing instrument rather than develop a new one with no opportunity to assess its validity. There are several questions to consider in assessing the suitability of existing instruments:

- Is the outcome of interest clearly linked to the goal of the study (e.g. intervention)?
- Is the conceptual basis of any instrument clear?
- Does it match the outcome of interest?
- Does the measure have face validity (as assessed by the local research team, not the originators)?
- What evidence of criterion and predictive validity is there?
- Are the criteria used to assess the instrument meaningful and theoretically valid?
- Is there evidence that the measure is reliable?

Formal claims about content validity have little meaning in the absence of evidence of criterion or predictive validity. However, they may be of relevance in selecting items for a battery of questions (see above) or a battery of outcome measures. We identified above that in some cases the outcomes to be assessed follow directly and logically from the goal of the intervention. In many cases, this may not be clear-cut. Few interventions have a single object. Even the treatment of life-threatening disease aims to do more than simply save life, and the 'outcome', or effectiveness, of treatment has many dimensions and can be defined differently from different perspectives.

In many research studies, a 'battery' of measures and outcomes are used, and researchers must select a range of outcomes to measure. Certainly, theory should inform the selection of measures. Increasingly, people who have experienced care themselves are involved in identifying appropriate domains of outcome measurement. However, simply measuring all possible outcomes is not an acceptable approach because there are problems associated with using multiple measures. The burden of measurement (on research participants and researchers) is a vital consideration. Furthermore, taking multiple measures risks the possibility of making type 1 errors where it is concluded that a result is 'statistically significant' even when it is the product of chance alone. Such chance relationships occur due to random variation in the measurements or because of chance variation between groups. Such errors occur with a known frequency when one outcome is measured: the frequency of errors is 5 times in 100 when statistical significance is set at 0.05. However, if a study includes tests of several outcomes that are independent of each other, the probability of making a type I error increases dramatically since each relationship tested carries an additional chance of error and so the overall chance of making at least one such error is increased.

Reflection activity

Consider the advantages and disadvantages of developing a new instrument for pressure sore grading with respect to validation and reliability testing. How might this compare with such testing for an existing tool?

OTHER CONSIDERATIONS IN IDENTIFYING OUTCOMES

It is likely that a given study will have several outcomes. In such cases, it is important to clearly identify a *primary* outcome – that is, the single most important outcome. Earlier, we described a hypothetical relaxation intervention for reducing post-operative pain. If pain relief was the main goal, this would be the most appropriate primary outcome with outcomes such as relaxation and recovery time identified as secondary outcomes. The primary outcome should be identified before the study commences. Defining a single primary outcome has a number of purposes. It identifies for future readers what the researcher saw as the most important *question* before data began to provide answers, which is important in maintaining objectivity. Procedures to assess the required sample size should be based upon the primary outcome. Emphasis on the results from the primary outcome in framing conclusions helps to avoid making type 1 errors because conclusions based on secondary outcomes alone should be more tentative as the risk of these errors is higher.

There is little point in identifying a primary outcome that is not sufficiently sensitive to change to show a difference in a study. For example, many studies show a relationship between levels of nurse staffing and mortality, but it is unlikely that introducing a new nurse on one ward would show a measurable difference in death rates. A study on a single ward would be destined to fail unless a meaningful primary outcome could be identified (perhaps impact upon staff sense of well-being and effectiveness).

Another issue to consider is the timing of outcome assessment. Often, the same outcome will be assessed at several different time periods. It is often easy to demonstrate an immediate effect of an intervention, but such immediate effects are often of less interest than longer-term ones. Researchers need to decide how long benefit must be sustained in order to be truly important. For example, studies of relaxation therapy may show a reduction in anxiety and blood pressure. However, unless this reduction is sustained beyond the immediate period of relaxation, the outcome may be relatively trivial if the concern is (say) hypertension, although such short-term benefits may be sufficient if the therapy is designed to help people cope with a transient stress, such as undergoing a painful procedure. In deciding the primary outcome, the appropriate follow-up period must also be defined.

Relevance of the outcome is another factor to consider. Current health policy can affect the impact of a research project in terms of the attention that is paid and the perception of how useful results are. For example, assessments of mortality are one of the main indicators for the NHS Outcomes Framework (Department of Health 2013). Recent nursing policy focuses on care, compassion, competence, communication, courage and commitment (Department of Health 2012). Researchers identifying outcome measures for these areas may help to develop the evidence base for those policies and so improve the use that is made of their research.

USING CLINICAL DATA AND OTHER ROUTINELY COLLECTED DATA IN RESEARCH

Clinical records and many administrative systems contain data that can be used in research. In England, the Hospital Episode Statistics (HES) contain details of all admissions to NHS hospitals based on an abstract from the medical record. Each HES record contains a wide range of information about an individual patient admitted to hospital. For example:

- clinical information about diagnoses and operations
- information about the patient (such as age group, gender and ethnic category)
- administrative information, such as time waited and date of admission
- geographical information on where the patient was treated and the area in which they lived

Some of this information is readily available in aggregated forms and under some circumstances detailed information is available to researchers. The

RESEARCH EXAMPLE

33.2 Using Routinely Collected Data in Research

Rafferty AM, Clarke SP, Coles J, Ball J, James P, McKee M, Aiken LH (2007) Outcomes of variation in hospital nurse staffing in English hospitals: cross-sectional analysis of survey data and discharge records. *International Journal of Nursing Studies* **44**(2): 175–182.

There is an increasing body of research in nursing that has used routinely collected patient and/or workforce data to assess the impact of variation in nurse staffing on patient outcomes. The authors explored whether English hospitals in which nurses care for fewer patients have better outcomes, building on growing evidence from the United States. They used hospital administrative data to look at patient mortality and failure to rescue (mortality risk for patients with complicated stays). They also conducted a survey to explore nurse job dissatisfaction, burnout and nurse-rated quality of care. The use of existing data meant that 118,752 patients in 30 English acute trusts could contribute. They found that patients and nurses in the quartile of hospitals with the most favourable staffing levels (the lowest patient-to-nurse ratios) had consistently better outcomes than those in hospitals with less favourable staffing. Patients in the hospitals with the highest patient-to-nurse ratios had 26% higher mortality (95% CI, 12–49%); the nurses in those hospitals were approximately twice as likely to be dissatisfied with their jobs, to show high burnout levels and to report low or deteriorating quality of care on their wards and hospitals.

Reflection activity

What factors might encourage you to utilise routinely collected data versus generating new data to measure outcomes in a given study?

NHS Information Centre also provides detailed information on NHS staffing, which can be accessed for research. Local administrative systems and audits can give even richer data from the medical and nursing records. Some influential research has been undertaken using these sorts of data including a series of studies linking nurse staffing to patient outcomes (see Research Example 33.2).

However, use of these data is not without problems. Although researchers can access data on a scale that they would not otherwise be able to do, these data was not gathered for research purposes. Before embarking on such a study, researchers need to consider the quality of the data. While some objective outcomes, such as mortality or place of discharge, are likely to be accurately recorded, others are not. For example, a study of pressure ulcer incidence using nursing records would be dependent upon accurate and timely identification of the ulcer and accurate, timely and correct recording and classification of ulcer severity using one of several systems. Researchers would not have the opportunity to train observers and so issues of unreliability and bias in observations could be severe. Errors and inconsistencies in recording would add further to both error and bias.

CONCLUSION

There are many issues to be considered when selecting outcome measures for a study. Careful thought and selection of measures prior to commencing a study can do much to enhance the usefulness of the findings by reducing error and ensuring a valid measure of outcome is offered. Researchers should be wary of accepting the previous use of a measure as evidence of its reliability, validity or utility for a particular study. Nursing care has the potential to make significant changes in people's lives, and it is a key task for research to measure and demonstrate those changes properly.

References

Beckstead JW (2009) Content validity is naught. *International Journal of Nursing Studies* **46**(9): 1274–1283.

Bergstrom N, Demuth PJ, Braden BJ (1987) A clinical trial of the Braden Scale for predicting pressure sore risk. *Nursing Clinics of North America* **22**(2): 417–428.

Bland JM, Altman DG (2010) Statistical methods for assessing agreement between two methods of clinical measurement. *International Journal of Nursing Studies* **47**(8): 931–936.

Brennan P, Silman A (1992) Statistical methods for assessing observer variability in clinical measures. *British Medical Journal* **304**(6840): 1491–1494.

Cohen S, Kamarck T, Mermelstein R (1983) A global measure of perceived stress. *Journal of Health And Social Behavior* **24**(4): 385–396.

Department of Health (2012) *Compassion in Practice: nursing midwifery and care staff, our vision and strategy*. Leeds, Department of Health.

Department of Health (2013) *The NHS Outcomes Framework 2014–2015*. London, Department of Health.

Donabedian A (1978) The quality of medical care. *Science* **200**(4344): 856–864.

Griffiths, P, Murrells T (2010) Reliability assessment and approaches to determining agreement between measurements: classic methods paper. *International Journal of Nursing Studies* **47**(8): 937–938.

Griffiths P, Jones S, Maben J, Murrells T (2008) *State of the Art Metrics for Nursing: a rapid appraisal*. London, King's College London.

Griffiths P, Richardson A, Blackwell R (2012) Outcomes sensitive to nursing service quality in ambulatory cancer chemotherapy: systematic scoping review. *European Journal of Oncology Nursing* **16**(3): 238–246.

Kane R, Shamliyan T, Mueller C, Duval S, Wilt T (2007) The association of registered nurse staffing levels and patient outcomes: systematic review and meta-analysis. *Medical Care* **45**(12): 1195–1204.

Kazanjian A, Green C, Wong J, Reid R (2005) Effect of the hospital nursing environment on patient mortality: a systematic review. *Journal of Health Services Research and Policy* **10**: 111A–117A.

Linacre J, Heinemann A, Wright B, Granger C, Hamilton B (1994) The structure and stability of the functional independence measure. *Archives of Physical Medicine and Rehabilitation* **75**(2): 127–132.

Maas ML, Johnson M, Moorhead S (1996) Classifying nursing-sensitive patient outcomes. *Journal of Nursing Scholarship* **28**(4): 295–302.

Mahoney FI, Barthel DW (1965) Functional evaluation: the Barthel Index. *Maryland State Medical Journal* **14**: 61–65.

Pancorbo-Hidalgo PL, Garcia-Fernandez FP, Lopez-Medina IM, Alvarez-Nieto C (2006) Risk assessment scales for pressure ulcer prevention: a systematic review. *Journal of Advanced Nursing* **54**(1): 94–110.

Pedley GE (2004) Comparison of pressure ulcer grading scales: a study of clinical utility and inter-rater reliability. *International Journal of Nursing Studies* **41**(2): 129–140.

Rafferty AM, Clarke SP, Coles J, Ball J, James P, McKee M, Aiken LH (2007) Outcomes of variation in hospital nurse staffing in English hospitals: cross-sectional analysis of survey data and discharge records. *International Journal of Nursing Studies* **44**(2): 175–182.

Rosenberg M (1979) *Conceiving the Self.* New York, Basic Books.

Spielberger CD, Gorsuch RL, Lushene R (1970) *STAI Manual.* Palo Alto, CA, Consulting Psychologists Press.

The EuroQol Group (1990) EuroQol-a new facility for the measurement of health-related quality of life. *Health Policy* **16**: 199–208.

Ware JE, Sherbourne CD (1992) The MOS 36-item short-form health survey (SF-36). *Medical Care* **30**(6): 473–483.

Wen S, Kramer M, Hoey J, Hanley J, Usher R (1993) Terminal digit preference, random error, and bias in routine clinical measurement of blood pressure. *Journal of Clinical Epidemiology* **46**(10): 1187.

Zigmond AS, Snaith RP (1983) The hospital anxiety and depression scale. *Acta Psychiatrica Scandinavica* **67**(6): 361–370.

Further reading

Doran D (2003) *Nursing-Sensitive Outcomes: state of the science*. Sudbury, MA, Jones and Bartlett.

McDowell I (2006) *Measuring Health: a guide to rating scales and questionnaires*, 3rd edition. New York, Oxford University Press.

Waltz C, Strickland O, Lenz E (2005) *Measurement in Nursing and Health Research.* New York, Springer Publishing Company.

SECTION 5

Making Sense of Data

Section 5 is short, but the processes it describes are of critical importance in any research study. Without analysis of data, it would be impossible to convey with any clarity or precision what exactly the research has discovered. It is also the stage in the research process that is often most taxing and confusing, as the researcher wades through a mass of statistical or narrative data and wonders how to bring order out of the seeming chaos.

Chapter 34 tackles qualitative data analysis. Many of the chapters dealing with qualitative methods have already given some guidelines for analysis, but here a clear overview of the broad principles of qualitative analysis is presented, with the aim of getting the novice researcher started. A choice can then be made between major methods such as narrative analysis, framework analysis and grounded theory. The chapter builds on the earlier chapters in Section 3 (Chapters 14–17), and the reader is encouraged to use these five chapters in parallel and to pursue the suggestions for further reading in particular areas as necessary.

Chapters 35 and 36 are designed to be read together, as they are written by the same authors and use a consistent worked example throughout. Chapter 35, however, may be sufficient for some readers who only need to be able to present and describe quantitative data in a basic way. For those wishing to test hypotheses or analyse relationships in data, Chapter 36 takes them further into statistical analysis and provides some basic methods of making inferences from data. Recommendations for further reading are given for students who wish to pursue statistical analysis further.

The Research Process in Nursing, Seventh Edition. Edited by Kate Gerrish and Judith Lathlean.

Companion Website: www.wiley.com/go/gerrish/research

CHAPTER 34

Qualitative Analysis

Judith Lathlean

Key points

- There are a number of different approaches to qualitative analysis depending on the research design and nature of the data.
- Qualitative data analysis is usually ongoing and iterative throughout the research process; as such, it can inform the research design as well as provide an interpretation of the findings.
- The validity of the analysis, triangulation and reflexivity are all important concepts when undertaking qualitative analysis.
- Different frameworks, matrices, procedural steps and software packages exist to assist in the practical process of qualitative data analysis.

INTRODUCTION

For the qualitative researcher, the process of analysing data is not necessarily linear or even predictable. Qualitative research studies do not follow the traditional route of hypothesising or identifying a research problem, doing a literature review to clarify what is already known about the proposition or problem, collecting some data and only then analysing these data. Indeed, the actual analytical process can start at the very beginning and inform all the aspects and stages of the research. Furthermore, there is no one 'right' way of doing the analysis and no standard recipe for success. It depends as much on what one wants to achieve as the view of what would lead to the production of a rich account and a deep understanding about the phenomena being studied. Despite the relative lack of prescription, much has been written about qualitative data analysis, and there is general agreement that there are some helpful principles to consider as well as some tried and tested schematic approaches and practical aids. This chapter explores these principles and discusses several more popular methods of analysis in some detail. It also looks at the practicalities of qualitative data handling and analysis including the use of software packages.

The Research Process in Nursing, Seventh Edition. Edited by Kate Gerrish and Judith Lathlean.

Companion Website: www.wiley.com/go/gerrish/research

PRINCIPLES OF QUALITATIVE ANALYSIS

Objectivity or subjectivity?

In thinking about the nature of qualitative research, the discussions have frequently been presented as dichotomous choices. Are objective or subjective data being generated and are the analytical processes lending themselves to objective or subjective descriptions? Is the aim for replication (i.e. if a finding holds true in one setting, does it also in another comparable setting) or for authenticity (is this an authentic and credible portrait of what is being examined)? Is the aim to study representative samples or is there more interest in purposely selected samples? Is the ability to generalise conclusively being sought or is it accepted that all situations are unique and therefore only tentative theoretical generalisations are possible? In reality, these distinctions are not clear-cut, although the qualitative analyst will tend to lean more towards the right-hand position in these dichotomies.

Building and developing theory

Qualitative researchers almost invariably agree that theory (or theorisation) should be the primary goal of research. Nevertheless, they frequently reject the formulation of theories in advance of their fieldwork, considering this to be unduly constraining. The process of developing and testing theory is often said to proceed in tandem with data collection, and the main methods of analysis, such as analytic induction and grounded theory, offer fruitful strategies for theory building. So, for example, in analytic induction, the analyst tries to formulate generalisations that hold true across all of their data, and when adopting a grounded theory approach, the theory is inductively derived from the study of the phenomenon it represents.

Eisenhardt (1989) described how to build theories from case study research. In doing so, she drew on grounded theory building and the analytical methods described by Miles and Huberman (1994). Her logical step-by-step approach to developing theory includes tips on entering the field, analysing within-case data, searching for cross-case patterns, shaping hypotheses, comparing emergent concepts and theory with the existing literature and reaching closure (the point when the analyst ceases to add cases and stops going back and forth between theory and data).

> **Reflection activity**
>
> What is the researcher aiming for in attempting to analyse qualitative data? Is striving for objectivity the aim? What part can theory play in the analytical process?

Pope *et al.* (2013) is an example of a research study that uses the idea of applying theory to the findings as part of the analysis, in order to understand and generalise them on a wider basis (see Chapter 13, Research Example 13.4). The researchers selected three settings to compare the implementation of a single computer decision support system and then used a Normalization Process Theory framework to explain their findings.

Concurrent data collection and analysis

It is common in qualitative research for data that are analysed early on in research to inform the rest of the data collection, the research design and sometimes even the actual research questions. This is illustrated by a study I undertook of the implementation and development of lecturer practitioner roles in nursing (Lathlean 1997). At the outset, I had anticipated using an action research approach where I tried to find out 'how' these new roles should be developed and what processes were necessary to enhance their effectiveness. Following initial data collection and analysis, it quickly became obvious that the prime question was not to do with 'how' but rather 'what', that is, 'what is the nature and reality of the job of lecturer practitioner?' So I chose an ethnographic research design with a number of different stages, each being thoroughly analysed before proceeding to the next one.

Another reason for analysing data as a study progresses is to identify when the data have reached 'theoretical' saturation (see Chapter 14 on grounded theory).

Validation by respondents or researchers

In qualitative research, the distinction is sometimes made between internal validity (the extent to which research findings represent reality) and external validity (the extent to which abstractions and concepts are applicable across groups). The qualitative analyst has strategies that can be used to ensure or at least facilitate both. These include giving the original data (e.g. an interview transcript) to the interviewee and asking them to clarify the meaning of their responses. Participant observation (which is common in ethnographic studies) allows data to be collected over a prolonged period, and this is accompanied by continual data analysis. In this way, constructs can be refined and checked out with participants.

A crucial test of qualitative research accounts is whether those people whose beliefs and behaviour are supposedly presented in the accounts actually recognise the validity of the accounts. However, it is necessary to be cautious about the process of respondent validation, since it cannot be assumed that any actor is a privileged commentator on his or her actions, in the sense that the intentions, motives and beliefs involved are accompanied by a *guarantee* of truth. In addition, if the researcher asks the respondent to 'check' the data produced, it could be argued that if there is a subsequent view expressed by the latter, this in effect presents a second order or level of data. This then provides a challenge for the analyst; how are these 'views', which may be at variance with the original, subsequently handled?

Triangulation

Data-source triangulation (Denzin 1970) involves the comparison of data relating to a phenomenon, which have been derived, for example, from separate phases of the fieldwork or from the accounts of various participants including the researcher. The claim is that if different kinds of data lead to the same conclusion, this increases confidence in the conclusions. This approach should not be confused with '*methodological* triangulation' when methods either from within the same paradigm or across paradigms are used to study the same phenomena. This type of triangulation has relevance to mixed methods research where, for example, the results of interviews are compared with the researcher's observations or with data from very structured questionnaires relating to the same phenomenon. This can be problematic, however, since it assumes that there is a single 'reality' that is waiting to be discovered, a suggestion that is anathema to most qualitative researchers.

In my research on lecturer practitioners, the presentation of my accounts of their lives to the participants was a way of 'validating' those accounts and a form of triangulation (Lathlean 1997). The accounts generated at the three different stages over 3 years were compared and contrasted for each participant as well as being examined for consistency across cases. However, I needed to be careful to distinguish between differences that occurred as a result of the way the data had been collected (e.g. the interviews may have thrown up different points about the experiences of the lecturer practitioners than I gleaned in my role as observer), and differences that were the result of real disparities in their lives at separate points in time.

Following the ethnographic study, I surveyed the perspectives of all lecturer practitioners who were in post in one health authority at that time, using a structured questionnaire. Conducting this separate study could have been construed as a form of triangulation as the intention was to achieve a fuller and more penetrating understanding of the lecturer practitioners. But I had to be cautious about interpreting the results. A match or mismatch between the perceptions of the participants in the survey and the 'reality' of the lecturer practitioners as observed in the ethnographic study did not necessarily confirm or put into question the validity of either study. Rather, it could simply mean that there were

Reflection activity

In order to increase the 'validity' or 'authenticity' of the analysis, what steps and strategies can be taken? Why do we have to be careful about 'respondent validation' and triangulating the analyses arising from different data collection methods? What can we claim if the results show up differences of perception?

differences between the lives of lecturer practitioners and other people's understandings of those lives.

Reflexivity

Qualitative research stresses the importance of reflexivity whereby the researcher recognises that he or she has a social identity and background that has an impact on the research process. Reflexivity is especially relevant in nursing research because often the researcher is also a nurse. In such circumstances, the researcher needs to think carefully – to reflect – on the impact that being a member of the same professional group as study participants may have on all aspects of the research process especially interpretation of research findings. So, for example, in a qualitative study that was undertaken of community mental health nurses' experience of taking part in a clinical trial of treatment for patients with common mental health problems (see Simons *et al.* 2008), the researcher – a nurse herself – had to make a conscious effort to expose and make clear what biases she brought to the research so that the analyses could be viewed in that light. Simons' use of narrative analysis in her study, with its emphasis on the nurses' talk itself and the *way* they told their stories, was also helpful in this respect.

EXAMPLES OF METHODS OF ANALYSIS

Two particular overarching strategies for analysis are frequently cited in texts, such as Bryman (2012: 564). These are analytic induction and grounded theory. In addition, there are other approaches that are especially suited to more open-ended forms of textual data such as discourse, conversation and narrative analysis. Another analytical tool, which tends to suit policy and applied research, is referred to as 'Framework' analysis, derived to order and synthesise data (Ritchie & Lewis 2003). Similarly, 'Template Analysis' (King 2004) also provides a matrix that can be of use at an early stage of qualitative data analysis. Embedded within both Framework and Template Analysis, and indeed much qualitative analysis in general, is the derivation of 'themes', thus leading to a discussion as to whether 'thematic analysis' is a distinct form of analysis in its own right.

Analytic induction

Analytic induction is a process of analysing data where the researcher tries to find explanations by carrying on with the data collection until no cases (referred to as deviant or negative cases) are found that are inconsistent with a hypothetical explanation of a phenomenon. The process of analytic induction is illustrated in Box 34.1.

From this brief description, it can be seen that the analytic induction method shares attributes of 'positivism' or a 'realist' stance in research, for example, the setting up of a 'hypothesis' and the confirmation or refutation of that hypothesis. However, it is based on a case study research design, whereby cases are not selected to be representative and therefore theoretical rather than statistical generalisation occurs.

Box 34.1 Steps in analytic induction

1 Set up a definition of a problem
2 Provide a hypothetical explanation of the problem
3 Investigate a number of cases
   a. Find that these cases are in line with the hypothesis – hypothesis is confirmed
   b. Find cases that deviate from hypothesis
      i. reformulate hypothesis and go back to step 3 or
4 Redefine hypothetical explanation to exclude deviant cases and end data collection

Furthermore, the final explanations that result from analytic induction may specify the conditions that are *sufficient* for a phenomenon to occur, but rarely those that are *necessary*. So, for example, studies have shown that certain people in particular circumstances become drug or alcohol dependent, but analytic induction will not shed light on why other people with the same characteristics in similar circumstances do *not* become addicted. Also, in analytic induction, there are no hard and fast rules as to how many cases need to be investigated before the absence of negative cases and the validity of the hypothesis can be confirmed.

Reflection activity

In what types of research are we trying to gain inductive knowledge and in what circumstances would a grounded theory approach to research be the chosen design? When would we choose just grounded theory analytical methods as opposed to a complete grounded theory methodology? You might want to look at Chapter 14 – Grounded Theory – to answer this question.

Grounded theory

For a detailed discussion of grounded theory, see Chapter 14. However, it is referred to briefly here since it is one of the most widely cited approaches to the analysis of qualitative data. While there is some disagreement about the precise nature of the grounded theory approach, most consider that there are usually four aspects in the analytical process: theoretical sampling, coding, theoretical saturation and constant comparison (see Box 34.2).

Some studies claim to be using a grounded theory methodology when what they really mean is that they are employing some of the stages or principles of analysis such as theoretical saturation or constant comparison. This is not necessarily a problem, but in these instances, it needs to be recognised that only parts of the approach are being adopted.

Analysing narrative

The most common approaches to analysing narrative are conversation analysis, discourse analysis and narrative analysis. Conversation analysis is based on an attempt to describe people's methods

Box 34.2 Key aspects in a grounded theory approach to analysis

Theoretical sampling – this is the process of data collection for generating theory whereby the researcher jointly collects, codes and analyses the data and decides what data to collect next in order to develop the emerging theory (Glaser & Strauss 1967).

Coding – this is where data are broken down into component parts and names are given to the parts.

Theoretical saturation – this refers to the point when no further coding is necessary because no new instances are required to confirm a category, and/or when no new data collection is required as there is sufficient confidence about the nature of the emerging concepts.

Constant comparison – this is the process whereby the data and the subsequent conceptualisations from it are compared to ensure that there is a good fit. This happens throughout data analysis.

for producing orderly social interaction and has a relatively long history. It is concerned with the sequential organisation of talk – how talk overlaps and the lengths of pauses in a conversation are key attributes. Silverman (1998) suggested that it is important in conversation analysis to try to identify sequences of related talk, to examine how speakers take on certain roles or identities through their talk, such as 'client–professional', and to look for particular outcomes in talk such as laughter and then work back from there to see how it was produced. For an introduction to conversation analysis, see Heritage (2004).

Discourse analysis is very similar to conversation analysis in that it seeks to analyse the activities present in talk. However, unlike conversation analysis, discourse analysis possesses the following three features:

- It is concerned with a far broader range of activities such as gender relations or social control.
- It does not always use analysis of ordinary conversation as a baseline for understanding talk in organisational settings.
- It works with far less precise transcripts than conversation analysis.

Greenhalgh *et al.* (2012) used discourse analysis to map how different stakeholders understood telehealth and telecare technologies. This study was based on the analysis of a sample of 68 publications (academic, policy, service, commercial and lay) and field notes from knowledge-sharing events. It concluded that there were four conflicting discourses, which only engaged minimally with one another's arguments. Another study has used discourse analysis to investigate what happens in patient forums on the Internet and has found that patients are prepared to share knowledge about a range of topics using language that might not feature in more formal interviews (De Simoni 2014).

Research Example 34.1 illustrates the use of a particular approach known as critical discourse analysis (CDA). This study by Schofield *et al.* (2011) examined how nurses work with older people with delirium in hospital. In the presentation of the research, care was taken to provide substantial data extracts followed by detailed linguistic analysis in order to overcome the criticism of some that discourse analytic studies are a little different from studies that use thematic analysis. The aim was to uncover the kinds of knowledge that informs nurses' care and to explicate the basis of that knowledge by the use of CDA. This is underpinned with the premise that powerful interests in society shape how we construct and talk about practices. In this study, it was then the role of the analytical process to make these discourses transparent.

RESEARCH EXAMPLE

34.1 Critical Discourse Analysis

Schofield I, Tolson D, Fleming V (2011) How nurses understand and care for older people with delirium in the acute hospital: a critical discourse analysis. *Nursing Inquiry* **19**(12): 165–176.

This study examined nurses' day-to-day practice of nursing patients with delirium. The aim was to uncover the kinds of knowledge that informs nurses' care and to make clear the basis of that knowledge. Critical discourse analysis is underpinned by the premise that powerful interests within society mediate how social practices are constructed. Links were made between the language nurses used in interviews and naturalistic settings. Findings indicated that nurses were influenced by major discourses of risk reduction and safety, and they talked about patients with delirium as 'risk objects'. The philosophy of person-centred and dignified care advocated in the nursing literature and government policy is an emerging discourse, though was little evident in the data.

RESEARCH EXAMPLE

34.2 Narrative Analysis

Brown J, Addington-Hall J (2008) How people with motor neurone disease talk about living with their illness: a narrative study. *Journal of Advanced Nursing* **62**(2): 200–208.

This study was based on longitudinal narrative interviews conducted at 3-monthly intervals over 18 months with 13 people suffering from motor neurone disease. Narrative case studies were used, with the unit of analysis being the person (patient) in their own home or a care home. The interviews were analysed by focusing on the form and content of the narrative. Four types of narrative or storyline were found: sustaining (relating to living life and keeping active); enduring (where a person feels disempowered and unable to fight); preserving (where the essence is survival); and fracturing (with its concern with loss and fear of what is to come). The paper concluded that 'storylines' help make sense of complex narratives by encouraging listening – on the part of the 'interviewer' – as well as being organising threads to assist professionals and families to better understand what it is like for someone to live with motor neurone disease. The paper also includes a useful diagram of the iterative process for analysis of narratives including the stages of immersion, analysis of narratives, trial framework, framework mapping and narrative types and storylines.

There are numerous definitions and conceptualisations of narrative research (see Chapter 17) and narrative analysis, which leads to differing views and methods of analysis. Leiblich *et al.* (1998) suggested the dimensions of holism and category as important differentiations wherein the first approach analyses a narrative in its entirety and the latter supports the extraction of text for thematic classification. Reissman (2008), in a useful source book, offers four approaches including thematic, structural, visual and performative analysis. Smith and Sparkes (2008) presented a helpful typology of narrative analysis predicated by the use of systematic and rigorous strategies and techniques designed to identify, explain and think about the features of the story. They divide story analysis between investigating the 'whats' and 'hows'. This involves questions being asked of the stories such as why was the narrative told in that way and in that order? How is the narrator located in relation to other characters and to the audience? What are the identity claims and how are these performed?

Bingley *et al.* (2008) claimed that qualitative analysis methods applied to narratives and narrative analysis are distinct approaches. In the former, general methods of qualitative analysis such as thematic, discourse and conversation analysis may be applied to the interpretation of narratives as well as other sources of data. In the latter, specific analytic techniques have been developed that are devoted to narratives. Bingley *et al.* paper offers a summary table of different narrative analysis approaches when the emphasis is on content, structure and/or form.

A commonality across narrative analysis methods is that the focus of inquiry lies on the narrative, regardless of whether the emphasis is on content, structure and/or form. An example of the use of form in narrative is found in the study investigating how patients talk about living with motor neurone disease (Brown & Addington-Hall 2008) (see Research Example 34.2).

Reflection activity

How do narrative approaches to analysis differ from other types? What are the practical implications for transcription and presentation of data in narrative studies? Look at the examples given and the practical considerations later in this chapter.

Framework analysis

Ritchie and Spencer (2004) developed 'Framework' as a method of data analysis particularly suited to policy and applied research. It involves a number of distinct though interconnected stages (see Box 34.3). An example of a project in nursing where Framework analysis was used is a study of infection control and clinical placements by Ward (2010, 2012). In Research Example 34.3, Ward *et al.* (2013) demonstrate the five stages of the analytical process that were used in analysing the data from this study. Another helpful source is Gale *et al.* (2013), which explains the procedures for using it in multidisciplinary health research teams. A worked example of how codes are attached and how a coding framework is developed when adopting this strategy is given in Research Example 34.4.

Box 34.3 Five key stages of data analysis in the 'Framework' approach

Familiarization – immersion in the data (listening to tapes, reading transcripts, studying notes etc.) to get an initial feel for the key ideas and recurrent themes.

Identifying a thematic framework – the process of identifying key issues, concepts and themes and the setting up of an index or framework. This can be used for sifting and sorting data including a priori issues (used to inform the focus of the research and the data collection guides), emergent themes raised by respondents and analytical themes which are evident through recurring patterns in the data.

Indexing – the process of systematically applying the index or framework to the text form of the data, by annotating the text with codes in the margin.

Charting – data are 'lifted' from their original context and rearranged according to themes in chart form. There may be separate charts for each major subject or theme and they will contain data from several different respondents. This process involves considerable synthesis and abstraction.

Mapping and interpretation – the charts are used to define concepts, map the range and nature of phenomena, create typologies, and find associations between themes in order to provide explanations for the findings. This process is guided by the original research questions as well as themes and relationships emerging from the data.

RESEARCH EXAMPLE

34.3 Framework Analysis

Ward DJ, Furber C, Tierney S, Swallow V (2013) Using Framework analysis in nursing research: a worked example. *Journal of Advanced Nursing* **699**(11): 2423–2431.

This article usefully presents the processes that the researchers went through in analysing the data from an interview study of infection control in clinical placements, which involved nursing students and mentors. The five stages of the Framework Approach (see Box 34.3) are carefully explained using worked examples. Suggestions are made to guide researchers through the key steps in undertaking the analysis and the benefits and limitations of the approach are discussed. The study findings are reported elsewhere (see for example Ward 2010, 2012).

RESEARCH EXAMPLE

34.4 Illustrative Example of Analysis Using the Framework Approach

As part of a study of out-of-hours health services (Lattimer *et al.* 2005) a postal survey of patient satisfaction with the services was undertaken, resulting in both quantitative and qualitative data. The qualitative data were in the form of open-ended comments which were analysed using the Framework approach. First, extracts from 3 comments related to the telephone contact are presented with codes attached. Second, an excerpt is given from the coding frame and third, the chart shows how these can be compared across different sites.

Comment A: "I was quite happy with phone service;	*generally satisfied (2.1)*
I'd seen notices about it in the doctor's surgery and I read about it in the local paper;	*well advertised (2.1.1)*
but there was one small aspect that I found irritating and it could be improved – different people asking the same questions *(balanced - 1.1)*	*repeated questioning (2.2.1)*
Comment B: Can't fault [the phone service]; got to speak to nurse immediately which was good *(all positive - 1.3)*	*put straight through to nurse/ doctor (2.1.7)*
Comment C: Didn't realise that I'd have to phone GP and NHS Direct as well; so I was not pleased and then the operator spoke so fast I couldn't take it in *(all negative - 1.2)*	*ringing doctor and then NHSD (2.1.10) person spoke too fast*

Extract from coding framework (with examples of codes)

Balance of comments overall	1
Balanced comments	1.1
All negative comments	1.2
All positive comments	1.3
Theme: ease of access over the phone	2
Positive	2.1
General	
Well advertised	2.1.1
Good recommendation of other services	2.1.2
Continuity of information between services	2.1.3 etc.
Waiting time	
Put straight through to nurse/doctor	2.1.7 etc.
Negative	2.2
Questioning	
Repetitive questioning	2.2.1
Repetitive questioning causing delay	2.2.2
Perceived irrelevant questioning	2.2.3 etc
Clarity of process	
Ringing doctor and then NHSD	2.2.10
Emergency doctors with no access to information	2.2.11 etc.
Communication problems	
Person spoke too fast	2.2.19
Difficulty communicating with call handler	2.2.20 etc.

Extract from chart comparing responses across sites

	Code	Site 1		Site 2		Site 3	
		n	%	n	%	n	%
Balance of comments	1						
Mixed comments	1.1	47	29.4	31	26.1	30	29.1
All negative comments	1.2	47	29.4	35	29.4	27	26.2
All positive comments	1.3	66	41.3	53	44.5	46	44.7
All comments coded		160		119		103	
Returned questionnaires		332		274		249	
Theme: Ease of access over the phone	2						
Positive	2.1	23	35.9	9	25.0	7	35.0
Negative	2.2	41	64.1	27	75.0	13	65.0
Total		64	40.0	36	30.3	20	19.4

RESEARCH EXAMPLE

34.5 Template Analysis

McCluskey S, Brooks J, King N, Burton K (2011) The influence of 'significant others' on persistent back pain and work participation: a qualitative exploration of illness perceptions. *BMC Musculoskeletal Disorders* **12**: 236.

A convenience sample of disability benefit claimants and significant others (such as partners) were recruited from the Lancashire Condition Management Programme (CMP) in the North-West of England. Individual semi-structured interviews based on the chronic pain version of the revised Illness Perceptions Questionnaire (IPQ-R) were conducted. The interview schedule included the same or similar questions to those making up the nine subscales of the IPQ-R: illness identity; timeline (acute/chronic); timeline (cyclical); consequences of illness; personal control over illness; treatment control over illness; emotional representations; illness coherence; and beliefs about causality. Template Analysis was chosen because it allows a-priori themes to be used to help develop an initial version of the coding template – in this case, these nine subscales. Claimant interview data were then mapped onto the initial template, modifying it further until all relevant data were coded satisfactorily. The process was concluded by applying the final version of the template to the data as a whole, and a-priori themes were redefined or discarded if they did not prove to be helpful in capturing key meanings in the data.

Template Analysis

Nigel King has promoted a qualitative data analysis method he has called Template Analysis (King 2004, 2012). It is a form of thematic analysis where the researcher identifies themes or codes that summarise and integrate important ideas, actions, experiences and concepts from the data. These are presented as a structured matrix, which can then be used as the basis for writing about the themes.

King's empirical work has been in primary health-care settings, and interests include the experience of chronic illness, professional identities in health and social care and paranormal beliefs and experiences. It is within these fields that he has most commonly used Template Analysis. (See Research Example 34.5, which uses Template Analysis in a study of disability benefit claimants by McCluskey *et al.* 2011.)

PRACTICALITIES

Recording and transcribing data

In order to be able to analyse data from interviews, a verbatim record of the interview should be obtained. By far, the best approach is to digitally record the interaction and then to transcribe the recording. Some researchers use a transcription service, but wherever possible, it is better for the interviewer to do this themselves, since it is a good opportunity to start the process of 'immersion' in the data. The extent to which every single word is extracted, and every pause and emphasis is noted, will depend on the particular approach to analysis. So, for example, if thematic analysis is chosen, then pauses are not essential to record, whereas with discourse and narrative analyses, there are conventions that must be followed in preparing the transcript. Transcription is a very lengthy process, with a 60-minute interview needing several hours for transcription.

Field notes in observation can follow a structure, according to the purpose of the observation, or they can be more free-flowing. If a structure is used, this can form the basis for the analysis. On the other hand, a predetermined structure may be unduly constraining. Sometimes, it is a good idea to take a few notes during an interview as well, even when it is being recorded. This can be helpful both as prompts for further questioning in a relatively unstructured or semi-structured interview and as a backup, should the recording fail.

Doing qualitative analysis

Despite the frequency of mention in papers and texts, thematic analysis is relatively under-developed as a way of actually doing the analysis. Some specifications or steps are available; the structure provided by Braun and Clarke (2006) is a useful one (see Box 34.4). In this, themes are generally regarded as a category, identified by the researcher from their data, relating to the research topic and often the research question(s) and a basis for the theoretical understanding of the data.

Within a theme, the most usual way of condensing or grouping data is to attach codes to it. These codes may have been decided upon in an a priori way or they may emerge as the fieldwork unfolds. Different

Box 34.4 Steps in thematic analysis adapted from Braun and Clarke (2006)

Step 1	Familiarisation with the data
Step 2	Generation of initial codes
Step 3	Searching for themes
Step 4	Reviewing the themes
Step 5	Defining and naming the themes

approaches to analysis use the word 'code' to mean slightly different things, so the best plan when following one particular type of analysis is to be clear about what constitutes a 'code' in that approach.

A thematic analysis process is illustrated by a study of prisoners' views of a telepsychiatry service, conducted by Sarah Leonard (2004). She undertook 20 tape-recorded semi-structured interviews with prisoners after they had participated in an experimental telepsychiatry initiative. The questioning focused on the experience of the prisoners being assessed in terms of their mental health by a video-recorded link with a remote psychiatrist in a setting far from the prison. While their feelings about the experience of assessment using this process were central to the interview, the prisoners also talked graphically about their lives in prison.

These interviews were analysed using the stages outlined by John Creswell, first presented in 2007, and now updated as Creswell (2013). First, each interview was transcribed by the researcher herself and the transcription was then shared with the interviewee. This was to check out with them her understanding of the language they used – which tended to rely quite heavily on prison 'jargon' – rather than to 'validate' the transcripts. She then imported the text of the transcripts into a software package (see section on Using computer software). The second stage involved familiarisation with the range, depth and diversity of the data by listening to the tapes, reading the transcripts several times and reflecting on each interview. During this 'immersion' in the data, 'memos' – consisting of initial impressions, key ideas and recurring themes – were written in the margins of the transcript. The next stage entailed description, the identification of codes and the clustering of similar ones under theme headings. Examples relating to the prisoners' life in prison included 'lack of structure and meaningful activity', 'routines and lack of change' and 'rigid system' and 'predictability'. Finally, the data clustered under these themes were again scrutinised and presented within a framework of main headings. Thus, the aforementioned became sub-themes under the main heading of 'factors that help or hinder adaptation' to prison life. Verbatim comments were used to provide evidence of the participants' experience.

EXAMPLES OF ANALYSES

As referred to previously, different types of analytical approaches require the transcribed data to be presented in particular ways. Two contrasting examples are given to illustrate this – a narrative analysis (Research Example 34.6) and a piece of analysis using the 'Framework' approach (Research Example 34.4). Whereas these are quite different strategies – for example, the narrative analysis requires the data to be presented with every single utterance, repetition and pause and with lines identified, while the Framework analysis works on chunks of verbatim quotes with undue repetition left out – there are similarities. The analyst in both works from the transcripts, identifying key concepts and producing an analytical framework, which can then be used to compare across other cases.

Analysing qualitative data is never easy, despite the impression given by many published studies that the results flow effortlessly from an obvious process and it is often not possible to stick slavishly to one particular approach. A helpful sourcebook of methods is that of Miles and Huberman (1994). They define analysis as 'consisting of three concurrent flows of activity: data reduction, data display, and conclusion drawing/verification' (Miles & Huberman 1994: 10). Data reduction refers to the process of selecting, focusing, simplifying, abstracting and transforming the data found in field notes and transcriptions and occurs throughout the project, not just at the end of a data collection period. The second type of activity is data display, which can mean the presentation of extended quantity of text, or at the very least copious snippets of verbatim quotes. Miles and Huberman provide examples of different types of display such as charts, graphs, matrices and networks, which can work well to begin to show relationships and connections. The third 'stream' of activity is that of conclusion drawing and verification. This process starts in the data collection stage when the researcher begins to note possible patterns, explanations and propositions. However, 'final' conclusions may not be apparent until data collection is completed. Then the conclusions need to be 'tested' and 'verified' lest the analyst is left with

RESEARCH EXAMPLE

34.6 Illustrative Example of Narrative Analysis

This example is from Lucy Simons' qualitative study of community mental health nurses' experiences of treating patients with common mental health problems within a randomised trial (Simons *et al.* 2008). It is in three parts: first a story described by Len about his experience, presented using the conventions of narrative analysis, see Reissman (2002); second, the detailed analysis of this story and third, the template that this story is placed in so that it can be compared and contrasted with the other narratives in the study.

The story: 'Len, the most rewarding of all'	*Line No.*
Er:::m (1) but I think actually one of the most rewarding ones was	*105*
the e:r (,) um was a relatively young guy (.) who worked in a local Bank	*106*
who um (1) lived I think with his sister so a single guy um (.) and um	*107*
who actually not only told me that his problems were resolved by the end	*108*
but actually said you know how how he now understood about tackling his	*109*
future problems you know in view of you know (.) that he not only not	*110*
only resolved his current problems but had learnt had learnt a way of	*111*
tackling (.) um how he perceives things in the future you know um which I	*112*
I find that (.) actually the most rewarding of all um (.) erm: you know	*113*
because hopefully you know not only has it resolved during the time	*114*
that I saw him but he will be able to do it himself next time which is	*115*
what of course was said on the on the course itself but um (.) he	*116*
actually he actually came out with that himself and when he when he did	*117*
it um you know that was quite encouraging.	*118*
- - - - - - - - - - - - - -	
I think like	508
I said it was great when that guy said to me you know that he got	509
something he got something (.) for himself for the future he could use	510
you know and how to perceive things differently if you know I think that	511
was ur extremely good.	512

The detailed analysis of the story

Narrative characters and how Len wants them to be known

Len provided an introduction to the patient at the start of this narrative. He is constructed as a single young man who held a respectable job and lived with his sister (lines 106–107). Within this narrative Len hardly features and little is learnt about his character. This narrative featured some time into the interview and Len had already made identity claims earlier on.

Social positioning

The patient has the most dominant social position in this narrative in that all the actions that take place are attributed to him. The patient's actions are related to what he tells Len about the outcome of the encounter – that his problems were resolved (line 108) and that he had learnt to manage better in the future (lines 109–110). These ideas were then repeated twice (lines 110–112, 114–115). The patient had also offered this information to Len without prompting (line 117). When Len returned to the narrative much later in the interview the actions taken were still the patients' actions of telling Len that he had learnt for the future (lines 509–510).

In contrast Len did not attribute any actions to himself during the narrative. He described how he felt about the encounter: it was 'rewarding' (line 105), which he found 'quite encouraging' (line 118) and 'extremely good' (line 512), but it was not clear what actions Len had actually taken to help bring about the problem resolution and the skills that the patient told him he had acquired. Len was the passive recipient in this narrative, as the patient told him what the outcome of the encounter was and even where Len refers to the problem-solving training course he frames this as what was said to him rather than what he learnt (line 116).

Although the patient was the most active and agentic character in the narrative the activity attributed to him is about telling Len the result of the treatment encounter. The problems were described as being 'resolved' (lines 108, 111, 114) by the end of the encounter without any clear idea who or what was responsible for this outcome.

Other narrative/discursive devices

Repetition

Len repeated the main idea of the narrative on three occasions throughout the whole narrative but rather than build on or add detail to the idea at each repetition he simply restated what happened.

Analytical framework

Who are the characters in the story?	Patient (dominant): young, single guy
Are they dominant or subordinate?	Len (subordinate): on receiving end of action
Type of story	Change achieved and possibly successful PST[1]
What action takes place?	*Patient*: 108: told Len problems were resolved 109: told Len understood how to tackle problems 111: had resolved current problems 117: identified learning from the encounter 509: told Len what he had got from the encounter *Len*: none
Does the patient achieve change?	Yes, problems resolved
Social positioning of characters	*Patient* 108: problems resolved (no action taken) 110-2: resolved problems (taken action) and learnt how to in future 114: resolved during the time (no action) 115: future action indicated *Len*: 108, 117, 509: informed by patient 118, 512; encouraged by events of this encounter
Other narrative devices used	Repetition Main idea returned to much later in interview
Blame (if no change achieved)	N/A

(*Problem solving technique used to treat patients randomised to this intervention)

an interesting story of what happened but one of unknown truth and utility.

USING COMPUTER SOFTWARE FOR QUALITATIVE DATA ANALYSIS

The use of dedicated software packages for analysing qualitative data has become increasingly popular. The early software of the late 1980s was designed mainly for the analysis of text. However, more recently, they have been developed to handle a variety of data, including visual and multimedia non-numerical material. They also have many more functions than initially, such as both coding and retrieval, and theory building categories. Computer-assisted qualitative data analysis software (CAQDAS) provides tools to identify and code themes, concepts, processes and contexts to build theories or enlarge upon existing theories. Two of the most popular packages currently are ATLAS.ti7 (http://www.atlasti.com/index.html) and QSR NVivo10 (http://www.qsrinternational.com).

Bryman (2012: 590) discusses CAQDAS in relation to the use of NVivo and presents helpful plates, visually describing how it works as an approach to computerised qualitative analysis. He also provides a balanced account of the positive and negative aspects. Silver and Lewins (2014) provide a useful guide to assist the choice of the most appropriate package for a study and illustrate a wide range of tasks and processes in the data management and analysis process.

Above all, software packages can help with the process of analysing data, but they are not shortcuts to rigorous analysis and they still require the researcher to make decisions about categorisation. As such, they are tools to facilitate the analytical process, but many would say that they are no substitute for immersing oneself in the data and really getting a feel for the nature of the data and the interrelationships between different aspects. They are well suited to medium-sized to larger projects where there are reasonable amounts of data. Conversely, where the beginning researcher has a few short interviews, they can provide learning opportunities for use in future projects.

Reflection activity

What are the advantages and challenges of using a computer-assisted approach to analysing qualitative data? In what circumstances might it be helpful? Does it mean that further interpretation of the data are not necessary?

CONCLUSION

In conclusion, qualitative data analysis in nursing and health-care research is a complex, creative process, which is ongoing, interactive, inductive and reflexive. It occurs throughout the study from the initial conception of the idea to the production of the final report or account. While it can be quite different from the processes used to analyse quantitative data, nevertheless, it still needs to be rigorous, systematic and transparent.

References

Bingley AB, Thomas C, Brown JB, Reeves J, Payne S (2008) Developing narrative research in supportive and palliative care: the focus on illness narratives. *Palliative Medicine* **22**(5): 653–658.

Braun V, Clarke V (2006) Using thematic analysis in psychology. *Qualitative Research in Psychology* **3**(2): 77–101.

Brown JB, Addington-Hall J (2008) How people with motor neurone disease talk about living with their illness: a narrative study. *Journal of Advanced Nursing* **62**(2): 200–208.

Bryman A (2012) *Social Research Methods*, 4th edition. Oxford, Oxford University Press.

Creswell JW (2013) *Qualitative Inquiry and Research Design: choosing among five approaches*, 3rd edition. Thousand Oaks, Sage.

Denzin NK (1970) *The Research Act in Sociology: a theoretical introduction to sociological methods.* London, Butterworth.

De Simoni A, Shanks A, Mant J, Skelton J (2014) Making sense of patients' internet forums: a systematic method using discourse analysis. *British Journal of General Practice* **64**(620): 178–180.

Eisenhardt K (1989) Building theories from case study research. *Academy of Management Review* **14**(4): 532–550. Reprinted in Huberman AM, Miles MB (eds) (2002) *The Qualitative Researcher's Companion*. Thousand Oaks, Sage, pp 5–35.

Gale N, Heath G, Cameron E, Rashid S, Redwood S (2013) Using the framework method for the analysis of qualitative data in multi-disciplinary health research. *BMC Medical Research Methodology* **13**: 117.

Glaser B, Strauss A (1967) *The Discovery of Grounded Theory*. Chicago, Aldine.

Greenhalgh T, Procter R, Wherton J, Sugarhood P, Shaw S (2012) The organising vision for telehealth and telecare: discourse analysis. *BMJ Open* **2**: e001574.

Heritage J (2004) Conversation analysis and institutional talk: analysing data. In: Silverman D (ed) *Qualitative Research: theory, method and practice*. London, Sage, pp 161–182.

King N (2004) *Template Analysis – What is Template Analysis?* University of Huddersfield, Huddersfield. Available at http://www2.hud.ac.uk/hhs/research/template_analysis/ (accessed 14 April 2014).

King N (2012) Doing template analysis. In: Symon G, Cassell C (eds.) *Qualitative Organizational Research: core methods and current challenges*. London, Sage, pp 426–450.

Lathlean J (1997) *Lecturer Practitioners in Action*. Oxford, Butterworth-Heinemann.

Lattimer V, Turnbull J, Burgess A, Surridge H, Gerard K, Lathlean J, Smith H, George S (2005) Effect of introduction of integrated out-of-hours care in England: observational study. *British Medical Journal* **331**: 81–84.

Leonard S (2004) The successes and challenges of developing a prison telepsychiatry service. *Journal of Telemedicine and Telecare* **10**: 69–71.

Lieblich A, Tuval-Mashiach R, Zilber T (1998) *Narrative Research: reading, analysis and interpretation*. Thousand Oaks, Sage.

McCluskey S, Brooks J, King N, Burton K (2011) The influence of 'significant others' on persistent back pain and work participation: a qualitative exploration of illness perceptions. *BMC Musculoskeletal Disorders* **12**: 236.

Miles MB, Huberman AM (1994) *Qualitative Data Analysis: an expanded sourcebook*, 2nd edition. Thousand Oaks, Sage.

Pope C, Halford S, Turnbull J, Prichard J, Calestani M, May C (2013) Using computer decision support systems in NHS emergency and urgent care: ethnographic study using normalization process theory. *BMC Health Services Research* **13**: 111.

Reissman CK (2002) Narrative analysis. In: Huberman AM, Miles MB (eds.) *The Qualitative Researcher's Companion*. Thousand Oaks, Sage, pp 217–270.

Reissman CK (2008) *Narrative Methods for the Human Sciences*. Thousand Oaks, Sage.

Ritchie J, Lewis J (2003) *Qualitative Research Practice: a guide for social science students and researchers*, 1st edition. Thousand Oaks, Sage.

Ritchie J, Spencer L (1994) Qualitative data analysis for applied policy research. In: Huberman AM, Miles M B (eds.) *The Qualitative Researcher's Companion*. Thousand Oaks, Sage, pp 305–331.

Schofield I, Tolson D, Fleming V (2011) How nurses understand and care for older people with delirium in the acute hospital: a critical discourse analysis. *Nursing Inquiry* **19**(12): 165–176.

Silver C, Lewins A (2014) *Using Software in Qualitative Research: a step-by-step guide*, 2nd edition. London, Sage.

Silverman D (1998) *Harvey Sacks and Conversation Analysis*. Cambridge, Polity Press.

Simons L, Lathlean J, Squire C (2008) Shifting the focus: sequential methods of analysis with qualitative data. *Qualitative Health Research* **18**(1): 120–132.

Smith B, Sparkes AC (2008) Narrative and its potential contribution to disability studies. *Disability and Society* **2**(1): 17–28.

Ward D (2010) Infection control in clinical placements: experiences of nursing and midwifery students. *Journal of Advanced Nursing* **66**(7): 1533–1542.

Ward D (2012) Attitudes towards infection prevention and control: an interview study with nursing students and nurse mentors. *BMJ Quality and Safety* **21**(4): 301–306.

Ward DJ, Furber C, Tierney S, Swallow V (2013) Using Framework Analysis in nursing research: a worked example. *Journal of Advanced Nursing* **69**(11): 2423–2431.

Further reading

Pope C, Ziebland S, Mays N (2006) Analysing qualitative data. In: Pope C, Mays N (eds.) *Qualitative Research in Health Care*. Oxford, Blackwell, pp 63–81.

Ritchie J, Lewis J, McNaughton Nicholls C, Ormston R (2013) *Qualitative Research Practice: a guide for social science students and researchers*, 2nd edition. Thousand Oaks, Sage.

Silverman D (2006) *Interpreting Qualitative Data: methods for analyzing talk, text and interaction*, 3rd edition. Thousand Oaks, Sage.

Websites

http://caqdas.soc.surrey.ac.uk – CAQDAS Networking Project – University of Surrey, ESRC Researcher Development Initiative Project including Qualitative Innovations in CAQDAS (QUIC) programme. It provides:

- Training and support in using a range of CAQDAS packages
- Comprehensive bibliography relating to use of CAQDAS packages
- Links to online journals and articles
- Links to software development and distributor sites, including free and low cost packages
- Reports on funded research

http://onlineqda.hud.ac.uk – Online CAQDAS and Qualitative Data Analysis. University of Huddersfield and University of Surrey, ESRC Research Methods Project, Online QDA is a set of learning materials which address common issues of undertaking qualitative data analysis (QDA) and beginning to use Computer Assisted Qualitative Data AnalysiS (CAQDAS) packages. The authors aim to complement courses run by, for example, the CAQDAS Networking project, many independent trainers and the large number of undergraduate and postgraduate social sciences research methods training courses.

http://www.hud.ac.uk/hhs/research/template-analysis/what-is-template-analysis/ – University of Huddersfield Template Analysis website, updated April 2014 and designed to be used as a resource for those using – or considering using – an approach to qualitative data analysis known as 'Template Analysis'.

CHAPTER 35

Descriptive Analysis of Quantitative Data

Stephen J. Walters and Jenny Freeman

Key points

- Different types of quantitative data need to be handled, presented and described in appropriate ways.
- Data checking and cleaning are essential first steps in recording and entering data for analysis.
- Tables and graphs are commonly used to display data, but attention needs to be paid to presentation.
- Summary statistics such as means, medians and standard deviation are used to describe quantitative data.

INTRODUCTION

The prospect of collecting and analysing quantitative data can be daunting, especially the first time. However, it need not be, and the purpose of this and the next chapter is to demystify the process and introduce some basic statistical ideas, so that when preparing to conduct a study, the tools with which to proceed are available. This chapter describes the basic data types encountered in quantitative analysis together with some simple ways of describing and displaying them. The following chapter introduces the concept of hypothesis testing and describes some basic methods for testing hypotheses. In order to provide continuity, data from the same study will be used throughout both chapters to illustrate key concepts. This study is described in Research Example 35.1, but briefly, it is a randomised controlled trial (see Chapter 18) of community versus hospital rehabilitation followed by telephone or conventional follow-up in 161 patients with the lung condition chronic obstructive pulmonary disease (COPD). Patients were assessed at entry to the study, 8 weeks after randomisation and then at six-monthly intervals until the final follow-up at 18 months. Outcome measures included exercise capacity, health-related quality of life and use of health-care resources.

The Research Process in Nursing, Seventh Edition. Edited by Kate Gerrish and Judith Lathlean.

Companion Website: www.wiley.com/go/gerrish/research

RESEARCH EXAMPLE

35.1 Case Study of a Randomised Controlled Trial

Waterhouse JC, Walters SJ, Oluboyede Y, Lawson RA (2010) The CoHoRT study: a randomised 2×2 trial of community versus hospital rehabilitation followed by telephone or conventional follow up; impact on quality of life, exercise capacity and use of health care resources. *Health Technology Assessment* **14**(6): 1–140.

This study comprised a randomised controlled trial to test whether pulmonary rehabilitation undertaken in a community setting was more effective than that undertaken in a hospital setting (standard care), as assessed by exercise capacity and health-related quality of life. It also looked at whether a further telephone follow-up produced a greater persistence of effect of pulmonary rehabilitation compared to standard care.

Two hundred and forty patients with chronic obstructive pulmonary disease (COPD) were randomised to receive pulmonary rehabilitation in either a community ($n=111$) or hospital setting ($n=129$). Following standardised pulmonary rehabilitation for 6 weeks, patients were followed up over 18 months (with assessments post-rehabilitation approximately 8 weeks post-randomisation and 6, 12 and 18 months after rehabilitation). Analysable data were obtained for exercise capacity post-rehabilitation for 161 patients, 85/129 (66%) in the hospital group and 76/111 (68%) in the community group. Patients were further randomised to telephone or standard follow-up, with analysable data for $n=40$, 34, 25 and 36, respectively, in hospital rehabilitation/telephone follow-up, hospital rehabilitation/standard follow-up, community rehabilitation/telephone follow-up and community rehabilitation/no telephone follow-up groups.

The primary outcome was distance walked post-rehabilitation on the endurance shuttle walk test. The mean baseline endurance shuttle test walking distance was 280.5 and 278.9 m for the community and hospital groups, respectively. Post rehabilitation, the mean distance walked was 496.6 and 557.7 m for the community and hospital groups, respectively. The baseline-adjusted mean difference in walking distance immediately post-rehabilitation was not significantly different at 67.8 m in favour of the hospital group (95% CI −41.8 to 176.6 m, $p=0.22$). Over the long-term 18 months post-rehabilitation follow-up, the mean difference in endurance shuttle walking test distance between the hospital and community groups, after adjustment for baseline distance walked time and factorial design, was not significantly different at 52.3 m (95% CI −31.7 to 136.3, $p=0.22$). Furthermore, there was no significant difference in endurance shuttle walking distance in telephone versus standard follow-up groups, with a mean difference, after adjustment for baseline distance walked, time and factorial design, in post-rehabilitation walking time of 65.1 m (95% CI −19.4 to 149.6, $p=0.131$).

DATA TYPES

In order to collect and analyse data as part of the research process, it is necessary to understand what the different types of data are. Figure 35.1 shows a basic hierarchy of data types. Data are either *quantitative* or *categorical*. Quantitative variables can be either count or continuous. *Count* data are also known as discrete data and occur when the data can only take whole numbers, such as the number of children in a family or the number of visits to a GP in a year. *Continuous* data are data that can be measured, and they can take any value on the scale on which they are measured; they are limited only by the scale of measurement, and examples include height, weight, blood pressure and distance walked.

Data are described as *categorical* when they can be categorised into distinct groups, such as ethnic

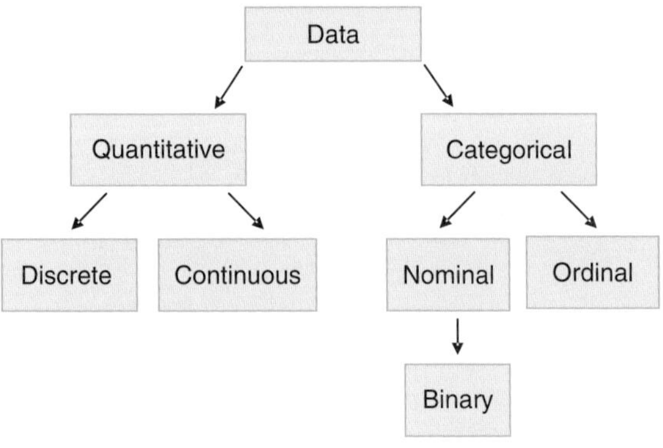

Figure 35.1 Types of data

Reflection activity

Consider the different types of data you routinely collect, interpret and use in your work setting or data you could collect linked to a research study that you would like to take forward. Would you classify this data as categorical or quantitative?

group or disease severity. Although categorical data may be coded numerically, for example, gender may be coded 1 for male and 2 for female, these codes have no intrinsic numerical value; it would be nonsense to calculate an average gender. Categorical data can be divided into either *nominal* or *ordinal*. Nominal data have no natural ordering, and examples include eye colour, marital status and area of residence. *Binary* data is a special subcategory of nominal data, where there are only two possible values (e.g. male/female, yes/no, treated/not treated). Ordinal data occurs when there can be said to be a natural ordering of the data values, such as better/same/worse, grades of breast cancer or social class.

RECORDING DATA

When collecting data, either *forms* or *questionnaires* may be used. Forms are used to record factual information such as a subject's age, ethnic group or blood pressure. They are often completed by the study investigator(s) and thus need to be clearly laid out and familiar to all investigators. Although questionnaires may ask about basic demographic information, they are generally used to measure more personal, subjective attributes such as attitudes and opinions or levels of pain. When designing the layout of questionnaires, it is usual for the data to be recorded in a series of boxes, as this will aid data entry.

In addition to collecting data using forms and questionnaires, a *data coding sheet* may be useful. This document is a link between the data collected on paper and the data stored on a computer as it contains information about how the individual variables are to be named, labelled and coded in the chosen computer package or spreadsheet. It should also have details of any special codes that are to be used for data that are missing or not applicable. It is a common convention when coding data to reserve 9, 99, 999, etc. as codes for missing data. Table 35.1 is an example of a data coding sheet.

Use of spreadsheets and statistical packages

Once the data have been collected and the questionnaires and forms completed, the information recorded can then be input directly onto the computer ready for analysis. Two of the most commonly used packages for data storage and basic statistical analysis are Excel and Statistical Package for the Social Sciences (SPSS®). Both are Windows packages with easy-to-follow pull-down menus. Excel is a spreadsheet with some statistical functions. It also has good facilities for producing graphs. However, if more than the most basic statistical analyses are planned, it is better to use SPSS as this has more comprehensive and flexible statistical analysis and data management facilities. Data can be entered into either package, and most usefully, it is possible to transport files and data between the two, should this be necessary. SPSS will read Excel files, whilst it is possible to save SPSS files as Excel files. As stated previously, all data should be coded numerically when being entered into the computer, unless it is free text. Free text is

Table 35.1 Example of data coding sheet

Variable	Label	Values	
ID	Patient ID number		
Age	Age (years)	999	Missing
Sex	Sex	0	Male
		1	Female
		9	Missing
Height	Height (metres)	999	Missing
Weight	Weight (kg)	999	Missing
BMI	Body mass index	999	Missing
Group	Rehabilitation group	1	Community
		2	Hospital
Withdrawn	Withdrawn from study	0	No
		1	Yes
Reason2	Reason for withdrawal	String	
Reason2	Recoded reason for withdrawal	1	Completer
		2	Deceased
		3	Lost to follow-up
		4	Now unsuitable
		5	Protocol violator
		6	Withdrawn

data that is entered as a string of words. For example, in the rehabilitation trial, for those patients who withdrew, information was recorded on their reason for withdrawal. These would have been entered into a single variable as a string of words, which could then be recoded into numeric categories. In SPSS, it is possible to label both variables and the individual values of a categorical variable to ensure that all output is appropriately labelled and readily understandable.

Data entry and data storage

When entering data onto the computer either into a spreadsheet or a statistical package, it is conventional for each column to represent a different variable and each row to represent the data for an individual subject. For categorical variables, the different categories should be input as distinct numerical values. This is because the standard statistical packages can have problems handling non-numerical data; they are not able to test for a difference between the two groups 'male' and 'female'; they would however be able to test for a difference between groups 1 and 2. Figure 35.2 shows the data view window of SPSS for the rehabilitation trial data (see Research Example 35.1). Each row contains the data for a particular patient, identified by their (unique) patient ID number (STUDYNUMBER), and each column contains the data for a particular variable; for example, the first column contains patient ID number (STUDYNUMBER), the second column contains information on the group the patient was randomised to (GROUP01) and so on. Although the

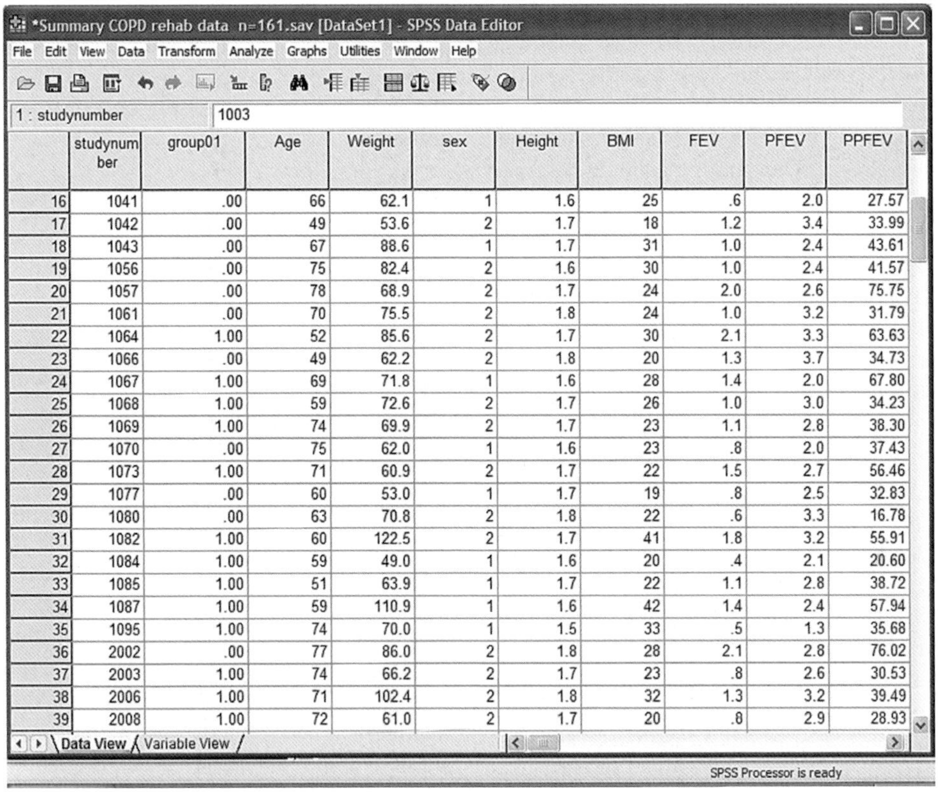

*Summary COPD rehab data n=161.sav [DataSet1] - SPSS Data Editor

File Edit View Data Transform Analyze Graphs Utilities Window Help

1 : studynumber 1003

	studynumber	group01	Age	Weight	sex	Height	BMI	FEV	PFEV	PPFEV
16	1041	.00	66	62.1	1	1.6	25	.6	2.0	27.57
17	1042	.00	49	53.6	2	1.7	18	1.2	3.4	33.99
18	1043	.00	67	88.6	1	1.7	31	1.0	2.4	43.61
19	1056	.00	75	82.4	2	1.6	30	1.0	2.4	41.57
20	1057	.00	78	68.9	2	1.7	24	2.0	2.6	75.75
21	1061	.00	70	75.5	2	1.8	24	1.0	3.2	31.79
22	1064	1.00	52	85.6	2	1.7	30	2.1	3.3	63.63
23	1066	.00	49	62.2	2	1.8	20	1.3	3.7	34.73
24	1067	1.00	69	71.8	1	1.6	28	1.4	2.0	67.80
25	1068	1.00	59	72.6	2	1.7	26	1.0	3.0	34.23
26	1069	1.00	74	69.9	2	1.7	23	1.1	2.8	38.30
27	1070	.00	75	62.0	1	1.6	23	.8	2.0	37.43
28	1073	1.00	71	60.9	2	1.7	22	1.5	2.7	56.46
29	1077	.00	60	53.0	1	1.7	19	.8	2.5	32.83
30	1080	.00	63	70.8	2	1.8	22	.6	3.3	16.78
31	1082	1.00	60	122.5	2	1.7	41	1.8	3.2	55.91
32	1084	1.00	59	49.0	1	1.6	20	.4	2.1	20.60
33	1085	1.00	51	63.9	1	1.7	22	1.1	2.8	38.72
34	1087	1.00	59	110.9	1	1.6	42	1.4	2.4	57.94
35	1095	1.00	74	70.0	1	1.5	33	.5	1.3	35.68
36	2002	.00	77	86.0	2	1.8	28	2.1	2.8	76.02
37	2003	1.00	74	66.2	2	1.7	23	.8	2.6	30.53
38	2006	1.00	71	102.4	2	1.8	32	1.3	3.2	39.49
39	2008	1.00	72	61.0	2	1.7	20	.8	2.9	28.93

Data View / Variable View

SPSS Processor is ready

Figure 35.2 Example of the data view window in SPSS

latest version of SPSS will allow variable names longer than eight characters, in general, statistical packages including older versions of SPSS restrict the length of variable names to eight characters. Thus, the data coding form can be useful in linking the variable names on the computer to a longer more informative label.

Data checking

Errors in recorded data are common. Errors can be made when measurements are taken (data collection), when the data are originally recorded, when they are transcribed from the original source (such as from hospital notes) or when being typed into a computer (data transfer). It is not always possible to know what is correct and so attention must be restricted to making sure that the recorded values are plausible. The data should be scrutinised for potential errors and omissions, and if possible, these should be corrected, either by checking the original questionnaire or remeasuring the variable. This process is known as *data checking* (or *data cleaning*). Since the data will be analysed on a computer, this checking should take place after the data have been entered on the computer.

Initial checks should be made that the values are logical and that there are no missing or clearly implausible values. For categorical variables, this can be as basic as tabulating the values (i.e. calculating the frequency for each value and putting these into a table) and checking that they are all possible. If for example, sex can only take the numerical values 1 (male), 2 (female) and 9 (missing), then any values outside of these three are clearly wrong.

For continuous measurements, it should be possible to specify lower and upper limits on what is reasonable for the variable concerned. For example, for age, limits of 0 and 100 may be used. Age values above 100 should be checked, because although these are possible, they are unlikely. Equally, if adults are being studied, values below 18 should be checked. Values that lie away from the main body of the data are known as *outliers*. They may be genuine observations from individuals with extreme values of the measurement, or they may be erroneous. As with all error checking, once outliers have been checked, they should only be changed if they are known to be wrong, and values remaining outside a pre-specified range must be left as they are or recorded as 'missing'. Values should never be removed from the dataset simply because they are higher or lower than would be expected although the presence of these outlying values may influence the choice of statistical technique used (as outlined in the following chapter). One method for ensuring few errors occur during data entry is to enter the data twice and compare the two datasets. This technique is known as double entry, and any values that are not the same can be checked against the original source. The disadvantage of this approach is that it can be expensive and time-consuming, particularly for large datasets. However, this must be balanced against the fact that the errors that can occur in data entry will have been minimised. It is important to note that this method should never be used as a substitute for the logic and range checking described earlier once the data have been entered.

A by-product of data cleaning is that any missing observations will be identified. As stated earlier, it is usual to use codes such as 9, 99, 999 or 99.9, according to the nature of the variable, although some computer programs, such as SPSS, allow a full stop (.) to indicate a missing observation. If a numeric value is used in SPSS, it is essential to identify the value as a 'user-defined' missing value before analysing the data. It is easy to forget that one or two values are missing, perhaps coded as 999, when carrying out an analysis and the effects on the subsequent results can be severe.

As a final point, it is worth considering why the data are missing. In particular, is there a reason related to the nature of the study? If this is the case, it can have serious implications for the generalisability of the study results. Frequently, however, values are missing essentially at random for reasons not related to the study. As with impossible values, it may be possible to check with the original source of the information that missing observations are really missing.

PRESENTING DATA IN GRAPHS

As a first step to any analysis, it is useful to plot the data and examine them visually. This will show any extreme observations (outliers) together with any interesting patterns. In addition to being a useful preliminary step to analysis, information can also be displayed pictorially when summarising the data and reporting results. Graphs are useful as they can be read quickly and help particularly when presenting information to an audience. However, when using graphs for presentation purposes, care must be taken to ensure that they are not misleading. A graph should have a title explaining what is displayed and axes should be clearly labelled. A fundamental principle, for both graphs and tables, is that they should maximise the amount of information presented for the minimum amount of ink used (Tufte 1983). Gridlines should be kept to a minimum as they act as a distraction and can interrupt the flow of information. All the graphs and tables covered in the following sections were drawn using data from the rehabilitation trial as described in Research Example 35.1.

Basic graphs for categorical data

Categorical data may be displayed using either a *bar chart* or a *pie chart*. Figure 35.3 shows a bar chart of the level of breathlessness of the rehabilitation patients. On the horizontal axis are the different breathlessness categories, whilst on the vertical axis is percentage. Each bar represents the percentage of the total population in that category. For example, examining Figure 35.3, it can be seen that the percentage of rehabilitation participants who walked slower than their contemporaries on level ground due to breathlessness was about 30%. Figure 35.4 shows the same data displayed as a pie chart. Generally, pie

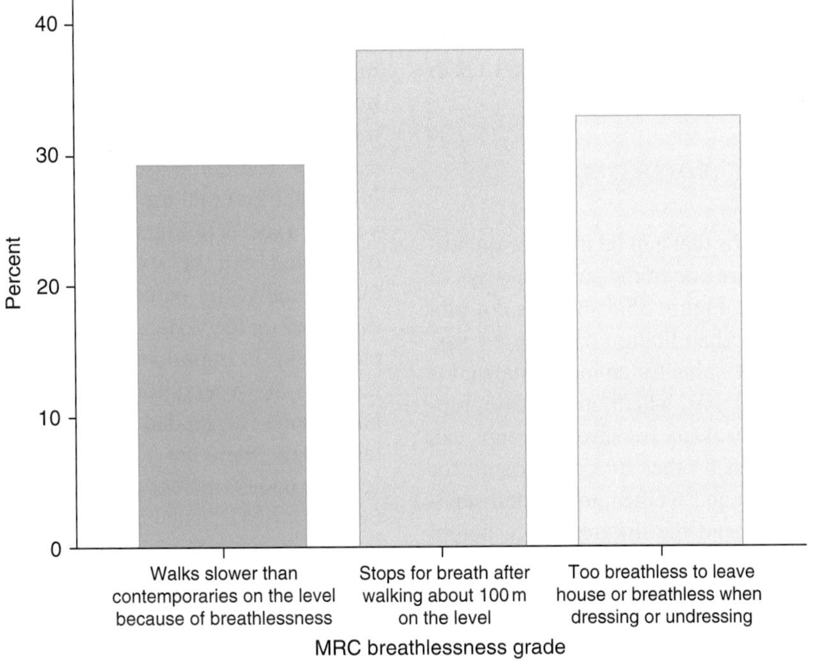

Figure 35.3 Bar chart of breathlessness status for the rehabilitation patients (n = 161)

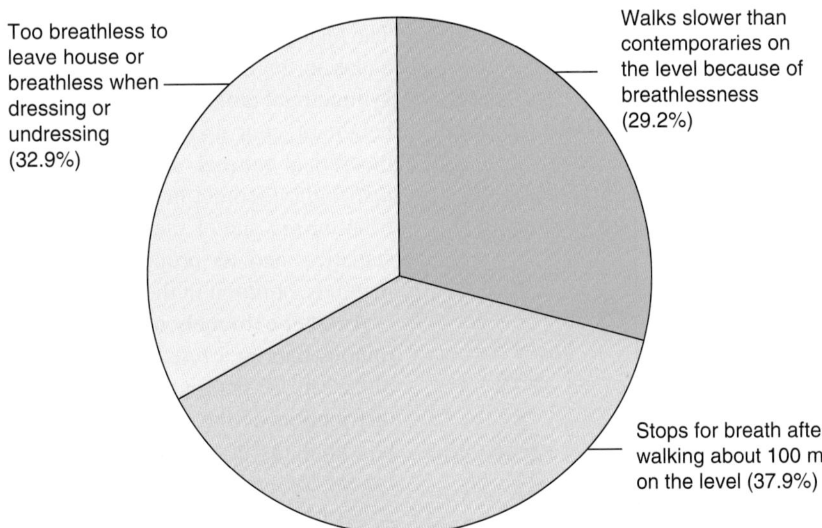

Figure 35.4 Pie chart of breathlessness status for the rehabilitation patients (n = 161)

charts are to be avoided as they can be difficult to interpret particularly when the number of categories becomes greater than 5. In addition, unless the percentages in the individual categories are displayed (as here), it can be much more difficult to estimate them from a pie chart than from a bar chart. For both chart types, it is important to include the number of observations on which it is based, particularly when comparing more than one chart. And finally, neither of these charts should be displayed as 3-D as these are especially difficult to read and interpret (Huff 1991; Freeman *et al.* 2008).

Basic graphs for quantitative data

There are several graphs that can be used for quantitative data. *Dot plots* are one of the simplest ways of displaying all the data. Figure 35.5 shows a dot plot of the heights for the rehabilitation patients, by sex. Each dot represents the value for an individual and is plotted along a vertical axis, which, in this case, represents height in metres. Data for several groups can be plotted alongside each other for comparison; for example, data for men and women are plotted separately in Figure 35.5, and the differences in height between men and women can clearly be seen.

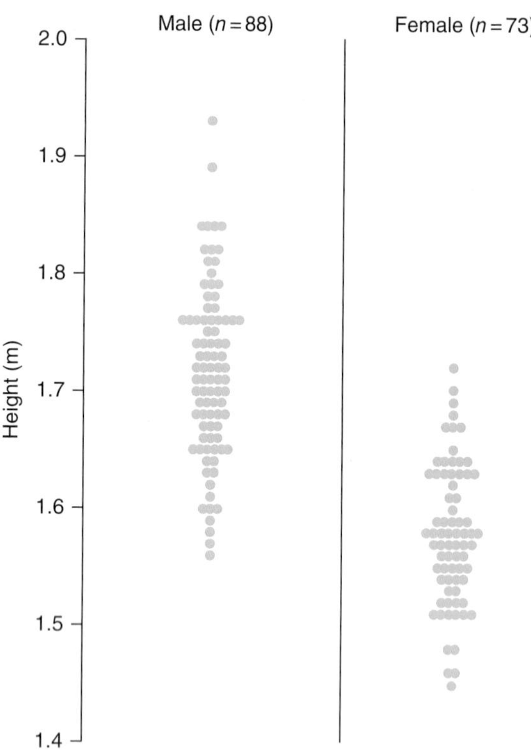

Figure 35.5 Dot plot of height by sex for (n = 161) rehabilitation patients

The most common method for displaying continuous data is a *histogram*. In order to construct a histogram, the data range is divided into several non-overlapping categories of equal length and the number of observations falling into each category counted. The categories are then displayed on the horizontal axis and the frequencies displayed on the vertical axis, as in Figure 35.6. The way that data are distributed can be examined using a histogram. Occasionally, the percentages in each category are displayed on the vertical axis rather than the frequencies, and it is important that if this is done, the total number of observations that the percentages are based upon is included in the chart. For the rehabilitation data, there are a total of 161 observations (73 females and 88 males), and it is conventional to write this as '$n=161$'. The choice of number of categories is important: too few categories and much important information is lost, and too many and any patterns are obscured by too much detail. Usually, between 5 and 15 categories will be enough to gain an idea of the distribution of the data. One useful feature of a histogram is that it makes it possible to see whether the distribution of the data is approximately *normal*. The histogram of normally distributed data will have a classic 'bell' shape, with a peak in the middle and symmetrical tails, such as those in Figure 35.6 for the height of men and women, displayed here with a theoretical normal distribution curve. The *normal distribution* (sometimes known as the Gaussian distribution) is one of the fundamental distributions of statistics, and its properties underpin many of the methods explored in the following chapter.

Another extremely useful method of plotting continuous data is a *box-and-whisker* or *box plot*. Box plots can be particularly useful for comparing the distribution of the data across several groups. The box contains the middle 50% of the data, with the lowest 25% of the data lying below it and the highest 25% of the data lying above it. In fact, the upper and lower edges represent a particular quantity called the interquartile range (IQR) (described later; see Box 35.2). The median is shown by the horizontal line across the box (this is described later; see Box 35.1), but briefly, it is the value such that half of the observations lie below this value and half lie above it. The whiskers extend to the largest and

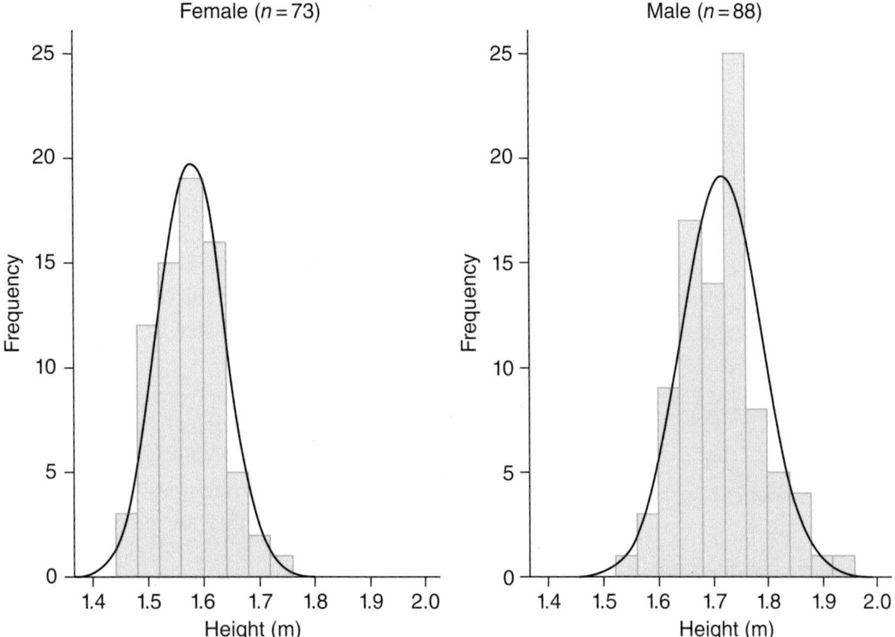

Figure 35.6 Histograms of height for male and female rehabilitation patients

Box 35.1 Measures of location

Mode Most common observation.

Median Middle observation, when the data are arranged in order of increasing value. If there is an even number of observations, the median is calculated as the average of the middle two observations.

Mean $\frac{\text{Sum of all observations}}{\text{Number of observations}}$.

For example, consider the ages (in years) of five patients recruited to the rehabilitation trial: 82, 72, 81, 85 and 58.

The most common observation is 82 or 72 or 81 or 85 or 58. Unfortunately, multiple modes exist in this example, so there is no unique **mode.**

The five ages in ascending order are 58, 72, 81, 82 and 85. The **median** is the middle or third value of the ranked or ordered ages, that is, 81 years.

The **mean** is 82+72+81+85+58=378 divided by the number of observations, 5, that is, 75.6 years.

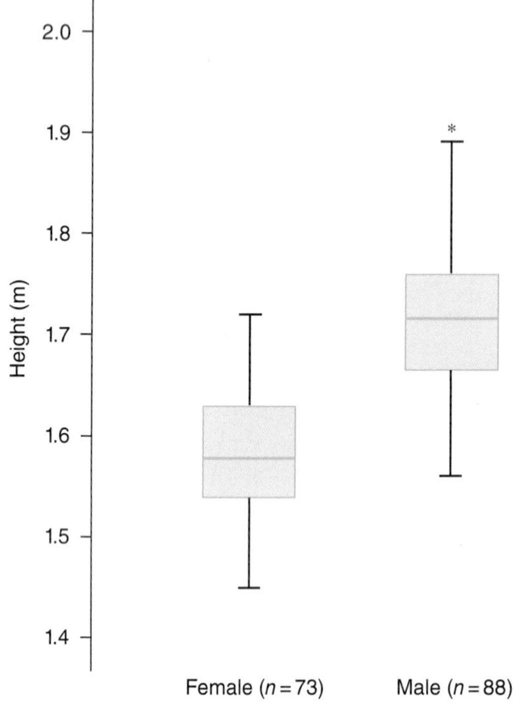

Figure 35.7 Box plot of height for men and women

smallest values excluding the outlying values. The outlying values are those values more than 1.5 box lengths from the upper or lower edges and are represented as the dots outside the whiskers. Figure 35.7 shows box plots of the heights of the men and women in the rehabilitation trial. The gender differences in height are immediately obvious from this plot, and this illustrates the main advantage of the box plot over histograms when looking at multiple groups. Differences in the distributions of data between groups are much easier to spot with box plots than with histograms.

The association between two continuous variables can be examined visually by constructing a *scatter plot*. The values of one variable are plotted on the horizontal axis (sometimes known as the x-axis) and the values of another are plotted on the vertical axis (y-axis). If it is known (or suspected) that the value of one variable (independent) influences the value of the other variable (dependent), it is usual to plot the independent variable on the horizontal axis and the dependent variable on the vertical axis (the reason for this will be explained in the following chapter). Figure 35.8 shows the scatter plot of forced expiratory

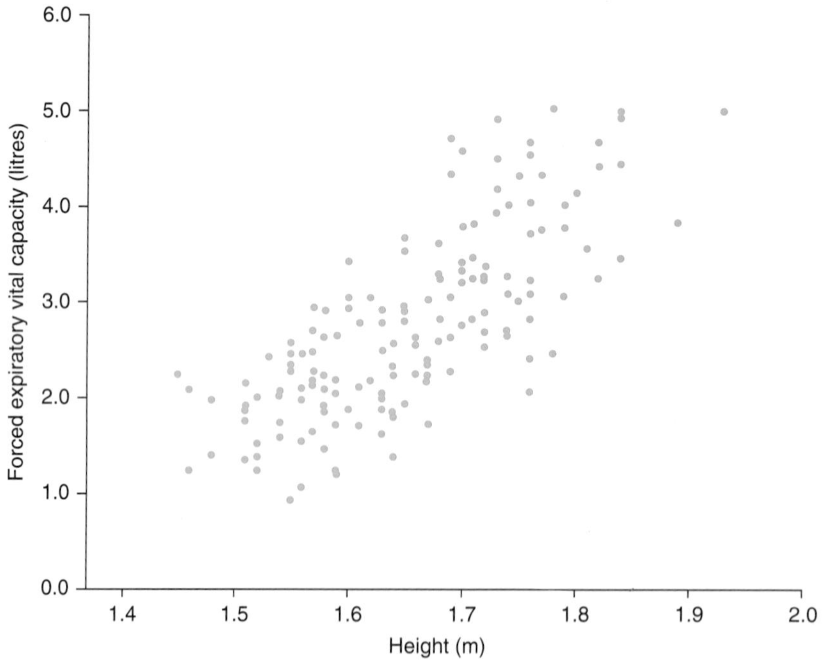

Figure 35.8 Scatterplot of height and forced expiratory vital capacity for 161 rehabilitation patients

vital capacity (in litres) against height (in metres), and each dot represents the height and forced expiratory vital capacity values for an individual. As height determines forced expiratory vital capacity, to an extent, and not the other way around, it is plotted on the horizontal axis, although the variables could legitimately be plotted the other way around.

Reflection activity

Consider the different types of categorical and quantitative data you routinely collect, interpret and use in your work setting or data you could collect linked to a research study that you would like to take forward. Reflect on the advantages and disadvantages of different ways of presenting this data graphically. What do you think are the most appropriate ways of presenting this data graphically? Explain and justify your reasons for this choice?

DESCRIBING DATA

Describing categorical data

A first step to analysing categorical data is to count the number of observations in each category and express them as percentages of the total sample size. For example, as part of the rehabilitation trial, the participants were asked about their level of breathlessness. There were three categories as displayed in Table 35.2. The first column shows category names, whilst the second shows the number of individuals in each category together with its percentage contribution to the total. In addition to tabulating each variable separately, it might be of interest to compare two categorical variables at the same time, and in this case, the data can be *cross-tabulated*. Table 35.3 shows the distribution of level of breathlessness by study group; in this case, it can be said that breathlessness status has been cross-tabulated with the study group. Table 35.3 is an example of a contingency table with three rows (representing level of breathlessness) and two columns

Table 35.2 Level of breathlessness for the rehabilitation trial patients ($n = 161$)

MRC breathlessness grade	*n*	%
Walks slower than contemporaries on the level because of breathlessness	47	(29.2)
Stops for breath after walking about 100 m on the level	61	(37.9)
Too breathless to leave house or breathless when dressing or undressing	53	(32.9)

Table 35.3 Level of breathlessness for the rehabilitation trial patients, by study group ($n = 161$)

	Community group N (%)	**Hospital group N (%)**
MRC breathlessness grade		
Walks slower than contemporaries on the level because of breathlessness	20 (26.3)	27 (31.8)
Stops for breath after walking about 100 m on the level	29 (38.2)	32 (37.6)
Too breathless to leave house or breathless when dressing or undressing	27 (35.5)	26 (30.6)
Total	76 (100)	85 (100)

(representing treatment group). This table suggests that the distribution of breathlessness status is broadly similar between the two study groups, and in the following chapter, this will be formally tested.

Describing quantitative data

As it can be difficult to make sense of a large set of numbers, an initial approach would be to calculate summary measures, to describe the *location* (a measure of the 'middle value') and the *spread* (a measure of the dispersion of the values) of each variable. These are of great interest, particularly if a comparison between groups is to be made or the results of the study are to be generalised to a larger group, and so it is necessary to find reliable ways of determining their values.

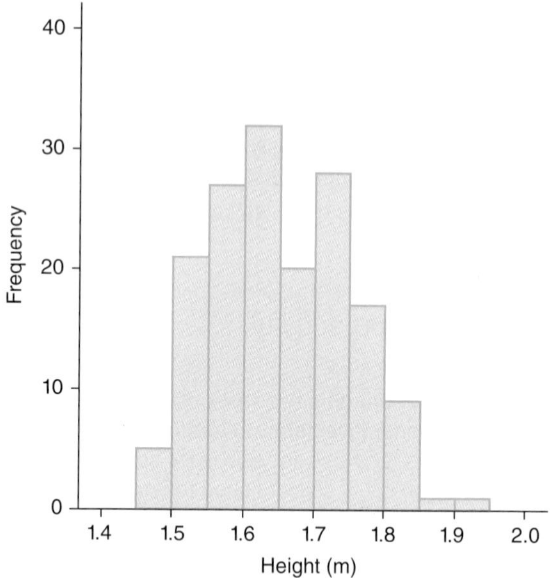

Figure 35.9 Histogram of height, sexes combined, for 161 rehabilitation patients

Measures of location

There are several commonly used measures of location, as summarised in Box 35.1. The simplest is the *mode*. This is the most common observation and is the highest bar of the histogram. Looking at the histograms (Figure 35.6) for height, 1.70–1.75 m is the modal height category for men as this is the height category with the highest bar on the histogram, and 1.55–1.60 m is the modal category for women. However, the mode is rarely used since its value depends upon the accuracy of the measurement. If, for example, the height intervals were 10 cm wide rather than 5 cm, the mode would change to 1.60–1.70 m. In addition, it can be difficult to determine if there is more than one distinct peak such as that for the height of all patients (Figure 35.9). In this case, the presence of two peaks is a reflection of the differing distribution of height between men and women.

Two other more useful and commonly calculated measures are the *median* and the *mean*. The median is the middle observation, when the data are arranged in order of increasing value. It is the value that divides the data into two equal halves. If there is an even number of observations, then the median is calculated as the average of the two middle observations. For example, if there are 11 observations, the median is simply the 6th observation, but if there are 10 observations, the median is the average of the 5th and 6th observations: (5th + 6th observation)/2. The median is not sensitive to the behaviour of outlying data; thus, if the smallest value was even smaller, or the largest value even bigger, it would have no impact on the value of the median.

Generally, the most useful measure of the central value of a set of data is the *mean*. It is calculated as the sum of all observations divided by the total number of observations. Each observation makes a contribution to the mean value, and thus, it is sensitive to the behaviour of outlying data; as the largest value increases, this causes the mean value to increase, and conversely, as the value of the smallest observation becomes smaller, the value of the mean decreases.

Both the mean and median can be useful, but they can give very different impressions when the distribution of the data is *skewed*, because of the relative contributions (or lack of, in the case of the median) of the extreme values. Skewed data are data that are not symmetrical. This is best illustrated by examining the shape of the histogram for the percentage of rehabilitation sessions attended (Figure 35.10). There are few observations at the lower end of the scale, whilst the majority of observations are clustered at the top end of the scale, showing clearly that the majority of participants attended most of their

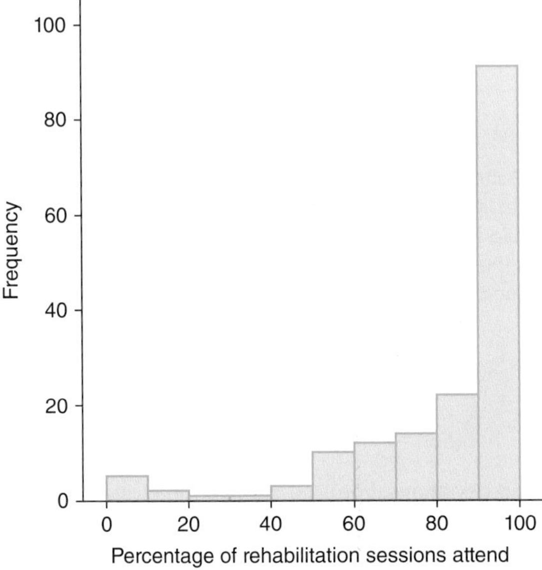

Figure 35.10 Histogram of the percentage of rehabilitation sessions attended showing negative skew of the percentage for this sample (long tail of lower percentages and clustering of values at the higher percentages) for 161 rehabilitation patients

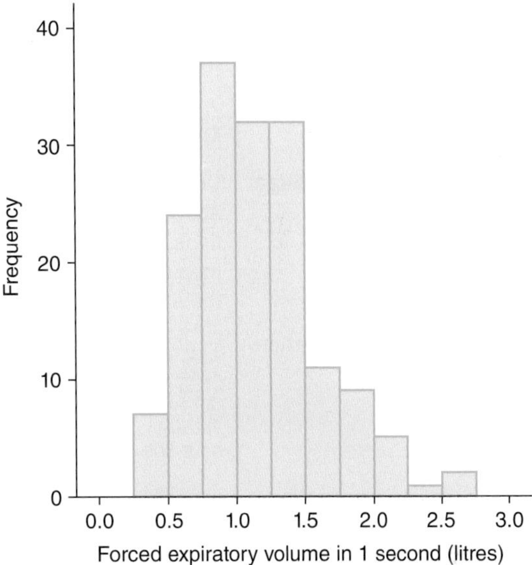

Figure 35.11 Histogram of forced expiratory volume in 1 second in litres for 160 rehabilitation patients showing positive skew

rehabilitation sessions. This is described as being negatively skewed, as there is a long left-hand tail at lower values. Data that have a long right-hand tail of higher values, but where the majority of observations are clustered at lower values, are called positively skewed. The forced expiratory volume data in Figure 35.11 are an example of positively skewed data. There are no firm rules about which to use, but when the distribution is symmetrical, it is usual to use the mean. However, if data are skew, then it is better to use the median, as this is not influenced by the extreme values and may not be as misleading as the mean.

Measures of spread

In addition to finding measures to describe the location of a dataset, it is also necessary to be able to describe its spread. Just as with the measures of location, there are both simple and more complex possibilities (as summarised in Box 35.2). The simplest is the *range* of the data, from the smallest to the largest observation. The range of age for the rehabilitation patients is 49–86 years (or 36 years as a single number). The advantage of the range is that it is easily calculated, but its drawback is that it is vulnerable to *outliers*, extremely large and extremely small observations. A more useful measure is to take the median value as discussed earlier and further divide the two data halves into halves again. These values are called the quartiles, and the difference between the bottom (or 25% percentile) and top quartile (or 75th percentile) is the IQR. This is the observation below which the bottom 25% of the data lie and the observation above which the top 25% lie. The middle 50% of the data lie between these limits. Unlike the range, it is not as sensitive to the extreme values. The IQR for the age of the 161 patients involved in the rehabilitation trial is 63–75 years or 12 years. Strictly speaking, the range and IQR are single numbers, but frequently, the two values, minimum and maximum, or the 25 and 75% percentiles, respectively, are reported as this can be more informative.

However, the most common measure of the spread of the data is the standard deviation (see Box 35.2). It provides a summary of the differences of each observation from the mean value. The standard deviation

Box 35.2 Measures of spread

Range Minimum observation to the maximum observation

Interquartile range Observation below which the bottom 25% of data lie and the observation above which the top 25% of data lie. If the value falls between two observations, for example if 25th centile falls between 5th and 6th observations then the value is calculated as the average of the two observations (this is the same principle as for the median)

Standard deviation $\sqrt{\frac{\sum_{i=1}^{n}(x_i-\bar{x})^2}{n-1}}$ where $\bar{x}$ is the sample mean, x_i is the ith observation, n is the sample size and the notation $\sum_{i=1}^{n}$ represents the addition or summing up of all the squared deviations from the sample mean from the first ($i=1$) to the last (nth) observation

For example, consider the ages (in years) of five patients recruited to the rehabilitation trial: 82, 72, 81, 85 and 58.

The **range** of the data is from 58 to 85 years or 27 years.

The five ages in ascending order are 58, 72, 81, 82, and 85. The bottom 25% of data, falls somewhere between the 1st and 2nd ordered observations, that is 58 and 72, so we can take the average of these two observations 58+72=130/2=65.0. The top 25% of data, falls somewhere between the 4th and 5th ordered observations, that is 82 and 85. So the 75th percentile is the average of the 2 observations 82+85=167/2=83.5. Hence the **interquartile** range is 65.0 to 83.5 years or 18.5 years.

The **standard deviation** is calculated by first working out the squared deviation of each observation from the sample mean of 75.6 years that is

$$(82-75.6)^2+(72-75.6)^2+(81-75.6)^2+(85-75.6)^2+(58-75.6)^2=481.2\,years^2.$$

This result is divided by the number in the sample minus one (i.e. 5−1=4) that is 481.2/4=120.30 years^2. Finally, we take the square root of this number to give us a standard deviation of 10.97 years.

has units on the same scale as the original measurement (e.g. metres if height is being measured).

As with the measures of location, when deciding which measure of spread to present, it is necessary to know whether the data are skewed or not. This will also have a bearing on how the data will be analysed subsequently, as will be seen in the following chapter. When the distribution is symmetrical, it is usual to use the standard deviation. However, if data are skew, then it is better to use the range or IQR.

PRESENTING DATA AND RESULTS IN TABLES

Some basic graphs for displaying data have been described earlier in this chapter. As stated, plotting data can be a useful first stage to any analysis, as this will show extreme observations together with any interesting patterns. Graphs are useful as they can be read quickly and are particularly helpful when

Reflection activity

Consider the different types of quantitative data you routinely collect, interpret and use in your work setting or quantitative data you could collect linked to a research study that you would like to take forward. For these quantitative data, what do you think are the most appropriate summary (and easily understandable and interpretable) measures of location and spread? Explain and justify your reasons for this choice.

presenting information to an audience such as in a seminar or conference presentation. Although there are no hard and fast rules about when to use a graph and when to use a table, when presenting the results in a report or a paper, it is often best to use tables so that the reader can scrutinise the numbers directly. Tables can be useful for displaying information about many variables at once, whilst graphs can be useful for showing multiple observations on groups or individuals (such as a dot plot or a histogram). As with graphs, there are a few basic rules of good presentation:

- Numerical precision should be consistent throughout, and summary statistics such as means and standard deviations should not have more than one extra decimal place compared to the raw data. (Spurious precision should be avoided, although when certain measures are to be used for further calculations or when presenting the results of analyses, greater precision may be necessary.)
- Gridlines can be used to separate labels and summary measures from the main body of the data in a table. However, their use should be kept to a minimum, particularly vertical gridlines, as they can interrupt eye movements and thus the flow of information. Elsewhere, white space can be used to separate data, for example, different variables from each other.

Reflection activity

Consider the different types of quantitative data you routinely collect, interpret and use in your work setting or quantitative data you could collect linked to a research study that you would like to take forward. Do you think these quantitative data are best presented in a table or a graph? Explain and justify your reasons for this decision.

- The information in tables is easier to comprehend if the columns (rather than the rows) contain like information, such as means and standard deviations, as it is easier to scan down a column than across a row.
- Tables should be clearly labelled, and a brief summary of the contents of a table should always be given in words, either as part of the title or in the main body of the text.

When summarising categorical data, both frequencies and percentages can be used, but if percentages are reported, it is important that the denominator (i.e. total number of observations) is given.

For summarising numerical data, the mean and standard deviation may be used, or if the data have a skewed distribution, the median and range or IQR. As with categorical data, the number of observations should be stated.

CONCLUSION

This chapter has looked at the different types of data encountered in quantitative analysis, together with ways of displaying these different data types. Basic summary measures of both location and spread have been discussed, and advice has been given on the best way of presenting these statistics. In the next chapter, some basic approaches to the analysis of these types of data will be examined.

References

Freeman JV, Walters SJ, Campbell MJ (2008) *How to Display Data*. Oxford, BMJ Books, Blackwell.

Huff D (1991) *How to Lie With Statistics*. London, Penguin Books.

Tufte ER (1983) *The Visual Display of Quantitative Information*. Connecticut, Graphics Press.

Waterhouse JC, Walters SJ, Oluboyede Y, Lawson RA (2010) A randomised 2×2 trial of community versus hospital pulmonary rehabilitation, followed by telephone or conventional follow-up: impact on quality of life, exercise capacity and use of health care resources. *Health Technology Assessment* **14**(6): 1–140.

Further reading

Altman DG, Machin D, Bryant TN, Gardner MJ (2000) *Statistics with Confidence. Confidence Intervals and Statistical Guidelines*, 2nd edition. London, BMJ Books.

Bland M (2000) *An Introduction to Medical Statistics*, 3rd edition. Oxford, Oxford Medical Publications.

Campbell MJ, Machin D, Walters SJ (2007) *Medical Statistics: A text book for the health sciences*, 4th edition. Chichester, Wiley.

Campbell MJ, Swinscow TDV (2009) *Statistics at Square One*, 11th edition. London, BMJ Books.

Field A (2013) *Discovering Statistics Using IBM SPSS Statistics*, 4th edition. London, Sage.

Gray CD, Kinnear PR (2012) *IBM SPSS Statistics 19 Made Simple*. Hove, Psychology Press.

Hart A (2001) *Making Sense of Statistics in Healthcare*. Oxford, Radcliffe Medical Press.

Marston L (2010) *Introductory Statistics for Health and Nursing Using SPSS*. London, Sage.

Petrie A, Sabin C (2013) *Medical Statistics at a Glance Text and Workbook*, 3rd edition. Oxford, Wiley-Blackwell.

Walters SJ (2009) *Quality of Life Outcomes in Clinical Trials and Health Care Evaluation: a practical guide to analysis and interpretation*. Chichester, Wiley.

Websites

http://www.statsoftinc.com/textbook/stathome.html – StatSoft Electronic Textbook. An electronic Statistics Textbook offering training in the understanding and application of statistics

http://www.bmj.com/education/endgames – Series of questions aimed at helping junior doctors with the postgraduate exam preparation but contains some useful statistics questions and answers

http://peltiertech.com/Excel/Charts/statscharts.html#BoxWhisker – Excel charts (Biostatistics/Charting and Graphing Data/Charting Data/Excel Charting Tutorials/Charts for Statistics/Box and Whiskers Plots)

http://msor.rsscse.org.uk/leaflets/ssim/Supporting%20stats%20MEDEV.pdf – Supporting Statistics in Medicine facts and formula leaflet

CHAPTER

36 Examining Relationships in Quantitative Data

Jenny Freeman and Stephen J. Walters

Key points

- There are two basic approaches to statistical analysis: hypothesis testing using P-values and estimation using confidence intervals.
- Appropriate statistical methods for analysing relationships in quantitative data include tests for differences between groups and tests for relationships between variables.
- When choosing the correct statistical test for the purpose of the study, the nature of the research question and the type of data collected are crucially important.

INTRODUCTION

The previous chapter looked at the different types of data encountered in quantitative analysis, together with ways of displaying them. Basic summary measures of both location and spread were discussed and advice given on the best ways of presenting these statistics. This chapter will examine the two basic approaches to statistical analysis – *hypothesis testing* (using P-values) and *estimation* (using confidence intervals) – and consider some elementary approaches to analysing the types of data outlined in the previous chapter, including the use of statistical techniques for investigating differences between groups. Example outputs from SPSS will be shown, but formulae and mathematical detail will be kept to a minimum, and the interested reader is referred to the more advanced texts, as listed at the end of Chapter 35 and this chapter. As with the previous chapter, all the example analyses will be based upon data from the COPD rehabilitation trial as outlined in Research Example 35.1 of Chapter 35.

STATISTICAL ANALYSIS

It is rarely possible to obtain information on an entire population, and usually, data are collected on a sample of individuals from the population of interest. The main aim of statistical analysis is to use the information from the sample to draw conclusions (*make inferences*) about the population of interest.

The Research Process in Nursing, Seventh Edition. Edited by Kate Gerrish and Judith Lathlean.

Companion Website: www.wiley.com/go/gerrish/research

For example, it would not be feasible to randomise all individuals with COPD to one of the two interventions, and thus, the rehabilitation trial (see Research Example 35.1) was conducted on a sample of individuals with COPD in order to estimate the effect of community compared to hospital rehabilitation for patients with COPD. The two main approaches to statistical analysis, hypothesis testing and estimation, are outlined in the following section.

Hypothesis testing (using P-values)

Before examining the different techniques available for analysing data, it is essential to understand the process of hypothesis testing and its key principles, such as what a P-value is (and what it is not) and what is meant by the phrase 'statistical significance'. Figure 36.1 describes the steps in the process of hypothesis testing. At the outset, it is important to have a clear research question and know what the outcome variable to be compared is. Once the research question has been stated, the null and alternative hypotheses can be formulated. The null hypothesis (H_0) assumes that there is no difference in the outcome of interest between the study groups. The study or alternative hypothesis (H_1) states that there is a difference between the study groups. In general, the direction of the difference (e.g. that treatment A is better than treatment B) is not specified. For the rehabilitation trial, the research question of interest is as follows:

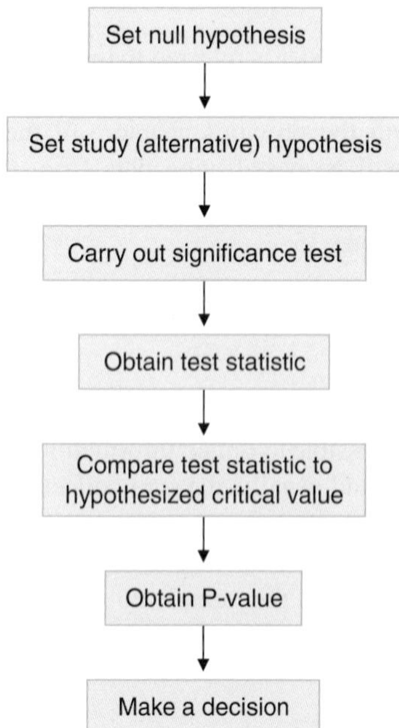

Figure 36.1 Hypothesis testing: the main steps

> For patients with COPD, does rehabilitation in a community setting rather than rehabilitation in a hospital affect exercise capacity (distance walked on an endurance shuttle test)?

The null hypothesis, H_0, is as follows:

> There is no difference in exercise capacity (distance walked on an endurance shuttle test) between the hospital and community rehabilitation groups.

And the alternative hypothesis, H_1, is as follows:

> There is a difference in exercise capacity (distance walked on an endurance shuttle test) between the hospital and community rehabilitation groups.

Having set the null and alternative hypotheses, the next stage is to carry out a significance test. This is done by first calculating a *test statistic* using the study data. This test statistic is then used to obtain a P-value. For the aforementioned comparison, patients in the hospital group could, on average, walk 65.7 m more post-rehabilitation than the community group, and the P-value associated with this difference was

Reflection activity

Assume that you plan to undertake a study to answer the following research question: For patients with gastric reflux, does a new management protocol have an impact on the amount of medication that they take? What are the null and alternative hypotheses for this study?

0.292. The final and most crucial stage of hypothesis testing is to make a decision, based upon the P-value. In order to do this, it is necessary to understand first what a P-value is and what it is not and then understand how to use it to make a decision about whether to reject or not reject the null hypothesis.

So what does a P-value mean? *A P-value is the probability of obtaining the study results (or results more extreme) if the null hypothesis is true*. Common misinterpretations of the P-value are that it is either the probability of the data having arisen by chance or the probability that the observed effect is not a real one. The distinction between these incorrect definitions and the true definition is the absence of the phrase 'when the null hypothesis is true'. The omission of 'when the null hypothesis is true' leads to the incorrect belief that it is possible to evaluate the probability of the observed effect being a real one. The observed effect in the sample is genuine, but what is true in the population is not known. All that can be known with a P-value is, if the null hypothesis is true, how likely is the result obtained (from the study data). For the current example, the null hypothesis is that there is no difference in the distance walked; thus, the P-value tells us how likely it is that we would have found a difference at least as large as the one that we have got, if there truly was no difference in the distance walked between the two rehabilitation groups.

It is important to remember that a P-value is a probability, and its value can vary between 0 and 1. A 'small' P-value, say, close to zero, indicates that the results obtained are unlikely when the null hypothesis is true, and in this case, the null hypothesis is rejected. Alternatively, if the P-value is 'large', then the results obtained are likely when the null hypothesis is true, and in this case, the null hypothesis is not rejected. *But how small is small?* Conventionally, the cut-off value or *significance level* for declaring that a particular result is *statistically significant* is set at 0.05 (or 5%). Thus, if the P-value is less than this value, the null hypothesis (of no difference) is rejected, and the result is said to be statistically significant at the 5% or 0.05 level (Box 36.1). For the previous example of the difference in the distance walked, the P-value is 0.292. As this is more than the cut-off value of 0.05, the difference in exercise capacity is said to be not statistically significant between the two groups at the 5% level.

If we were to ignore the effect of the type of rehabilitation (hospital/community) and instead ask the question 'does rehabilitation affect the exercise capacity of an individual with COPD?', we have the following null and alternative hypotheses:

Null hypothesis: *Rehabilitation makes no difference to the exercise capacity of patients with COPD.*

Box 36.1 Statistical significance

We say that our results are statistically significant if the P-value is less than the significance level (α) set at 5% or 0.05.

	$P \leq 0.05$	$P > 0.05$
Result is	Statistically significant	Not statistically significant
Decide	That there is sufficient evidence to reject the null hypothesis and accept the alternative hypothesis	That there is insufficient evidence to reject the null hypothesis

We cannot say that the null hypothesis is true, only that there is not enough evidence to reject it.

Alternative hypothesis: *Rehabilitation makes a difference to the exercise capacity of patients with COPD.*

When we compare the results in exercise capacity, as measured by distance walked, from before rehabilitation to after, there is a mean difference of 251 m. Before rehabilitation, on average, patients could only walk 280 m, whereas after rehabilitation, the distance walked had increased to 531 m and the P-value associated with this change was less than 0.001. As this is less than 0.05, we can conclude that there is a statistically significant change in the distance walked following rehabilitation at the 5% level.

Though the decision to reject or not reject the null hypothesis may seem clear-cut, it is possible that a mistake may be made, as can be seen from the shaded cells of Table 36.1. Whatever is decided, this decision may correctly reflect what is true in the population: the null hypothesis is rejected, when it is in fact false; or the null hypothesis is not rejected, when in fact it is true. Alternatively, it may not reflect what is true in the population: the null hypothesis is rejected, when it is in fact true (*false-positive* or *type I error*, α); or the null hypothesis is not rejected, when in fact it is false (*false-negative*, *type II error*, β).

The probability that a study will be able to detect a difference, of a given size, if one truly exists is called the *power* of the study and is the probability of rejecting the null hypothesis when it is actually false. It is usually expressed in percentages, so for a study that has 80% power, there is a likelihood of 80% of being able to detect a difference, of a given size, if there genuinely is a difference of at least this size in the population.

Reflection activity

Consider the study outlined previously about the effect that rehabilitation has on the exercise capacity of patients with COPD. Assume that the study has measured the distance walked by the two groups at the end of the trial. How might you explain the results that give a P-value of 0.2 to a patient? How might you explain results that give a P-value of 0.02 to a patient?

Estimation (using confidence intervals)

*Statistical significance does not necessarily mean the result obtained is clinically significant or of any practical importance***.** A P-value will only indicate how likely the results obtained are when the null hypothesis is true. It can only be used to decide whether the results are statistically significant or not, it does not give any information about the likely effect size. Much more information, such as whether the result is likely to be of clinical importance can be gained by calculating a *confidence interval.* A confidence interval may be calculated for any estimated quantity (from the sample data), such as the mean, median, proportion or even a difference, for example, the mean difference in distance walked between the two rehabilitation groups. It is a measure of the precision (accuracy) with which the quantity of interest is estimated (in this case, the mean difference, between

Table 36.1 Making a decision

		The null hypothesis is actually	
		False	**True**
Decide to	Reject the null hypothesis	Correct	Type 1 error (α) (false-positive error)
	Not reject the null hypothesis	Type 2 error (β) (false-negative error)	Correct

the community and hospital groups, in exercise capacity – the distance walked post-rehabilitation).

Technically, the 95% confidence interval is the range of values within which the true population quantity would fall 95% of the time if the study were to be repeated many times. Crudely speaking, the confidence interval gives a range of plausible values for the quantity estimated; although not strictly correct, it is usually interpreted as the range of values within which there is 95% certainty that the true value in the population lies. For the aforementioned rehabilitation trial, the quantity estimated was the mean difference in the distance walked between the hospital and community groups following rehabilitation, 65.7 m (see Figure 36.3, explained fully in the following section 'Independent samples *t*-test for continuous outcome data'). The 95% confidence interval for this difference was –56.9 to 188.2 m. Thus, whilst the best available estimate of the mean difference was 65.7 m, it could be as low as –56.9 m or as high as 188.2 m, with 95% certainty. This range clearly does include the value for no difference (in this case 0). So the confidence interval is consistent with there being no difference in distance walked post-rehabilitation between the groups. The P-value associated with this difference was 0.292, and in the previous section, it was concluded that this difference was not statistically significant at the 5% level. Whilst the P-value will give an indication of whether the result obtained is statistically significant or not, it gives no other information. The confidence interval is more informative as it gives a range of plausible values for the estimated quantity. Provided this range *does not* include the value for no difference (in this case 0), it can be concluded that there is a difference between the groups being compared.

Statistical versus clinical significance

So far, we have considered both the process of hypothesis testing and estimation. However, in addition to statistical significance, it is useful to consider the concept of clinical significance. Whilst a result may be statistically significant, it may not be clinically significant (relevant/important), and conversely, an estimated difference that is clinically important may not be statistically significant. For the example earlier, whilst there is no statistically significant difference between the two rehabilitation groups in terms of the distance walked, the confidence interval for the difference is rather large; it ranges from –56.9 to 188.2 m. Thus, it is possible that the difference could be as great as 188 m, a difference that could be (clinically) important to some individuals with COPD. In order to conclude that there truly was no difference between the two groups, we would want a confidence interval that not only included 0, but was also narrow enough to exclude any difference of importance. For example, if we were to decide that a difference of more than 30 m was clinically important, then in order to state that there was no clinically important difference between the groups, we would want to see that not only did the confidence interval include 0 but that it lay between the limits –0.30 and 30 m.

> **Reflection activity**
>
> Why might a large difference not be statistically significant? Does this mean that there is actually no difference?

This is not simply a trivial point. Often in presentations or papers, P-values alone are quoted and inferences are made based on this one statistic. It may be possible to have a P-value greater than the magic 5% for there to be a genuine difference between groups. Conversely, statistically significant P-values may be masking the fact that differences have little clinical importance: absence of evidence is not evidence of absence.

CHOOSING THE STATISTICAL METHOD

The type of statistical analysis to be carried out depends on the answer to five key questions (Box 36.2). Once these questions have been answered, an appropriate approach to the statistical analysis of

Box 36.2 Five key questions to ask

1 What are the aims and objectives?
2 What is the hypothesis to be tested?
3 What type of data are the outcome data?
4 How are the outcome data distributed?
5 What is the summary measure for the outcome data?

Box 36.3 Three most common problems in statistical inference

1 Comparison of independent groups, for example, groups of patients given different treatments
2 Comparison of the response for paired observations, for example, in a crossover trial, or for matched pairs of subjects
3 Investigation of the relationship between two variables measured on the same sample of subjects

the data collected can be decided upon. The type of statistical analysis depends fundamentally on what the main purpose of the study is. In particular, what is the main question to be answered? The data type for the outcome variable will also govern how it is to be analysed, as an analysis appropriate to continuous data would be completely inappropriate for binary data. In addition to what type of data the outcome variable is, its distribution is also important, as is the summary measure to be used. Highly skewed data require a different analysis compared to data that are *Normally* distributed.

The choice of method of analysis for a problem depends on the comparison to be made and the data to be used. This chapter outlines the methods appropriate for the three most common problems in statistical inference as outlined in Box 36.3. Before beginning any analysis, it is important to examine the data, using the techniques described in Chapter 35; adequate description of the data should precede and complement the formal statistical analysis. For most studies and for RCTs in particular, it is good practice to produce a table or tables that describe the initial or baseline characteristics of the sample.

Comparison of two independent groups

Before comparing two independent groups, it is important to decide what type of data the outcome is and how it is distributed, as this will determine the most appropriate analysis. This section describes, for different types of data, the statistical methods available for comparing two independent groups, as outlined in Figure 36.2.

Independent samples *t*-test for continuous outcome data

The independent samples *t*-test is used to test for a difference in the mean value of a continuous variable between two groups. For example, one of the main questions of interest in the rehabilitation trial was whether there was a difference in distance walked post-rehabilitation between the hospital and the community groups. As the distance walked is continuous data and there are two independent groups (i.e. the two randomised groups), assuming the data are Normally distributed in each of the two groups, then the most appropriate summary measure for the data

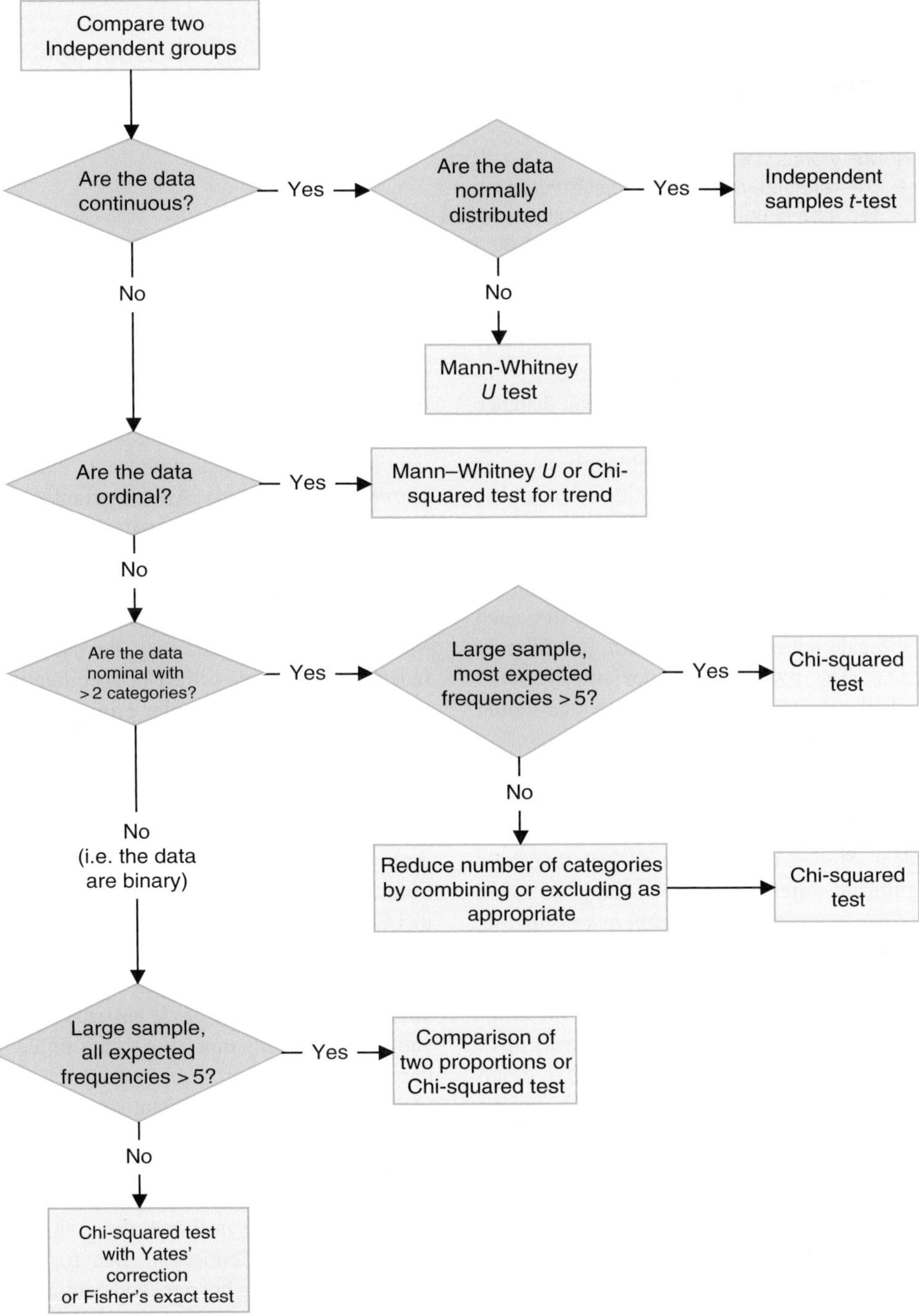

Figure 36.2 Statistical methods for comparing two independent groups or samples

Box 36.4 The assumptions underlying the use of the independent samples *t*-test

1 The groups are independent.
2 The variables of interest are continuous.
3 The data in both groups have similar standard deviations.
4 The data are Normally distributed in both groups.

is the sample mean, and the best comparative summary measure is the difference in the mean distance walked post-rehabilitation between the two groups.

When conducting any statistical analysis, it is important to check that the assumptions that underpin the chosen method are valid. The assumptions underlying the two-sample *t*-test are outlined in Box 36.4. The assumption of Normality can be checked by plotting two histograms, one for each sample; these do not need to be perfect, just roughly symmetrical. The two standard deviations should also be calculated, and as a rule of thumb, one should be no more than twice as large as the other.

Figure 36.3 shows the SPSS output for comparing distance walked post-rehabilitation (endurance shuttle walk test) between the two groups using the two independent samples *t*-test. It can be seen that there is no significant difference between the groups; *the 95% confidence interval for the difference* suggests that on average patients in the hospital group might be able to walk up to 188.2 m further than patients in the community group; equally, patients in the community group might, on average, be able to walk up to 56.9 m further than patients in the hospital group (with 95% certainty), and the best estimate is a mean difference of 65.7 m. Clearly, the confidence interval includes a zero difference and the result is equivocal.

Mann–Whitney *U* test

There are several possible approaches when at least one of the requirements for the *t*-test is not met. The data may be transformed (e.g. the logarithm transformation can be useful particularly when the variances are not equal) or a *non-parametric method* can be used. Non-parametric or distribution-free methods do not involve distributional assumptions, that is, making assumptions about the manner in which the data are distributed (e.g. that the data are *Normally* distributed). An important point to note is that it is the test that is parametric or non-parametric, not the data.

When the assumptions underlying the *t*-test are not met, then the non-parametric equivalent, the Mann–Whitney *U* test, may be used. Whilst the independent samples *t*-test is specifically a test of the null hypothesis that the groups have the same mean value, the Mann–Whitney *U* test is a more general test of the null hypothesis that the distribution of the outcome variable in the two groups is the same. It is possible for the outcome data in the two groups to have similar measures of central tendency or location, such as mean and medians, but different distributions. The Mann–Whitney *U* test requires all the observations to be ranked as if they were from a single sample. From this, the statistic *U* is calculated; it is the number of all possible pairs of observations comprising one from each sample for which the value in the first group precedes a value in the second group. This test statistic is then used to obtain a P-value.

Examining the output from the Mann–Whitney *U* test in SPSS (Figure 36.4), there is insufficient evidence to *reject the null hypothesis* that there is no difference in distribution of data for the distance walked between the hospital and community groups.

In the majority of cases, it is reasonable to treat *discrete data*, such as number of children in a family or number of visits to the GP in a year, as if they were continuous, at least as far as the statistical analysis

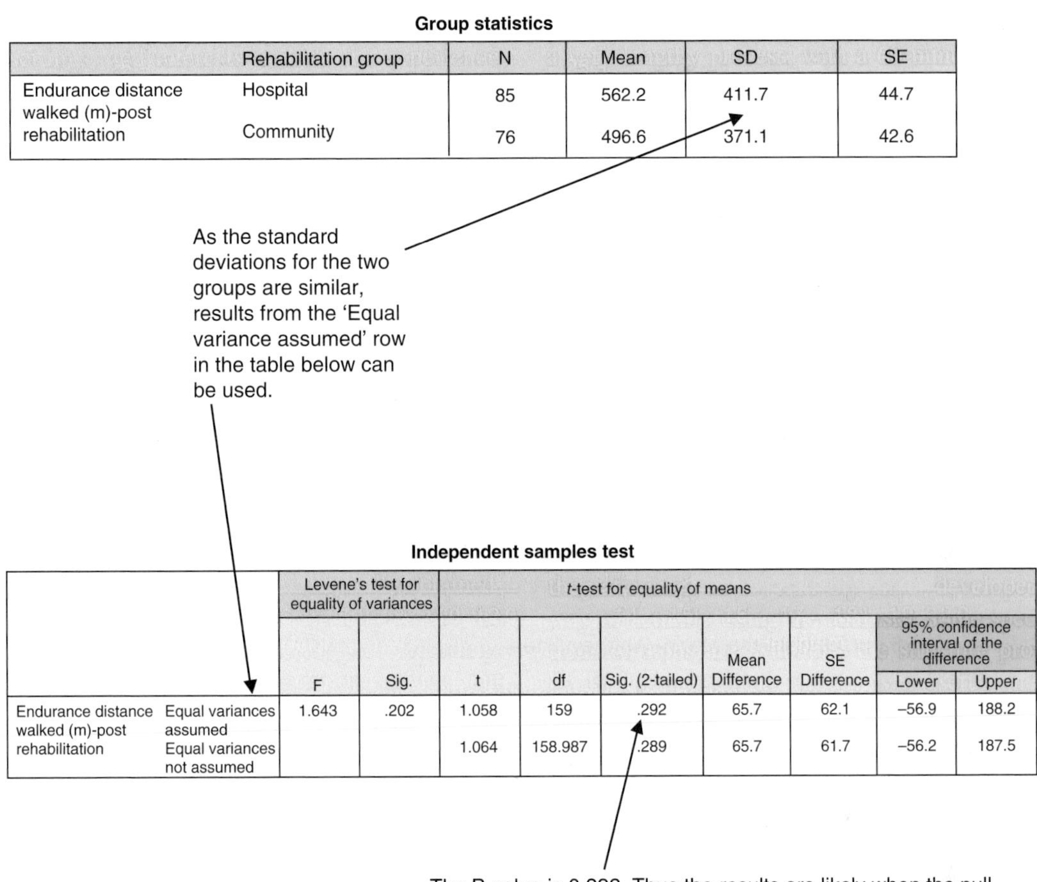

Group statistics

	Rehabilitation group	N	Mean	SD	SE
Endurance distance walked (m)-post rehabilitation	Hospital	85	562.2	411.7	44.7
	Community	76	496.6	371.1	42.6

Independent samples test

		Levene's test for equality of variances		*t*-test for equality of means					95% confidence interval of the difference	
		F	Sig.	t	df	Sig. (2-tailed)	Mean Difference	SE Difference	Lower	Upper
Endurance distance walked (m)-post rehabilitation	Equal variances assumed	1.643	.202	1.058	159	.292	65.7	62.1	–56.9	188.2
	Equal variances not assumed			1.064	158.987	.289	65.7	61.7	–56.2	187.5

As the standard deviations for the two groups are similar, results from the 'Equal variance assumed' row in the table below can be used.
The P-value is 0.292. Thus the results are likely when the null hypothesis (that there is no difference between the groups) is true. The result is said to be *not statistically significant* because the P-value is greater than the significance level (α) set at 5% or 0.05 and there is insufficient evidence to reject the null hypothesis and accept the alternative hypothesis that there is a difference in mean distance walked between the hospital and community rehabilitation groups.

Figure 36.3 SPSS output from the independent samples *t*-test

goes. Ideally, there should be a large number of different possible values, but in practice, this is not always necessary. However, where ordered categories are numbered such as stage of disease or social class, the temptation to treat these numbers as statistically meaningful must be resisted. For example, it is not sensible to calculate the average social class or stage of cancer, and in such cases, the data should be treated in statistical analyses as if they are ordered categories.

Comparing more than two groups

The methods outlined earlier can be extended to more than two groups. For the independent samples *t*-test, the analogous method for more than two groups is called the *analysis of variance (ANOVA)*, and the assumptions underlying it are similar. The non-parametric equivalent for the method of ANOVA when there are more than two groups is called the *Kruskal–Wallis test*. A fuller explanation of these

NPar tests
Mann-Whitney test

Ranks

	Rehabilitation group	N	Mean rank	Sum of ranks
Endurance Distance Walked (m) - post-rehabilitation	Community	76	77.76	5910.00
	Hospital	85	83.89	7131.00
	Total	161		

Test statistics[a]

	Endurance distance walked (m)-post rehabilitation
Mann-Whitney *U*	2984.000
Wilcoxon W	5910.000
Z	–.833
Asymp. Sig. (2-tailed)	.405

[a] Grouping variable: rehabilitation group

P-value: probability of observing the test statistic under the null hypothesis. As the value of 0.405 is greater than the significance level (α) set at 0.05 or 5% this means that the result obtained is likely when the null hypothesis is true and it is said to be not statistically significant. Thus there is insufficient evidence to reject the null hypothesis and accept the alternative hypothesis that there is a difference in the distribution of endurance distance walked after rehabilitation between the hospital and community and groups.

Figure 36.4 SPSS output from the Mann–Whitney *U* test

Table 36.2 Cross-tabulation of treatment group versus post-treatment increase in exercise capacity

	Treatment group		
	Community rehabilitation	**Hospital rehabilitation**	**Total**
Increase in exercise capacity:			
No change or deteriorated	22 (28.9%)	17 (20.0%)	39 (24.2%)
Improved	53 (71.1%)	68 (80.0%)	122 (75.8%)
Total	76	85	161

methods is beyond the scope of this chapter, and the interested reader is referred to the more advanced statistical textbooks listed at the end of this chapter and Chapter 35.

Chi-squared test for categorical outcome data

Sometimes, when comparing two independent groups, the outcome variable is categorical rather than continuous. For example, in the rehabilitation trial, it was of interest to know whether patients increased their exercise capacity after rehabilitation or if it remained the same or deteriorated and if there was a difference between the groups with respect to the proportions with increased exercise capacity post-rehabilitation. With two independent groups (hospital and community) and a binary (exercise capacity increased vs. no change/decreased) rather than a continuous outcome, the data can be cross-tabulated as in Table 36.2. This is an example of a 2×2 contingency table with 2 rows (for treatment) and 2 columns (for outcome), that is, 4 cells in total. The most appropriate summary measure is simply the proportion in the sample whose exercise capacity increased and the best comparative

Box 36.5 Guidelines for the chi-squared test to be valid

1 At least 80% of cells should have expected frequencies greater than 5.
2 All cells should have expected frequencies greater than 1.

summary measure is the difference in proportions with increased exercise capacity between the two groups. The most appropriate hypothesis test, assuming a large sample and all expected frequencies greater than 5, is the *chi-squared test*.

The null hypothesis is that the two classifications (e.g. *group and increased exercise capacity*) are unrelated in the relevant population (*patients with COPD*). More generally, the null hypothesis, H_0, for a contingency table is that there is no association between the row and column variables in the table, that is, they are independent. The general alternative hypothesis, H_1, is that there is an association between the row and column variables in the contingency table, that is, they are not independent or unrelated. For the chi-squared test to be valid, two key assumptions need to be met, as outlined in Box 36.5. If these are not met, Fisher's exact test can be used for 2×2 tables.

Figure 36.5 shows the results of analysing Table 36.2 in SPSS. The P-value of 0.255 indicates that there is little evidence of a difference in the proportion of patients with increased exercise capacity post-rehabilitation between the community and hospital groups.

Two groups of paired observations

When there is more than one group of observations, it is vital to distinguish the case where the data are paired from that where the groups are independent. Paired data may arise when the same individuals are studied more than once, usually in different circumstances, or when individuals are paired as in a case–control study. For example, as part of the rehabilitation trial, data were collected on exercise capacity (distance walked on the endurance shuttle test) at baseline and post-rehabilitation (~8 weeks post-baseline). We have already demonstrated that there is no statistically significant difference in distance walked between the hospital and community groups. However, Figure 36.5 shows that 75.8% (122/161) of the combined sample increased their exercise capacity. Suppose we want to test whether the change in distance walked pre- to post-rehabilitation is different from zero, that is, that rehabilitation makes a difference to exercise capacity, irrespective of where it is delivered. Methods of analysis for paired samples are summarised in Figure 36.6.

Paired *t*-test

Distances walked at baseline and post-rehabilitation are both continuous variables, and the data are paired as measurements are made on the same individuals at baseline and post-rehabilitation (approximately 8 weeks). Therefore, the interest is in the mean of the differences, not the difference between the two means. If we assume that the paired differences are *Normally* distributed, then the most appropriate comparative summary measure is the mean of the paired difference in distance walked between baseline and post-rehabilitation. Given the null hypothesis (H_0) that there is no difference (or change) in mean distance walked at baseline and post-rehabilitation follow-up, the most appropriate test is the paired *t*-test.

There were 161 patients with both pre- and post-rehabilitation distance walked data. Examining the SPSS output for the comparison of distance walked for these 161 patients pre- and post-rehabilitation shows that the result is statistically significant (Figure 36.7). *The 95% confidence interval of the difference* suggests that we are 95% confident that distance walked has changed. It has increased by between 196.9 and 306.2 m between baseline and post-rehabilitation, and the best estimate is a mean change of 251.6 m.

The assumptions underlying the use of the paired *t*-test are outlined in Box 36.6. If these are not met, a

Cross tabs

Increase in exercise capacity post-rehabilitation * Rehabilitation group crosstabulation

			Rehabilitation group		Total
			Hospital (n=85)	Community (n=76)	
Increase in exercise capacity post-rehabilitation	No change or deteriorated	Count	17	22	39
		% within rehabilitation group	20.0%	28.9%	24.2%
	Yes	Count	68	54	122
		% within rehabilitation group	80.0%	71.1%	75.8%
Total		Count	85	76	161
		% within rehabilitation group	100.0%	100.0%	100.0%

Chi-Square tests

	Value	df	Asymp. Sig. (2-sided)	Exact Sig. (2-sided)	Exact Sig. (1-sided)
Pearson Chi-square	1.750[b]	1	.186		
Continuity correction[a]	1.296	1	.255		
Likelihood ratio	1.750	1	.186		
Fisher's exact test				.202	.127
Linear-by-Linear Association	1.739	1	.187		
N of Valid cases	161				

[a] Computed only for a 2 × 2 table

[b] 0 cells (.0%) have expected count less than 5. The minimum expected count is 18.41.

To improve the approximation for a 2 × 2 table, Yates' correction for continuity is sometimes applied. Altman (1991) recommends the use of Yates' correction for all chi-squared tests on 2 × 2 tables. In a 2 × 2 table when expected cell counts are less than 5, or any are less than 1 even Yates' correction does not work and thus Fisher's exact test is used. When comparing frequencies amongst groups that have an ordering (e.g. group by pain score), any difference among the groups would be expected to be related to the ordering and the Mantel-Haenszel test for linear association or trend can be carried out. Although the Mantel-Haenszel statistic is displayed, it should not be used for purely nominal data, like we have here.

This suggests that the chi-squared test is valid as all the expected counts are greater than 5.

The P-value of 0.255 indicates that the results obtained are likely if the null hypothesis (of no association between the rows and columns of the contingency table above) is true. Thus there is insufficient evidence to reject the null hypothesis and the results are said to be not statistically significant.

Figure 36.5 SPSS output for cross-tab procedure and chi-squared test

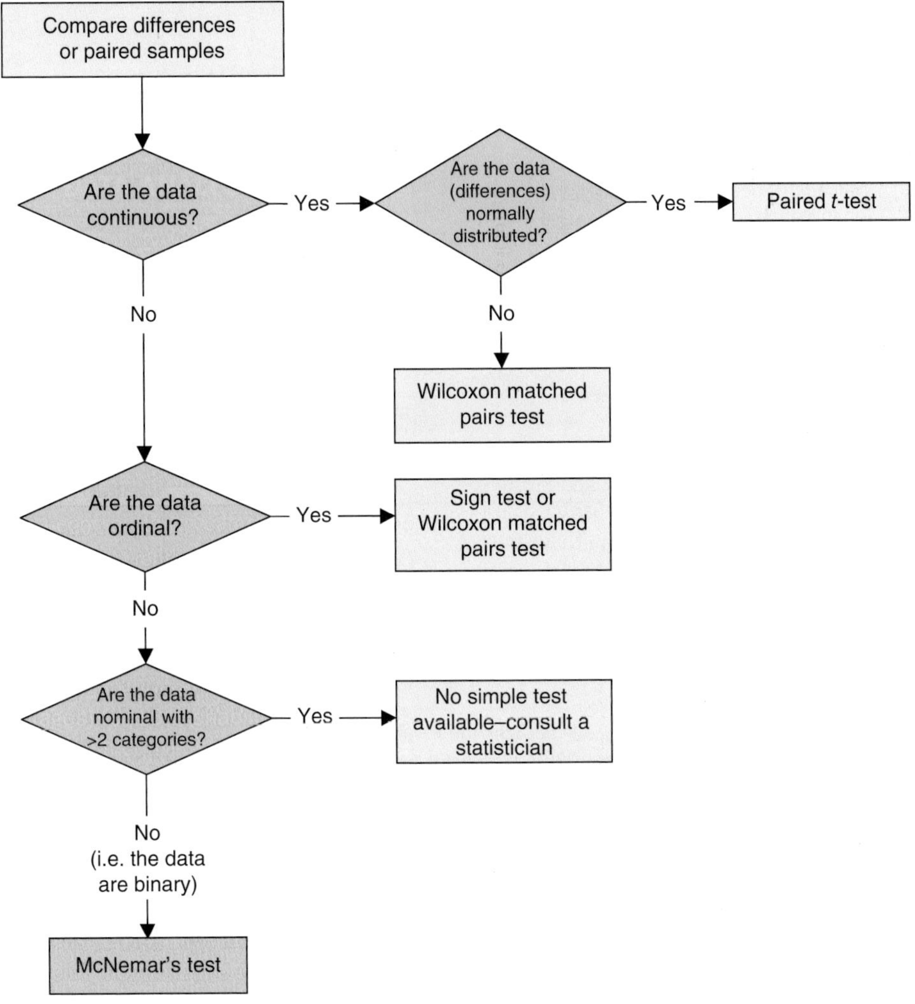

Figure 36.6 Statistical methods for differences or paired samples

non-parametric alternative, the *Wilcoxon signed-rank sum test*, can be used.

THE RELATIONSHIP BETWEEN TWO CONTINUOUS VARIABLES

Many statistical analyses are undertaken to examine the relationship between two continuous variables within a group of subjects (Table 36.3). Two of the main purposes of such analyses are as follows:

- To assess whether the two variables are associated. There is no distinction between the two variables and no causation is implied, simply *association*.
- To enable the value of one variable to be predicted from any known value of the other variable. One variable is regarded as a *response* to the other *predictor (explanatory)* variable, and the value of the predictor variable is used to *predict* what the response would be.

For the first of these, the statistical method for assessing the association between two *continuous* variables

T-Test

Paired samples statistics

		Mean	N	SD	SE Mean
Pair 1	Endurance Distance Walked (m): baseline	279.7	161	138.3	10.9
	Endurance distance Walked (m)-post rehabilitation	531.2	161	393.2	31.0

Paired samples test

		Paired differences							
					95% Confidence interval of the difference				
		Mean	SD	SE Mean	Lower	Upper	t	df	Sig. (2-tailed)
Pair 1	Endurance Distance Walked (m): baseline - Endurance Distance Walked (m)-post rehabilitation	251.6	351.1	27.7	196.9	306.2	-9.091	160	.000

In SPSS if the P-value is less than 0.001, it is written as 0.000, thus here the P-value is < 0.001 (not 0.000 as could be mis-interpreted from this table), indicating that the results obtained are unlikely when the null hypothesis is true. The result is statistically significant because the P-value is less than the significance level (α) set at 0.05 or 5% and there is sufficient evidence to reject the null hypothesis. The alternative hypothesis, that there is a difference in distance walked before and after rehabilitation is accepted.

Figure 36.7 SPSS output for paired *t*-test

Box 36.6 The assumptions underlying the use of the paired *t*-test

1. The paired differences are plausibly Normally distributed (it is not essential for the original observations to be Normally distributed).
2. The paired differences are independent of each other.

is known as *correlation*, whilst the technique for the second, prediction of one continuous variable from another is known as *regression*. Correlation and regression are often presented together, and it is easy to get the impression that they are inseparable. In fact, they have distinct purposes, and it is relatively rare that one is genuinely interested in performing both analyses on the same set of data. However, when preparing to analyse data using either technique, it is always important to construct a scatter plot of the values of the two variables against each other. By drawing a scatter plot, it is possible to see whether or not

Table 36.3 Statistical methods for relationships between two variables measured on the same sample of subjects

	Continuous, Normal	Continuous, non-Normal	Ordinal	Nominal	Binary
Continuous	Regression Correlation: Pearson's *r*	Regression Rank correlation: Spearman's r_s	Rank correlation: Spearman's r_s	One-way analysis of variance	Independent samples *t*-test
Continuous, non-Normal		Regression Rank correlation: Spearman's r_s	Rank correlation: Spearman's r_s	Kruskal–Wallis test	Mann–Whitney *U* test
Ordinal			Rank correlation: Spearman's r_s	Kruskal–Wallis test	Mann–Whitney *U* test Chi-squared test for trend
Nominal				Chi-squared test	Chi-squared test
Binary					Chi-squared test Fisher's exact test

there is any visual evidence of a straight line or linear association between the two variables.

Correlation

As stated previously, as part of the rehabilitation trial, distance walked on the endurance shuttle test was measured at baseline (pre-rehabilitation) and follow-up (post-rehabilitation). Plotting the distanced walked at baseline and follow-up indicates that there is a positive linear relationship between baseline and follow-up distance walked (Figure 36.8). Unsurprisingly, distance walked post-rehabilitation is generally related to distance walked pre-rehabilitation, that is, short distances walked at baseline generally correspond with shorter distances walked after rehabilitation. Conversely, longer distances walked at baseline seem to correspond with greater distances at follow-up. In order to examine whether there is an association between the two variables, the *correlation coefficient* can be calculated. At this point, no assumptions are made about whether the relationship is causal, that is, whether one variable is influencing the value of the other variable. The standard method (often ascribed to Karl Pearson) leads to a statistic called *r*. In essence, *r* is a measure of the scatter of the points around an underlying *linear trend*: the closer the spread of points to a straight line, the higher the value of the correlation coefficient; the greater the spread of points, the lower the correlation. Pearson's correlation coefficient *r* must be between −1 and +1, with −1 representing a perfect negative correlation, +1 representing perfect positive correlation and 0 representing no linear trend.

The assumptions underlying the validity of the hypothesis test associated with the correlation coefficient are outlined in Box 36.7. The easiest way to check the validity of the hypothesis test is by examining a scatter plot of the data. This plot should be produced as a matter of routine when correlation coefficients are calculated, as it will give a good indication of whether the relationship between the two variables is roughly linear and thus whether it is appropriate to calculate a correlation coefficient. If the data do not have a Normal distribution, a non-parametric correlation coefficient, Spearman's rho (r_s), can be calculated.

From Figure 36.9, it can be seen that the Pearson correlation coefficient between pre- and post-rehabilitation distance walked on the endurance shuttle test is 0.46, and this is statistically significant.

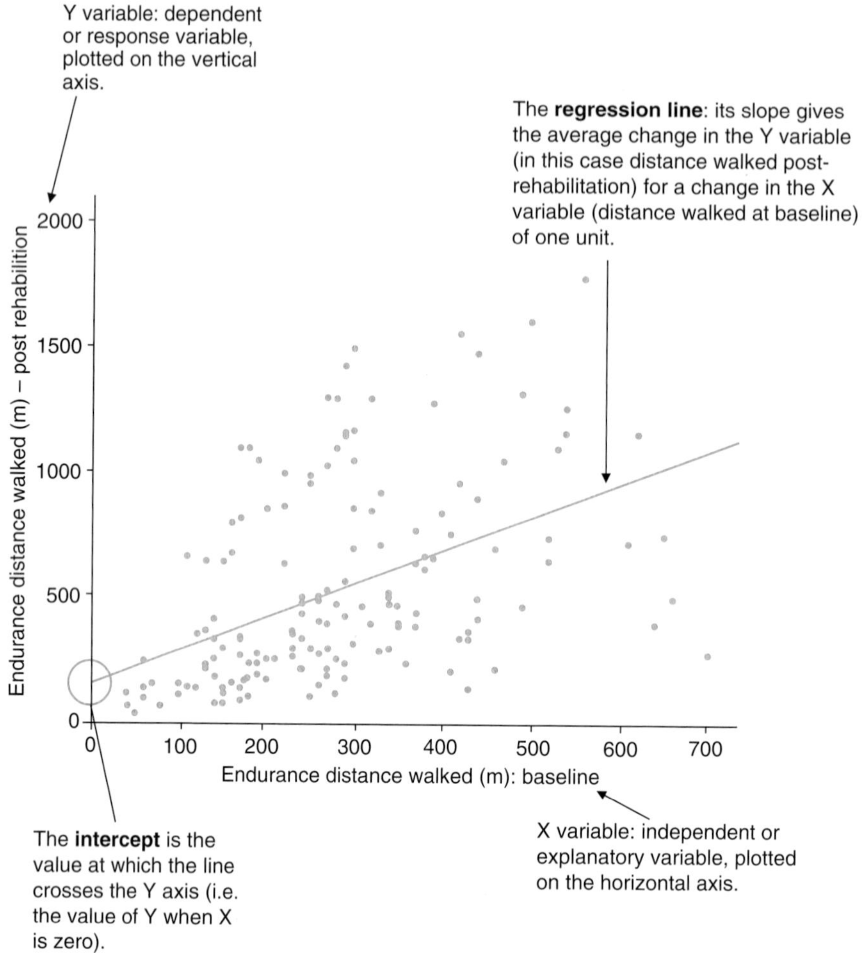
Y variable: dependent or response variable, plotted on the vertical axis.
The **regression line**: its slope gives the average change in the Y variable (in this case distance walked post-rehabilitation) for a change in the X variable (distance walked at baseline) of one unit.
Endurance distance walked (m) – post rehabilition
2000
1500
1000
500
0
0
100
200
300
400
500
600
700
Endurance distance walked (m): baseline
The **intercept** is the value at which the line crosses the Y axis (i.e. the value of Y when X is zero).
X variable: independent or explanatory variable, plotted on the horizontal axis.

Figure 36.8 Scatter plot of pre- (baseline) and post-rehabilitation distance walked on endurance shuttle test for 161 patients with COPD

Box 36.7 The assumptions underlying the validity of the hypothesis test associated with the correlation coefficient

1. The two variables are observed on a random sample of individuals.
2. The data for at least one of the variables should have a Normal distribution in the population.
3. For the calculation of a valid confidence interval for the correlation coefficient, both variables should have a Normal distribution.

Correlations

		Endurance Distance Walked (m): baseline	Endurance distance walked (m) - post rehabilitation
Endurance Distance Walked (m): baseline	Pearson Correlation	1	.464**
	Sig. (2-tailed)		.000
	N	161	161
Endurance Distance Walked (m) - post rehabilitation	Pearson Correlation	.464**	1
	Sig. (2-tailed)	.000	
	N	161	161

** Correlation is significant at the 0.01 level (2-tailed).

The pearson correlation coefficient between distance walked at baseline and distance walked post-rehabilitation is 0.464. Its associated P-value is given underneath it; in this case its value is 0.000 indicating that the result is statistically significant and there is sufficient evidence to reject the null hypothesis of no linear relationship between distance walked at baseline and post-rehabilitation. It can be concluded that the two are correlated.

Correlations

			Endurance Distance Walked (m): baseline	Endurance Distance Walked (m) - post rehabilitation
Spearman's rho	Endurance Distance Walked (m): baseline	Correlation Coefficient	1.000	.558**
		Sig. (2-tailed)	.	.000
		N	161	161
	Endurance Distance Walked (m) - post rehabilitation	Correlation Coefficient	.558**	1.000
		Sig. (2-tailed)	.000	.
		N	161	161

** Correlation is significant at the 0.01 level (2-tailed).

The Spearman correlation coefficient is 0.558 (P-value = 0.000). This is similar to the results for the Pearson correlation coefficient, though this will not always be the case.

Figure 36.9 Output of correlation analysis in SPSS

Regression (including multiple regression)

Often, it is of interest to quantify the relationship between two continuous variables and, given the value of one variable for an individual, to predict the value of the other variable. This is not possible from the correlation coefficient as it simply indicates the strength of the association as a single number; in order to describe the relationship between the values of the two variables, a technique called *regression* is used. Thus, using regression, the value of baseline distance walked could be used to predict the post-rehabilitation distance walked. Baseline pre-rehabilitation distance walked is regarded as the

Box 36.8 Assumptions underlying regression analysis

1 The values of the response variable Y should have a Normal distribution for each value of the explanatory variable X.
2 The variance (or standard deviation) of Y should be the same at each value of X, that is, there should be no evidence that as the value of Y changes, the spread of the X values changes.
3 The relationship between the two variables should be linear.

X variable; it is also called the independent predictor or explanatory variable, and it should be plotted on the horizontal axis of the scatter plot. Post-rehabilitation distance walked is regarded as the Y variable; it is also known as the dependent or response variable and is plotted on the vertical axis of the scatter plot (Figure 36.8). Three important assumptions underlie regression analysis as outlined in Box 36.8.

Regression slopes can be used to predict the response of a new patient with a particular value of the predictor/explanatory/independent variable. However, it is important that the regression model is not used to predict outside of the range of observations. In addition, it should not be assumed that just because an equation has been produced it means that X causes Y. The results of regressing post-rehabilitation distance walked on baseline distance walked are displayed in Figure 36.10. Looking at the table for the coefficients at the bottom of the figure, it can be seen that the slope coefficient for baseline distance walked is 1.32 (P-value=0.000), indicating that baseline distance walked has a significant effect on post-rehabilitation distance walked. For every metre that an individual could walk at baseline, they were able to walk an additional 1.32 times further after rehabilitation, that is, $1.32 \times 1 = 32$ cm. The value of r^2 is often quoted in published articles and indicates the proportion (sometimes expressed as a percentage) of the total variability of the outcome variable that is explained by the regression model fitted. In this case, 21.5% of the total variability in post-rehabilitation distance walked is explained by pre-rehabilitation distance walked.

Regression, as described previously, involves the investigation of the effect of a single explanatory variable on the outcome of interest. However, there is usually more than one possible explanatory variable influencing the values of the outcome variable, and the method of regression can be extended to investigate the influence of more than one variable. In this case, it is referred to as *multiple regression*, and the influence of several explanatory variables on the outcome of interest is investigated simultaneously. For example, in the rehabilitation trial, apart from baseline distance walked, age and gender may have a role to play in post-rehabilitation distance walked and these may be fitted into the model to examine what their influence on distance walked is, over and above that exerted by baseline distance walked. Figure 36.11 shows the results of this multiple regression analysis. Age and gender are not significantly associated with post-rehabilitation distance walked, so the simpler model of Figure 36.10, with baseline distance walked as the only predictor variable, is to be preferred.

Regression or correlation?

Regression is more informative than correlation. Correlation simply quantifies the degree of linear association (or not) between two variables. However, it is often more useful to *describe* the relationship between the two variables or even *predict* a value of one variable for a given value of the other, and this is done using regression. If it is

Variables entered/removed[b]

Model	Variables entered	Variables Removed	Method
1	Endurance Distance Walked (m): baseline[a]	.	Enter

[a] All requested variables entered.
[b] Dependent variable: Endurance eistance walked (m) - post rehabilitation

Model Summary

Model	R	R square	Adjusted R square	Std. Error of the estimate
1	.464[a]	.215	.210	349.4431

[a] Predictors: (Constant), Endurance Distance Walked (m): baseline

R^2 is a number which gives the percentage of variability explained by the predictor variable, X, and gives an indication of how well the model explains the data.

Anova[b]

Model		Sum of Squares	df	Mean square	F	Sig.
1	Regression	5321185	1	5321184.728	43.577	.000[a]
	Residual	2E+007	159	122110.483		
	Total	2E+007	160			

[a] Predictors: (Constant), Endurance distance walked (m): baseline
[b] Dependent Variable: Endurance distance walked (m) - post rehabilitation

Coefficients[a]

		Unstandardized coefficients		Standardized coefficients			95% Confidence Interval for B	
Model		B	Std. Error	Beta	t	Sig.	Lower bound	Upper bound
1	(Constant)	162.465	62.284		2.608	.010	39.455	285.476
	Endurance Distance Walked (m): baseline	1.319	.200	.464	6.601	.000	.924	1.713

[a]Dependent Variable: Endurance Distance Walked (m) - post rehabilitation

Regression coefficient for the value of the intercept. The value of 162.465 indicates that when distance walked at baseline is zero, distance walked post rehabilitation is 162.465 m.

Regression coefficient for the slope of distance walked at baseline. The value of 1.319 indicates for every increase of a metre in distance walked at baseline, there is an increase in distance walked post rehabilitation of 1.319 m.

The P value for the intercept is 0.010, which indicates that the value of the intercept (162.465) is unlikely when the null hypothesis (that the true value is zero) is true. Thus the result is said to be statistically significant. This is also the case for the regression coefficient for the slope: distance walked at baseline.

Figure 36.10 SPSS output from regression analysis

Model summary

Model	R	R Square	Adjusted R Square	Std. Error of the Estimate
1	.474[a]	.225	.210	349.5416

[a] Predictors: (Constant), Gender, Age (years), Endurance distance walked (m): baseline

Coefficients[a]

Model		Unstandardized coefficients		Standardized coefficients	t	Sig.	95% confidence interval for B	
		B	Std. error	Beta			Lower bound	Upper bound
1	(Constant)	320.995	280.860		1.143	.255	−233.756	875.746
	Endurance Distance Walked (m): baseline	1.211	.215	.426	5.646	.000	.787	1.635
	Age (years)	−3.305	3.697	−.065	−.894	.373	−10.608	3.998
	Gender	63.635	57.511	.081	1.106	.270	−49.960	177.231

[a] Dependent variable: Endurance distance walked (m) - post rehabilitation

Figure 36.11 SPSS output from multiple regression analysis

Reflection activity

A mobile phone app for managing weight loss has been developed. A group of patients are randomised to either use the app or be given standard advice about diet and exercise. Assuming that the main outcome of interest is the amount of weight lost over a 6-month period, use the information in Table 36.3, Figure 36.2 and Figure 36.6 to decide on the most appropriate method for analysing the results of this study.

sensible to assume that one variable may be causing a response in the other, then regression analysis should be used.

CONCLUSION

This chapter has outlined the process of testing hypotheses and emphasised the usefulness of confidence intervals when drawing conclusions from the results of studies. In addition, it has covered some of the basic statistical tests for the types of data outlined in the previous chapter. Armed with this information, for a given set of such data, it should be possible to decide upon the most appropriate analysis, carry out the chosen method and draw conclusions from the results.

Further reading

Huff D (1991) *How to Lie with Statistics*. London, Penguin Books.

Gray CD, Kinnear PR (2012) *IBMSPSS 19 Statistics Made Simple*. Hove, Psychology Press.

See Chapter 35 for further references.

SECTION 6

Putting Research into Practice

The final section of this book moves on from the practical process of doing research to consider how research can make a difference to nursing and health care practice.

Chapter 37 deals with the very important stage of moving a research study on from an investigation into a piece of new knowledge, accessible to other members of the profession and the wider public. It is a practical guide to writing research reports, journal articles, presenting at conferences and other means of dissemination.

Chapters 38 and 39 take the next logical step of considering how health care practice integrates (or does not) the new knowledge generated by research. These two chapters are designed to be read together, but each also stands complete in itself. Chapter 38 looks at the theory underpinning evidence-based practice and assesses different models of research utilisation relevant to nursing. Chapter 39 builds on this foundation to discuss knowledge translation and the different ways in which research products can be used in practice. The difficult process of change implementation is fundamental to this process and is given some consideration in the last section of the chapter.

The book ends with a chapter, Chapter 40, which continues the discussion begun in Chapter 1 on the context of nursing research. It examines some key trends of nursing research that are likely to influence nurse researchers in the coming years. The increasing emphasis on the importance of research addressing societal expectations challenges nurse researchers to think very carefully about the relevance of their research to nursing policy, practice and education and what its ultimate impact might be at local, national and even international levels. Moreover, the continuing growth of digital technologies is set to present nurse researchers with expanding opportunities to use such technologies to enhance their research. Ultimately, the success or otherwise of their endeavours will impact upon patient outcomes, and it is this which underlines the value of nursing research.

The Research Process in Nursing, Seventh Edition. Edited by Kate Gerrish and Judith Lathlean.

Companion Website: www.wiley.com/go/gerrish/research

CHAPTER 37

Disseminating Research Findings

Kate Gerrish

Key points

- Research findings need to be disseminated in various formats for different audiences.
- Journal articles and research reports are the main written forms of dissemination, and each needs to be written in an appropriate style.
- Presentations at conferences, verbally or in poster format, are effective ways of disseminating results and networking with other researchers.
- Social media, websites and workshops can be used by researchers to tell others about their work.

INTRODUCTION

Although research may be an interesting and intellectually satisfying activity in its own right, there is little point in carrying out research unless it is disseminated to those who can make use of the new knowledge generated. Public funding of research by bodies such as the Department of Health, Research Councils and charities is done on the understanding that results will be made known to the public and, where appropriate, used to improve healthcare. Having said this, many research reports never get very far beyond the desk of those carrying out the study and those funding it. Even publication in a journal does not guarantee that the appropriate community, professional or public, gets to hear about the research. So how do we ensure optimum communication from the research community to the professionals involved in healthcare, to users of healthcare and to the wider public?

COMMUNICATING WITH DIFFERENT AUDIENCES

The same piece of research may be disseminated in different ways. Firstly, a report is likely to be written as a permanent record of the research and to satisfy the needs of those commissioning, funding and

The Research Process in Nursing, Seventh Edition. Edited by Kate Gerrish and Judith Lathlean.

Companion Website: www.wiley.com/go/gerrish/research

supporting the study. If the research was undertaken as part of an education programme, the report will take the form of a dissertation or thesis.

The research may also be reported as an article in a high-status academic journal such as the *Journal of Advanced Nursing* or the *British Medical Journal*, where it is likely to be read primarily by nurses and other healthcare professionals in academic roles and by some students and practitioners. Such journals have strict guidelines for the reporting of research (see, e.g. http://onlinelibrary.wiley.com/journal/10.1111/(ISSN)1365-2648 and www.bmj.com) that should be followed. The research findings may even be picked up from high-profile journals and reported in the media, if it is of public interest or controversial.

Research findings may also be written up, perhaps in a different form, in a professional journal such as *Nursing Standard*. Here, a wider range of practising nurses who are not necessarily engaged in academic study will read about the research. Furthermore, there is an increasing expectation that research findings should be disseminated to those who participated in the study. A succinct summary written in a suitable language may need to be prepared for patients and the wider public.

Researchers often communicate their work as an oral or poster presentation at international, national and local conferences, workshops and seminars and research interest groups in the workplace.

Increasingly, information technology, in particular social media, is being used to disseminate research findings, and this is set to grow as new technologies emerge. Whereas dedicated websites have been used for some time to disseminate information about ongoing research and ultimately the findings, other technologies such as Twitter, YouTube, Vimeos, webinars and podcasts are increasingly used by research teams to ensure rapid dissemination of research findings to a wide audience. Chapter 6 provides more detail on the use of digital technologies to support the dissemination of research findings.

Each of these ways of disseminating research findings requires a different style and different resources and serves a different audience. These various means of dissemination will be examined in turn.

Reflection activity

Consider the various ways in which research findings can be communicated to different audiences that are identified earlier. What do you think are the strengths and limitations of each approach? What factors might influence researchers when deciding how to communicate their research?

THE RESEARCH REPORT

A research study is not complete until a report has been written and submitted to interested parties. The report serves as a complete record of what was done, how it was undertaken, details of results and conclusions. Implications for practice may also be included where relevant. The report will provide an account of the research to those who commissioned and funded it but can also become a means of dissemination to those who can make use of the findings. The length and style of a research report is highly variable. Where research is conducted for an education degree, the report is the dissertation or thesis, written in academic language and, in the case of a doctoral thesis, running to 100,000 words or more. In contrast, a small project carried out in clinical practice may be reported in 20 pages or less. Whatever the length and style, however, the content is likely to be similar in format. It should be noted that universities produce guidelines on the presentation and content of a thesis and these should be adhered to.

The writing of a research report follows conventions that closely mirror the research process itself. These are outlined in Box 37.1. Sections of the report will vary according to the intended audience.

WRITING AN ARTICLE FOR PUBLICATION

Publishing research in an academic or professional journal provides a means of disseminating the findings to a wide, possibly international, audience.

Box 37.1 Sections of a research report

Abstract or executive summary

This should orientate the reader to the whole study. It is best written at the end after the detailed report is complete.

Introduction

This section describes the background to the study and the context in which it was undertaken.

Aims of the research

The aims, research questions and any hypotheses to be tested should be stated clearly.

Literature review

A comprehensive literature review will set out the available knowledge before the research commenced. The length and depth of this review will depend on the audience of the report. An academic dissertation requires a substantial section critically appraising the available literature, whereas policymakers are likely to require a more concise summary.

Research design

A clear description is required of the conceptual framework used, the methodology adopted and data collection methods selected in order to give the reader an understanding of the research design.

Access and ethical approval

All research conducted in a healthcare context should have obtained ethical and research governance approval, and a statement to this effect should be included. Other access negotiations and procedures for recruiting and gaining consent from research participants will be given. Copies of consent forms and information sheets may be included in an appendix.

Sampling

This section will provide details of how sampling was done, sample size calculations and the composition and characteristics of the sample obtained.

Data collection

A full account of how data were collected, data collection tools and outcome measures used will be given.

Data analysis

A detailed description of how data were analysed is necessary. In a quantitative study, reference should be made to the statistical tests employed. Qualitative studies should provide a description of the various steps in analysis to demonstrate how the researcher moved from transcripts and/or field notes to develop themes and categories.

Results

A full presentation of the results should be made. For quantitative research, this will be in the form of tables and figures, with a narrative commentary. For qualitative research, the results will be presented in words, with verbatim quotations from interviews, field notes, etc. as supporting evidence. Qualitative research reports may include some discussion within the presentation of the results, rather than keeping the two sections separate as suggested below.

Discussion and conclusion

This section gives the researcher the opportunity to reflect upon the findings in the light of previous literature in order to draw out the contribution to knowledge that the research has made. Implications for practice, suggested further research and any limitations of the study are commonly included. The report should end with a concise conclusion.

Authors also gain considerable personal satisfaction to see their work in print.

A published article on a research study will generally follow the same structure as a research report referred to in the previous section, albeit in a more condensed format. However, the content of the paper and writing style will vary according to the target audience for the journal. An academic journal normally requires a detailed account of the research in which the author demonstrates rigour in carrying out the study as well as showing how the research contributes to advancing knowledge in the field. The style of writing tends to be formal. By contrast, the account of the research methodology in a professional journal is normally concise with more emphasis placed on the findings and implications for policy and practice. A journalistic approach that seeks to engage the reader's attention may be used.

Preparing an article for submission

Selecting an appropriate journal for publication requires careful groundwork. The first step is to become familiar with the journal by reading some previous issues. This will provide insight into the types of article the editor seeks to publish, the intended audience and the writing style. Most journals provide detailed guidance for contributors, and this may be published in the journal or on the journal's website. This guidance frequently provides information on the aims and scope of the journal to help authors decide whether their work is appropriate for a particular journal. A very useful website run by the Medical College of Ohio provides an index of all instructions for authors for nursing and healthcare journals at http://mulford.meduohio.edu/instr/ http://mulford.utoledo.edu/instr/.

Once familiar with the type of articles published in different journals, a decision can be made about which one to pursue. This decision should be informed by an objective appraisal of the match between the type of article published in the journal and the nature of the research to be reported. If in doubt, advice should be sought from someone who is experienced at writing for publication or from the journal editors themselves.

The guidelines for authors normally provide details of the expected content and format of the

Box 37.2 General criteria used to review an article

Relevance of topic to journal aims
Potential interest to readership
Originality and contribution to knowledge and/or practice
Scientific rigour
Clarity and coherence of the article
Style of writing, angle, level of presentation

article and should be followed closely. Most journals require electronic submission via a manuscript tracking system that enables the publication process to be managed electronically and provides the opportunity for authors to check on progress with their paper.

Having decided on the journal and studied the guidance for authors, writing can begin. A novice will find it beneficial to co-author with someone with a track record of publication. Once a draft version of the paper has been written, it is advisable to seek feedback from colleagues who can provide constructive advice on how it might be improved. A paper is likely to require several revisions before it reaches the stage where it is ready for submission. Before submitting the paper, it is important to undertake a final proofread, check all references are correctly cited in the text and the reference list and ensure that it is presented in the required format.

The review process

All papers submitted to editors undergo some form of assessment in order to ascertain whether they are suitable for publication in a particular journal. Academic journals and an increasing number of professional journals seek an independent review (peer review) of the paper by one or more people who are judged to be experts in the field. Before a decision is made to send a paper for review, the editor usually undertakes an initial assessment, and it may be that the paper is considered unsuitable and rejected at this stage. Usually, a paper is reviewed 'blind'; in other words, the reviewer does not know the identity of the author, and the feedback from the reviewer to the author is anonymised. However, there is a move towards a more open review process, and some editors now make authors and reviewers aware of each other's identity.

Many journals provide guidance to reviewers on the areas they should consider when assessing a paper. Whereas journals differ in terms of their aims and readership, the criteria used to assess a paper are often similar. An example of general criteria used by reviewers is given in Box 37.2.

It will normally take several weeks for an author to receive feedback from the editor. The reviewers' comments are usually sent to authors together with an editorial decision. In exceptional circumstances, the paper may be accepted as submitted. However, it is more common for authors to be asked to revise their paper on the basis of the feedback from reviewers. Where a paper is rejected outright, the reviewers' feedback should provide an indication as to why it was considered unsuitable. Suggestions may also be made on how to develop the paper for publication elsewhere.

When revising a paper, the author should give serious consideration to the reviewers' recommendations. Where an author disagrees with a reviewer, the editor needs to be informed of the reasons why the author has not taken the recommendations on board. Indeed, many journals ask authors to submit a separate report providing details of how they have responded to the reviewers' comments. A revised paper may need to be sent out for further review, so authors should anticipate a time delay.

The publication process

Once a paper has been accepted for publication, the editor will notify the author and may provide an indication of the anticipated publication date. Many journals now publish articles 'online early' some months before they appear in the printed version of the journal. Before the paper is published, authors will be asked to sign a copyright declaration form that assigns the copyright of the article to the publisher. Whereas assigning copyright imposes certain restrictions on the author's future use of the material, it is designed to protect the interests of the author, for example, should others plagiarise their work.

Shortly before publication, the author is sent the page proofs to check. These are presented in the format in which the article will appear in the journal. It is important that authors check the page proofs carefully for accuracy. However, only essential changes can be made at this stage as more extensive editing is costly and will delay publication. Authors need to be aware that minor changes may have been made to their original manuscript. Usually, this is to correct minor errors, but some editors of professional journals may make more significant changes. If an author is unhappy with any changes that have been made to the article, it is essential that the editor is informed. After all, it is the author's work, and they have the right to decide the ultimate content of the article.

Many journals are now published in electronic, as well as paper format, and some are only produced electronically. These 'e-journals' appear on the Internet, and articles can be downloaded, but they never appear in print form. This form of publication reduces the time taken for an article to be published. Many e-journals have a stringent system of ensuring quality, just as print journals do.

E-journals are often 'open access', which means that they have no subscription system so that anyone can download the article. However, authors may be asked to pay for publication of their article. *BioMed Central (BMC) Nursing* is an example of such a journal, running since 2002 (http://www.aahperd.org/iejhe/). Increasingly, research funders require researchers to publish their findings in open-access journals. As a result, many subscription-based journals now offer authors the opportunity for their paper to be 'open access' if they pay a fee associated with the publication.

Political issues in the publication process

It may be necessary to seek permission to publish from the funding body that has commissioned the research. This requirement is usually written into the research contract. The research funder may wish to see the paper before it is sent for publication and may require a disclaimer to be included, which states that the views expressed in the paper are those of the authors and not the research funding body.

It is also good practice to acknowledge those who have contributed to the research but are not co-authors of the paper. This may include the funding body, individuals who have granted special permissions, for example, agreeing to a questionnaire they have developed being used in the study, or who have provided particular support, such as a supervisor or Project Advisory Group members.

Where a team has undertaken a study, it is generally appropriate for all members to be co-authors of the article. This should be agreed in advance, as there can be difficulties if a member of the research team feels they were not given an opportunity to contribute to a paper. Disagreements about whose name will appear first are likely if this is not made clear from the outset. Supervisors often co-author papers with their students, and normally, the student's name appears as first author. Anyone who co-authors a paper should have made a significant contribution to the research study and to writing the paper. Increasingly, editors require each author to sign a declaration confirming their contribution.

Researchers who are based in academic institutions in the United Kingdom may be required to submit their publications as part of the Research Excellence Framework (REF). This is a periodic assessment by national and international experts of the quality of research in a particular discipline, for example, nursing. The quality of published research is the main criterion used to judge the overall quality of research within a university. Numerical ratings of research quality ranging from 1×(national significance) to 4×(world leading) are linked to funding allocations, and therefore, universities take the REF most seriously. High-status academic journals are regarded by many disciplines as the most appropriate avenue for research outputs to be included in the REF. The quality of such journals is reflected in their impact factor: a numerical measure based on the average number of citations to recent articles published in the journal. Journals with a high impact factor are considered to be more important than those with lower ones. Novice researchers would do well to seek advice from more experienced colleagues on the most suitable journals in which to publish.

PREPARING A REPORT FOR THE PUBLIC

Increasingly, researchers are expected to feed back their findings to those who have participated in the study and to make their findings more widely accessible to the general public. Whereas researchers will still need to present an account of what they set out to achieve, how they went about undertaking the study, what they found and what conclusions they were able to draw, the traditional headings of 'aims', 'methodology', 'results' and 'conclusions' may not be easily understandable to the general public who have little knowledge of the research process. Instead, researchers should write a summary, in plain English, which gives a clear overview of the study. It should be written in a style that engages the reader. Technical terms should be avoided, or where these are necessary, an explanation should be given. It may be helpful to ask lay members of a Project Advisory Group, or even family and friends to comment on a draft to ensure that it is readily understandable to the general public. Details of the full project report or links to a website for further information may also be included for people who are interested in finding out more.

PRESENTING RESEARCH AT A CONFERENCE

Presenting research at a conference helps to disseminate the findings more quickly than is possible by publication. Research findings can be presented in the form of an oral presentation or a poster at national or international conferences. Increasingly, healthcare organisations host conferences that provide the opportunity to disseminate research across the local health community and facilitate networking with colleagues who share similar interests. Such conferences provide an ideal opportunity for the novice presenter to hone their skills. Many national and international conferences focus on a particular area of nursing, for example, clinical practice, management or education, and presentations need to address the conference theme. However, some conferences, such as the Royal College of Nursing Annual International Nursing Research Conference, focus specifically on research and invite presentations on a broad range of topics.

Whereas conference organisers may invite lead researchers to present their work, most researchers are required to submit an abstract for an oral or poster presentation for consideration by a selection panel. When deciding where to submit an abstract, it is worth considering the material to be presented and the intended audience. For example, a study examining a new form of treatment for the management of leg ulcers by community nurses might form the basis of an abstract for a conference on community nursing, wound management or a research conference. If the intention is to disseminate the findings to a large number of clinical nurses, then a conference related to a particular area of nursing may be most suitable. Research conferences, by contrast, provide the opportunity to discuss aspects of the research process as well as the findings with an audience who have a particular interest in research.

Writing a conference abstract

A major factor in having an abstract accepted for presentation is whether the author has followed the guidelines in the published 'call for abstracts'. This normally specifies:

- the conference themes
- the deadline date for submission
- the format and content of the abstract, including the maximum word length
- whether there is an option to present the work as an oral presentation or a poster
- the criteria by which the abstract will be judged

Box 37.3 Abstract submission checklist

Royal College of Nursing of the United Kingdom

Annual International Nursing Research Conference

Abstract submission checklist

Abstracts submitted to the RCN's Annual International Nursing Research Conference are peer reviewed by an international panel. The criteria against which reviewers make their recommendations are detailed in the online abstract submission form. These criteria are listed here in the form of a checklist for you to use prior to submitting your abstract. If you have any ticks in the 'No' column, you can then amend your abstract before you submit it and hence increase the potential for your abstract to be accepted and included in the conference programme.

		Yes	No	N/a
1	The abstract must be about a research project or a critical reflection on a research-related issue (e.g. policy or a methodological issue).			
2	Material presented in abstracts must be concise and coherent, with the focus of the abstract and its relevance to an international audience stated clearly, for example, a local study needs to be placed in some generalised context.			
3	The authors must make explicit what they intend to present.			
4	The abstract title should be short and clearly declare the content of the abstract			
5	Abstracts of empirical studies must outline the research process and the focus of the analysis; they must indicate the month(s) and year(s) when the data were collected and provide an indication of the results. (NB An abstract will not be accepted if data has not already been collected.)			
6	Abstracts reporting on the results of research studies should be structured: background, aims, methods, results, discussionand conclusions. Statistics including sample size and sampling method used must be supplied where appropriate.			
7	Abstracts relating to methodological papers should include background to the method, debate, topic, etc. including definition of technical terms, aims of the paper, methodological discussion/presentation and a conclusion that summarises the contribution of the paper.			
8	Relevant contextual information including definitions of specialist terms must be given.			

		Yes	No	N/a
9	Authors must consider and specify how their paper contributes to the development of a generalised knowledge base, for example, a service evaluation is likely to be of little interest to an audience unless its contribution to theory policy or future practice in different settings is made clear.			
10	All abstracts must be written in English. NB All accepted abstracts will be published 'as submitted'. It is therefore incumbent upon the author to ensure that the spelling, grammar and syntax are of an academic publishing standard.			
11	The word limit must be adhered to and authors are required to declare that their abstract is within the limit: (a) For **concurrent** and **poster** submissions, the word limit is 300 (excluding references). (b) For **symposium** submissions, the word limit is 300 for each of the individual papers to be included in the symposium (excluding references, authors' details and principal authors' CV).			
12	Abstracts for poster and concurrent presentations must not contain information that could identify the author(s), as these are reviewed blind.			
13	For poster and concurrent presentations, up to three references may be cited, and these must be provided using the Harvard referencing system.			
14	Symposium and workshop abstracts must be accompanied by a CV demonstrating the principal author's competence to deliver.			

Reproduced with Permission from the RCN Research Society and R&D Co-ordinating Centre

The abstract provides the only information that a selection panel has to make its decision about whether a proposed presentation is relevant and of suitable quality. It is essential to present information in a concise and informative way that grabs the interest of the reviewer and ultimately the conference delegate. Box 37.3 gives an example of the criteria by which an abstract may be judged.

Abstracts that exceed the word length or that do not use the specified headings may be automatically rejected. Despite these constraints, it is possible to convey a considerable amount of information in relatively few words. For example, consider the following: 'A survey by self-completed questionnaire was undertaken with a random sample of ward-based nurses working in a large teaching hospital in England. Content validity and reliability of the questionnaire were established. Of a random sample of 700 nurses, 563 responded'. This covers the design, method, sample and setting in just 40 words. An example of an abstract is given in Research Example 37.1.

Deciding whether to present an oral paper or a poster is to some extent a matter of personal choice. Whereas novice presenters may feel more comfortable with a poster presentation, they should not underestimate the considerable effort and resources required to produce a high-quality poster as well as

RESEARCH EXAMPLE

37.1 A Conference Abstract

Capturing the impact of nurse consultant roles in the United Kingdom

Background: Following the introduction in 2000 of nurse consultants in the United Kingdom, there has been growing interest in demonstrating their impact, although robust evidence of impact is lacking. Existing frameworks for evaluating the impact of advanced practice roles do not cover the four dimensions of the nurse consultant role (clinical practice, leadership, education and research) sufficiently.

Aim: To develop a framework to evaluate the impact of nurse consultants on patient, professional and organisational outcomes and identify associated indicators of impact.

Methods: Individual case studies of six nurse consultants in England were undertaken. Each case study involved interviews with the nurse consultant, healthcare staff, managers, patients and carers (a total of 58 participants). Interviews explored participants' perceptions of the impact of the nurse consultant and indicators of actual and/or potential impact. Data were analysed using Framework approach.

Results: Three domains of impact of nurse consultant roles were identified: clinical significance, professional significance and organisational significance. Each domain included three to four indicators of impact. All nurse consultants showed some evidence of impact in each domain although the primary focus varied across different nurse consultants. Due to the wide diversity in nurse consultant roles there was little commonality in the specific indicators of impact across all nurse consultants.

Conclusion: The framework for capturing the impact of nurse consultants can be used by researchers and by nurse consultants to demonstrate their impact. Further research is required to assess the suitability of the framework for capturing the impact of other advanced practice roles.

(250 words – maximum allowed)

(Oral presentation at the International Nurse Practitioner Conference, Helsinki, 2014 by K Gerrish, A McDonnell, F Kennedy)

the time required during the conference to be available to discuss the poster. Although the idea of an oral presentation may appear daunting, with careful planning and the opportunity to practise by presenting the paper to colleagues beforehand, the novice researcher can get an enormous amount of personal satisfaction from delivering an oral presentation.

Oral presentations

The communication confirming acceptance of an oral presentation will normally include information on the time allocated for the paper, where it appears on the conference programme and what audiovisual facilities will be available.

Novice presenters may feel that they need to read verbatim from a paper. Whereas this provides the opportunity to produce a coherent, well-constructed presentation, it can be difficult for the audience to concentrate on someone reading for any length of time. A presenter who uses notes or written prompt cards for guidance and who maintains eye contact with the audience is more likely to keep their attention.

The key to presenting a successful paper is to be realistic on how much information can be included within the time available. If planning to read a paper verbatim, a reasonable conversion rate is to consider 500 words as equivalent to 5 min speaking time. If using PowerPoint slides, it is appropriate to prepare one slide per 2 min of presentation. This means that only limited information on some aspects of a research study can be included.

Deciding what to include is probably the most difficult task. Delegates at a conference that attracts clinical nurses will be interested in research findings and their implications for practice, whereas those attending a research conference are likely to be interested in the methodology used. Many conferences request that presenters allow time at the end of their paper for the audience to ask questions. Ensure that this is planned into the allotted time. When planning to use a PowerPoint presentation, it is essential to check which version of the software is available. Animation features available in the most recent version may not work with older versions. Assistance on preparing audiovisual aids may be available locally in healthcare organisations or universities and can also be found on the Internet.

Once the presentation has been prepared, it is beneficial to rehearse, preferably in front of friendly colleagues. Keeping to time should be the most important priority. Conference programmes often run to a tight schedule, and it can be frustrating for delegates when a paper is cut short because the presenter has run out of time.

Once at the conference, check out the venue and the audiovisual facilities as far in advance of the presentation as possible, seeking assistance from a technician if required. In terms of the actual delivery, it is important to consider:

- posture, movement and hand actions – face the audience, stand rather than sit, avoid excessive movements and fiddling with paper clips, etc.
- eye contact and facial expression – look at the audience, adopt a relaxed facial expression and try to smile!
- voice – aim to achieve clarity and variety, speak clearly, slowly and use appropriate intonation by raising, lowering and altering the tone of voice.

Poster presentations

Preparing a poster requires considerable time, so it is essential to think about the presentation well in advance of the conference. Many healthcare organisations and universities have departments that can assist with both design and production. The cost of producing a poster ranges from a few pounds to several hundred. Whereas a professionally presented poster produced with the assistance of a graphic designer is impressive, there is no reason why someone with a more modest budget cannot produce a very effective poster. Advice on designing posters is readily available via the Internet. Computer software (such as MS Word, PowerPoint and Desktop publishing) can all be used to produce posters.

Details indicating the amount of space available will accompany the correspondence that confirms acceptance of the abstract. It is essential that the poster fits the parameters given. A poster should not be overcrowded with information as this will detract from its impact. The noise and bustle of a poster viewing hall is rarely conducive to a serious read! Text should be sufficiently large to be read easily from a distance of at least 1 m although the title should be larger to attract interest from a distance. There should be a balance between text and other visual stimuli such as graphs, figures or photographs. Material should be sequenced in a logical manner with the reader clearly guided through the content. Numbered headings or arrows can assist here.

There is a tendency when planning the content of a poster to be overambitious in terms of content. The key is to present information succinctly – short phrases rather than full sentences will often suffice. The title needs to be short and snappy to attract attention. The name and contact details of members of the research team should be included. It is usual to provide a brief introduction to the project before moving on to provide information about the aims, sample, methods, findings and conclusions. Supporting materials that delegates can take away can also be produced. For example, a scaled-down version of the poster can be printed on A4 paper or alternatively a more detailed written account of the research project prepared as a handout.

When designing a poster on a tight budget, there may be a tendency to take the easy option of printing out a series of A4 PowerPoint slides and mounting these on the poster board. Whereas this kind of display can convey the essential information, its visual impact is not as great as a large poster. Many computer software packages allow for a larger format than A4 to be designed. Once the poster has been designed on the computer, it may be possible to have it printed within a local healthcare organisation or university. Alternatively, a number of high street print companies will produce the poster from a USB stick onto suitably sized paper and laminate it for a reasonable price. However, before the material is taken for printing, it is essential to proofread carefully as errors cannot be rectified.

Consideration should be given to transporting the poster to the conference. It is recommended that it is taken as hand luggage in a waterproof container. Although conference organisers may provide materials to mount the poster on the presentation board, it is advisable to take an 'emergency kit', including Velcro, double-sided tape, drawing pins and scissors.

Finally, remember that presenters are normally required to spend time beside the poster discussing it with interested parties. This is often during meal breaks, and presenters need to think about how to manage their time. When it is necessary to leave a poster unattended during a specified conference viewing time, it is helpful to leave a note beside the poster indicating when the presenter will be available to answer questions, together with a phone number or email address.

Reflection activity

Consider a research project you have been involved with or another initiative linked to your practice that you think others would be interested to learn about. Identify an audience to whom you wish to communicate the work – this may be researchers, practitioners, managers or patients and the wider public. Sketch out the key content you wish to include in the poster. How has your consideration of the audience you wish to communicate with influenced what you plan to include in your poster?

SOCIAL MEDIA AND NETWORKING OPPORTUNITIES

In addition to the more traditional means of dissemination through publication and conference presentations, there are several other ways of disseminating research.

Websites

Large-scale, funded research projects often have a dedicated website that will include regular updates with progress of the study, and researchers may post interim findings before they are disseminated more widely. The website for a university department or healthcare organisation may provide the opportunity for a synopsis of ongoing or recently completed research to be posted. Websites allow more visual and interactive communication than paper-based formats and so provide opportunities for creative presentation of research findings to different audiences.

Social media

Social media is increasingly being used to promote rapid and widespread communication of information in general and carries considerable potential to facilitate the timely dissemination of research findings. Social media offer a range of tools that researchers can use to communicate their findings. Some of the most familiar include Twitter, YouTube and WordPress. However, it is beyond the scope of this chapter to consider these in any detail, but the reader's attention is drawn to the potential for using social media. Chapter 6 provides a more detailed account of how social media can be used to support research.

Research funding organisations such as the National Institute for Health Research, as well as individual research teams, may use Twitter to share headline news about the latest research findings and create links to further information (e.g. websites, webinars, etc.), which provide more detailed information. Researchers may also choose to share their findings through video. There are several video libraries where these can be hosted, for example, YouTube and Vimeo, or they can be incorporated within a website. Webinars and podcasts provide the opportunity to present an oral account of research findings.

When using social media to disseminate research findings, it is important to consider the audience. Social media can generally be accessed by anyone – this includes peers, research subjects and the public at large. Consideration needs to be given to an appropriate writing style through which to convey the message so that it is engaging.

It is also important to consider whether there are any intellectual property or copyright implications of making findings available using websites and social media to disseminate findings. Academic journals will only publish original research that has not been published elsewhere. Placing a research report or dissertation on a university website that is open access may be viewed by journal editors as a form of publication. If a researcher then reproduces this work for a journal article, it may be considered by the editor to have already been published. Many academic journals carry out plagiarism checks before publication, and duplication of content with research reports accessible via websites will most likely be identified. If in doubt, contact the journal editor.

Workshops and seminars

Universities and healthcare organisations may have research interest groups that meet regularly to provide a forum for local researchers to present their work. A seminar, in which the audience is encouraged to discuss a paper in some detail, calls for a more participatory form of presentation than a traditional conference paper. Workshops may also be provided that enable participants to engage more actively in discussion and contribute their own ideas, often through working on specific tasks in small groups. This can be particularly useful for researchers who wish to work with potential 'users' of their research, such as patient groups, healthcare providers, educators and policymakers in order to consider the implementation of their findings.

Reflection activity

Consider a research study that you have been involved with or that you plan to undertake. Develop a dissemination plan for your study by identifying the different audiences to whom you want to communicate your findings and select the different approaches you will use to communicate with these audiences, for example, journal articles, conference and social media. What factors have influenced your selection of the different approaches?

CONCLUSION

Dissemination of research, while it is being undertaken and after its completion, is essential if the knowledge generated is going to be used by the nursing profession. Dissemination also gives an opportunity for researchers to learn from one another's experience and to engage in networks with others working in a similar field. There are many forms of communication available to researchers ranging from academic journal articles to informal local discussion groups, and researchers need to consider their different audiences (peers, healthcare professionals, research subjects, patient and the public) when deciding on an appropriate form of communication.

Further reading

Briggs DJ (2009) A practical guide to designing a poster for presentation. *Nursing Standard* **23**(34): 35–39.

Cann A, Dimitriou K, Hooley T (2011) *Social Media: a guide for researchers*. Research Information Network.

Available at http://www.rin.ac.uk/our-work/communicating-and-disseminating-research/social-media-guide-researchers (accessed 30 Aug 2014).

Canter D, Fairbairn G (2006) *Becoming an Author: advice for academics and other professionals*. Buckingham, Open University Press.

Hand H (2010) Reflections on preparing a poster presentation. *Nurse Researcher* **17**(2): 52–59.

Hardicre J, Devitt P, Coad J (2007) Ten steps to successful poster presentation. *British Journal of Nursing* **16**(7): 398–401.

Holland K, Watson R (eds) (2012) *Writing for Publication in Nursing and Healthcare: getting it right*. Chichester, Wiley-Blackwell.

Johnstone M (2004) *Effective Writing for Health Professionals: a practice guide to getting published*. Oxford, Routledge.

Murray R (2006) *How to Write a Thesis*. Buckingham, Open University Press.

Murray R (2008) *Writing Up Your University Assignments and Research Projects*. Buckingham, Open University Press.

Murray R (2009) *Writing for Academic Journals*, 2nd edition. Buckingham, Open University Press.

Oermann MH, Hays J (2011) *Writing for Publication in Nursing*, 2nd edition. New York, Springer.

Webb C (2009) *Writing for Publication: an easy to follow guide for any nurse thinking of publishing their work*. Oxford, Wiley-Blackwell. Available at http://www.nurseauthoreditor.com/WritingforPublication2009.pdf (accessed 30 Aug 2014).

Websites

http://mulford.meduohio.edu/instr/ – The Medical College of Ohio website that lists all instructions for authors for journals in the health and medical sciences.

http://www.rcn.org.uk/development/researchanddevelopment/dissemination – The RCN Research and Development Co-ordinating Centre contains tips and advice on getting published and information on different nursing and health journals with links to their websites.

https://www.vitae.ac.uk – The researchers' portal of the 'vitae realising the potential of researchers' website provides practical advice on presenting research for different audiences and on publishing research findings.

http://www.rin.ac.uk/our-work/communicating-and-disseminating-research/social-media-guide-researchers – A useful site for information about the use of social media in research – including dissemination.

CHAPTER 38

Evidence-Based Practice

Kate Gerrish

Key points

- Evidence-based practice involves integrating the best available research evidence with professional expertise while also taking account of patient preferences, the patient's state, setting and circumstances and health-care resources.
- Evidence-based practice is a complex undertaking that involves identifying and appraising different sources of evidence, translating evidence into clear guidance for practice, implementing and finally evaluating the impact of change.
- Research findings may be applied directly to practice in the form of clinical protocols or practice guidelines, be used indirectly to inform nurses' understanding of practice or can be used persuasively to present a case for change in policy or practice.
- Barriers to achieving evidence-based practice relate to the nature of the evidence, the ways in which the evidence is communicated, the knowledge and skills of the individual nurse and the organisational context.

INTRODUCTION

Evidence-based practice has become a major concern of health-care policymakers, care providers and professional groups. Nurses, alongside other health-care practitioners, recognise that high-quality care is dependent on being able to use robust evidence to underpin clinical interventions. Yet achieving evidence-based care is a complex undertaking. It requires considerable skill in identifying and appraising evidence in order to decide whether it is appropriate to use. The evidence then needs to be translated into guidance that can be understood and used by practitioners, before being introduced into everyday practice. However, introducing change is far from straightforward. Commitment is needed from individual nurses together with support from colleagues within the multidisciplinary team and from managers. Finally, the impact of the change in practice needs to be evaluated. It requires appropriate resources and should take place in an environment

The Research Process in Nursing, Seventh Edition. Edited by Kate Gerrish and Judith Lathlean.

Companion Website: www.wiley.com/go/gerrish/research

where practitioners are comfortable with questioning practice and are willing to embrace change.

This chapter examines the concept of evidence-based practice. The debates about what constitutes 'good' evidence are explored and consideration given to different models of research utilisation and factors influencing evidence-based practice. This sets the scene for the following chapter that examines the implementation of evidence-based practice.

THE NATURE OF 'EVIDENCE'

There is debate within the nursing literature about whether the 'evidence' in evidence-based practice should relate solely to research evidence or if a broader definition is more appropriate bearing in mind that there may be insufficient research evidence to support some nursing interventions. The potential contribution of different forms of evidence is identified in one of the earliest and most frequently used definitions of evidence-based practice: Sackett *et al.* (1996) define evidence-based medicine as follows:

> The conscientious, explicit and judicious use of current best evidence in making decisions about the care of individual patients. The practice of evidence-based medicine means integrating individual clinical expertise with the best available external evidence from systematic research.

Although this definition refers to evidence-based *medicine*, it has been applied to nursing and health-care practice more generally. Whereas the definition focuses on the care required by individual patients, the concept of evidence-based practice can be extended to groups of patients, health-care services and policy initiatives (Muir Gray 2004; Sigma Theta Tau 2008).

It is worth examining the above definition in more detail. The emphasis on *current best evidence* draws attention to the changing nature of evidence. As more research is undertaken on a topic, a body of knowledge is built up; however, this knowledge is constantly evolving. Nurses need to keep up to date with new research findings in order to provide the best possible care. The reference to *external evidence from systematic research* implies that research evidence should be in the public domain and accessible. Furthermore, the process whereby the evidence was generated should be clearly stated and open to scrutiny. Sackett *et al.*'s definition also emphasises the part that *clinical expertise* should play in making decisions about appropriate care. This is particularly important in situations where research evidence is lacking or the findings are inconclusive or contradictory. Clinical expertise is the proficiency that practitioners gain through experience and is reflected in effective assessment and in thoughtful and compassionate use of individual patient's preferences in making decisions about their care (Sackett *et al.* 1996).

The early definitions of evidence-based practice have been criticised by Bucknall and Rycroft-Malone (2010) as being overly simplistic in that they do not take account of the complexity of clinical judgement and or contextual issues such as the patients' health status and the organisational resource available to support change. More recent models of evidence-based practice, such as that developed by DiCenso *et al.* (2005), take an expanded view and include five key components:

- Research evidence
- Clinical expertise
- Patient preferences and actions
- The patient's clinical state, setting and circumstances
- Health-care data and resources

Let us consider the different components of evidence-based practice.

Research evidence

As the previous chapters of this book have demonstrated, the systematic nature of research means that it should be possible to use research findings with a reasonable degree of confidence. However, all research has limitations. It is essential, therefore, that research reports are subject to critical scrutiny in order to decide whether or not the quality of the research is sufficient to support the conclusions drawn. Chapter 8 provides guidance on how to critically appraise published research. However, the skills of critical appraisal cannot be viewed in isolation from knowledge of the research process. In order to review a research report thoroughly, it is essential to understand different research designs, methods of data collection and analysis as well as ethical considerations.

Evidence provided from a single research study is generally considered insufficient grounds to justify changing practice. Rather, a body of research evidence on a particular topic needs to be established. Ideally, a systematic review (as outlined in Chapter 25) should be undertaken in order to draw an overall conclusion about the cumulative evidence. This activity is time consuming and requires a sound understanding of research methodologies. It is therefore beyond the scope of many nurses unless undertaken as part of an education course. However, there are several organisations that publish systematic reviews of clinical interventions that can be accessed by nurses or that translate the information provided from systematic reviews into evidence-based guidelines (see Box 38.1).

Even when a systematic review has been published, it may still not provide conclusive evidence to guide practice, for example, the NICE guidance on oral nutrition support of adults based many of the recommendations on best practice, as there was insufficient robust research evidence (NICE 2006). In the United Kingdom, the NICE has collated and published information about the uncertainties associated with the effects of some treatments (Database of Uncertainties about the Effects of Treatments (DUET), http://www.library.nhs.uk/duets). The information draws upon patients' and clinicians' questions about the effects of treatments, recommendations in reports of systematic reviews of existing research and clinical guidelines where knowledge gaps have been identified, and ongoing research. Identifying the uncertainties about the evidence base for treatments enables patients and clinicians to make informed decisions and can guide researchers and research funders to focus their efforts and resources where needed.

In concluding this section, it should be acknowledged that although the evidence base for some interventions may be well founded, such as a meta-analysis across a number of clinical trials that finds a consistent effect, other interventions are not underpinned by this level research evidence (Dopson 2007). Moreover, as Bucknall (2007) points out,

Box 38.1 Organisations publishing information to support evidence-based practice

Systematic reviews and knowledge summaries

Bandolier – http://www.medicine.ox.ac.uk/bandolier

Cochrane Collaboration – http://www.cochrane.org

NIHR Centre for Reviews and Dissemination – http://www.york.ac.uk/inst/crd

National Institute for Health and Care Excellence (NICE) clinical knowledge summaries – http://cks.nice.org.uk

Joanna Briggs Institute – http://joannabriggs.org

Nursing+Best Evidence for Nursing Care – http://plus.mcmaster.ca/np/Default.aspx

Evidence-based guidelines

National Clinical Guideline Centre (UK) – http://www.ncgc.ac.uk

scientific facts derived through research only become evidence when the practitioner decides that the information is relevant to a particular situation.

Professional expertise

There is debate in the nursing literature as to whether professional expertise should be considered 'evidence'. Closs (2003), for example, argues that although clinical expertise is essential to the delivery of high-quality care, it does not constitute evidence per se. From her perspective, evidence is derived from research findings that have been validated through the process of peer review and resulted in publication. She also cautions against assuming that experience will lead to excellence in practice. Although experienced nurses may be able to predict problems and needs that other nurses may not, they may hold personal opinions that have no factual basis and that do not form reliable evidence.

Other commentators take a broader view of evidence derived from professional experience. Eraut (1994) describes this form of evidence as 'practical knowledge' and differentiates it from the 'technical' or 'propositional knowledge' derived from research. It is the knowledge that is embedded in practice and that is often tacit or intuitive. Nurses acquire such knowledge by working alongside role models or others considered experts. Research has highlighted the extent to which nurses draw upon the knowledge gained experientially in the workplace, for example, from specialist nurses, members of the multidisciplinary team and professional networks (Thompson *et al.* 2001; Milner *et al.* 2005; Gerrish *et al.* 2011). Indeed, nurses draw upon these sources of knowledge more frequently than formal sources of knowledge such as published research reports (Gerrish *et al.* 2008).

Liaschenko and Fisher (2009) provide a useful way of conceptualising the knowledge that nurses use within the context of evidence-based practice. They identify three different forms of knowledge:

- *Scientific knowledge* is largely biomedical knowledge derived from research and includes, for example, nurses' knowledge of disease processes and treatment regimes.
- *Patient knowledge* includes knowledge about how an individual becomes identified as a patient, how the person responds to treatment, how to get things done for the patient and who else may be involved in providing services for the patient. Nurses use this practical 'know-how' knowledge gained through experience, alongside research-based knowledge to guide their practice.
- *Person knowledge* is gained through viewing a patient as an individual with a personal biography and who occupies a particular social space. Knowing a person means understanding something of what living with the disease or disability is like for the individual and seeing that individual as more than a patient in a health-care system.

Liaschenko and Fisher indicate that experienced nurses draw upon these different forms of knowledge, especially when there may be conflict between an individual patient's preferences and the opinions of health professionals or among the professionals themselves. For example, they use it to justify an alternative approach to disease management and to defend their actions to support an individual patient's choice, even when this may conflict with established biomedical or institutional practices.

The experiential forms of knowledge (patient and person) identified earlier can have a reciprocal, reinforcing relationship with scientific evidence. Ferlie *et al.* (1999) have shown that research evidence is more influential when it tallies with clinical

Reflection activity

Identify an example where you, or a more senior nurse you have been working with, have drawn upon the three types of knowledge that Liaschenko and Fisher have identified to inform decisions about the care of a patient. How did the different forms of knowledge influence the decisions that were made?

experience; conversely, when research evidence and clinical experience do not match, its use in practice can be variable. They describe how the use of a drug was influenced by the beliefs of a group of orthopaedic surgeons that were based on their experience. There was a disparity between the research evidence and clinical expertise, and as a result, the uptake of the new drug was 'patchy'.

Reflection activity

From your experience, are patients engaged in decisions concerning their care? To what extent do you share knowledge about the best available evidence with patients to help them make decisions? Are there things that you could do differently?

Patient experience

Farrell and Gilbert (1996) draw a distinction between *individual* and *collective* involvement of patients and carers in health care that provides a useful means of viewing patient experience in the context of evidence-based practice. *Individual* involvement concerns individual patients and their contact with particular practitioners during episodes of care, whereas *collective* involvement entails the participation of groups or communities in health-care planning or service delivery.

In order to involve *individual* patients and their carers effectively in decisions about their care, their views and preferences should be taken into account. Patients and carers will draw upon their knowledge of their physical and psychological 'self', their social lives and their previous experiences of care. Integrating the experiential knowledge of patients with scientific knowledge requires considerable skill. It is generally accepted that health professionals should share their knowledge of research findings underpinning clinical interventions with patients so that patients understand the appropriateness of the intervention and can exercise an informed choice when there are alternative courses of action available. Patients are also becoming more informed about health care. Access by the general public to health information has increased significantly in recent years, supported by government initiatives and consumer organisations that provide information via the Internet. Some initiatives, for example, healthtalkonline (http://healthtalkonline.org/), link patients' experiences with research information. However, nurses may encounter a mismatch between the research evidence and patient preferences. Rycroft-Malone *et al.* (2004) provide an example whereby robust research evidence that recommends the use of compression bandaging to treat venous leg ulcers may not tally with a patient's experience of discomfort caused by the bandaging. The individual practitioner's skills in identifying these issues and negotiating the most appropriate course of action are essential to improving patient outcomes.

There are various means whereby a *collective* view of patient and carer perspectives can inform evidence-based practice. For example, at a national level, the NICE ensures patient and carer representation on its committees and involvement in the development of national guidelines. At a local level, patient satisfaction surveys undertaken by health-care organisations provide a means whereby a collective view of patient perspectives can be gleaned through patient feedback.

The patient's state, setting and circumstances

The patient's state, the setting in which they are receiving care and their circumstances may each influence evidence-based practice. In some situations, a patient's state (e.g. severity of illness, cognitive state, physical (dis)ability) may mean that a particular evidence-based intervention is inappropriate and alternatives need to be considered. Furthermore, although it may be feasible to implement some evidence-based interventions in a hospital setting where there are skilled nurses at hand, it may be more difficult to continue with the same intervention once the patient is discharged into the

Research evidence
Compression bandaging has improved healing rates compared to treatments using no compression
Compression therapy is more cost-effective because the faster healing rates saved nurses time.
High compression achieves better healing rates than low compression
Multi-layer compression systems are more effective than single layer systems.

Clinical expertise
Practitioner is:
- Informed of benefits of compression bandaging
- Trained in applying compression bandaging
- Skilled in patient education to promote patient understanding of leg ulcer management and concordance with treatment regime

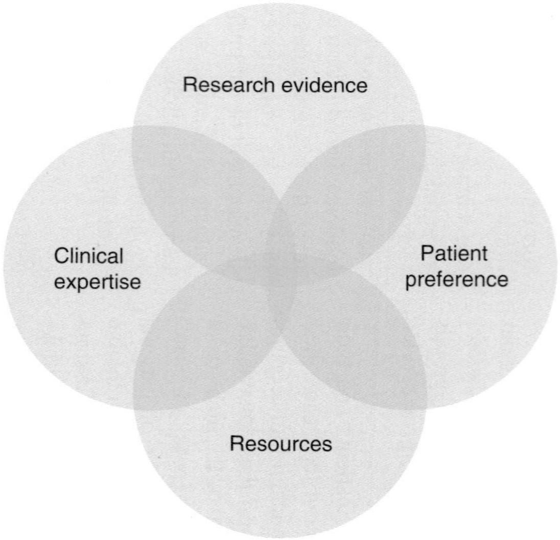

Patient preference, state, setting, circumstances
Willingness to try techniques offered
Readiness to comply with treatment regime
Experience of other treatment programmes
Able to adopt a lifestyle to prevent ulcer reoccurrence (mobility, leg elevation, skin care, avoiding trauma)
Understands rationale for care and can tolerate compression bandages for length of time prescribed

Resources
Access to:
- Doppler screening for accurate diagnosis
- Compression bandaging

On-going patient follow-up every 6–12 months following healing

Research evidence drawn from:
NICE Clinical Knowledge Summary Leg ulcers – venous (2012) http://cks.nice.org.uk/leg-ulcer-venous
Royal College of Nursing (2006)The nursing management of patients with venous leg ulcers, London, RCN

Figure 38.1 An example of the interrelationship between the elements of evidence-based practice

community if professional support is less readily available. A patient's circumstances may also influence the extent to which they are able to adhere to an evidence-based intervention: for example, a review of evidence undertaken for the NICE identified that a person who is homeless and suffering from TB is likely to find it much harder to complete the arduous medication regimen required to treat the disease (O'Mara *et al.* 2010).

Health-care information and resources

There are various sources of information in addition to those identified earlier that can inform evidence-based practice. These include clinical audit data, resource management data, policy and strategy information and information from public sources (such as media sources) (Sigma Theta Tau 2008). Some of this information is produced nationally; for example, in the United Kingdom, the Audit Commission (www.audit-commission.gov.uk) undertakes external audits of the NHS and publishes its findings. There are also national initiatives to help organisations monitor their performance on important aspects of care. For example, the Health and Social Care Information Centre (www.hscic.gov.uk/home) provides information and data to help health-care organisations monitor standards in evidence-based care, including a number of nurse-sensitive indicators, such as pressure ulcers and patient falls. However, much of this type of information is produced locally by health-care organisations and therefore can be particularly helpful in informing local decision-making by mangers and practitioners about evidence-based care. There may be situations where decision-makers may conclude that the potential benefits of a particular evidence-based intervention are outweighed by the costs associated with it. However, such decisions should not be taken lightly, and decision-makers need to consider both the benefits and risks to patients as well as the health-care organisation (DiCenso *et al.* 2005).

In summary, evidence-based practice requires a blending of the research-based and experiential knowledge of professionals with the individualised personal knowledge of patients and their carers while taking account of the patients' state, setting and circumstances and health-care information and resources available. Figure 38.1 illustrates how these elements of evidence-based practice are interrelated in regard to the use of compression bandages to treat venous leg ulcers. Where there is a lack of congruence, for example, between the research evidence, the practitioner's skills to apply the bandages correctly and the patient's willingness to try a new treatment, the outcomes for the individual patient are likely to be affected.

HIERARCHIES OF EVIDENCE

If it is accepted that evidence-based practice involves drawing upon the different types of evidence outlined earlier, how then are decisions made about what constitutes the 'best' evidence? Muir Gray (1997) provides a classification that groups different sources of research evidence into five categories and ranks them in order of the strength of the evidence (see Box 38.2). This form of classification, commonly known as a 'hierarchy of evidence', ranks different research designs in terms of the extent to which they prevent bias from influencing the research findings. The randomised controlled trial (RCT) in which the researcher seeks to minimise the effects of bias is judged to be the most robust form of evidence, whereas expert opinion and descriptive studies are considered to be weaker.

Hierarchies of evidence are important in guiding systematic reviews undertaken by the Cochrane Collaboration and the National Institute for Health Research (NIHR) Centre for Research and Dissemination and in informing the guidance produced by the NICE. However, this approach has been criticised for devaluing the contribution of qualitative and participatory forms of research. Whereas some criticism may be justified, it is important to recognise that the hierarchy of evidence was developed to help judge the robustness of evidence examining the *outcomes* of different clinical interventions and treatments, and in this respect, it is a useful tool for deciding which sources of evidence are best able to link cause and effect. If a district nurse wants to

Box 38.2 Hierarchies of evidence

I Randomised controlled trial
II Non-randomised trials
III Non-experimental studies
IV Descriptive studies, expert committees

(Muir Gray 1997)

know which type of dressing is most effective in healing venous leg ulcers, then an RCT that compares different types of dressing while at the same time seeking to reduce the effect of other factors that might influence wound healing will clearly provide more robust evidence than the professional opinion of nurses who have used different dressings.

However, where evidence is sought to provide guidance on an aspect of care that is not focused on measurable outcomes, the hierarchy of evidence is inappropriate. For example, if a nurse wants to understand what the transition from independence to dependence is like for an older person in order to provide sensitive and compassionate care, then qualitative studies are likely to provide appropriate evidence to inform practice. Guidance is now available on how to judge the robustness of evidence derived from this approach and use it to inform the development of clinical guidelines (see Chapters 8 and 25).

What needs to be emphasised is the value of different research methodologies in providing guidance for practice and the need to acknowledge the contribution of different sources of knowledge where research evidence is lacking.

RESEARCH UTILISATION

The different forms of evidence identified in the hierarchy of evidence lend themselves to different models of research utilisation. Much of the literature on evidence-based practice focuses on the direct application of research findings to practice often in the form of clinical protocols, practice guidelines or care pathways. Estabrooks (1998) refers to this as *instrumental* research utilisation. Quantitative research, and in particular the RCT, is most suited to direct application. The hierarchy of evidence is generally used to determine the robustness of evidence used in this model of research utilisation.

An alternative model of research utilisation is proposed by Weiss and Bucuvalas (1980) who suggest that research findings may be used but not necessarily always in a direct way that the instrumental model implies. Research findings may exert an influence through a process of subliminal diffusion that informs a person's understanding. In this model of *indirect* research use, practitioners become aware of research findings, internalise them and use them to inform their practice in ways that are often not explicit (Estabrooks 1998). Qualitative research findings tend to be used more indirectly.

Research findings may also be used persuasively to argue for a change in policy or practice. Florence Nightingale's collation of epidemiological data during the Crimean War, which she then used to persuade government officials of the need for radical reform in the British military, is an example of the persuasive use of research at a macro level. However, nurses use research as a means of persuasion in much more modest ways. For example, Gerrish *et al.* (1999) describe how a team of nurses in the operating theatre department in the hospital in which they worked used research examining the risk assessment of pressure damage to change surgeons' perceptions and gain support for the introduction of new theatre mattresses to minimise such risk.

The three models of research utilisation referred to earlier are helpful in thinking about different approaches to evidence-based practice. The instrumental model of research utilisation is reflected in the standard linear process of evidence-based practice outlined in Box 38.3, whereas the other two models identify how evidence can be used in more subtle ways to inform practice.

Box 38.3 The stages of evidence-based practice

- Identify a problem or issue from practice
- Formulate an answerable question
- Identify the available evidence
- Appraise the evidence
- Develop guidance for practice
- Plan strategy for introducing change
- Implement change
- Evaluate the impact of change

Reflection activity

Think about your own area of practice and try to identify examples of where research has been used directly (instrumentally), indirectly (conceptually) and persuasively. Which model of research utilisation is most common? Why do you think this is the case?

THE PROCESS OF EVIDENCE-BASED PRACTICE

As Box 38.3 shows, there are several stages involved in evidence-based practice. Guidance on how to achieve the first 4 stages can be found in earlier chapters of this book (Chapter 7, 8 and 25), whereas Chapter 39 deals with the implementation of evidence-based practice in more detail. Although individuals or small groups of nurses may choose to take forward evidence-based initiatives using these stages, the implementation of evidence-based practice often involves a large-scale organisational initiative in which evidence-based guidelines are implemented across particular patient pathways or in throughout a clinical setting.

This approach to evidence-based practice is concerned primarily with *process*, which is ensuring that practitioners use the best available evidence to inform their practice, rather than with the outcome of that evidence for the patient. However, to use evidence to underpin practice and not to evaluate its effect on patients is short sighted. Clinically effective practice can only occur when practitioners use the best available evidence to maximise patient outcomes. Evaluation is essential to monitoring outcomes of care.

BARRIERS TO ACHIEVING EVIDENCE-BASED PRACTICE

Translating the aspirations of evidence-based practice into reality is far from straightforward, and nurses need to appreciate what is involved. Barriers to achieving evidence-based practice need to be overcome, and certain conditions are necessary for the successful implementation of evidence-based practice. These will be considered in turn.

Several research studies have identified barriers to evidence-based practice by using an anglicised version of the Barriers to Research Utilisation Scale developed by Funk *et al.* (1991) in the United States (see Kajermo *et al.* (2010) for a review of 60 studies). Other researchers have developed specific instruments to examine different barriers to evidence-based practice (e.g. McKenna *et al.* 2004; Upton & Upton 2006; Gerrish *et al.* 2007). Many, although not all, of these studies have focused on research use rather than other forms of evidence. The collective findings from these studies have identified barriers that can be grouped into four categories.

The nature of the evidence

Although the amount of research conducted by nurses and/or examining nursing practice has grown considerably, some nursing interventions still lack robust research evidence. Researchers have been accused of not asking questions that are relevant to clinical practice, and there is a plethora of small-scale studies that focus on local need and lack generalisability, as opposed to large-scale definitive studies. Nursing research also varies considerably in terms of its quality: not all published research may have been undertaken sufficiently rigorously.

The way the evidence is communicated

Research is often published in academic journals rather than professional journals that clinical nurses are more likely to read. Evidence suggests that nurses tend not to read research journals (Bostrom *et al.* 2008; Gerrish *et al.* 2008), preferring instead to access research information via a third party, such as specialist nurses and medical staff, or through attending in-service training and conferences (Gerrish *et al.* 2008; Gerrish & Cook 2013). However, opportunities for practising nurses to attend conferences where up-to-date research is presented are limited.

The language of research can also act as a barrier. Research papers often use complex terminology and are written in a style that is not particularly accessible. Researchers may fail to draw out the implications of their research for practice, leaving it to the reader to do the hard work. Practising nurses perceive that research reports lack clinical credibility and fail to provide sufficient clinical direction (Thompson *et al.* 2005). Researchers, therefore, need to pay attention to how best communicate their findings to those who may use them in practice.

Knowledge and skills of the individual nurse

Although nurses may be willing to use research, they may lack the skills to do so. Studies examining barriers to research utilisation have consistently identified that nurses do not know how to access and appraise research information. In the past, the main concern was whether nurses could use library resources effectively. The increasing availability of evidence-based information on the Internet means that nurses now need to be competent in using IT in the workplace. Yet, research has shown that nurses lag behind other professional groups in their use of IT in the workplace (Estabrooks *et al.* 2003; Bertulis 2008). One of the challenges of using the Internet is coping with information overload. A seemingly straightforward search may result in a baffling array of research and other sources of evidence, some of which may be contradictory. Making sense of all this information is a daunting task even for the most determined practitioner.

Nurses have also been shown to lack skills in evaluating different sources of evidence and in drawing out the implications of research findings for practice. As Chapter 8 has shown, critical appraisal of research findings demands considerable knowledge about the research process and is very time consuming. Whereas these skills now form part of both pre- and post-registration nurse education, many nurses still do not consider themselves to be competent in this area (Pravikoff *et al.* 2005; Gerrish *et al.* 2007).

The organisation

Major obstacles that nurses encounter in implementing evidence-based practice relate to insufficient time to access and review research reports together with lack of authority and support to implement findings. Organisational factors have been identified as a major impediment to achieving evidence-based practice. In particular, lack of support from managers and doctors, problems with dissemination of information within the organisation, difficulties in the management of innovations including the time necessary to implement change and resource constraints all hinder the successful implementation of evidence-based practice (Meijers

Reflection activity

Think about your own area of practice. What do you see as the main barriers to achieving evidence-based practice? How might these barriers be overcome?

et al. 2006; Ploeg *et al.* 2007). Additionally, practitioners may experience restricted local access to information, for example, library resources or the Internet. Encouragingly, progress is being made in overcoming some of these organisational barriers although there remains much to be achieved (Gerrish *et al.* 2008).

IMPLEMENTING EVIDENCE-BASED PRACTICE

Whereas there is general consensus about what the barriers to evidence-based practice are, there is less agreement about how they might be overcome. Evidence-based practice requires complex actions on the part of organisations to facilitate its implementation including high-level management commitment, putting in place systems for managing information and innovation and for individual skills development (Estabrooks *et al.* 2008). Kitson *et al.* (1998) propose that the implementation of evidence-based practice depends on three factors. First, the nature of the evidence is important, and this has been discussed earlier in this chapter. Second, structures and mechanisms are required to facilitate change. External and internal change agents can support the process of change although consideration should be given to the personal characteristics of the facilitator, the style of facilitation and the role of the facilitator in terms of authority. Finally, consideration of the context draws attention to the importance of the ward/team culture in terms of patient centeredness, valuing team members and promoting a learning environment, the leadership styles of senior clinical nurses and the audit and review procedures in place. Successful implementation of evidence-based practice is also dependent upon the resources available. These are many and varied and include the availability and access to library and IT resources, finances to support new treatments, an adequate number of nurses with appropriate skills, sufficient time for gathering and appraising research evidence and implementation activities and finally co-operation from peers, managers and other professionals.

CONCLUSION

It is crucial that nurses use the best available evidence to inform their practice in order to provide high-quality patient care. Evidence derived from rigorous research is fundamental to the process of evidence-based practice but is not sufficient in its own right. Research evidence may be lacking or the findings may be inconclusive or contradictory. In recognising that knowledge derived from research is never absolute, nurses need to draw upon their own expertise and that of more experienced nurses to inform decisions about patient care. Clinical expertise should not been seen as a substitute for research evidence but rather as contributing to the decision-making process. It should be remembered that evidence-based practice is about providing care to patients and both patients and their carers will have their own views about the care they wish to receive. Therefore, nurses have a responsibility to share their knowledge of the best available evidence with patients in order to help them to make informed choices.

Achieving evidence-based practice is a complex undertaking that involves identifying and appraising different sources of evidence, translating evidence into clear guidance for practice, implementing change and finally evaluating the impact of change. The following chapter considers how evidence can be implemented in practice.

References

Bertulis R (2008) Barriers to accessing evidence-based information. *Nursing Standard* **22**(36): 35–39.

Boström AM, Kajermo K, Nordström G, Wallin L (2008) Barriers to research utilization and research use among registered nurses working in the care of older people: does the BARRIERS Scale discriminate between research users and non-research users on perceptions of barriers? *Implementation Science* **3**: 24. DOI: 10.1186/1748-5908-3-24.

Bucknall T (2007) A gaze through the lens of decision theory toward knowledge translation science. *Nursing Research* **56**: S60–S66.

Bucknall T, Rycroft-Malone J (2010) Evidence-based practice: doing the right thing for patents. In: Rycroft

Malone J, Bucknall T (eds) *Models and Frameworks for Implementing Evidence-Based Practice: linking evidence to action*. Oxford, Wiley-Blackwell, pp 1–21.

Closs SJ (2003) Evidence and community-based nursing practice. In: Bryer R, Griffiths J (eds) *Practice Development in Community Nursing*. London, Arnold, pp 33–56.

DiCenso A, Ciliska D, Guyatt G (2005) *Evidence-Based Nursing: a guide to clinical practice*. Philadelphia, Elsevier/AMA Press.

Dopson S (2007) A view from organisational studies. *Nursing Research* **56**: S72–S77.

Eraut M (1994) *Developing Professional Knowledge and Competence*. London, Falmer Press.

Estabrooks C (1998) Will evidence-based nursing practice make practice perfect? *Canadian Journal of Nursing Research* **30**: 15–36.

Estabrooks C, O'Leary K, Ricker K, Humphrey C (2003) The Internet and access to evidence: how are nurses positioned? *Journal of Advanced Nursing* **42**: 73–81.

Estabrooks C, Scott, S, Squires J, Stevens B, O'Brien-Pallas L, Watt-Watson J, Profetto-McGrath J, McGilton K Golden-Biddle K, Lander J, Donner G, Boschma G, Humphrey C Williams J (2008) Patterns of research utilisation on patient care units. *Implementation Science* **3**:31. DOI: 10.1186/1748-5908-3-31.

Farrell C, Gilbert H (1996) *Health Care Partnerships*. London, Kings Fund.

Ferlie E, Wood M, Fitzgerald L (1999) Clinical effectiveness and evidence-based medicine: Some implementation issues. In: Lugon M, Secker-Walker J (eds) *Clinical Governance: making it happen*. London, The Royal Society of Medicine, pp 49–60.

Funk S, Champagne M, Weise R, Tornquist E (1991) BARRIERS: the barriers to research utilisation scale. *Applied Nursing Research* **4**: 39–45.

Gerrish K, Ashworth P, Lacey A, Bailey J, Cooke J, Kendall S, McNeilly E (2007) Factors influencing the development of evidence-based practice: a research tool. *Journal of Advanced Nursing* **57**: 328–338.

Gerrish K, Ashworth P, Lacey A, Bailey J (2008) Developing evidence-based practice: experiences of senior and junior clinical nurses. *Journal of Advanced Nursing* **62**: 62–73.

Gerrish K, Clayton J, Nolan M, Parker K, Morgan L (1999) Promoting evidence-based practice: managing change in the assessment of pressure damage risk. *Journal of Nursing Management* **7**: 355–362.

Gerrish K, Cook J (2013) Factors influencing evidence-based practice among community nurses. *Journal of Community Nursing* **27**(4): 98–101.

Gerrish K, McDonnell A, Nolan M, Guillaume L, Kirshbaum M, Tod A (2011) The role of advanced practice nurses in knowledge brokering as a means of promoting evidence-based practice among clinical nurses. *Journal of Advanced Nursing* **67**: 2004–2014.

Kajermo KN, Bostrom AM, Thompson D, Hutchinson A, Estabrooks CE, Wallin L (2010) The BARRIERS scale: the barriers to research utilisation scale: a systematic review. *Implementation Science* **5**: 32.

Kitson A, Harvey G, McCormack B (1998) Enabling the implementation of evidence-based practice: a conceptual framework. *Quality in Health Care* **7**: 149–158.

Liaschenko J, Fisher A (2009) Theorising the knowledge that nurses use in the conduct of their work. In: Reed P, Crawford Shearer N (eds) *Perspectives on Nursing Theory*, 5th edition. Philadelphia, Wolters Kluwer, Lippincott Williams and Wilkins, pp 129–138.

Maijers J, Janssen M, Cummings G, Wallin L, Estabrooks C, Halfens R (2006) Assessing the relationship between contextual factors and research utilisation: a systematic review. *Journal of Advanced Nursing* **55**: 622–635.

McKenna H, Ashton S, Keeney S (2004) Barriers to evidence-based practice in primary care. *Journal of Advanced Nursing* **45**: 178–189.

Milner M, Estabrooks C, Humphrey C (2005) Clinical nurse educators as agents for change: increasing research utilisation. *International Journal of Nursing Studies* **42**: 899–914.

Muir Gray JA (1997) *Evidence-Based Health Care*. Edinburgh, Churchill Livingstone.

Muir Gray JA (2004) Evidence-based policy making. *British Medical Journal* **329**: 988–989.

NICE (2006) *Nutrition support in adults: oral nutrition support, enteral tube feeding and parenteral nutrition*. Clinical Guideline, Volume **32**. London, NICE.

O'Mara A, Marrero-Guillamón I, Jamal F, Lehmann A, Cooper C, Lorencet T (2010) *Tuberculosis Evidence Review 1: review of barriers and facilitators*. London, National Institute for Health and Clinical Excellence (NICE), Matrix Knowledge Group.

Ploeg J, Davies B, Edwards N, Gifford W, Miller PE (2007) Factors influencing best-practice guidelines implementation: lessons learned from administrators, nursing staff and project leads. *Worldviews on Evidence-Based Nursing* **4**(4): 210–219.

Pravikoff D, Tanner A, Pierce S (2005) Readiness of US nurses to evidence-based practice: many don't understand or value research and have had little or no training to help them find evidence on which to base their practice. *American Journal of Nursing* **105**(9): 40–51.

Rycroft-Malone J, Seers K, Titchen A, Harvey G, Kitson A, McCormack B (2004) What counts as evidence in evidence-based practice? *Journal of Advanced Nursing* **47**(1): 81–90.

Sackett DL, Rosenburg WM, Muir Gray JA, Haynes RB, Richardson WS (1996) Evidence-based medicine: what it is and what it isn't. *British Medical Journal* **312**: 71–72.

Sigma Theta Tau International (2008) Sigma Theta Tau International position statement on evidence-based practice. *Worldviews on Evidence-Based Nursing* **5**(2): 57–59.

Thompson C, McCaughan D, Cullum N, Sheldon T, Mullhall A, Thompson D (2001) The accessibility of research-based knowledge for nurses in United Kingdom acute care settings. *Journal of Advanced Nursing* **36**: 11–22.

Thompson C, McCaughan D, Cullum N, Sheldon T, Raynor P (2005) Barriers to evidence-based practice in primary care nursing: why viewing decision-making as context is helpful. *Journal of Advanced Nursing* **52**: 432–444.

Upton D, Upton, P (2006) Development of an evidence-based practice questionnaire for nurses. *Journal of Advanced Nursing* **53**: 454–458.

Weiss C, Bucuvalas M (1980) *Social Science Research and Decision Making*. New York, Columbia University Press.

Further reading

Cullum N, Ciliska D, Hayes B, Marks S (2008) *Evidence-Based Nursing: an introduction*. Oxford, Blackwell.

Rycroft-Malone J, Bucknal T (2010) *Models and Frameworks for Implementing Evidence-Based Practice: linking evidence to action*. Oxford, Wiley-Blackwell.

Websites

http://plus.mcmaster.ca/np/Default.aspx – Nursing+ Best Evidence for Nursing Care based at McMaster University's Health Information Research Unit provides access to current research evidence to support evidence-based clinical decisions.

http://www.evidence.nhs.uk/about-evidence-services – An online resource comprising a range of evidence services that provide access to high-quality evidence and best practice in health, social care and public health services.

http://www.cochrane.org/index.htm – The Cochrane Collaboration is an international organisation that makes up-to-date, accurate information about the effects of health care readily accessible. It produces and disseminates systematic reviews of health-care interventions.

CHAPTER 39

Translating Research Findings into Practice

Kate Gerrish

Key points

- Translating evidence into clinical practice at the point of care is a complex and challenging process.
- Clinical guidelines are recommendations on the most appropriate care of people with specific conditions, based on the best available evidence: they provide a means of translating research findings into practice.
- Where possible, existing published guidelines should be adapted for local use. Published guidelines should be appraised in order that an assessment can be made of their quality and appropriateness for the local context.
- Strategies for translating research findings into practice should be carefully planned and executed. There are several frameworks and tools that can assist at different stages of the process in order to enhance the likelihood of success.

INTRODUCTION

As discussed in the previous chapter, evidence-based practice involves practitioners in making decisions about the care they provide based on the integration of research evidence with clinical expertise and the patients' preferences and circumstances while taking account of the local context. It is a complex undertaking that involves identifying and appraising different sources of evidence, translating the evidence into clear guidance for practice, implementing change and finally evaluating the impact of that change. Despite a strong commitment towards evidence-based practice in nursing, the uptake of research findings in practice continues to be challenging (Gerrish *et al.* 2007; Harrison & Graham 2012). This problem has led to increased recognition that the process of translating research findings into practice is complex. Attempts have been made to understand how it might be achieved and strategies developed to increase its success.

The term 'knowledge translation' is used increasingly to describe the complex process of moving

The Research Process in Nursing, Seventh Edition. Edited by Kate Gerrish and Judith Lathlean.

Companion Website: www.wiley.com/go/gerrish/research

what is learned through undertaking research to applying such knowledge in a variety of practice settings and circumstances (Sudsawad 2007). Whereas evidence-based practice is concerned with using the best available evidence to inform what practitioners actually do, knowledge translation is a much broader concept and encompasses the whole of the research process. The Canadian Institutes of Health Research (CIHR) is attributed with first using the term knowledge translation and define it as

> 'a dynamic and iterative process that includes synthesis, dissemination, exchange and ethically-sound application of knowledge to improve the health of *Canadians*, provide more effective health services and products and strengthen the health care system'. (CIHR 2013)

There is often a tendency to assume that knowledge translation occurs at the end of a project, once the findings are known. However, the CIHR (2012) proposes that researchers should consider a more integrated approach to knowledge translation with interactions between researchers and users of research spanning the whole of the research process. This approach is also known as collaborative research, action research and co-production of knowledge. As Box 39.1 shows, there are several opportunities within the research cycle during which interactions between researchers and knowledge users can facilitate the transfer of knowledge into practice. These range from defining research questions, selecting appropriate research methods, conducting the research, disseminating the findings and applying the research to resolve practice problems. Chapter 4 has outlined strategies that can be used to engage the users of research more actively in the research process. The focus in this chapter is on how research findings can be applied in practice.

Knowledge generated by a particular research study contributes to the overall knowledge base about a specific topic or issue. However, before the findings can be applied in practice, they need to be considered within the context of what is already known about the topic. For example, do the findings support or refute current knowledge, or do they provide new insights into practice that indicate the need for change? Systematic reviews provide a mechanism for integrating knowledge from several studies on a particular topic, and this is an important step in contextualising knowledge. However, before the findings of a systematic review can be applied, there is a need to consider the context in which the findings will be implemented. This involves taking account of individual and organisational sociocultural norms that may influence how the findings might be used. Research findings that reflect closely current practice are more readily accepted and incorporated into everyday practice than findings that challenge existing practice and indicate the need for significant change. Once research findings have been contextualised, there is a need to think about how they can most readily be applied in practice. Relying solely on practitioners to apply research findings to practice is unrealistic. Practitioners may interpret the implications for practice arising from research study differently, and this will lead to variability in the standard of care. In order to avoid such inconsistencies, research findings need to be translated into research tools and products that can be applied in practice.

Box 39.1 Opportunities for knowledge translation within the research process

1. Development or refinement of the research questions
2. Selection of the methodology
3. Data collection and tools development
4. Selection of outcome measures
5. Interpretation of the findings
6. Crafting of the message and dissemination of the results

(CIHR 2012)

TRANSLATING RESEARCH FINDINGS INTO RESEARCH PRODUCTS

In most instances, it is inappropriate to change practice based on the findings from a single study. Rather, the findings from several studies on the same topic need to be evaluated and brought together in the form of a systematic review (see Chapter 25). Where there is a range of sources of evidence (not just research), then a realist synthesis (Chapter 26) may be undertaken. Whichever approach is used, the intention is to provide a comprehensive account of the knowledge on a particular topic, which will include a statement of the strength of the evidence as a quality indicator. The next step is to translate the evidence synthesis into a 'product' that practitioners can use to inform their practice. Clinical guidelines are the most common research product used by nurses and other health-care professionals.

CLINICAL GUIDELINES

Clinical guidelines are systematically developed statements to assist practitioner and patient decisions about appropriate health care for specific clinical circumstances (Lohr & Field 1992). Guidelines are based on the best available evidence and make recommendations for the treatment and care of patients by nurses and other health-care professionals. Guidelines can also be used to help patients make informed decisions about their care and improve communication between the patient and health-care professionals. However, guidelines do not replace practitioner's knowledge and skills (NCGC 2010). Developing robust clinical guidelines requires considerable expertise and resources, so where possible, existing guidelines should be adapted for local use.

Several government agencies and professional organisations in the United Kingdom and internationally develop clinical guidelines through a structured process of reviewing and synthesising international research literature, drawing upon renowned experts in the field and conducting a meta-analysis to generate guidelines based on the best available evidence. In the United Kingdom, the National Clinical Guideline Centre (NCGC) hosted by the National Institute for Health and Care Excellence (NICE) and the Scottish Intercollegiate Guidelines Network (SIGN) produce guidelines on a range of clinical topics, and professional bodies such as the Royal College of Nursing and several of the medical royal colleges also develop guidelines. There are equivalent organisations in many other countries, some of which focus on nursing topics such as the Joanna Briggs Institute in Australia.

There may be several guidelines on the same topic produced by different organisations. When planning to introduce a guideline, it is worthwhile undertaking a thorough search to identify relevant ones. Guideline developers may make their guidelines available via the Internet as this facilitates timely dissemination and enables rapid updating as new evidence becomes available. The websites of organisations such as the NCGC, NICE, SIGN, Royal College of Nursing and medical royal colleges are a useful starting point for locating existing guidelines. The National Guideline Clearinghouse in the United States also has a large collection of clinical guidelines that can be accessed easily. It can be helpful to search the Internet for guidelines using search engines such as Google. However, there is no guarantee that guidelines published on the Web will have been developed through the same rigorous approach adopted by the NCGC or SIGN. Moreover, even where national guidelines have been produced by one of the organisations identified earlier, it cannot be assumed that they can be applied directly to the local context. It is important that guidelines are evaluated in order that an

Reflection activity

What criteria would you use to judge whether a guideline produced outside your organisation is appropriate to use locally? Why are these criteria important? Once you have read the remainder of this section, compare your criteria to those listed in Box 39.2.

Box 39.2 The Appraisal of Guidelines Research and Evaluation II (AGREE II) instrument quality criteria

Scope and purpose

1 The overall objective(s) of the guidelines is (are) specifically described
2 The health question(s) covered by the guideline is (are) specifically described
3 The population (patients, public, etc.) to whom the guideline is meant to apply is specifically described

Stakeholder involvement

4 The guideline development group includes individuals from all the relevant professional groups
5 The views and preferences of the target population (patients, public, etc.) have been sought
6 The target users of the guideline are clearly identified

Rigour of development

7 Systematic methods were used to search for evidence
8 The criteria for selecting the evidence are clearly described
9 The strengths and limitations of the body of evidence are clearly described
10 The methods used for formulating the recommendations are clearly described
11 The health benefits, side effects and risks have been considered in formulating the recommendations
12 There is an explicit link between the recommendations and the supporting evidence
13 The guideline has been externally reviewed by an expert panel prior to publication
14 A procedure for updating the guideline is provided

Clarity and presentation

15 The recommendations are specific and unambiguous
16 The different options for management of the condition or health issue are clearly presented
17 Key recommendations are easily identifiable

Applicability

18 The guideline describes facilitators and barriers to its application
19 The guideline provides advice and/or tools on how the recommendations can be put into practice
20 The potential resource implications of applying the recommendations have been considered
21 The guideline presents monitoring and/or audit criteria

Editorial independence

22 The views of the funding body have not influenced the content of the guideline
23 Competing interests of guideline development group members have been recorded and addressed

(AGREE Research Trust 2009)

assessment can be made of their quality and appropriateness for use locally.

There are several guideline appraisal tools that can help in the process. However, the Appraisal of Guidelines Research and Evaluation II (AGREE II) instrument (AGREE Research Trust 2009) is generally accepted as the gold standard for guideline appraisal (Graham & Harrison 2008). It was developed by an international group of researchers to assess the quality of clinical guidelines by considering the process of guideline development and the extent to which the process has been reported. Whereas the instrument provides an assessment of the likelihood that the guideline will achieve its intended outcome, it does not assess the impact of the guideline on patient outcomes. It can be used to assess guidelines developed by local, national or international groups and applied to new guidelines or when updating existing guidelines. Ideally, at least two reviewers should independently appraise the guideline.

The AGREE instrument comprises 23 items grouped into six domains with each domain addressing a separate dimension of guideline quality. Each item is rated on a 7-point Likert scale ranging from 'strongly disagree' to 'strongly agree', which measures the extent to which the item has been addressed. The reviewer is also required to provide an overall assessment of the quality of the guideline taking each of the appraisal criteria into account and decide whether they would recommend use of the guideline. The AGREE II quality criteria are shown in Box 39.2.

Once a guideline has been appraised and recommended for use, it may be appropriate to adopt it as it stands or it may require some adaptation for the local context. For example, some recommendations may not apply to the types of patients seen in the practice setting; alternatively, contextual factors or resource considerations may make it impractical to implement some of the recommendations (Graham & Harrison 2008).

Guideline adaptation involves taking the most appropriate recommendations and repackaging them to form a new local guideline. Modifications to evidence-based recommendations should not be made unless the supporting evidence has changed since the guideline was first developed. Where modifications are made, the rationale for such changes needs to be made explicit (Harrison *et al.* 2010). Ensuring that a rigorous process in guideline adaptation is employed is essential. Research Example 39.1 outlines the ADAPTE process that provides a systematic step-by-step approach to adapting guidelines for use in other settings.

Following adaptation, the guideline should be reviewed by local practitioners and other stakeholders, such as managers and patients, to test out its relevance to the local context in which it will be implemented. The people who will ultimately use the guideline will be able to comment on how relevant the content is to the local setting and factors that may influence its uptake. Final adjustments can then be made to the guideline and decisions made as to when and how it will be reviewed and updated before it is officially endorsed by the organisation. Many healthcare organisations have mechanisms set up to approve guidelines prior to implementation and to oversee the review process.

In situations where there are no national guidelines that can be adapted, it may be necessary to develop a local guideline. The work involved in developing a guideline cannot be underestimated, and it is important that as rigorous a method as possible is used. A guideline development group should be formed to take collective ownership for the development and subsequent implementation of the guideline (Eccles *et al.* 2012). The composition of the group will vary depending on the clinical topic, but as a general principle, it is beneficial to involve members of the multidisciplinary team. For example, if developing a nursing care guideline to provide oral nutrition support for patients at risk of malnutrition, it would be prudent to involve nurses who will be involved in using the guideline, a dietitian, a medical consultant with expertise in nutrition and a speech and language therapist with expertise in dysphagia. Consideration should also be given as to how the patient perspective can be incorporated. This might be through involving a patient representative in the guideline development group or through consulting with relevant patient groups at key points in the development process (Eccles *et al.* 2012).

Developing local guidelines has been made easier by the availability of high-quality published systematic reviews. However, there are a limited number of systematic reviews on specific nursing topic, partly

RESEARCH EXAMPLE

39.1 Adapting Clinical Guidelines to Local Settings

Harrison M, Legare F, Graham I, Fervers B (2010) Adapting clinical practice guidelines to local context and addressing barrier to their use. *Canadian Medical Association Journal* **182**(2): 78–84.

Customising a clinical guideline to a particular setting can improve its uptake into practice. Active involvement of the people who will ultimately use the guideline in the process of adapting it to the local context is more likely to lead to changes in practice. The authors of this article outline a systematic approach – the ADAPTE process – to adapting guidelines to local contexts by involving end users. The process involves three stages:

- The *set-up phase* outlines the tasks to be completed before the process of adaptation, including the necessary skills and resources required and the panel that should include relevant end users of the guidelines, for example, clinicians, managers and patients.
- The *adaptation phase* involves retrieving and appraising existing guidelines. Guidelines are appraised for quality, currency, acceptability and applicability. This evaluation forms the basis for informed and transparent decision-making concerning the selection and modification of the guideline. This may result in minor changes being made to the guideline, such as updating a single recommendation and more significant changes being made, or to the production of a customised guideline based on various guidelines as sources.
- The *finalisation phase* involves external review of the guidelines, feedback from relevant stakeholders, establishing a process for updating the adapted guidelines and producing the final version of the guideline.

because robust research evidence to inform some nursing interventions is lacking. Where there is insufficient research evidence, it will be necessary to rely more heavily on expert professional opinion, for example, from members of the multidisciplinary team with specialist expertise in the clinical area. In such situations, it is important to acknowledge limitations that may arise from the nature of the evidence upon which the guideline is based and the process whereby the guideline was developed (Woolf *et al.* 2012).

As the preceding discussion has shown, there are several steps involved in developing or adapting clinical guidelines. The Practice Guidelines Evaluation and Adaptation Cycle developed by Graham and colleagues (2005) captures each of these steps and provides a useful framework to guide clinical guideline development (Figure 39.1). An example of how the cycle can be applied to the adaptation of national and international clinical guidelines on leg ulcer management for local use is given in Research Example 39.2.

Once a guideline has been formally approved by the organisation, consideration should to be given to how it will be implemented. This is unlikely to be straightforward. As discussed in Chapter 38, there are many barriers to implementing research findings in practice.

There are several factors that influence the adoption of clinical guidelines. Francke *et al.* (2008) identify the following considerations:

- The characteristics of the guideline – Guidelines that are easy to understand, can easily be tried out and do not require specific resources have a greater chance of implementation.
- The attributes of the health-care professionals – For example, awareness of the existence of the guideline and familiarity with its content will promote uptake.
- The characteristics of patients – For example, co-morbidity reduces the chance that guidelines are followed.

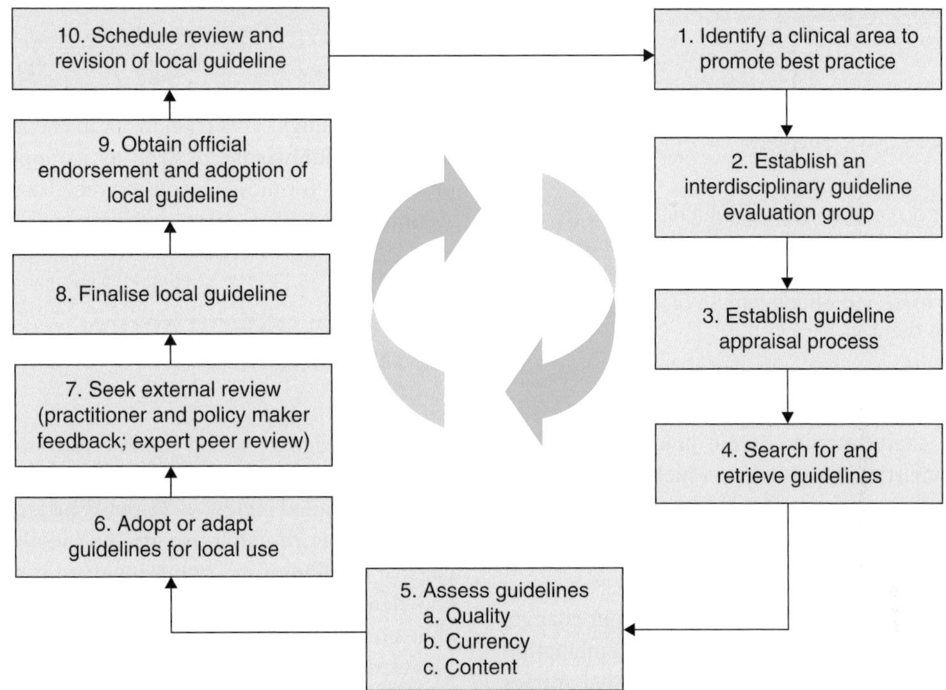

Figure 39.1 Practice Guidelines Evaluation and Adaptation Cycle
This figure was published in Graham I, MB Harrison, Brouwers M (2003) Evaluating and adapting practice guidelines for local use: a conceptual framework. In: Pickering S, Thompson J, (eds) *Clinical Governance and Best Value*, p 215. Copyright Churchill Livingstone. Reproduced with permission from Churchill Livingstone–Elsevier.

RESEARCH EXAMPLE

39.2 Adapting Guidelines on Leg Ulcer Management for Local Use

Graham *et al.* (2005) Adapting national and international leg ulcer practice guidelines for local use: the Ontario Leg Ulcer Community Care Protocol. *Advances in Skin and Wound Care* **18**(6): 307–318.

The increasing need to devote resources to individuals requiring community care for leg ulcers led to the development of a dedicated community-based leg ulcer service in Ontario, Canada. In order to provide up-to-date evidence-based care, existing leg ulcer clinical practice guidelines were identified and appraised for quality and suitability for the new service. The Practice Guidelines Evaluation and Adaptation Cycle was used to guide the development of a local protocol for leg ulcer care. This involved (i) systematically searching for practice guidelines, (ii) appraising the quality of identified guidelines using a validated guideline appraisal instrument, (iii) conducting a content analysis of guideline recommendations, (iv) selecting recommendations to include in the local protocol and (v) obtaining practitioner and external expert feedback on the proposed protocol. Only guidelines that were treatment focused, written in English and developed after 1998 were included. Of the 19 guidelines developed, only 5 met the inclusion criteria. Of these, 3 were fairly well developed and made similar recommendations. The level of evidence supporting specific recommendations ranged from randomised clinical trials to expert opinion. The guidelines were assessed for quality and content and a consensus reached regarding recommendations appropriate for local application.

Reflection activity

What do you think are the main barriers to the implementation of clinical guidelines in your area of practice? Why do these barriers exist and what might be done to overcome them?

- The characteristics of the practice setting or organisational context in which the guideline is to be implemented – For example, a lack of support from peers or superiors, as well as insufficient staff and time.

Bearing in mind the complexity of behaviour change, there is growing recognition that implementation activities should be guided by a conceptual framework (Rycroft-Malone & Bucknall 2010).

KNOWLEDGE TRANSLATION FRAMEWORKS

There are several frameworks that can help guide the translation of research findings into practice. Five of the most common ones are outlined in Box 39.3. The Diffusion of Innovations theory (Rogers 2003), the Promoting Action on Research Implementation in Health Services (PARIHS) (Kitson *et al.* 1998; Rycroft-Malone 2010), the Diffusion of Innovations in Service Organisation (Greenhalgh *et al.* 2004) and the Consolidated Framework for Implementation Research (Damschroeder *et al.* 2009) vary in their level of complexity and focus. However, they all share a common purpose in clarifying the many and varied factors to be considered when seeking to implement research findings in practice. A limitation of these frameworks is that although they describe comprehensively the factors that may influence the uptake of research evidence, they do not in themselves provide guidance on how change might best be achieved. By contrast, the Knowledge to Action framework (Graham *et al.* 2006; Graham & Tetroe 2010) provides a series of interrelated stages to progress through in order to seek to implement research findings. This framework also considers the creation of knowledge as well as its application to practice. It is for these reasons that the Knowledge to Action framework is discussed in more detail.

THE KNOWLEDGE TO ACTION FRAMEWORK

The Knowledge to Action framework (Graham *et al.* 2006; Graham & Tetroe 2010) was developed following a detailed review of 31 published frameworks for promoting research use and provides a comprehensive account of the stages involved in translating knowledge derived from research through to sustainable change in practice. It has two components: knowledge creation and an action cycle, and each component has several phases (see Figure 39.2).

Knowledge creation – Within the framework, 'knowledge' includes not just knowledge derived from research but also the tacit knowledge held by patients and the procedural knowledge derived from clinical expertise. The process of moving from research findings to research products and tools suitable for application is depicted as an inverted funnel where multiple sources of knowledge are reduced in number through knowledge synthesis and then developed into an even a smaller number of tools or products to facilitate implementation in practice.

The *action cycle* depicts the activities needed for the successful application of knowledge. It starts with a problem or issue being identified by an individual or group who then seek out knowledge relevant to solving the problem and appraise it in terms of its validity and usefulness. Alternatively, an individual or group may start by identifying the new knowledge (e.g. a clinical guideline) and then decide whether there is a knowledge–practice gap that needs bridging. 'Generic' knowledge (such as that derived from a systematic review) is seldom taken directly off the shelf and applied without some tailoring to the local context. The knowledge is therefore assessed regarding its usefulness in the particular setting and circumstances and then adapted to fit the local context. The next step is to

Box 39.3 Common frameworks for knowledge translation

Diffusion of Innovations (Rogers 2003)

First developed in the 1950s, Rogers draws upon the broader principles of communication theory to propose four main elements that influence the spread of ideas. These are (i) the characteristics of the innovation, (ii) the channels of communication, (iii) the time it takes individuals to accept new ideas and (iv) the characteristics of the social system, including the role of opinion leaders and change agents and whether the decisions around the innovation are voluntary or imposed.

Promoting Action on Research Implementation in Health Services framework (Kitson et al. 1998; Rycroft-Malone 2004)

According to the Promoting Action on Research Implementation in Health Services (PARIHS) framework, successful implementation of research findings into practice is a function of the interplay of three core elements: (i) the level and nature of the evidence used, (ii) the context or environment in which the research is to be placed and (iii) the method by which the research implementation process is facilitated. Evidence is defined as a combination of research, clinical experience, patient experience and local information. Context refers to the setting in which the proposed change is to be implemented. The framework specifies three themes under context: (i) culture, (ii) leadership and (iii) evaluation. Facilitation has a key role in helping individuals and teams understand what and how they need to change to apply evidence to practice. According to the framework, there are three aspects of facilitation: (i) purpose, (ii) roles and (iii) skills and attributes.

Knowledge to Action process (Graham et al. 2006)

The Knowledge to Action framework has two components. Knowledge creation involves knowledge inquiry, knowledge synthesis and the production of knowledge tools or products. The action cycle involves a set of eight logically interrelated steps: (i) identifying the problem that needs addressing; (ii) identifying, reviewing and selecting knowledge relevant to the problem; (iii) adapting the knowledge to the local context; (iv) assessing barriers to using the knowledge; (v) designing transfer strategies to promote the use of knowledge; (vi) monitoring how the knowledge diffuses throughout the user group; (vii) evaluating the impact of the users' application of the knowledge; and (viii) sustaining the ongoing use of knowledge by users.

Determinants of Diffusion, Dissemination and Implementation of Innovations in Health Service Delivery and Organisations (Greenhalgh et al. 2004)

Greenhalgh and colleagues undertook a systematic review examining the spread and sustainability of innovations in health service organisation and delivery. The complex model identifies eight determinants affecting the diffusion, dissemination and implementation of innovations. These include (i) the characteristics of the innovation, (ii) the process of adoption by individuals,

continued

(iii) assimilation of the innovation into the health-care system, (iv) the process of diffusion and dissemination, (v) the characteristics of the organisation (both structural and cultural), (vi) the readiness of the system for innovation, (vii) the external context in terms of external networks and collaborations and (viii) implementation and routinisation.

Consolidated Framework for Implementation Research (Damschroeder et al. 2009)

Damscroeder and colleagues undertook a detailed review of existing frameworks to support implementation of research findings. They subsequently developed a comprehensive framework, the Consolidated Framework for Implementation Research (CFIR), which encapsulates the key components of the various frameworks. The CFIR is composed of five domains: intervention characteristics, outer setting, inner setting, characteristics of the individuals involved and the process of implementation. Eight constructs were identified related to the intervention (e.g. evidence strength and quality), four constructs were identified related to outer setting (e.g. patient needs and resources, peer pressure), twelve constructs were identified related to inner setting (e.g. culture, leadership engagement, learning culture), five constructs were identified related to individual characteristics (e.g. knowledge and beliefs about the intervention), and eight constructs were identified related to process (e.g. use of opinion leaders and champions).

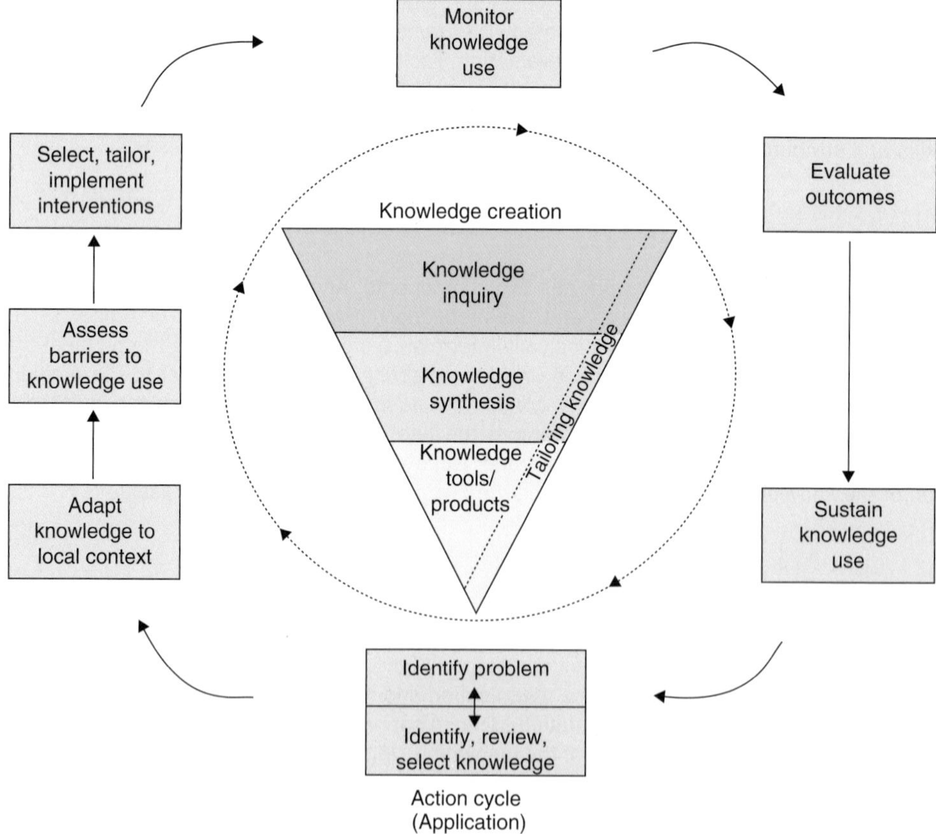

Figure 39.2 The Knowledge to Action process
From Graham I *et al.* (2006) Lost in knowledge translation: time for a map. *Journal of Continuing Education in the Health Professions* **26**(1): 13–24, 19. Reprinted with permission from John Wiley & Sons Inc.

RESEARCH EXAMPLE

39.3 Example of Knowledge Translation

Graham K, Logan J (2004) Using the Ottawa model of research use to implement a skin care programme. *Journal of Nursing Care Quality* **19**(1): 18–24.

The authors used the Ottawa model of research use to guide the implementation of clinical guidelines on skin care intended to prevent the development of decubitus ulcers in a surgical setting of a large hospital in Canada. Existing clinical guidelines were appraised and adapted for local use. An assessment was made of the knowledge, skills, attitudes and motivation of health-care practitioners together with their receptiveness to change. In addition, potential barriers and facilitators to implementation of the guidelines in the practice environment were identified. With the information gleaned, strategies to address the barriers and implement the guidelines were developed. A range of outcome measures were used to evaluate the impact of the guidelines at the level of the patient, practitioner and health-care system. The authors identified that although the evaluation demonstrated positive results, adoption took longer than anticipated. They concluded that there is a tendency to underestimate the time taken to change practice in complex care environments.

assess potential barriers that may impede or limit uptake of the knowledge so that these barriers may be targeted and hopefully overcome or diminished by intervention strategies. Attempts should also be made to identify enablers that can be taken advantage of. This information is then used to develop and implement interventions to promote awareness and uptake of the knowledge. The next step involves monitoring knowledge use in order to determine the effectiveness of the intervention strategies in promoting the uptake of knowledge and whether the interventions have brought about the desired change or whether new interventions may be required.

The impact of using the knowledge should be evaluated in order to determine whether application of the knowledge has actually made a difference in terms of positive outcomes for patients, practitioners or the health-care system. In recognising that barriers to ongoing knowledge use may be different to the barriers that needed to be addressed when the knowledge was first introduced, a plan should be drawn up to sustain the change over time. Although the action phases in Figure 39.2 are depicted as a cyclical process, in reality, they may occur sequentially or simultaneously, and the knowledge phases may influence all the action phases.

Reflection activity

Assume that you are responsible for leading the implementation of a new clinical guideline in your practice setting. Why might it be helpful to use a framework, such as the Knowledge to Action framework, to guide the implementation process?

Research Example 39.3 provides an example of knowledge translation, albeit using a different framework to guide the implementation process.

INTERVENTIONS TO PROMOTE BEHAVIOURAL CHANGE

Translating research findings into practice requires practitioners to change their behaviour so that they adopt and use research-based knowledge. However, changing behaviour can be notoriously difficult to achieve. As the Knowledge to Action framework

Box 39.4 Interventions to promote behavioural change (Adapted from Cochrane Effective Practice and Organisation of Care Group)

Intervention	Description
Audit and feedback	Any written or verbal summary of clinical performance of health-care professionals over a specified period of time. The summary may also include recommendations for clinical action
Education outreach visits	Use of a trained person who meets with professionals in their practice setting to provide information with the intent of improving practice
Educational materials	Distribution of published or printed recommendations for clinical care, including clinical guidelines, audiovisual materials and electronic publications
Interactive educational meetings	Participation of professionals in workshops that include discussion
Local consensus processes	Inclusion of participating professionals in discussion to ensure that they agree that the chosen clinical problem was important and the approach to managing the problem was appropriate
Local opinion leaders	Use of providers nominated by their colleagues as 'educationally influential'
Multifaceted interventions	A combination that includes two or more of audit and feedback, reminders, local consensus processes and patient-mediated interventions
Reminders	Any intervention, manual or computerised, that prompts professionals to perform a clinical action
Tailoring	An intervention tailored to address prospectively identified barriers to change

From O'Brien MA (2008) Closing the gap between nursing research and practice. In: Cullum N, Ciliska D, Haynes RD, Marks S (eds) *Evidence Based Nursing: an introduction*. p 246, Reproduced with permission from Blackwell Publishing.

identifies, there is a need to select appropriate interventions to implement change. Interventions may be many and varied and where possible should be evidence based. Box 39.4 identifies nine of the most common approaches that have been identified by the Effective Practice and Organisation of Care Group (EPOC). This group is part of the Cochrane Collaboration and produces systematic reviews of educational, behavioural, financial, regulatory and organisational interventions designed to improve the practice of health-care professionals and the organisation of health-care services.

There are many studies that have examined the effectiveness of different implementation strategies to promote behavioural change, and several systematic reviews of these studies have been conducted. Bero *et al.* (1998) undertook an overview of 18 systematic reviews on this topic published between 1989 and 1995. The authors grouped interventions into three types based on how effective the interventions were in promoting behavioural change:

- *Consistently effective interventions* – These included educational outreach visits, manual or computerised reminders, multifaceted interventions that comprised two or more approaches of audit and feedback, reminders and interactive educational meetings.
- *Interventions of variable effectiveness* – These included audit and feedback and the use of local opinion leaders, local consensus processes and patient-mediated interventions.
- *Interventions that have little or no effect* – These included the passive dissemination of educational materials and didactic educational meetings.

The authors concluded that specific implementation strategies are needed to promote changes in practice, and the more concerted the effort, the more successful it is likely to be. A subsequent overview of 41 systematic reviews undertaken by Grimshaw *et al.* (2001) confirmed that passive approaches were generally ineffective and unlikely to lead to behavioural change although they could be useful in raising awareness. Multifaceted interventions that targeted several barriers to change were more likely to be effective than single interventions. Audit and feedback and the use of local opinion leaders were of variable effectiveness, whereas educational outreach and reminders were more likely to be effective. The review concluded that most of the interventions were effective under some circumstances; however, none were effective under all circumstances. A more recent overview of systematic reviews on effective implementation of research into practice (Boaz *et al.* 2011) confirmed that single interventions such as audit and feedback, computerised decision-making and opinion leaders were less effective in changing professional behaviour than multifaceted interventions.

ACHIEVING CHANGE

So far, this chapter has focused on translating research findings into research products such as clinical guidelines and considering implementation strategies that can be used to facilitate the uptake of research products into everyday practice. Implementation strategies are intended to lead to a change in how practitioners provide care. In order to select appropriate strategies, an understanding of the principles underpinning successful change is necessary.

Any plan for introducing change must seek to overcome barriers to its successful implementation. It is important, therefore, to identify potential barriers to change in the local context. The most common barriers to implementing research-based change are summarised by Pearson *et al.* (2007):

- *Staff information and skills deficits* include lack of knowledge regarding current recommendations and guidelines or results of clinical research and lack of skills in accessing and applying research finding to practice
- *Psychosocial barriers* include attitudes, beliefs, values and previous experience that affect practice and an individual's willingness to change.
- *Organisational barriers* include systems and processes that may create an organisational culture that is not responsive to change.
- *Resource barriers* include a lack of required tools, equipment, staff and other resources needed to achieve change.

The Knowledge to Action framework presented earlier draws attention to the need to assess barriers to implementing change and plan accordingly. Attempts to overcome or at least reduce some of the barriers should be undertaken before introducing the change. For example, before a malnutrition screening tool and accompanying clinical guidelines can be introduced, it may be necessary to overcome the following potential barriers:

- *Staff information and skills deficits*: Nurses may not have sufficient knowledge about malnutrition screening and support and may lack the skills to use the screening tool and implement the clinical guideline.
- *Psychosocial barriers*: Nurses may feel that existing practice is satisfactory and therefore there is no need to change, or they may be

reluctant to take on new responsibilities as it is seen as extra work.

- *Organisational barriers:* Other priorities may take precedence over nutrition support that could lead to a lack of managerial commitment to making the change happen, communication systems may be lacking that means that dissemination of information about the new initiative may be poor, etc.
- *Resource barriers*: Clinical areas may not have appropriate, calibrated, well-maintained equipment to weigh and measure the patient's height accurately, new nursing documentation may need to be introduced to record the results of the screening and care plan, additional staff may be required to facilitate the introduction, etc.

Once barriers have been identified, consideration needs to be given as to how change might be achieved. There is a wealth of literature accumulated over the past 50 years that describes a wide range of approaches to change management. The evidence is derived from different organisations, not just the health-care sector, and by using a broad range of methodologies (Cameron *et al.* 2001). It is beyond the scope of this chapter to explore the different theoretical perspectives on change management. Iles and Sutherland (2001) produced a comprehensive review of different models of change management in order to help health-care practitioners and managers access the literature and consider the evidence available about different approaches to change. Additional related publications provide practical guidance on developing change management skills based on selected change management theories (Iles & Cranford 2004) and making informed decisions on change (Cameron *et al.* 2001). These three publications can be downloaded free of charge (www.evidence.nhs.uk). The NICE also produce generic and guidance-specific implementation tools that support the implementation of all types of NICE guidance, which can be useful more broadly, and a generic guide on 'how to change practice' (NICE 2007). These are available via the NICE website. Finally, Grol *et al.* (2013) have produced an informative text on the implementation of change in health care.

Reflection activity

Identify an aspect of practice from your own setting where you think change is needed. What are the staff information and skills, psychosocial, organisational and resource barriers that might be encountered when introducing the proposed change? How might these barriers be overcome?

CONCLUSION

Translating research findings into practice is a complex undertaking that involves identifying and evaluating different sources of evidence, translating evidence into clear guidance for practice, implementing change and finally evaluating the impact of change. It is important that those who want to implement clinical research findings draw upon the evidence base about the effectiveness of implementation strategies to inform their plans. In the same way that a research study should be undertaken in a systematic and rigorous manner, the process of translating research findings into practice should be carefully planned and executed. There are several frameworks and tools that can assist at different stages of the process in order to enhance the likelihood of success.

References

AGREE Research Trust (2009) *The Appraisal Guidelines for Research and Evaluation II (AGREE II) instrument.* London, The AGREE Trust.

Bero L, Grilli R, Grimshaw J, Harvey E, Oxman A, Thomson M (1998) Closing the gap between research and practice: an overview of systematic reviews of interventions to promote the implementation of research findings. *British Medical Journal* **317**: 465–468.

Boaz A, Baeza J, Fraser A (2011) Effective implementation of research into practice: a overview of systematic reviews of the health literature. *BMC Research Notes* **4**:212. DOI: 10.1186/1756-0500-4-212.

Cameron M, Cranfield S, Iles V, Stone J (2001) *Making Informed Decisions on Change*. London, London School of Hygiene and Tropical Medicine.

Canadian Institutes of Health Research (2012) *Guide to Knowledge Translation Planning at CIHR: integrated and end of grant approaches*. Ottawa, Canadian Institutes of Health Research (http://www.cihr-irsc.gc.ca/e/documents/kt_lm_ktplan-en.pdf; accessed 14 April 2014).

Canadian Institutes of Health Research (2013) *More about Knowledge Translation at CIHR*. Ottawa, Canadian Institutes of Health Research (http://www.cihr-irsc.gc.ca/e/39033.html#Two-Types-2; accessed 14 April 2014).

Damschroeder L, Aron D, Keith R, Kirsh S, Alexander J, Lowery J (2009) Fostering implementation of health services research findings into practice: a consolidated framework for advancing implementation science. *Implementation Science* **4**:50. DOI: 10.1186/1748-5908-4-50.

Eccles MP, Grimshaw JM, Shekelle P, Schunemann HJ, Woolf S (2012) Developing clinical practice guidelines: target audiences, identifying topics for guidelines, guideline group composition and functioning and conflicts of interest. *Implementation Science* **7**:60. DOI: 10.1186/1748-5908-7-60

Francke AL, Smit MC, de Veer AJE, Mistiaen P (2008) Factors influencing the implementation of clinical guidelines for health care professionals: a systematic meta-review. *BMC Medical Informatics and Decision Making* **8**:38. DOI: 10.1186/1472-6947-8-38.

Gerrish K, Ashworth P, Lacey A, Bailey J (2007) Developing evidence-based practice: experiences of senior and junior clinical nurses. *Journal of Advanced Nursing* **62**: 62–73.

Graham I, Harrison M (2008) Appraising and adapting clinical practice guidelines. In: Cullum N, Ciliska D, Haynes RB, Marks S (eds) *Evidence Based Nursing: an introduction*. Oxford, Blackwell, pp 219–230.

Graham I, Harrison M, Lorimer K, Piercianowski T, Friedberg E, Buchanan M, Harris C, (2005) Adapting national and international leg ulcer practice guidelines for local use: the Ontario leg ulcer community care protocol. *Advances in Skin and Wound Care* **18**(6): 307–318.

Graham K, Logan J (2004) Using the Ottawa model of research use to implement a skin care programme. *Journal of Nursing Care Quality* **19**(1): 18–24.

Graham I, Logan J, Harrison M, Strauss S, Tetroe J, Caswell W, Robinson N (2006) Lost in knowledge translation n: time for a map. *Journal of Continuing Education in the Health Professions* **26**(1): 13–24.

Graham I, Tetroe J (2010) The knowledge to action framework. In: Rycroft-Malone J, Bucknall T (eds) *Models and Frameworks for Implementing Evidence-Based Practice: linking evidence to action*. Chichester, Wiley-Blackwell, pp 207–221.

Greenhalgh T, Robert G, Macfarlane F, Bates P, Kyriakidou O (2004). Diffusion of innovations in service organizations: systematic review and recommendations. *Milbank Quarterly* **82**(4): 581–629.

Grimshaw J, Shirran L, Thomas R, Mowatt G, Fraser C, Bero L (2001) Changing provider behaviour: an overview of systematic reviews of interventions. *Medical Care* **39**(8 Suppl. 2) II-2–II-25.

Grol R, Wensing M, Eccles M, Davies D (2013) *Improving Patients Care: the implementation of change in health care*. 2nd edition. Oxford, Wiley-Blackwell.

Harrison M, Graham I (2012) Roadmap for a participatory research-practice partnership to implement evidence. *Worldview on Evidence-Based Nursing* **9**: 210–220.

Harrison M, Legare F, Graham I, Fervers B (2010) Adapting clinical practice guidelines to local context and assessing barriers to their use. *Canadian Medical Association Journal* **182**(2): 78–84.

Iles V, Cranfield S (2004) *Developing Change Management Skills: a resource for health care professionals and managers*. London, London School of Hygiene and Tropical Medicine.

Iles V, Sutherland K (2001) *Organisational Change: a review for health care managers, professionals and researchers. A resource for health care professionals and managers*. London, London School of Hygiene and Tropical Medicine.

Kitson A, Harvey G, McCormack B (1998) Enabling the implementation of evidence-based practice: a conceptual framework. *Quality in Health Care* **7**: 149–158.

Lohr K, Field M (1992) A provisional instrument for assessing clinical practice guidelines. In: Field MJ, Lohr KN (eds) *Guidelines for Clinical Practice: from development to use*. Washington, DC, Institute of Medicine, National Academy Press, pp 346–410.

National Clinical Guideline Centre (2010) *Development of the guideline*. National Clinical Guideline Centre (http://www.ncgc.ac.uk/Guidelines/Methodology/; accessed 14 April 2014).

NICE (2007) *How to Change Practice: understand, identify and overcome barriers to change*. London, National Institute for Health and Clinical Excellence.

O'Brien M (2008) Closing the gap between nursing research and practice. In: Cullum N, Ciliska D, Haynes

RB, Marks S (eds) *Evidence Based Nursing: an introduction*. Oxford, Blackwell, pp 244–252.

Pearson A, Field J, Jordan Z (2007) *Evidence-Based Clinical Practice in Nursing and Health Aare: assimilating research, experience and expertise*. Oxford, Blackwell.

Rogers E (2003) *Diffusion of Innovations*. 5th edition. New York, The Free Press.

Rycroft-Malone J (2004) The PARIHS framework: a framework for guiding the implementation of evidence-based practice. *Journal of Nursing Care and Quality* **19**: 297–304.

Rycroft-Malone J (2010) Promoting Action on Research Implementation in Health Services (PARIHS). In: Rycroft-Malone J, Bucknall T (eds) *Models and Frameworks for Implementing Evidence-Based Practice: linking evidence to action*. Chichester, Wiley-Blackwell, pp 109–13.

Rycroft-Malone J, Bucknall T (2010) Theory, frameworks and models: laying down the groundwork. In: Rycroft-Malone J, Bucknall B (eds) *Models and Frameworks for Implementing Evidence-Based Practice: linking evidence to action*. Chichester, Wiley-Blackwell, pp 23–50

Sudsawad P (2007) *Knowledge Translation: introduction to models, strategies and measures*. Wisconsin, National Centre for the Dissemination of Disability Research.

Woolf S, Schunemann HJ, Eccles MP, Grimshaw JM, Shekelle P (2012) Developing clinical practice guidelines: types of evidence and outcomes, values and economics, synthesis, grading, and presentation and deriving recommendations. *Implementation Science* **7**:61. DOI: 10.1186/1748-5908-7-61.

Further reading

Bick D, Graham ID (eds) (2010) *Evaluating the Impact of Implementing Evidence-Based Practice*. Chichester, Wiley-Blackwell.

Grol R, Wensing M, Eccles M, Davis D (eds) (2013) *Improving Patient Care: the implementation of change in health care*. 2nd edition, Oxford, Wiley Blackwell.

Rycroft-Malone J, Bucknall B (eds) *Models and Frameworks for Implementing Evidence-Based Practice: linking evidence to action*. Chichester, Wiley-Blackwell.

Strauss S, Tetroe J, Graham ID (2009) *Knowledge Translation in Health Care: moving evidence into practice*. Chichester, Wiley-Blackwell.

Websites

http://www.evidence.nhs.uk – This website hosted by the NICE provides the opportunity to search on key terms, for example, managing change, and will provide links to relevant publications, including those published by the National Institute for Health Research.

http://agreetrust.org – AGREE is an international collaboration of researchers and policymakers who seek to improve the quality and effectiveness of clinical practice guidelines by establishing a shared framework for their development, reporting and assessment.

http://www.cihr.ca/e/29418.html – The Canadian Institutes of Health Research website provides information on and tools of assist in knowledge translation. There are also knowledge translation learning modules that can be freely accessed at http://www.cihr.ca/e/39128.html.

http://www.nice.org.uk – The National Institute for Health and Care Excellence (NICE) is an independent organisation responsible for providing national guidance on promoting good health and preventing and treating ill health. It also publishes guidance on implementation strategies at https://www.nice.org.uk/article/pmg15/chapter/15-implementation-support-for-good-practice-guidance.

http://www.sign.ac.uk/about/introduction.html – The Scottish Intercollegiate Guidelines Network (SIGN) undertakes the development and dissemination of national clinical guidelines containing recommendations for effective practice based on current evidence.

http://www.ncgc.ac.uk – The National Clinical Guideline Centre is a multidisciplinary health services research team funded by the National Institute for Health and Care Excellence (NICE) that produces evidence-based clinical practice guidelines on behalf of the NICE.

http://www.guideline.gov/index.aspx – The National Guideline Clearinghouse that is part of the Agency for Healthcare Research and Quality in the United States is a public resource for evidence-based clinical practice guidelines.

http://plus.mcmaster.ca/KT – The KT+ knowledge translation website hosted by McMaster University, Canada, provides a range of resources to support the implementation of evidence into practice.

CHAPTER 40

Future Trends in Nursing Research

Kate Gerrish and Judith Lathlean

Key points

- There is increasing emphasis placed on the need for research addressing societal expectations.
- Nurse researchers should consider innovative ways to identify research priorities and undertake research of relevance to those who use healthcare services and those who provide such services.
- There is an increasing imperative to consider the impact of the research, whether through quantitative measures of effectiveness; qualitatively derived understanding of patients', consumers' and professionals' perspectives and experiences or the empowerment of individuals through action-orientated approaches.
- The influences of advancing technologies affect both the topics studied and the methods used in nursing research and will present new opportunities for nurse researchers in the future.

INTRODUCTION

In this final chapter, we consider some recent trends influencing nursing research that we anticipate will continue to gain momentum in coming years. Since the 6th edition of *The Research Process in Nursing* was published in 2010, research funders and policy makers have placed greater emphasis on the importance of research addressing societal expectations. In respect of nursing and healthcare research, there is a growing expectation that research will lead to demonstrable benefits to patients or to healthcare services within 5 years of the research having been completed. This in turn has required researchers to consider innovative approaches to identifying priorities and undertaking research of relevance to patients and those providing healthcare services in order to maximise the impact of their research.

Whereas national funding agencies, for example the National Institute for Health Research (NIHR), undertake consultation exercises inviting healthcare

The Research Process in Nursing, Seventh Edition. Edited by Kate Gerrish and Judith Lathlean.

Companion Website: www.wiley.com/go/gerrish/research

professionals, researchers and the public to contribute to research priority setting exercises, which then inform the commissioning of large-scale studies, we suggest that nurse researchers more generally should think carefully about how their research might address societal concerns relating to health and health care and subsequently impact on the health and well-being of patients and the population at large as well as influence healthcare delivery.

In addition to the need for researchers to address questions that are relevant to patients, the public and healthcare professionals and to consider the impact of their work, we also recognise the growing tendency for technology to influence both health care and research. As Chapter 6 has illustrated, social media and Web 2.0 technologies provide useful tools for researchers at all stages of the research process, and this trend is set to continue.

In the subsequent sections of this chapter, we draw upon examples from our own research and those of others to illustrate these trends and provide some pointers for researchers to consider in their own research.

ENSURING THE RELEVANCE OF RESEARCH

The overarching purpose of nursing, and indeed healthcare research, remains to develop knowledge that informs decision-making at all levels from the bedside, within the community or from a national or increasingly international perspective. How then might researchers ensure that the topics they choose to address are relevant to those who might benefit from the findings?

Many national organisations who fund research or who have an interest in research undertake work to identify research priorities. For example, the James Lind Alliance (www.lindalliance.org) works with health and research organisations to establish 'priority-setting partnerships' to identify research priorities to address health-related topics where there is a lack of evidence. Working with the Alzheimer's Society, they undertook an extensive consultation with people with dementia and their carers, healthcare and social care practitioners and organisations that represent these groups to identify 10 priorities (from a total of 4000 research questions proposed) for research on the prevention, diagnosis, treatment and care of dementia (see Box 40.1). Several of these priorities for dementia research are highly relevant to nurse researchers. Whereas research-funding organisations can commission studies to address such priorities, there is considerable scope for nurse researchers undertaking smaller-scale studies to focus their research on some of these topics and thereby make a valuable contribution to knowledge.

In addition to addressing priorities set nationally, nurse researchers can also seek to identify local priorities. Indeed, as discussed in Chapter 24 on practitioner research, nurses who work in practice settings are well placed to identify research questions of direct relevance to patients or the delivery of nursing care. Nurse researchers who are not directly involved in patient care can still engage in dialogue with practitioners, healthcare managers, patients and the public to identify research questions that are of local relevance.

Identifying research questions through engaging with those who might ultimately benefit from research is clearly an important step in ensuring the relevance of research. However, Chapter 39 introduced the concept of knowledge translation as a means of maximising the potential for research findings to be used in practice. Knowledge translation involves researchers, as knowledge producers, interacting with the users of research knowledge, be they managers, practitioners and/or patients, to facilitate

Reflection activity

How would you go about identifying local research priorities relevant to your area of practice? Which individuals or groups might you engage with to identify research topics and how will you consult with them? If they propose a number of priorities, how will you decide which one you might take forward in your own research?

Box 40.1 Priorities for research on the prevention, diagnosis, treatment and care of dementia

1. What are the most effective components of care that keep a person with dementia as independent as they can be at all stages of the disease in all care settings?
2. How can the best ways to care for people with dementia, including results from research findings, be effectively disseminated and implemented into care practice?
3. What is the impact of an early diagnosis of dementia and how can primary care support a more effective route to diagnosis?
4. What non-pharmacological and/or pharmacological (drug) interventions are most effective for managing challenging behaviour in people with dementia?
5. What is the best way to care for people with dementia in a hospital setting when they have acute health care needs?
6. What are the most effective ways to encourage people with dementia to eat, drink and maintain nutritional intake?
7. What are the most effective ways of supporting carers of people with dementia living at home?
8. What is the best way to care for people with advanced dementia (with or without other illnesses) at the end of life?
9. When is the optimal time to move a person with dementia into a care home setting and how can the standard of care be improved?
10. What are the most effective design features for producing dementia friendly environments at both the housing and neighbourhood levels?

Developed by the Dementia Priority Setting Partnership involving the Alzheimer's Society and James Lind Alliance (http://alzheimers.org.uk/site/scripts/documents_info.php?documentID=1804; accessed 24 April 2014)

the uptake of research findings into practice. Whereas knowledge translation has traditionally been undertaken once a research project has been completed, the Canadian Institutes of Health Research (2012) have promoted a model of *integrated knowledge translation* whereby researchers work collaboratively with the ultimate users of their research throughout the various stages of the research process. Clearly, if those who are likely to use the research are involved in defining the research questions, help to shape the plan of investigation and possibly engage in different aspects of data collection and analysis, as well as the interpretation of the findings, then research findings are more likely to be relevant to practice and thereby have greater impact. Chapter 4 identified how service users can become more actively involved in research; indeed, it is seen as a priority of many research funders. Whereas patient and public involvement might be relatively modest in terms of, for example, membership of a project advisory group, patients or members of the public can play a fuller role in different stages of the research process in line with an integrated model of knowledge translation. Such involvement can be beneficial in ensuring the relevance of research, thereby maximising the potential impact of the research on patients and the public.

As the responsibility for the implementation of research findings often falls on practitioners and healthcare managers, involving them in an integrated approach to knowledge translation can be extremely beneficial. Not only does this ensure that research tackles questions that are of concern to healthcare professionals but also the findings are likely to be

RESEARCH EXAMPLE

40.1 Integrated Knowledge Translation: Engaging Healthcare Professionals and Community Members in Research Examining TB in the Somali Community

Gerrish K, Naisby A, Ismail I (2012) The meaning and consequences of tuberculosis among Somali people in the United Kingdom. *Journal of Advanced Nursing* **68**(12): 2654–2663.
Gerrish K, Naisby A, Ismail I (2013b) Experiences of the diagnosis and management of tuberculosis: a focused ethnography of Somali patients and healthcare professionals in the United Kingdom. *Journal of Advanced Nursing* **69**(10): 2285–2294.

The researcher (KG) was initially approached by a TB physician and TB specialist nurse who expressed concern that the care that they were providing was not responsive to the needs of Somali patients with TB. They highlighted in particular the apparent stigma associated with TB, which they felt influenced how Somali patients with TB engaged with TB services and managed their illness. The researcher worked with the TB healthcare professionals and Somali community leaders to identify the specific research questions, plan the investigation and secure funding for the study. A collective decision was made to undertake a participatory ethnographic study in order to gain insight into the sociocultural factors that influenced an understanding of TB within the Somali community and identify the barriers and enablers to Somali patients engaging with the TB services.

The TB specialist nurse and Somali researcher became members of the research team and were actively involved in all stages of the research process. In addition, Somali community researchers were recruited and trained to undertake interviews with Somali community members. A wider group of healthcare professionals involved in providing TB services, general practitioners, TB patients and Somali community leaders became members of an advisory group that met on a regular basis to inform the various stages of the research.

The collaborative approach continued once the research was completed with the researcher working with the TB specialist nurse to disseminate the findings to healthcare professionals and use the key messages from the research to inform training for general practitioners in order to raise their awareness of TB to ensure timely diagnosis and provide ongoing support to patients with TB. The TB nurse also used findings to inform work undertaken by the TB specialist nursing team and hospital and outpatient services for Somali patients. The Somali researcher worked with local community leaders and the TB specialist nurse to disseminate the findings to the Somali community through hosting community meetings and engaging a Somali poet to share some of the findings in a culturally appropriate manner. Community leaders and healthcare professionals subsequently reported that they perceived that TB was viewed with less stigma and patients were more open in sharing information to help with contact tracing, thus reducing the potential spread of the disease.

highly relevant to practice. Research Example 40.1 provides an illustration of an integrated knowledge translation project that involved researchers working together with healthcare professionals and members of the Somali community to undertake a collaborative study that examined how TB was viewed among Somalis in order to identify and overcome barriers to the uptake of TB services among the Somali community. Following completion of the research, the researchers continued to work with the healthcare professionals and Somalis who had been involved in the project to facilitate the uptake of findings within the Somali community and among a wider group of healthcare professionals.

Reflection activity

What are the potential benefits of adopting an integrated approach to knowledge translation in research? What are the challenges that researchers may encounter in using an integrated knowledge translation approach?

Whereas an integrated approach to knowledge translation can operate within a single research project, there is potential for this model to be applied more widely. For example, within England, the NIHR has funded a number of collaborative partnerships between universities and healthcare organisations in a defined geographical location with a remit to undertake applied health research of relevance to local populations and facilitate the implementation of research findings into practice. Known as Collaborations for Leadership in Applied Health Research and Care (http://www.nihr.ac.uk/infrastructure/Pages/CLAHRCs.aspx), these partnerships have a remit to create a model for the conduct and application of research that links those who undertake research with those who use it in practice across the local health community and develop approaches to research, its dissemination and uptake that are specifically designed to take account of the way that health care is delivered across the geographical area (NIHR 2014). We envisage that closer collaboration between researchers and those who may ultimately use the research findings is a trend that will continue in coming years, and it provides an opportunity for nurse researchers to ensure the relevance of their research and to maximise its impact.

ENHANCING THE IMPACT OF RESEARCH

It is vital to ensure research is undertaken that represents value for money and that influences practice, policy and education. Traditionally, the quality of nursing research has been judged in terms of the scientific merit of academic publications arising from a study. However, research funders are placing increasing importance on the impact of research. For example, it is stressed in research assessment endeavours especially in the United Kingdom whereby institutions have been required to submit impact case studies as part of the 2014 Research Excellence Framework exercise (http://www.ref.ac.uk/). Australia too has its own system for monitoring research, referred to as Excellence in Research for Australia (ERA) (http://www.arc.gov.au/), which for the next round – in 2015 – is likely to expand the ERA framework to allow for additional measures of research application, knowledge exchange and collaboration.

There are different dimensions of non-academic impact in terms of benefits of research to the economy and to the society and issues for nurses to consider including economic, social, public policy, health, cultural, quality of life, etc. Whereas the research undertaken as part of an education programme at masters or doctoral level may be quite modest in terms of its impact on policy or practice, it is still important for nurse researchers to think about the nature and extent of a specific impact. Indeed, employers who provide support to enable nurses to undertake research often have expectations that the research will benefit the organisation in some way. Clearly, action research and practitioner research, which have been discussed in detail in earlier chapters of this book, are research approaches that are intended to impact on practice because they focus on the process of change. Moreover, the findings of a randomised controlled trial that clearly demonstrate the effectiveness of a new nursing intervention over standard treatment have the potential to achieve a significant impact if the findings are implemented. However, nurse researchers should consider the impact of research arising from a broad range of research approaches, whether through quantitative measures of effectiveness, qualitatively derived understanding of patients', consumers' and professionals' perspectives and experiences or the empowerment of individuals through action-orientated approaches.

Impact should be considered at a local level and more widely with the potential for national and even international impact. For example, the ethnographic study of TB within the Somali community outlined in Research Example 40.1 not only achieved

RESEARCH EXAMPLE

40.2 Enhancing the Impact of Research: Developing a Practical Toolkit to Enable Nurse Consultants to Evaluate Their Impact on Patients, Staff and the Organisation in Which They Work

Gerrish K, McDonnell A, Kennedy F (2011) *Capturing Impact: a practical toolkit for nurse consultants.* Sheffield, Sheffield Hallam University (available at http://research.shu.ac.uk/hwb/ncimpact/NC%20Toolkit%20final.pdf, accessed 24 April 2014).
Gerrish K, McDonnell A, Kennedy F (2013a) The development of a framework for evaluating the impact of nurse consultant roles in the United Kingdom. *Journal of Advanced Nursing* **69**(10): 2295–2308.

The overall aim of this research study was to develop a framework to evaluate the impact of nurse consultant roles on patient, professional and organisational outcomes and identify associated indicators of impact. In order to maximise the impact of the research, the researchers decided from the outset to develop, pilot and evaluate a practical toolkit that could be used by nurse consultants to evaluate their impact. Case studies of six nurse consultants were undertaken. Individual interviews were conducted with each nurse consultant, healthcare professionals with whom they worked, patients and family carers and senior nurses of the organisations in which the nurse consultants worked. Interviews explored participants' perceptions of the impact of the nurse consultant and indicators of actual and/or potential impact. Three domains of impact of nurse consultant roles were identified: clinical significance, professional significance and organisational significance. Each domain included three to four indicators of impact. A practical toolkit (Gerrish *et al.* 2011) based on the findings was developed and piloted with nurse consultants. The toolkit guides nurse consultants through various steps in order to identify their impact on patients, other healthcare staff and the organisation in which they work and includes a number of tools, such as questionnaires, that they can use to capture different aspects of their impact.

The toolkit was made freely available for download via the project website, and the research team provided workshops for nurse consultants in different parts of the United Kingdom on how to use the toolkit. They also sought feedback from nurse consultants who were using the toolkit in order to evaluate its impact.

significant local impact but was also cited in a review of research on the management of TB among 'hard-to-research groups' (O'Mara *et al.* 2010) undertaken to inform national guidance on the management of TB produced by NICE (2012).

Considering the potential impact of research should start at the beginning when identifying research topics and questions and in planning the research approach: it is not just something to consider once the research is completed. Key questions to consider include the following:

- *How far-reaching is the impact of the research?* Small-scale studies often impact on local services; however, consideration should be given for the potential for the impact to extend more widely at national or even international levels.
- *Who will benefit from the impact of the research?* Typically, nursing research has the potential to benefit patients, nurses and/or other healthcare professionals, but there may be other groups who could benefit. Identifying the full range of individuals and groups will help guide actions to maximise impact.
- *In what way might the benefits of the research be felt?* It is important to consider how the research might impact on those with the

Reflection activity

Think of a research project you are undertaking or are interested in carrying out in the future. What steps can you take to maximise the impact of the findings? How will you subsequently judge whether your research has had an impact?

potential to benefit from the findings. For example, the research might lead to improved patient outcomes or enhance the patient experience of health care or quality of life. Alternatively, the research could result in changes to how care is delivered, thereby enhancing the quality of patient care and patient safety.

Research Example 40.2 provides an illustration of how a research team planned for wider impact of their study into assessing the impact of nurse consultant roles. The research aims sought to derive and validate a conceptual framework for assessing the impact of nurse consultants and also to develop a practical toolkit to help nurse consultants assess the impact of their role. The resultant toolkit was made freely available via the project website and has been used extensively by nurse consultants and other advanced practice nurses across the United Kingdom and beyond.

THE EVOLVING ROLE OF DIGITAL TECHNOLOGY

As outlined in Chapter 6, digital literacy is a vital skill for all nurse researchers and this is likely to increase over the next decade as digital technologies continue to develop. Social media and the related Web 2.0 tools are an integral aspect of everyday life and for researchers they provide a way to engage with clinicians and professionals, service users, communities, policy makers and research funders. They also pave the way to more creative approaches to collaborative international research and assist communication across international boundaries. For example, an Australian researcher (Tracy Levett-Jones) had the idea for a research study of the factors facilitating the learning of nursing students in clinical placements. She was introduced to a potential UK doctoral supervisor (Judith Lathlean) to discuss the possibility of an international PhD study. Owing to the development of technological communication such as email, video links and an online survey, she was able with relative ease to conduct a comparative project between Australia and the United Kingdom, resulting in a penetrating mixed methods study that revealed the outcomes as in part due to the different arrangements for nurse education in the two countries (see Levett-Jones & Lathlean 2009a,b).

Technology has also enabled the better dissemination of research and the sharing of tools developed from studies. Research Example 40.3 shows how a tool to measure belongingness in nurse education that was one of the outcomes of the aforementioned study (see Levett-Jones *et al.* 2009) was flagged up to researchers worldwide through an international online research network, ResearchGate, and a national university repository, e-Prints. Facilitated by these and other mechanisms for the setting up, conduct and dissemination of research, collaborative international projects are now commonplace and enable knowledge gained to be truly global in application.

As traditional boundaries are broken down through the use of digital technology, even novice researchers can build global links. International supervisory teams for doctoral students are increasingly common, as in the example aforementioned, and enable students to draw upon much wider expertise on their topic of interest and their chosen methodology. Moreover, novice researchers are able to build global networks with fellow students as well as academic researchers. For example, the International Network for Doctoral Education in Nursing (http://nursing.jhu.edu/excellence/inden) provides a number of resources for students and academic staff involved in doctoral supervision together with networking opportunities to support professional advancement. Such collaboration for

RESEARCH EXAMPLE

40.3 Dissemination Aided by Technology

Levett-Jones T, Lathlean J, McMillan M, Higgins I (2009) Development and psychometric testing of the Belongingness Scale – Clinical Placement Experience: an international comparative study. *Collegian* **16**(3): 153–324.

This paper describes a study that was conducted across three nursing education programmes – two in Australia and one in the United Kingdom. One of the outcomes was the production of a validated 'tool' to measure the level of belongingness experienced by nursing students in these programmes. This tool was reproduced in the paper. The journal was not one that is commonly known about outside of Australia, yet the requests to use and trial the tool have been numerous and from nurses and others around the world. This has been largely as a result of two technological developments in recent years – the establishment of online researcher networks (in this case ResearchGate) to which all of the authors subscribe, and which are gaining in popularity, and to a university repository in the United Kingdom, e-Prints.

Reflection activity

What are the benefits of establishing an international network to support your research endeavours? Do you see any potential drawbacks to engaging with other researchers globally? How might you manage these challenges to ensure you gain from such networking opportunities?

established as well as novice researchers is set to increase as digital technologies advance.

The past decade has seen an exponential growth in digital technology that has been incorporated into health care, both to support nurses and other health professionals to deliver care and to assist patients in managing their conditions. As a result, the use of digital technologies in health care is rising in popularity as a topic for nursing and healthcare research. A systematic review of 112 studies in the field of gerontology included telecare technologies (representing half the studies); electronic health records; decision support systems; web-based packages for patients and/or family care givers and assistive information technologies (Vedel *et al.* 2013). The review concluded that the most consistent finding was the positive outcomes of health information technology in terms of clinical processes. Although less frequently studied, positive impacts were also found on patients' health, productivity, efficiency and costs, clinicians' satisfaction, patients' satisfaction and patients' empowerment. Research Example 40.4 provides an illustration of one such study that examined how nurses use technology to support their decision-making and how nurses' experience impacted on their use of such technology.

As we look to the future, the growth in eHealth is likely to create new opportunities for nursing research. The term eHealth refers to health services and information delivered through the Internet and integrates the fields of medical informatics and public health. It allows health data to be rapidly shared across settings and geography, reducing delays and overcoming the disconnection between healthcare practitioners, hospitals and other healthcare facilities. Whereas there are major challenges in terms of information security, confidentiality and managing levels of authorised access, there is considerable potential for the data generated to be used for research purposes. For example, clinical databases and registries have become potent instruments for observing and understanding patterns of care received by patients, the effectiveness of care, patient responses to treatment and the monitoring of patient safety during treatment. Provided appropriate ethical

RESEARCH EXAMPLE

40.4 Nurses' Use of Technology

Dowding D, Mitchell N, Randell R, Foster R, Lattimer V, Thompson C (2009) Nurses' use of computerised clinical decision support systems: a case site analysis. *Journal of Clinical Nursing* **18**(8): 1159–1167.

This study explored how nurses use computerised clinical decision support systems in clinical practice and the factors that influence this. A multiple case study design, with four sites, was chosen, and data were collected by non-participant observation of nurse/patient consultations (n=115) and interviews with nurses (n=55). This elicited information about staff experience, technology used and decisions supported by the technology.

The study found that computerised decision support systems were used in a variety of ways by nurses, including recording information, monitoring patients' progress and confirming decisions that had already been made. Nurses' experience with the decision and the technology affected how they used a decision support system and whether or not they overrode recommendations made by the system. The ability of nurses to adapt the technology to 'fit' with local clinical practice also affected its use.

RESEARCH EXAMPLE

40.5 Using Digital Technologies to Engage Citizen Scientists and the Wider Public in Data Analysis

Cancer Research UK has created a genomics-driven predictor for cancer prognosis using citizen scientists and non-scientists. A computer gaming company worked with cancer research scientists to develop 'Play to Cure: Genes in space', an Internet-based and mobile game that enlists citizen scientists in cancer research and the wider public by competing in a space mission to collect a fictional substance dubbed Element Alpha, which represents genetic cancer data that might underpin certain types of cancer. Players fly through space, mapping their route thought the densest areas of Element Alpha, avoiding and destroying asteroids along the way in order to progress to the next level of Alpha collection. In playing the game, participants are analysing large amounts of genetic data and helping scientists spot patterns in the data from thousands of tumours that would take a considerable amount of time to analyse by traditional methods.

http://www.cancerresearchuk.org/support-us/play-to-cure-genes-in-space

and legal requirements are met, such databases provide a valuable means for researchers to access large amounts of data.

Chapter 6 referred to the emerging use of crowdsourcing to fund research; however, there are other ways in which crowdsourcing can be capitalised on by researchers. Crowdsourcing is a process whereby the collective power of a large number of people can be harnessed to achieve feats that were once the province of a specialised few (Howe 2006). It involves motivating large numbers of people to contribute their intelligence and ideas to collectively solve problems, process data and create outputs, and it opens up the opportunity for 'citizen scientists' to contribute to research in new and innovative ways. Research Example 40.5 is an illustration of a

Reflection activity

How might digital technologies be used to help you identify priorities for research and be used to enhance the impact of your research? You may find it helpful to refer to Chapter 6 when undertaking this activity.

crowdsourcing research project led by a national charity, Cancer Research UK, which seeks to engage the collective force of the public in contributing to the analysis of real genetic data through engaging them in a free mobile game – providing a very different perspective on patient and public involvement in research! Whereas such projects are currently only feasible for established research teams with significant funding to take forward, nurse researchers should be open to the potential for future technological developments to be used creatively in research.

CONCLUSION

This chapter has considered some current trends influencing nursing and healthcare research that are likely to continue for some time to come. The funders of research, the potential users of research findings and the public at large increasingly expect nursing and healthcare research not only to contribute to knowledge but also to address questions that have the potential to improve the health and well-being of patients and populations and lead to improvements in health care. Addressing societal expectations requires researchers to engage in identifying research priorities and undertake research of relevance to patients, clients and consumers. Linked with this is the increasing imperative to consider the impact of research, be it local, national or international, on the users of healthcare services and those who provide such services. The anticipated advancement in digital technologies will provide new opportunities for nurse researchers to use these technologies in their research and to enhance the impact of their research.

References

Canadian Institutes of Health Research (2012) *Guide to Knowledge Translation Planning at CIHR: integrated and end of grant approaches*. Ottawa, Canadian Institutes of Health Research. http://www.cihr-irsc.gc.ca/e/documents/kt_lm_ktplan-en.pdf (accessed 14 April 2014).

Dowding D, Mitchell N, Randell R, Foster R, Lattimer V, Thompson C (2009) Nurses' use of computerised clinical decision support systems: a case site analysis. *Journal of Clinical Nursing* **18**(8): 1159–1167.

Gerrish K, McDonnell A, Kennedy F (2011) *Capturing Impact: a practical toolkit for nurse consultants*. Sheffield, Sheffield Hallam University.

Gerrish K, McDonnell A, Kennedy F (2013a) The development of a framework for evaluating the impact of nurse consultant roles in the United Kingdom. *Journal of Advanced Nursing* **69**(10): 2295–2308.

Gerrish K, Naisby A, Ismail I (2012) The meaning and consequences of tuberculosis among Somali people in the United Kingdom. *Journal of Advanced Nursing* **68**(12): 2654–2663.

Gerrish K, Naisby A, Ismail I (2013b) Experiences of the diagnosis and management of tuberculosis: a focused ethnography of Somali patients and healthcare professionals in the United Kingdom. *Journal of Advanced Nursing* **69**(10): 2285–2294.

Howe J (2006) Crowdsourcing: a definition. Crowdsourcing: why the power of the crowd is driving the future of business blog. http://crowdsourcing.typepad.com/cs/2006/06/crowdsourcing_a.html, accessed 24 April 2014).

Levett-Jones T, Lathlean J (2009a) 'Don't rock the boat': Nursing students' experiences of conformity and compliance. *Nurse Education Today* **29**(3): 342–349.

Levett-Jones T, Lathlean J (2009b) The 'Ascent to Competence' conceptual framework: an outcome of a study of belongingness. *Journal of Clinical Nursing* **18**: 2870–2879.

Levett-Jones T, Lathlean J, McMillan M, Higgins I (2009) Development and psychometric testing of the Belongingness Scale-Clinical Placement Experience: an international comparative study. *Collegian* **16**(3): 153–324.

National Institute for Health and Clinical Excellence (2012) *Identifying and Managing Tuberculosis Among Hard-to-Reach Groups*. Public Health Guidance PH 37, London, NICE.

National Institute for Health Research (2014) *Collaborations for Leadership in Applied Health Research and Care (CLAHRCs)*. London, NIHR. http://www.nihr.ac.uk/about/collaborations-for-leadership-in-applied-health-research-and-care.htm (accessed 24 April 2014).

O'Mara A, Marrero-Guillamón I, Jamal F, Lehmann A, Cooper C, Lorencet T (2010) *Tuberculosis Evidence Review 1: review of barriers and facilitators*. London, National Institute for Health and Clinical Excellence (NICE), Matrix Knowledge Group.

Vedel I, Akhlaghpour S, Vaghefi I, Bergman H, Lapointe L (2013) Health information technologies in geriatrics and gerontology: a mixed systematic review. *Journal of the American Medical Informatics Association* **20**: 1109–1119.

Glossary

Abstract A concise summary of a research study, journal article or conference presentation, often limited to 200–300 words. It is usually found at the beginning of a research article or report and may be used alone in indexes and conference proceedings.

Action research Research that is characterised by the active participation of the researcher in the study. It may be carried out as part of a change process. It has a strong emphasis on context and the participation of non-researchers. Research methods are often **qualitative** but can also include **quantitative** data.

Altmetrics Measures of impact that are an alternative to journal impact factors, such as article citations, views and downloads or mentions in social and traditional media.

Analytic induction A process of data analysis where the researcher tries to find explanations by continuing data collection until no cases are found that are inconsistent with a hypothetical explanation of a phenomenon. (See **Induction**.)

Audit A rigorous procedure for measuring and improving the quality of care or clinical outcomes against an agreed standard at local or national level.

Bias The systematic influence of factors other than those being investigated. Bias should be eliminated or minimised, as it reduces the **validity** of the study.

Blended research See **Mixed Methods**.

Blinding The process, used in **experimental design**, whereby participants are unaware whether they are allocated to the experimental or control group. It may necessitate the use of a **placebo**. Data collectors and professional staff may also be blinded to the experimental group – this is known as **double blinding** and is used to reduce bias.

Blog A blog or 'Web log' is a self-published collection of short, regularly updated posts written by one or more authors that contain text, links, images and video.

Caldicott Guardian A person appointed to ensure the confidential, ethical and appropriate use of patient data for research purposes within an NHS organisation in the United Kingdom. May be a **gatekeeper** for access to patient data.

Care protocol See **clinical guideline**.

Case study The use of a single person, event or context in a research study in order to study a phenomenon in depth. Case study research may use multiple 'cases' to explore a subject area.

Clinical guideline or care protocol A document or resource that promotes best practice by incorporating the best available evidence into a written or electronic guide for the clinical care of patients with specific conditions or needs.

Clinical trial A rigorous form of research using experimental methods, usually used to test new

The Research Process in Nursing, Seventh Edition. Edited by Kate Gerrish and Judith Lathlean.

Companion Website: www.wiley.com/go/gerrish/research

drugs and clinical treatments. Clinical trials normally employ **randomised controlled trial** (RCT) methods.

Coding The stage of qualitative data analysis where categories and concepts are identified within the raw data and given individual codes.

Cohort study A form of research within the epidemiological tradition, where a group of research participants is recruited and followed up over time. Common examples are birth cohorts (all children born in a particular time period) and disease cohorts (all patients diagnosed in a particular year).

Computer-assisted qualitative data analysis (CAQDAS) A software system that provides tools to identify and code themes, concepts, processes and contexts to build theories or enlarge upon existing theories.

Conceptual framework An abstract set of concepts and theories that are related to one another and may be used to organise ideas and guide analysis within a study. A conceptual framework may be derived from a particular philosophical position.

Confidence interval A range within which the true value of a parameter (e.g. mean or proportion) is estimated to lie.

Consent form A legal document signed by a research participant who agrees to take part, or have data relating to them included, in a particular research project.

Control group A group of research participants recruited to be compared with an experimental or intervention group. The control group are not given the experimental treatment or condition, but may be given a placebo treatment or condition.

Correlation The extent to which variation in one variable is related to variation in another.

Covert observation A form of participant observation in which those being observed are not aware of the researcher's activity or intentions. Often involves some degree of deception and may therefore be considered unethical.

Cross tabulation A comparison, expressed in a table, of two or more categorical variables to show how they are related to one another, for example, age group, gender and smoking.

Crowdfunding 'Funding a project, by raising many small amounts of money from a large number of people, typically via the internet' (Oxford Dictionary).

Curation Collecting, filtering, organising and maintaining information. Additionally, using **Web 2.0** and social media platforms to share the curated collection for the benefit of others.

Data cleaning A process of examining data, once collected, to remove error and omissions. Usually applied to quantitative data once it has been entered into computer software for analysis.

Deduction The process of testing theories by the collection of data and analysis. Underlies much **quantitative research**, especially **experimental design**, and is opposed to **induction**.

Delphi technique A research method used to obtain a consensus of opinion of a group of experts by a series (or 'rounds') of intensive questionnaires interspersed with controlled feedback. It is a structured form of data collection that is usually used within a **quantitative research** framework.

Dependent variable The variable that forms the outcome of a study. Experimental studies are designed to explain changes in the dependent variable, possibly caused by an **independent variable**. In studies of nurse-related cross infection, wound sepsis might be the dependent variable, where handwashing technique is the independent variable.

Digital Using computer technology to use or store data or information.

Digital literacy The ability of digital technologies and networks to navigate, evaluate, communicate and create information.

Dissemination The process of informing others about the results of a particular research study. This may be by verbal, written, audiovisual or electronic means.

Emic The view from within a culture or research setting, recognised only by those who participate in that culture – opposed to **etic**.

Empirical That which can be observed, experienced and measured through the human senses, as opposed to theoretical, which is concerned with thought processes.

Emplotment A device used in narrative research to link together diverse events to form a plot that generates a coherent story.

Epidemiology The science of measuring the prevalence and incidence of disease and other phenomena in large populations.

Epistemology The philosophical theory of knowledge. Research approaches are based upon differing bodies of knowledge, known as their underlying epistemology.

Etic The view from outside a research setting or culture, whereby a researcher seeks to interpret the culture to a wider audience – opposed to **emic**.

Ethnicity A multifaceted biosocial concept that describes social groups in terms of their culture, race, identity, language or other shared characteristics. It can be a marker or proxy for a wide range of factors in a research study.

Ethnography An approach to qualitative research that focuses on culture and subcultures within a society. Ethnographers study behaviour, interaction, customs, rituals, values and institutions and attempt to interpret them in a narrative account.

Evaluation An attempt to assess the worth or value of something.

Evaluation research A type of research that has the purpose of assessing the worth or value of something (e.g. of practice, intervention, innovation or service).

Evidence-based practice Integrating the best available research evidence with professional expertise, taking into account patient or user preferences.

Experimental design A research design characterised by testing a **hypothesis** under controlled conditions. The method is **quantitative** and favoured in pure scientific and medical research.

Experimental group A group of research participants who are exposed to an experimental treatment or condition. Often called an **intervention** group. May be compared to a **control** group.

External validity The extent to which a research study can be **generalised** to other populations and contexts. Often called **generalisability**.

Factor analysis A statistical technique to describe variability among items in a questionnaire or measuring tool. The aim of factor analysis is to group together similar items and to reduce the number of variables being described.

Fieldwork Data collection that takes place in the everyday context of the research participants. Commonly used in **qualitative** research using interviews and **participant observation**.

Focus group A group of individuals assembled to take part in a group discussion, with the purpose of collecting data and observing the effect of group interaction. Often used in **qualitative** and market research.

Framework analysis A method of data analysis particularly suited to policy and applied research. Involves a number of distinct though interconnected stages.

Gatekeeper A term used for a person occupying a role that enables the researcher access to a setting or to research participants. May be a head teacher for access to schoolchildren or a practice manager for access to primary health-care facilities.

Generalisability The extent to which the findings from a research study can be applied to other populations and contexts. See **external validity**.

Grey literature Literature that has not been published in a formal book or journal (traditional or electronic) but still has value as a source of evidence. Grey literature includes conference proceedings, informal and local publications and transcripts of verbal communications.

Grounded theory A specific **inductive** methodology in **qualitative** research. Data collection and analysis take place simultaneously, with the ultimate goal of development of new theory.

Hawthorne effect A phenomenon observed in research, whereby the research participants change their behaviour purely as a result of taking part in an experiment. This effect is a threat to the **validity** of the study.

Health services research A broad term used to describe research into health-care systems, evaluation of health care and clinical effectiveness of interventions. Health service research uses a wide range of methodologies and is multidisciplinary in nature but excludes laboratory and biomedical research.

Hierarchy of evidence A representation of different research methodologies that suggests an order of preference for **evidence-based practice** in terms of rigour and reliability. The hierarchy is controversial, as it sees **randomised controlled trials** as the 'gold standard' against which other methods should be evaluated. Many qualitative researchers challenge the published hierarchy.

Hypothesis A statement about the relationship between two or more variables, which can be tested **empirically**.

Illness narratives The stories that sick people tell about their experiences.

Independent variable The variable that is thought to cause, or explain in some way, another variable, called the **dependent** variable. In studies of nurse-related cross infection, wound sepsis might be the dependent variable, where handwashing is the independent variable.

Induction The process of drawing conclusions and building theory from data that have been collected and analysed. Often used in **qualitative research** and opposed to **deduction**.

Inferential statistics Statistical techniques whereby hypotheses are tested and inference made from a sample to a wider population.

Informed consent The process of ensuring that research participants are fully aware of what the study involves and freely agree to take part. This usually requires a formal signature on a **consent form** after verbal and written information has been given.

In-depth interview An interview technique used in **qualitative** research in which the interviewer imposes minimal structure on the conversation in order to explore the perceptions or experience of the participant. Commonly used in **phenomenology** and **grounded theory** where little is known about the subject of interest.

Intellectual property rights Legal matters concerning the ownership of a new piece of knowledge or a research product such as a validated questionnaire or an item of technology.

Internal consistency A measure of how well items in a **questionnaire** or other data collection tool are related to, and agree with, one another.

Internal validity The extent to which effects observed in a research study are truly caused by the variables under study and not due to any **bias**, **unreliability** or other sources of error.

Interpretivism The belief that human beings continuously interpret and make sense of their environment, and so research into their behaviour and social processes must take the meaning of events into account. This approach underlies **qualitative** research methods and may be opposed to **positivism**.

Intervention group See **experimental group**.

Knowledge translation The process of moving what has been learned through research to the application of such knowledge in different practice settings and circumstances.

Likert scale A scale, usually used in **questionnaires**, where the respondent is asked to agree or disagree with a series of statements in order to measure an attitude or other variables.

Logic model Used to guide the gathering of data on the inputs, activities, outputs and outcomes or impacts in **evaluation research**.

Mean The statistical measure obtained by adding all scores for a variable together and dividing the sum by the number of items. Often known as a mathematical average.

Median The statistical measure that is the middle value when a range of scores are arranged in ascending or descending order.

Meta-analysis The statistical reanalysis of data from a number of studies to reach an interpretation of their combined data. Often found in **systematic reviews**. May also be attempted in a non-statistical form for **qualitative** studies.

Microblogging A very short message that may contain text, images or video links. Microblogs are posted on platforms such as Twitter or Tumblr or as status updates on platforms such as Facebook or LinkedIn.

Mixed methods A research study that integrates **quantitative** and **qualitative** methods in order to reflect and account for complexity. Sometimes known as **blended research**.

Mode The numerical value from a **frequency distribution** that occurs most often. This may have no relation to the middle value.

Narrative research A qualitative research approach that relies on the stories of participants about their experiences.

Non-probability sampling Refers to **sampling** that is not random. Includes quota, **purposive** and convenience sampling.

Null hypothesis A **hypothesis** written in negative terms for statistical testing. The null hypothesis usually states that there will be no difference between experimental groups.

Objectivity Observation or measurement that relies upon physical reality not amenable to individual interpretation. Examples would include temperature measurement and wound size. Can be argued that even such observations may be open to **subjectivity**.

Overt observation A form of observation where the researcher's intentions and actions are fully open to those being observed.

Paradigm A way of viewing reality, informed by a particular theoretical perspective, belief or set of assumptions.

Participant observation Used in **qualitative research**, the researcher takes part in the research context and may assume a role, for example, researcher becomes a nursing assistant in an A&E department in order to observe the interaction of patients and staff. May be **overt** (open) or **covert** (hidden).

Patient Information Sheet (PIS) A document given to research participants that explains to them, in lay language, what participation in the research project will involve. They are then asked to sign a **consent form**.

Peer review A system of assessing the quality of research proposals, conference presentations and journal articles, where respected researchers and other peers of the author are asked to comment critically upon the work.

Phenomenology An inductive approach to **qualitative** research that focuses on understanding the human experience from 'the inside'. Phenomenologists interpret the meaning of the 'lived experience' of study participants through their description.

Phenomenon An occurrence, circumstance, experience or fact that is perceptible to the senses.

Pilot study A preliminary study carried out before the full research to test out data collection instruments and other procedures.

Placebo A non-active substance or form of intervention used for the control group in experimental designs to avoid bias. Trial participants may be **blinded** to whether they are taking the active treatment or the placebo.

Population All possible participants or items that could be included in a sample. Sometimes called the target population. Might be all qualified nurses in an NHS trust or all patient records in a primary care practice. A **sample** is usually then selected from the population for study.

Positivism A theoretical position derived from 18th-century philosophy, believing that scientific truth can only be derived from that which is observable by the human senses. Positivists would apply the methods of traditional scientific enquiry to the study of human behaviour. **Quantitative** research methods rely on this tradition, rather than **interpretivism**.

Power calculation A statistical calculation that is carried out to determine sample size in a quantitative study to ensure enough participants or items are included to increase the probability of observing any real effects and reduce the probability of errors.

Practitioner research Any form of research that is conducted by, and for, practitioners in the clinical field.

Primary outcome The most important outcome variable being investigated in a study.

Principal investigator (PI) The lead researcher on a team and usually the most experienced member. The PI takes overall responsibility for ensuring accountability for the conduct of the research.

Probability sampling Random selection of units from a **population**. This ensures that all members of a target population have a known chance of being selected.

Psychometric analysis A statistical process to assess the **validity** and **reliability** of standardised **questionnaires**.

Purposive sampling The deliberate selection using **non-probability sampling** of individuals, events or settings that best illuminate the **phenomena** of interest.

Qualitative research The broad term used to denote research designs and methods that yield non-numerical data and are based upon an **interpretative** philosophy. Analysis is usually based on narrative and thematic methods.

Quantitative research The broad term used to denote research designs and methods that yield numerical data and are based upon a **positivist** philosophy. Analysis is usually based on statistical methods.

Quasi-experimental design A form of experiment where it is not possible or ethical to randomise participants to comparison groups.

Questionnaire A data collection tool, paper or Web based, where respondents are asked to complete a series of structured questions or items. Answers are often in 'tick box' format.

Random errors Errors that occur randomly in a sample as a result of under- or over-representation of certain groups.

Random sampling A form of sampling where units are chosen from a population in a systematic but random way to ensure each unit has an equal (and non-zero) chance of being selected.

Randomised controlled trial (RCT) An experimental design where participants are randomly allocated to comparison groups, sometimes using a **placebo**. Often referred to as the 'gold standard' for evaluating treatment and to form the basis for evidence-based practice. Most clinical trials of treatments use this design.

Realist evaluation/synthesis A newly emerging form of evidence review, based on realist philosophy, that is particularly appropriate for assessing the impact of complex interventions. It emphasises the context of interventions and unpacks how they work in particular settings, enabling theory development.

Reflexivity The process, used in **qualitative research**, whereby the researcher reflects continuously on how their own actions, values and perceptions impact upon the research setting and affect the data collection and analysis.

Regression Prediction of one continuous variable from another, using a particular statistical technique.

Reliability A measure of the consistency and accuracy of data collection. A data collection instrument may be said to be unreliable if it generates different readings on repeated measurements at the same time of the same person. Low reliability can cause a research study to lack **validity**, but high **reliability** does not necessarily ensure **validity**.

Representative sample A sample that contains a similar proportion of important variables (e.g. age, gender, medical condition) as the population from which it is drawn.

Research The attempt to produce generalisable new knowledge by addressing clearly defined questions with rigorous and systematic methods.

Research ethics committee (REC) A formal committee at local, national or international level that is charged with ensuring compliance with ethical standards for all research carried out within its geographical, organisational or specialist area.

Research Excellence Framework (REF) The system used by the funding council for higher education (HEFCE) in the United Kingdom to assess the quality of research undertaken in universities. The assessment is related to subject discipline and strength of research output, as measured by publications, external funding grants won, peer esteem and impact.

Research governance A system of regulation of research activity in health and social care organisations introduced in England and Wales in 2001 and updated in 2005.

Research infrastructure The structures and organisations that support research activity, such as research networks, research support and advice centres, information centres, clinical trials units and data processing facilities.

Research proposal A concise document that sets out what is to be done in a proposed piece of research, including aims and objectives, methods, sampling, analysis and costs. A proposal is normally written for funding applications or for permission from regulatory frameworks.

Response rate A measure, usually expressed as a percentage, of how many of the eligible sample members selected for a research study actually took part or completed all the data collection stages. Low response rates can affect the **validity** of the study and introduce **bias**.

Rigour The strength of a research design in terms of adherence to procedures, accuracy and consistency.

Sample A subset of a **population** drawn for the purpose of research. A sample may be made up of individuals, clinical material such as blood samples, organisations or events.

Sampling The process of selecting a **sample**. The sampling technique used will affect the **validity** of the research.

Sampling frame The list of units, individuals or organisations in a population, from which a sample is drawn. Common sampling frames are (for individuals) electoral rolls, GP registration lists, school registers and (for organisations) yearbooks of NHS organisations and mailing lists of university departments of nursing and midwifery in the United Kingdom.

Secondary analysis Reanalysis of data collected for another purpose or for a previous research study.

Semi-structured interview An interview technique whereby the interviewer uses predetermined topics and questions but retains the flexibility to follow-up ideas raised by the participant. Commonly used in **qualitative** research where there is a policy agenda, as in **health services research**.

Sensitivity The percentage of tests or cases where those who have the condition under investigation are correctly identified.

Social desirability The tendency of respondents to a survey or other study to give answers that they consider will meet with social approval.

Social media Websites and applications that enable users to create and share content or participate in **social networking**.

Social networking The use of dedicated websites and applications to create a public profile and communicate with other users. Social networks may consist of existing friendship groups or communities who share similar interests or beliefs.

Specificity The percentage of tests or cases where those who do not have the condition under investigation are correctly identified.

Stakeholder Someone in an organisation or other focus of a study who has an interest (stake) in the evaluation, or other research, and its outcomes. Includes participants, clients, workers and management.

Standard deviation A statistical measure of the spread of data in a sample. It measures dispersion from the **mean**.

Stratification The process of dividing a population into known strata by important variables (e.g. gender) before taking a **sample**.

Structured abstract A form of **abstract** where the information is given under prescribed headings (e.g. aim, method, results, conclusion). Some academic journals and conferences insist on presentation in this style.

Structured interview A form of interview where questions are preset both in topic and sequence. Commonly used in **quantitative** research.

Structured observation A form of observation used in **quantitative** research where events or actions being observed are recorded in predetermined categories, often using checklists or handheld computers as data collection tools.

Subjectivity Observation or measurement that is seen to be influenced by the perception of the individual. Examples would include the experience of pain or gender discrimination. Opposed to **objectivity**.

Survey A research design that collects information from a **sample** or **population** to obtain descriptive and **correlational** data. A whole **population** survey is called a census.

Systematic error Errors that usually occur as a result of inconsistencies in the **sampling frame**.

Systematic review A rigorous and systematic literature search, using a well-defined question and strict criteria for study inclusion and evaluation. It may also involve amalgamating statistical data from different studies in **meta-analysis**.

Template analysis A form of thematic analysis, presented as a structured matrix, where themes or codes are identified, which summarise and integrate important ideas, actions, experiences and concepts from the data.

Temporality The way that time is used and portrayed in a narrative account.

Think aloud A technique used for data collection whereby an individual's thinking and decision-making processes are recorded and used as data.

Transcription The process of transferring audio data (usually speech) to written data in narrative form for analysis.

Triangulation The use of two or more data sources, theoretical perspectives or methods in a research study to compare findings and hence achieve greater **validity**.

Thick description Detailed account of cultural behaviours and practices, described in context. Used particularly in **ethnography** and **narrative research**.

Validity The extent to which data, and their interpretation, reflect the phenomenon under investigation without **bias**. Studies and instruments used to collect data are unlikely to be **valid** unless they are also **reliable**. Some qualitative researchers prefer to use terms such as credibility and trustworthiness to describe this concept.

Vignettes Brief scenarios that can be given verbally or in writing to research participants to stimulate a response.

Visual analogue scale (VAS) A line on which a respondent is asked to rate the degree of some subjective variable, usually scored from 0 to 100. Pain is typically measured using a VAS, where 0 represents no pain and 100 represents the worst pain possible.

Web 2.0 The changing use of the Internet from static Web pages to **social media** and user-generated content.

Index

Page numbers in *italics* refer to illustrations; those in **bold** refer to tables

The Research Process in Nursing, Seventh Edition. Edited by Kate Gerrish and Judith Lathlean.

Companion Website: www.wiley.com/go/gerrish/research